Reviewers

Barbara Amendola, APN-C
Professor of Nursing
Ocean County College
Toms River, New Jersey

Judy A. Bourrand, RN, MSN
Assistant Professor (Course Coordinator, Psychiatric-
    Mental Health Nursing)
Samford University, Ida V. Moffett School of Nursing
Birmingham, Alabama

Janice Caie-Lawrence
Instructor
Henry Ford Community College
Dearborn, Michigan

Janet Niemi Chubb, MS, RN (DHSc candidate)
Assistant Professor of Nursing
North Georgia College and State University
Dahlonega, Georgia

Judith A. Collins, BSN, MA, ARNP, BC
Lecturer; Clinical Instructor
University of Iowa, College of Nursing
Iowa City, Iowa

Cindy Cunningham, MSN, APRN, BC
Nursing Instructor
Delaware Technical & Community College
Georgetown, Delaware

Jan Dalsheimer, MS, RN
Associate Clinical Professor
Texas Woman's University
Dallas, Texas

Karen S. Dearing
Assistant Professor
Brigham Young University
Provo, Utah

Leona F. Dempsey, RN, APNP, PhD
Assistant Professor
University of Wisconsin, Oshkosh and Medication
    Prescriber, Oshkosh Counseling and Wellness
    Center
University of Wisconsin Oshkosh
Oshkosh, Wisconsin

Jewel Diller, RN, MSEd, MSN, FNP
Associate Professor
Ivy Tech Community College of Indiana
Fort Wayne, Indiana

Denise Doliveira, RN MSN
Assistant Professor
Community College of Allegheny County, Boyce
    Campus
Monroeville, Pennsylvania

Janet Duffey, RN, MS, APRN, BC
Assistant Professor of Nursing
Napa Valley College
Napa, California

Allison Edmonds, MS, ARNP
Faculty Clinical Instructor
University of South Florida
College of Nursing
Tampa, Florida

Meredith Flood, PhD, APRN, BC
Assistant Professor
University of North Carolina at Charlotte
Charlotte, North Carolina

Gretchen Guhin, BSN, RN
Nurse Educator
Scott Community College
Davenport, Iowa

Mary Herda, MSN
Instructor
Kellogg Community College
Battle Creek, Michigan

Suzanne F. Lockwood, EdD, APRN
Professor of Nursing
Montana State University-Northern
Havre, Montana

Barbara A. May, PhD, APRN, BC
Professor of Nursing
Linfield College
Portland, Oregon

Debby A. Phillips, PhD, APRN, CS
Assistant Professor
Seattle University, College of Nursing
Seattle, Washington

iii

Kathy Quee, MScN
Instructor
British Columbia Institute of Technology
Vancouver, British Columbia
Canada

Karen Rich, PhD, RN
Instructor
The University of Southern Miss
Long Beach, Mississippi

Marilyn Siekierzynski, MSA, MSN, APRN-BC
Professor
Macomb Community College
Clinton Township, Michigan

Jeanne M. Soucy, MS, RN, CS, CAGS
Professor of Nursing
Mass Bay Community College
Framingham, Massachusetts

Preface

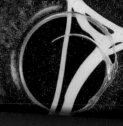

The fourth edition of *Psychiatric-Mental Health Nursing* maintains a strong student focus, presenting sound nursing theory, therapeutic modalities, and clinical applications across the treatment continuum. The chapters are short and the writing style direct in order to facilitate reading comprehension and student learning.

This text uses the nursing process framework and emphasizes assessment, therapeutic communication, neurobiologic theory, and pharmacology throughout. Interventions focus on all aspects of client care, including communication, client and family education, and community resources, as well as their practical application in various clinical settings.

This new edition is supported with a newly enhanced ancillary package designed to assist instructors with course planning and execution, and student evaluation; and to assist students with comprehensive knowledge synthesis.

ORGANIZATION OF THE TEXT

Unit 1: Current Theories and Practice provides a strong foundation for students. It addresses current issues in psychiatric nursing as well as the many treatment settings in which nurses encounter clients. It discusses thoroughly neurobiologic theories, psychopharmacology, and psychosocial theories and therapy as a basis for understanding mental illness and its treatment.

Unit 2: Building the Nurse–Client Relationship presents the basic elements essential to the practice of mental health nursing. Chapters on therapeutic relationships and therapeutic communication prepare students to begin working with clients both in mental health settings and in all other areas of nursing practice. The chapter on the client's response to illness provides a framework for understanding the individual client. An entire chapter is devoted to assessment, emphasizing its importance in nursing.

Unit 3: Current Social and Emotional Concerns covers topics that are not exclusive to mental health settings, including legal and ethical issues; anger, aggression, and hostility; abuse and violence; and grief and loss. Nurses in all practice settings find themselves confronted with issues related to these topics. Additionally, many legal and ethical concerns are interwoven with issues of violence and loss.

Unit 4: Nursing Practice for Psychiatric Disorders covers all the major categories identified in the *DSM-IV-TR*. Each chapter provides current information on etiology, onset and clinical course, treatment, and nursing care.

PEDAGOGICAL FEATURES

Psychiatric-Mental Health Nursing incorporates several pedagogical features designed to facilitate student learning:

- Learning Objectives focus the students' reading and study.

- Key Terms identify new terms used in the chapter. Each term is identified in bold and defined in the text.

- Application of the Nursing Process sections use the assessment framework presented in Chapter 8, so students can compare and contrast various disorders more easily.

- Critical Thinking Questions stimulate students' thinking about current dilemmas and issues in mental health.

- Key Points summarize chapter content to reinforce important concepts.

- Chapter Study Guides provide workbook-style questions for students to test their knowledge and understanding of each chapter

SPECIAL FEATURES

- Clinical Vignettes are provided for each major disorder discussed in the text to "paint a picture" for better understanding.

- Drug Alerts highlight essential points about psychotropic drugs.

- Cultural Considerations sections appear in each chapter, as a response to increasing diversity.

- Therapeutic dialogues give specific examples of nurse–client interaction to promote therapeutic communication skills.

- Internet Resources to further enhance study are located at the end of each chapter.

- Client/Family Teaching boxes provide information that help strengthen students' roles as educators.

- Symptoms and Interventions are highlighted for chapters in Units 3 and 4.

- Sample Nursing Care Plans are provided for chapters in Units 3 and 4.

- Self-Awareness features appear at the end of each chapter and encourage students to reflect on themselves, their emotions, and their attitudes as a way to foster both personal and professional development.

ENHANCED ANCILLARY PACKAGE FOR THE FOURTH EDITION

Faculty

This fourth edition comes with a newly revised collection of ancillary materials designed to help you plan class and clinical learning activities and evaluate students' learning. The Instructor Resource CD-ROM contains information and activities that will help you engage your students throughout the semester, including

- PowerPoint Slides
- Image Bank
- Test Generator

Additional content and technology resources are available online at thePoint—http://thepoint.lww.com—allowing instructors easy access to an extensive selection of materials for each chapter, including

- Pre-Lecture Quizzes
- Discussion Topics
- Written, Group, Clinical, and Web Assignments
- Guided Lecture Notes

Students

Free and bound in the book, the fourth edition CD-ROM supplies the following learning tools:

- **Movie Viewing Guides** highlighting films depicting individuals with mental health disorders and providing students the opportunity to approach nursing care related to mental health and illness in a novel way.

- **Clinical Simulations** on Schizophrenia, Depression, and the Acutely Manic Phase that walk students through case studies and put them in real-life situations.

- **Drug Monographs** of commonly prescribed psychotropic drugs.

These and other valuable student resources, including **NCLEX-style psychiatric nursing questions** designed to help students prepare to face exams armed with confidence and knowledge, are also available on thePoint– http://thepoint.lww.com.

ThePoint

ThePoint (http://thepoint.lww.com), a trademark of Wolters Kluwer Health, is a web-based course and content management system providing every resource that instructors and students need in one easy-to-use site. Advanced technology and superior content combine at thePoint to allow instructors to design and deliver online and off-line courses, maintain grades and class rosters, and communicate with students. Students can visit thePoint to access supplemental multimedia resources to enhance their learning experience, check the course syllabus, download content, upload assignments, and join an online study group.

In addition, ThePoint Solution package includes an **online eBook**, so students and instructors can search their text electronically, plus **journal articles** to aid student learning.

ThePoint . . . where teaching, learning, and technology click!

Acknowledgments

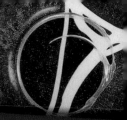

I am grateful to all the students in my classes who have taught me what I need to know to be a better teacher. Their continued input helps make this text practical, interesting, and focused on student learning.

I also want to thank the dedicated people at Lippincott Williams & Wilkins who provide all the assistance and resources I need to make this text a success. To Renee Gagliardi, Katherine Burland, Season Evans, Candice Davis, Mary Kinsella, and Margaret Zuccarini, I extend my appreciation for a job well done.

And as always, my friends continue to be a major part of my life—their support, encouragement, criticism, and loyalty help me in everything I do. My relationships with them help make this text possible.

Contents

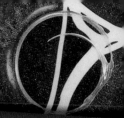

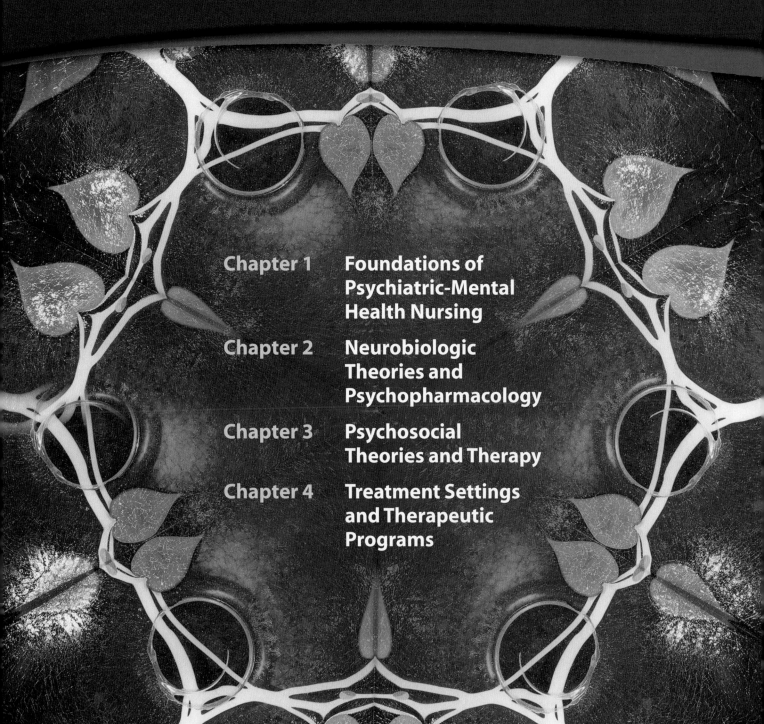

Unit 1

Current Theories and Practice

Foundations of Psychiatric-Mental Health Nursing

Key Terms

- asylum
- case management
- deinstitutionalization
- *Diagnostic and Statistical Manual of Mental Disorders, 4th edition, Text Revision (DSM-IV-TR)*
- managed care
- managed care organizations
- mental disorder
- mental health
- phenomena of concern
- psychotropic drugs
- self-awareness
- standards of care
- utilization review firms

Learning Objectives

After reading this chapter, you should be able to

1. Describe characteristics of mental health and mental illness.

2. Discuss the purpose and use of the American Psychiatric Association's *Diagnostic and Statistical Manual of Mental Disorders, 4th edition, Text Revision (DSM-IV-TR)*.

3. Identify important historical landmarks in psychiatric care.

4. Discuss current trends in the treatment of people with mental illness.

5. Discuss the American Nurses Association standards of practice for psychiatric-mental health nursing.

6. Describe common student concerns about psychiatric nursing.

As you begin the study of psychiatric-mental health nursing, you may be excited, uncertain, and even a little anxious. The field of mental health often seems a little unfamiliar or mysterious, making it hard to imagine what the experience will be like or what nurses do in this area. This chapter addresses these concerns and others by providing an overview of the history of mental illness, advances in treatment, current issues in mental health, and the role of the psychiatric nurse.

MENTAL HEALTH AND MENTAL ILLNESS

Mental health and mental illness are difficult to define precisely. People who can carry out their roles in society and whose behavior is appropriate and adaptive are viewed as healthy. Conversely, those who fail to fulfill roles and carry out responsibilities or whose behavior is inappropriate are viewed as ill. The culture of any society strongly influences its values and beliefs, and this in turn affects how that society defines health and illness. What one society may view as acceptable and appropriate, another society may see as maladaptive and inappropriate.

Mental Health

The World Health Organization defines health as a state of complete physical, mental, and social wellness, not merely the absence of disease or infirmity. This definition emphasizes health as a positive state of well-being. People in a state of emotional, physical, and social well-being fulfill life responsibilities, function effectively in daily life, and are satisfied with their interpersonal relationships and themselves.

No single universal definition of mental health exists. Generally, a person's behavior can provide clues to his or her mental health. Because each person can have a different view or interpretation of behavior (depending on his or her values and beliefs), the determination of mental health may be difficult. In most cases, mental health is a state of emotional, psychological, and social wellness evidenced by satisfying interpersonal relationships, effective behavior and coping, positive self-concept, and emotional stability.

Mental health has many components, and a wide variety of factors influence it. These factors interact; thus, a person's mental health is a dynamic, or ever-changing, state.

Factors influencing a person's mental health can be categorized as individual, interpersonal, and social/cultural. *Individual,* or personal, factors include a person's biologic makeup, autonomy and independence, self-esteem, capacity for growth, vitality, ability to find meaning in life, emotional resilience or hardiness, sense of belonging, reality orientation, and coping or stress management abilities. *Interpersonal,* or relationship, factors include effective communication, ability to help others, intimacy, and a balance of separateness and connectedness. *Social/cultural,* or environmental, factors include a sense of community, access to adequate resources, intolerance of violence, support of

diversity among people, mastery of the environment, and a positive, yet realistic, view of one's world. Individual, interpersonal, and social/cultural factors are discussed further in Chapter 7.

Mental Illness

The American Psychiatric Association (APA, 2000) defines a **mental disorder** as "a clinically significant behavioral or psychological syndrome or pattern that occurs in an individual and is associated with present distress (e.g., a painful symptom) or disability (i.e., impairment in one or more important areas of functioning) or with a significantly increased risk of suffering death, pain, disability, or an important loss of freedom" (p. xxxi). General criteria to diagnose mental disorders include dissatisfaction with one's characteristics, abilities, and accomplishments; ineffective or unsatisfying relationships; dissatisfaction with one's place in the world; ineffective coping with life events; and lack of personal growth. In addition, the person's behavior must not be culturally expected or sanctioned. However, deviant behavior does not necessarily indicate a mental disorder (APA, 2000).

Factors contributing to mental illness also can be viewed within individual, interpersonal, and social/cultural categories. Individual factors include biologic makeup, intolerable or unrealistic worries or fears, inability to distinguish

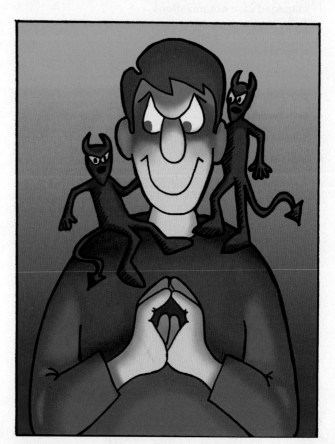

Possessed by demons

reality from fantasy, intolerance of life's uncertainties, a sense of disharmony in life, and a loss of meaning in one's life. Interpersonal factors include ineffective communication, excessive dependency on or withdrawal from relationships, no sense of belonging, inadequate social support, and loss of emotional control. Social/cultural factors include lack of resources, violence, homelessness, poverty, an unwarranted negative view of the world, and discrimination such as stigma, racism, classism, ageism, and sexism.

DIAGNOSTIC AND STATISTICAL MANUAL OF MENTAL DISORDERS

The *Diagnostic and Statistical Manual of Mental Disorders, 4th edition, Text Revision (DSM-IV-TR)* is a taxonomy published by the APA. The *DSM-IV-TR* describes all mental disorders, outlining specific diagnostic criteria for each based on clinical experience and research. All mental health clinicians who diagnose psychiatric disorders use the *DSM-IV-TR*.

The *DSM-IV-TR* has three purposes:

- To provide a standardized nomenclature and language for all mental health professionals
- To present defining characteristics or symptoms that differentiate specific diagnoses
- To assist in identifying the underlying causes of disorders

A multiaxial classification system that involves assessment on several axes, or domains of information, allows the practitioner to identify all the factors that relate to a person's condition:

- Axis I is for identifying all major psychiatric disorders except mental retardation and personality disorders. Examples include depression, schizophrenia, anxiety, and substance-related disorders.
- Axis II is for reporting mental retardation and personality disorders as well as prominent maladaptive personality features and defense mechanisms.
- Axis III is for reporting current medical conditions that are potentially relevant to understanding or managing the person's mental disorder as well as medical conditions that might contribute to understanding the person.
- Axis IV is for reporting psychosocial and environmental problems that may affect the diagnosis, treatment, and prognosis of mental disorders. Included are problems with the primary support group, the social environment, education, occupation, housing, economics, access to health care, and the legal system.
- Axis V presents a Global Assessment of Functioning, which rates the person's overall psychological functioning on a scale of 0 to 100. This represents the clinician's assessment of the person's current level of functioning; the clinician also may give a score for prior functioning (e.g., highest Global Assessment of Functioning in past year or 6 months ago).

All clients admitted to a hospital for psychiatric treatment will have a multiaxis diagnosis from the *DSM-IV-TR*. Although student nurses do not use the *DSM-IV-TR* to diagnose clients, they will find it a helpful resource to understand the reason for the admission and to begin building knowledge about the nature of psychiatric illnesses.

HISTORICAL PERSPECTIVES OF THE TREATMENT OF MENTAL ILLNESS

Ancient Times

People of ancient times believed that any sickness indicated displeasure of the gods and in fact was punishment for sins and wrongdoing. Those with mental disorders were viewed as being either divine or demonic, depending on their behavior. Individuals seen as divine were worshipped and adored; those seen as demonic were ostracized, punished, and sometimes burned at the stake. Later, Aristotle (382–322 BC) attempted to relate mental disorders to physical disorders and developed his theory that the amounts of blood, water, and yellow and black bile in the body controlled the emotions. These four substances, or humors, corresponded with happiness, calmness, anger, and sadness. Imbalances of the four humors were believed to cause mental disorders, so treatment was aimed at restoring balance through bloodletting, starving, and purging. Such "treatments" persisted well into the 19th century (Baly, 1982).

In early Christian times (1–1000 AD), primitive beliefs and superstitions were strong. All diseases were again blamed on demons, and the mentally ill were viewed as possessed. Priests performed exorcisms to rid evil spirits. When that failed, they used more severe and brutal measures, such as incarceration in dungeons, flogging, and starving.

During the Renaissance (1300–1600), people with mental illness were distinguished from criminals in England. Those considered harmless were allowed to wander the countryside or live in rural communities, but the more "dangerous lunatics" were thrown in prison, chained, and starved (Rosenblatt, 1984). In 1547, the Hospital of St. Mary of Bethlehem was officially declared a hospital for the insane, the first of its kind. By 1775, visitors at the institution were charged a fee for the privilege of viewing and ridiculing the inmates, who were seen as animals, less than human (McMillan, 1997). During this same period in the colonies (later the United States), the mentally ill were considered evil or possessed and were punished. Witch hunts were conducted, and offenders were burned at the stake.

Period of Enlightenment and Creation of Mental Institutions

In the 1790s, a period of enlightenment concerning persons with mental illness began. Phillippe Pinel in France and William Tukes in England formulated the concept of **asylum** as a safe refuge or haven offering protection at institutions where people had been whipped, beaten, and starved just because they were mentally ill (Gollaher, 1995). With this movement began the moral treatment of the mentally ill. In the United States, Dorothea Dix (1802–1887) began a crusade to reform the treatment of mental illness after a visit to Tukes' institution in England. She was instrumental in opening 32 state hospitals that offered asylum to the suffering. Dix believed that society was obligated to those who were mentally ill and promoted adequate shelter, nutritious food, and warm clothing (Gollaher, 1995).

The period of enlightenment was short-lived. Within 100 years after establishment of the first asylum, state hospitals were in trouble. Attendants were accused of abusing the residents, the rural locations of hospitals were viewed as isolating patients from their families and homes, and the phrase *insane asylum* took on a negative connotation.

Sigmund Freud and Treatment of Mental Disorders

The period of scientific study and treatment of mental disorders began with Sigmund Freud (1856–1939) and others, such as Emil Kraepelin (1856–1926) and Eugene Bleuler (1857–1939). With these men, the study of psychiatry and the diagnosis and treatment of mental illness started in earnest. Freud challenged society to view human beings objectively. He studied the mind, its disorders, and their treatment as no one had before. Many other theorists built on Freud's pioneering work (see Chapter 3). Kraepelin began classifying mental disorders according to their symptoms, and Bleuler coined the term *schizophrenia*.

Development of Psychopharmacology

A great leap in the treatment of mental illness began in about 1950 with the development of **psychotropic drugs**, or drugs used to treat mental illness. Chlorpromazine (Thorazine), an antipsychotic drug, and lithium, an antimanic agent, were the first drugs to be developed. Over the following 10 years, monoamine oxidase inhibitor antidepressants; haloperidol (Haldol), an antipsychotic; tricyclic antidepressants; and antianxiety agents, called benzodiazepines, were introduced. For the first time, drugs actually reduced agitation, psychotic thinking, and depression. Hospital stays were shortened, and many people were well enough to go home. The level of noise, chaos, and violence greatly diminished in the hospital setting (Trudeau, 1993).

Move Toward Community Mental Health

The movement toward treating those with mental illness in less restrictive environments gained momentum in 1963 with the enactment of the Community Mental Health Centers Construction Act. **Deinstitutionalization**, a deliberate shift from institutional care in state hospitals to community facilities, began. Community mental health centers served smaller geographic catchment, or service, areas that provided less restrictive treatment located closer to individuals' homes, families, and friends. These centers provided emergency care, inpatient care, outpatient services, partial hospitalization, screening services, and education. Thus, deinstitutionalization accomplished the release of individuals from long-term stays in state institutions, the decrease in admissions to hospitals, and the development of community-based services as an alternative to hospital care.

In addition to deinstitutionalization, federal legislation was passed to provide an income for disabled persons: Supplemental Security Income (SSI) and Social Security Disability Income (SSDI). This allowed people with severe and persistent mental illness to be more independent financially and to not rely on family for money. States were able to spend less money on care of the mentally ill than they had when these individuals were in state hospitals because this program was federally funded. Also, commitment laws changed in the early 1970s, making it more difficult to commit people for mental health treatment against their will. This further decreased the state hospital populations and, consequently, the money that states spent on them.

MENTAL ILLNESS IN THE 21ST CENTURY

The National Institute of Mental Health (NIMH) estimates that more than 26% of Americans aged 18 years and older have a diagnosable mental disorder—approximately 57.7 million persons each year (2006). Furthermore, mental illness or serious emotional disturbances impair daily activities for an estimated 10 million adults and 4 million children and adolescents. For example, attention deficit hyperactivity disorder affects 3% to 5% of school-aged children. More than 10 million children younger than 7 years grow up in homes where at least one parent suffers from significant mental illness or substance abuse, a situation that hinders the readiness of these children to start school. The economic burden of mental illness in the United States, including both health care costs and lost productivity, exceeds the economic burden caused by all kinds of cancer. Mental disorders are the leading cause of disability in the United States and Canada for persons 15 to 44 years of age. Yet only one in four adults and one in five children and adolescents requiring mental health services get the care they need.

Some believe that deinstitutionalization has had negative as well as positive effects. Although deinstitutionalization reduced the number of public hospital beds by 80%, the number of admissions to those beds correspondingly increased by 90%. Such findings have led to the term *revolving door effect*. Although people with severe and persistent mental illness have shorter hospital stays, they are admitted to hospitals more frequently. The continuous flow of clients being admitted and discharged quickly overwhelms general hospital psychiatric units. In some cities, emergency department visits for acutely disturbed persons have increased 400% to 500%.

Shorter hospital stays further complicate frequent, repeated hospital admissions. People with severe and persistent mental illness may show signs of improvement in a few days but are not stabilized. Thus, they are discharged into the community without being able to cope with community living. The result frequently is decompensation and rehospitalization. In addition, many people have a dual problem of both severe mental illness and substance abuse. Use of alcohol and drugs exacerbates symptoms of mental illness, again making rehospitalization more likely. Substance abuse issues cannot be dealt with in the 3 to 5 days typical for admissions in the current managed care environment.

Homelessness is a major problem in the United States today. The National Resource and Training Center on Homelessness and Mental Illness (2006) estimates that one third of adult homeless persons have a serious mental illness and that more than one half also have substance abuse problems. The segment of the homeless population considered to be chronically homeless numbers 200,000, and 85% of this group has a psychiatric illness or a substance abuse problem. Those who are homeless and mentally ill are found in parks, airport and bus terminals, alleys and stairwells, jails, and other public places. Some use shelters, halfway houses, or board-and-care rooms; others rent cheap hotel rooms when they can afford it. Homelessness worsens psychiatric problems for many people with mental illness who end up on the streets, contributing to a vicious cycle. North and colleagues (2004) found that rates of mental illness, particularly major depression, and substance abuse are increasing among the homeless population.

Many of the problems of the homeless mentally ill, as well as those who pass through the revolving door of psychiatric care, stem from the lack of adequate community resources. Money saved by states when state hospitals were

closed has not been transferred to community programs and support. Inpatient psychiatric treatment still accounts for most of the spending for mental health in the United States, so community mental health has never been given the financial base it needs to be effective. In addition, mental health services provided in the community must be individualized, available, and culturally relevant to be effective. Only 15% of people with mental illness appear to be getting minimally adequate treatment, that is, a prescription for medication and four or more visits with a psychiatrist or eight visits with any kind of mental health specialist (Wang, 2002).

In 1993, the federal government created and funded Access to Community Care and Effective Services and Support (ACCESS) to begin to address the needs of people with mental illness who were homeless either all or part of the time. The goals of ACCESS were to improve access to comprehensive services across a continuum of care, reduce duplication and cost of services, and improve the efficiency of services. Programs such as these provide services to people who otherwise would not receive them and have proved successful in treating psychiatric illness and in decreasing homelessness (Goldman et al., 2002).

Objectives for the Future

Unfortunately, only one in four affected adults and one in five children and adolescents receive treatment (Department of Health and Human Services [DHHS], 2002). Statistics like these underlie the Healthy People 2010 objectives for mental health proposed by the U.S. DHHS (2000; Box 1.1). These objectives, originally developed as Healthy People 2000, were revised in January 2000 to increase the number of people who are identified, diagnosed, treated, and helped to live healthier lives. The objectives also strive to decrease rates of suicide and homelessness, to increase employment among those with serious mental illness, and to provide more services for both juveniles and adults who are incarcerated and have mental health problems.

Community-Based Care

After deinstitutionalization, the 2,000 community mental health centers that were supposed to be built by 1980 had not materialized. By 1990, only 1,300 programs provided various types of psychosocial rehabilitation services. Persons with severe and persistent mental illness were either ignored or underserved by community mental health centers. This meant that many people needing services were, and still are, in the general population with their needs unmet. In a study comparing five countries, the United States had the largest percentage of mentally ill citizens (29.1%) and provided care for only one in three people who needed it (Bijl et al., 2003). Persons with minor or mild cases were most likely to receive treatment, whereas those with severe and persistent mental illness were least likely to be treated.

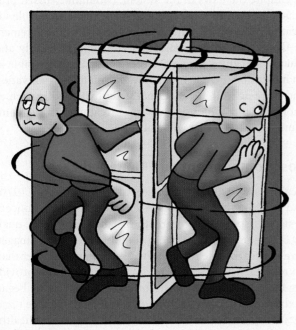

Revolving door

Box 1.1   HEALTHY PEOPLE 2010 MENTAL HEALTH OBJECTIVES

- Reduce suicides to no more than 6 per 100,000 people
- Reduce the incidence of injurious suicide attempts by 1% in 12 months for adolescents aged 14–17
- Reduce the proportion of homeless adults who have serious mental illness to 19%
- Increase the proportion of persons with serious mental illnesses who are employed to 51%
- Reduce the relapse rate for persons with eating disorders, including anorexia nervosa and bulimia nervosa
- Increase the number of persons seen in primary health care who receive mental health treatment screening and assessment
- Increase the proportion of children with mental health problems who receive treatment
- Increase the proportion of juvenile justice facilities that screen new admissions for mental health problems
- Increase the proportion of adults with mental disorders who receive treatment by 17%
  - Adults 18–54 with serious mental illness to 55%
  - Adults 18 and older with recognized depression to 50%
- Adults 18 and older with schizophrenia to 75%
- Adults 18 and older with anxiety disorders to 50%
- Increase the population of persons with concurrent substance abuse problems and mental disorders who receive treatment for both disorders
- Increase the proportion of local governments with community-based jail diversion programs for adults with serious mental illness
- Increase the number of states that track consumers' satisfaction with the mental health services they receive to 30 states
- Increase the number of states with an operational mental health plan that addresses cultural competence
- Increase the number of states with an operational mental health plan that addresses mental health crisis intervention, ongoing screening, and treatment services for elderly persons

U.S. Department of Health and Human Services. (2000). Healthy people 2010: National health promotion and disease prevention objectives. *Washington, DC: DHHS.*

Community support services programs were developed to meet the needs of persons with mental illness outside the walls of an institution. These programs focus on rehabilitation, vocational needs, education, and socialization as well as on management of symptoms and medication. These services are funded by states (or counties) and some private agencies. Therefore, the availability and quality of services vary among different areas of the country. For example, rural areas may have limited funds to provide mental health services and smaller numbers of people needing them. Large metropolitan areas, although having larger budgets, also have thousands of people in need of service; rarely is there enough money to provide all the services needed by the population. Chapter 4 provides a detailed discussion of community-based programs.

Unfortunately, the community-based system did not accurately anticipate the extent of the needs of people with severe and persistent mental illness. Many clients do not have the skills needed to live independently in the community, and teaching these skills is often time-consuming and labor-intensive, requiring a 1:1 staff-to-client ratio. In addition, the nature of some mental illnesses makes learning these skills more difficult. For example, a client who is hallucinating or "hearing voices" can have difficulty listening to or comprehending instructions. Other clients experience drastic shifts in mood, being unable to get out of bed one day and then unable to concentrate or pay attention a few days later.

Despite the flaws in the system, community-based programs have positive aspects that make them preferable for treating many people with mental illness. Clients can remain in their communities, maintain contact with family and friends, and enjoy personal freedom that is not possible in an institution. People in institutions often lose motivation and hope as well as functional daily living skills such as shopping and cooking. Therefore, treatment in the community is a trend that will continue.

Cost Containment and Managed Care

Health care costs spiraled upward throughout the 1970s and 1980s in the United States. **Managed care** is a concept designed to purposely control the balance between the quality of care provided and the cost of that care. In a managed care system, people receive care based on need rather than on request. Those who work for the organization providing the care assess the need for care. Managed care began in the early 1970s in the form of health maintenance organizations, which were successful in some areas with healthier populations of people.

In the 1990s, a new form of managed care, called **utilization review firms** or **managed care organizations**, was developed to control the expenditure of insurance funds by requiring providers to seek approval before the delivery of care. **Case management**, or management of care on a case-by-case basis, represented an effort to provide necessary services while containing cost. The client is assigned to a case manager, a person who coordinates all types of care needed by the client. In theory, this approach is designed to decrease fragmented care from a variety of sources, eliminate unneeded overlap of services, provide care in the least restrictive environment, and decrease costs for the insurers. In reality, expenditures are often reduced by withholding services deemed unnecessary or substituting less expensive treatment alternatives for more expensive care, such as hospital admission.

Psychiatric care is costly because of the long-term nature of the disorders. A single hospital stay can cost $20,000 to $30,000. Also, there are fewer objective measures of health or illness. For example, when a person is suicidal, the clinician must rely on the person's report of suicidality; no laboratory tests or other diagnostic studies can identify suicidal ideas. Mental health care is separated from physical health care in terms of insurance coverage: There are often specific dollar limits or permitted numbers of hospital days in a calendar year. When private insurance limits are met, public funds through the state are used to provide care. As states experience economic difficulties, the availability of state funds for mental health care decreases as well.

Mental health care is managed through privately owned behavioral health care firms that often provide the services and manage their cost. Persons without private insurance must rely on their counties of residence to provide funding through tax dollars. These services and the money to fund them often lag far behind the need that exists. In addition, many persons with mental illness do not seek care and in fact avoid treatment. These persons are often homeless or in jail. Two of the greatest challenges for the future are to provide effective treatment to all who need it and to find the resources to pay for this care.

The Health Care Finance Administration administers two insurance programs: Medicare and Medicaid. Medicare covers people 65 years and older, people with permanent kidney failure, and people with certain disabilities. Medicaid is jointly funded by the federal and state governments and covers low-income individuals and families. Medicaid varies depending on the state; each state determines eligibility requirements, scope of services, and rate of payment for services. Medicaid covers people receiving either SSI or SSDI until they reach 65 years of age, although people receiving SSDI are not eligible for 24 months. SSI recipients, however, are eligible immediately. Unfortunately, not all people who are disabled apply for disability benefits, and not all people who apply are approved. Thus, many people with severe and persistent mental illness have no benefits at all.

Another funding issue is mental health parity, or equality, in insurance coverage provided for both physical and mental illnesses. In the past, insurers had spending caps for mental illness and substance abuse treatment. Some policies placed an annual dollar limitation for treatment, whereas others limited the number of days that would be covered annually or in the insured person's lifetime (of the policy). In 1996, Congress passed the Mental Health Parity Act, which eliminated annual and lifetime dollar amounts for mental health care for companies with more than 50 employees. However, substance abuse was not covered by this law, and companies could still limit the numbers of days in the hospital or the number of clinic visits per year. Thus, parity did not really exist. This federal law was due to expire in 2002, but it has been extended while Congress continues to try to pass more effective parity legislation. In the meantime, some states have passed mental health parity laws; however, some of these laws are as limited as the federal law.

Cultural Considerations

The U.S. Census Bureau (2000) estimates that 62% of the population has European origins. This number is expected to continue to decrease as more U.S. residents trace their ancestry to African, Asian, Arab, or Hispanic origins. Nurses must be prepared to care for this culturally diverse population, which includes being aware of cultural differences that influence mental health and the treatment of mental illness. See Chapter 7 for a discussion of cultural differences.

Diversity is not limited to culture; the structure of families has changed as well. With a divorce rate of 50% in the United States, single parents head many families, and many blended families are created when divorced persons remarry. Twenty-five percent of households consist of a single person (U.S. Census Bureau, 2000), and many people live together without being married. Gay men and lesbians form partnerships and sometimes adopt children. The face of the family in the United States is varied, providing a challenge to nurses to provide sensitive, competent care.

PSYCHIATRIC NURSING PRACTICE

In 1873, Linda Richards graduated from the New England Hospital for Women and Children in Boston. She went on to improve nursing care in psychiatric hospitals and organized educational programs in state mental hospitals in Illinois. Richards is called the first American psychiatric nurse; she believed that "the mentally sick should be at least as well cared for as the physically sick" (Doona, 1984).

The first training of nurses to work with persons with mental illness was in 1882 at McLean Hospital in Belmont, Massachusetts. The care was primarily custodial and focused on nutrition, hygiene, and activity. Nurses adapted medical-surgical principles to the care of clients with psychiatric disorders and treated them with tolerance and kindness. The role of psychiatric nurses expanded as somatic therapies for the treatment of mental disorders were developed.

Treatments such as insulin shock therapy (1935), psychosurgery (1936), and electroconvulsive therapy (1937) required nurses to use their medical-surgical skills more extensively.

The first psychiatric nursing textbook, *Nursing Mental Diseases* by Harriet Bailey, was published in 1920. In 1913, Johns Hopkins was the first school of nursing to include a course in psychiatric nursing in its curriculum. It was not until 1950 that the National League for Nursing, which accredits nursing programs, required schools to include an experience in psychiatric nursing.

Two early nursing theorists shaped psychiatric nursing practice: Hildegard Peplau and June Mellow. Peplau published *Interpersonal Relations in Nursing* in 1952 and *Interpersonal Techniques: The Crux of Psychiatric Nursing* in 1962. She described the therapeutic nurse–client relationship with its phases and tasks and wrote extensively about anxiety (see Chapter 13). The interpersonal dimension that was crucial to her beliefs forms the foundations of practice today. Mellow's 1968 work, *Nursing Therapy*, described her approach of focusing on clients' psychosocial needs and strengths. Mellow contended that the nurse as therapist is particularly suited to working with those with severe mental illness in the context of daily activities, focusing on the here and now to meet each person's psychosocial needs (1986). Both Peplau and Mellow substantially contributed to the practice of psychiatric nursing.

In 1973, the division of psychiatric and mental health practice of the American Nurses Association (ANA) developed standards of care, which it revised in 1982, 1994, and 2000. **Standards of care** are authoritative statements by professional organizations that describe the responsibilities for which nurses are accountable. They are not legally binding unless they are incorporated into the state nurse practice act or state board rules and regulations. When legal problems or lawsuits arise, these professional standards are used to determine safe and acceptable practice and to assess the quality of care.

A two-part document, *Statement on Psychiatric-Mental Health Clinical Nursing Practice* and *Standards of Psychiatric-Mental Health Clinical Nursing Practice*, was jointly published in 1994 and revised in 2000 by the ANA, the American Psychiatric Nurses Association, the Association of Child and Adolescent Psychiatric Nurses, and the Society for Education and Research in Psychiatric-Mental Health Nursing (ANA, 2000). This document outlines the areas of concern and standards of care for today's psychiatric-mental health nurse. The **phenomena of concern** describe the 12 areas of concern that mental health nurses focus on when caring for clients (Box 1.2). The standards of care incorporate the phases of the nursing process, including specific types of interventions, for nurses in psychiatric settings and outline standards for professional performance: quality of care, performance appraisal, education, collegiality, ethics, collaboration, research, and resource utilization (Box 1.3). Box 1.4 summarizes specific areas of practice and specific interventions for both basic and advanced nursing practice.

Student Concerns

Student nurses beginning their clinical experience in psychiatric-mental health nursing usually find the discipline to be very different from any previous experience. As a result, they often have a variety of concerns; these concerns are normal and usually do not persist once the students have initial contacts with clients.

Box 1.2   PSYCHIATRIC-MENTAL HEALTH NURSING PHENOMENA OF CONCERN

Actual or potential mental health problems pertaining to

- The maintenance of optimal health and well-being and the prevention of psychobiologic illness
- Self-care limitations or impaired functioning related to mental and emotional distress
- Deficits in the functioning of significant biologic, emotional, and cognitive symptoms
- Emotional stress or crisis components of illness, pain, and disability
- Self-concept changes, developmental issues, and life process changes
- Problems related to emotions such as anxiety, anger, sadness, loneliness, and grief

- Physical symptoms that occur along with altered psychological functioning
- Alterations in thinking, perceiving, symbolizing, communicating, and decision making
- Difficulties relating to others
- Behaviors and mental states that indicate the client is a danger to self or others or has a severe disability
- Interpersonal, systemic, sociocultural, spiritual, or environmental circumstances or events that affect the mental or emotional well-being of the individual, family, or community
- Symptom management, side effects/toxicities associated with psychopharmacologic intervention, and other aspects of the treatment regimen

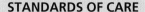

Box 1.3 STANDARDS OF PSYCHIATRIC-MENTAL HEALTH CLINICAL NURSING PRACTICE

STANDARDS OF CARE

Standard I. Assessment

The psychiatric-mental health nurse collects client health data.

Standard II. Diagnosis

The psychiatric-mental health nurse analyzes the data in determining diagnoses.

Standard III. Outcome Identification

The psychiatric-mental health nurse identifies expected outcomes individualized to the client.

Standard IV. Planning

The psychiatric-mental health nurse develops a plan of care that prescribes interventions to attain expected outcomes.

Standard V. Implementation

The psychiatric-mental health nurse implements the interventions identified in the plan of care.

Standard Va. Counseling

The psychiatric-mental health nurse uses counseling interventions to assist clients in improving or regaining their previous coping abilities, fostering mental health, and preventing mental illness and disability.

Standard Vb. Milieu Therapy

The psychiatric-mental health nurse provides, structures, and maintains a therapeutic environment in collaboration with the client and other health care providers.

Standard Vc. Self-Care Activities

The psychiatric-mental health nurse structures interventions around the client's activities of daily living to foster self-care and mental and physical well-being.

Standard Vd. Psychobiologic Interventions

The psychiatric-mental health nurse uses knowledge of psychobiologic interventions and applies clinical skills to restore the client's health and prevent further disability.

Standard Ve. Health Teaching

The psychiatric-mental health nurse, through health teaching, assists clients in achieving satisfying, productive, and healthy patterns of living.

Standard Vf. Case Management

The psychiatric-mental health nurse provides case management to coordinate comprehensive health services and ensure continuity of care.

Standard Vg. Health Promotion and Maintenance

The psychiatric-mental health nurse employs strategies and interventions to promote and maintain mental health and prevent mental illness.

(Interventions Vh–Vj are advanced practice interventions and may be performed only by the certified specialist in psychiatric-mental health nursing.)

Standard VI. Evaluation

The psychiatric-mental health nurse evaluates the client's progress in attaining expected outcomes.

STANDARDS OF PROFESSIONAL PERFORMANCE

Standard I. Quality of Care

The psychiatric-mental health nurse systematically evaluates the quality of care and effectiveness of psychiatric-mental health nursing practice.

Standard II. Performance Appraisal

The psychiatric-mental health nurse evaluates his or her own psychiatric-mental health nursing practice in relation to professional practice standards and relevant statutes and regulations.

Standard III. Education

The psychiatric-mental health nurse acquires and maintains current knowledge in nursing practice.

Standard IV. Collegiality

The psychiatric-mental health nurse contributes to the professional development of peers, colleagues, and others.

continued ···⟩

Box 1.3: Standards of Psychiatric-Mental Health Clinical Nursing Practice, cont.

Standard V. Ethics

The psychiatric-mental health nurse's decisions and actions on behalf of others are determined in an ethical manner.

Standard VI. Collaboration

The psychiatric-mental health nurse collaborates with the client, significant others, and health care providers in providing care.

Standard VII. Research

The psychiatric-mental health nurse contributes to nursing and mental health through the use of research.

Standard VIII. Resource Utilization

The psychiatric-mental health nurse considers factors related to safety, effectiveness, and cost in planning and delivering client care.

Reprinted with permission from the American Nurses Association. Scope and standards of psychiatric-mental health nursing practice. Copyright © 2000. Washington, DC: American Nurses Publishing, American Nurses Foundation/American Nurses Association.

Box 1.4   AREAS OF PRACTICE

BASIC-LEVEL FUNCTIONS

- Counseling
    - Interventions and communication techniques
    - Problem solving
    - Crisis intervention
    - Stress management
    - Behavior modification
- Milieu therapy
    - Maintain therapeutic environment
    - Teach skills
    - Encourage communication between clients and others
    - Promote growth through role modeling
- Self-care activities
    - Encourage independence
    - Increase self-esteem
    - Improve function and health
- Psychobiologic interventions
    - Administer medications
    - Teaching
    - Observations
- Health teaching
- Case management
- Health promotion and maintenance

ADVANCED-LEVEL FUNCTIONS

- Psychotherapy
- Prescriptive authority for drugs (in many states)
- Consultation
- Evaluation

Some common concerns and helpful hints for beginning students are as follows:

- *What if I say the wrong thing?*
  No one magic phrase can solve a client's problems; likewise, no single statement can significantly worsen them. Listening carefully, showing genuine interest, and caring about the client are extremely important. A nurse who possesses these elements but says something that sounds out of place can simply restate it by saying, "That didn't come out right. What I meant was. . . ."

- *What will I be doing?*
  In the mental health setting, many familiar tasks and responsibilities are minimal. Physical care skills or diagnostic tests and procedures are fewer than those conducted in a busy medical-surgical setting. The idea of "just talking to people" may make the student feel as though he or she is not really doing anything. The student must deal with his or her own anxiety about approaching a stranger to talk about very sensitive and personal issues. Development of the therapeutic nurse–client relationship and trust takes time and patience.

- *What if no one will talk to me?*
  Students sometimes fear that clients will reject them or refuse to have anything to do with student nurses. Some clients may not want to talk or are reclusive, but they may show that same behavior with experienced staff; students should not see such behavior as a personal insult or failure. Generally, many people in emotional distress welcome the opportunity to have someone listen to them and show a genuine interest in their situation. Being available and willing to listen is often all it takes to begin a significant interaction with someone.

- *Am I prying when I ask personal questions?*
  Students often feel awkward as they imagine themselves discussing personal or distressing issues with a client. It is important to remember that questions involving personal matters should not be the first thing a student says

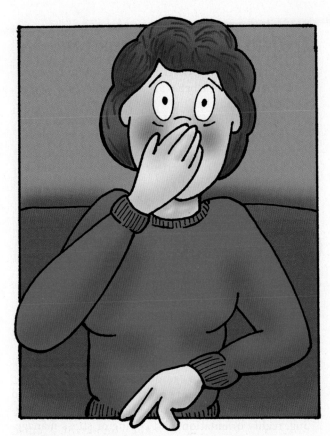

"What if I say the wrong thing?"

behavior, but with practice and the assistance of the instructor and staff, it becomes easier to manage. It is also important to protect the client's privacy and dignity when he or she cannot do so.

- *Is my physical safety in jeopardy?*
  Often students have had little or no contact with seriously mentally ill people. Media coverage of those with mental illness who commit crimes is widespread, leaving the impression that most clients with psychiatric disorders are violent. Actually, clients hurt themselves more often than they harm others. Staff members usually monitor clients with a potential for violence closely for clues of an impending outburst. When physical aggression does occur, staff members are specially trained to handle aggressive clients in a safe manner. The student should not become involved in the physical restraint of an aggressive client because he or she has not had the training and experience required. When talking to or approaching clients who are potentially aggressive, the student should sit in an open area rather than in a closed room, provide plenty of space for the client, or request that the instructor or a staff person be present.

- *What if I encounter someone I know being treated on the unit?*
  In any clinical setting, it is possible that a student nurse might see someone he or she knows. People often have additional fears because of the stigma that is still associated with seeking mental health treatment. It is essential in mental health that the client's identity and treatment be kept confidential. If the student recognizes someone he or she knows, the student should notify the instructor, who can decide how to handle the situation. It is usually best for the student (and sometimes the instructor or staff) to talk with the client and reassure him or her about confidentiality. The client should be reassured that the student will not read the client's record and will not be assigned to work with the client.

- *What if I recognize that I share similar problems or backgrounds with clients?*
  Students may discover that some of the problems, family dynamics, or life events of clients are similar to their own or those of their family. It can be a shock for students to discover that sometimes there are as many similarities between clients and staff as there are differences. There is no easy answer for this concern. Many people have stressful lives or abusive childhood experiences; some cope fairly successfully, whereas others are devastated emotionally. Although we know that coping skills are a key part of mental health, we do not always know why some people have serious emotional problems and others do not. Chapter 7 discusses these factors in more detail.

to the client. These issues usually arise after some trust and rapport have been established. In addition, clients genuinely are distressed about their situations and often want help resolving issues by talking to the nurse. When these emotional or personal issues are addressed in the context of the nurse–client relationship, asking sincere and necessary questions is not prying but is using therapeutic communication skills to help the client.

- *How will I handle bizarre or inappropriate behavior?*
  The behavior and statements of some clients may be shocking or distressing to the student initially. It is important to monitor one's facial expressions and emotional responses so that clients do not feel rejected or ridiculed. The nursing instructor and staff are always available to assist the student in such situations. Students should never feel as if they will have to handle situations alone.

- *What happens if a client asks me for a date or displays sexually aggressive or inappropriate behavior?*
  Some clients have difficulty recognizing or maintaining interpersonal boundaries. When a client seeks contact of any type outside the nurse–client relationship, it is important for the student (with the assistance of the instructor or staff) to clarify the boundaries of the professional relationship (see Chapter 5). Likewise, setting limits and maintaining boundaries are needed when a client's behavior is sexually inappropriate. Initially, the student might be uncomfortable dealing with such

SELF-AWARENESS ISSUES

Self-awareness is the process by which the nurse gains recognition of his or her own feelings, beliefs, and attitudes. In nursing, being aware of one's feelings, thoughts, and values is a primary focus. Self-awareness is particularly important in mental health nursing. Everyone, including nurses and student nurses, has values, ideas, and beliefs that are unique and different from others'. At times, a nurse's values and beliefs will conflict with those of the client or with the client's behavior. The nurse must learn to accept these differences among people and view each client as a worthwhile person regardless of that client's opinions and lifestyle. The nurse does not need to condone the client's views and behavior; he or she merely needs to accept them as different from his or her own and not let them interfere with care.

For example, a nurse who believes that abortion is wrong may be assigned to care for a client who has had an abortion. If the nurse is going to help the client, he or she must be able to separate his or her own beliefs about abortion from those of the client: the nurse must make sure personal feelings and beliefs do not interfere with or hinder the client's care.

The nurse can accomplish self-awareness through reflection, spending time consciously focusing on how one feels and what one values or believes. Although we all have values and beliefs, we may not have really spent time discovering how we feel or what we believe about certain issues, such as suicide or a client's refusal to take needed medications. The nurse needs to discover himself or herself and what he or she believes before trying to help others with different views.

Points to Consider When Working on Self-Awareness

- Keep a diary or journal that focuses on experiences and related feelings. Work on identifying feelings and the circumstances from which they arose. Review the diary or journal periodically to look for patterns or changes.
- Talk with someone you trust about your experiences and feelings. This might be a family member, friend, coworker, or nursing instructor. Discuss how he or she might feel in a similar situation, or ask how he or she deals with uncomfortable situations or feelings.
- Engage in formal clinical supervision. Even experienced clinicians have a supervisor with whom they discuss personal feelings and challenging client situations to gain insight and new approaches.
- Seek alternative points of view. Put yourself in the client's situation and think about his or her feelings, thoughts, and actions.
- Do not be critical of yourself (or others) for having certain values or beliefs. Accept them as a part of yourself, or work to change those values and beliefs you wish to be different.

KEY POINTS

- Mental health and mental illness are difficult to define and are influenced by one's culture and society.
- The World Health Organization defines health as a state of complete physical, mental, and social wellness, not merely the absence of disease or infirmity.
- Mental health is influenced by individual factors, including biologic makeup, autonomy and independence, self-esteem, capacity for growth, vitality, ability to find meaning in life, resilience or hardiness, sense of belonging, reality orientation, and coping or stress management abilities; by interpersonal factors, including effective communication, helping others, intimacy, and maintaining a balance of separateness and connectedness; and by social/cultural factors, including sense of community, access to resources, intolerance of violence, support of diversity among people, mastery of the environment, and a positive yet realistic view of the world.
- Historically, mental illness was viewed as demonic possession, sin, or weakness, and people were punished accordingly.
- Today, mental illness is seen as a medical problem with symptoms causing dissatisfaction with one's characteristics, abilities, and accomplishments; ineffective or unsatisfying interpersonal relationships; dissatisfaction with one's place in the world; ineffective coping with life events; and lack of personal growth.
- Factors contributing to mental illness are biologic makeup; anxiety, worries, and fears; ineffective communication; excessive dependence or withdrawal from relationships; loss of emotional control; lack of resources; and violence, homelessness, poverty, and discrimination.
- The *DSM-IV-TR* is a taxonomy used to provide a standard nomenclature of mental disorders, define characteristics of disorders, and assist in identifying underlying causes of disorders.
- A significant advance in treating persons with mental illness was the development of psychotropic drugs in the early 1950s.
- The shift from institutional care to care in the community began in the 1960s, allowing many people to leave institutions for the first time in years.

INTERNET RESOURCES

RESOURCE	INTERNET ADDRESS
• Center for the Study of the History of Nursing	http://www.nursing.upenn.edu/history
• Department of Health and Human Services	http://www.dhhs.gov
• National Alliance for the Mentally Ill	http://www.nami.org
• National Mental Health Association	http://www.nmha.org
• World Health Organization	http://www.who.int

- One result of deinstitutionalization is the revolving door of repetitive hospital admission without adequate community follow-up.
- It is estimated that one third of the homeless population have a mental illness and one half have substance abuse problems.
- The National Institute of Mental Health estimates that more than 26% of Americans 15 to 44 years of age have a diagnosable mental illness but that only one in four adults and one in five children and adolescents receive treatment.
- Community-based programs are the trend of the future, but they are underfunded and too few in number.
- Managed care, in an effort to contain costs, has resulted in withholding of services or approval of less expensive alternatives for mental health care.
- The population in the United States is becoming increasingly diverse in terms of culture, race, ethnicity, and family structure.
- Psychiatric nursing was recognized in the late 1800s, although it was not required in nursing education programs until 1950.
- Psychiatric nursing practice has been profoundly influenced by Hildegard Peplau and June Mellow, who wrote about the nurse–client relationship, anxiety, nurse therapy, and interpersonal nursing theory.
- The American Nurses Association has published standards of care that guide psychiatric-mental health nursing clinical practice.
- Common concerns of nursing students beginning a psychiatric clinical rotation include fear of saying the wrong thing, not knowing what to do, being rejected by clients, being threatened physically, recognizing someone they know as a client, and sharing similar problems or backgrounds with clients.
- Awareness of one's feelings, beliefs, attitudes, values, and thoughts, called self-awareness, is essential to the practice of psychiatric nursing.
- The goal of self-awareness is to know oneself so that one's values, attitudes, and beliefs are not projected to the client, interfering with nursing care. Self-awareness does not mean having to change one's values or beliefs, unless one desires to do so.

REFERENCES

American Nurses Association. (2000). *Scope and standards of psychiatric-mental health nursing practice.* Washington, DC: American Nurses Publishing, American Nurses Foundation/American Nurses Association.

American Psychiatric Association. (2000). *Diagnostic and statistical manual of mental disorders* (4th ed., text revision). Washington, DC: American Psychiatric Association.

Baly, M. (1982). A leading light. *Nursing Mirror, 155*(19), 49–51.

Bijl, R. V., de Graaf, R., Hiripi, E., et al. (2003). The prevalence of treated and untreated mental disorders in five countries. *Health Affairs, 22*(3), 122–133.

Department of Health and Human Services. (2000). *Healthy People 2010.* Washington, DC: Department of Health and Human Services.

Department of Health and Human Services. (2002). The Department of Health and Human Services on Mental Health Issues. Available: http://www.dhhs.gov.

Doona, M. (1984). At least well cared for . . . Linda Richards and the mentally ill. *Image, 16*(2), 51–56.

Goldman, H. H., Morrissey, J. P., Rosenheck, R. A., et al. (2002). Lessons from the evaluation of the ACCESS program. *Psychiatric Services, 53*(8), 967–969.

Gollaher, D. (1995). *Voice for the mad: The life of Dorothea Dix.* New York: Free Press.

McMillan, I. (1997). Insight into bedlam: One hospital's history. *Journal of Psychosocial Nursing, 3*(6), 28–34.

Mellow, J. (1986). A personal perspective of nursing therapy. *Hospital and Community Psychiatry, 37*(2), 182–183.

National Institute of Mental Health. (2006). Mental health statistics. Available: http://www.nimh.nih.gov.

National Resource and Training Center on Homelessness and Mental Illness. (2006). Get the facts. Available: http:/www.nrchmi.samhsa.gov/facts.

North, C. S., Pollio, D. E., Eyrich, K. M., et al. (2004). Are rates of psychiatric disorders in the homeless population changing? *American Journal of Public Health, 94*(1), 103–108.

Rosenblatt, A. (1984). Concepts of the asylum in the care of the mentally ill. *Hospital and Community Psychiatry, 35,* 244–250.

Trudeau, M. E. (1993). Informed consent: The patient's right to decide. *Journal of Psychosocial Nursing & Mental Health Services, 31*(6), 9–12.

U.S. Census Bureau. (2000). 2000 Census survey results. Available: http://www.census.gov.

Wang, P. S. (2002). Adequacy of treatment for serious mental illness in the United States. *American Journal of Public Health, 92*(1), 92–98.

ADDITIONAL READINGS

Forchuk, C., & Tweedell, D. (2001). Celebrating our past: The history of Hamilton Psychiatric Hospital. *Journal of Psychosocial Nursing, 39*(10), 16–24.

Spector, R. E. (2000). *Cultural diversity in illness and health* (5th ed.). Upper Saddle River, NJ: Prentice Hall Health.

Chapter Study Guide

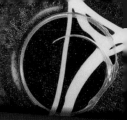

MULTIPLE-CHOICE QUESTIONS

Select the best answer for each of the following questions.

1. Approximately how many Americans have a diagnosable mental illness?
   A. 10%
   B. 19%
   C. 26%
   D. 35%

2. The Department of Health and Human Services estimates that of the 200,000 chronically homeless persons in the United States, the prevalence of mental illness and substance abuse is
   A. 25%
   B. 40%
   C. 70%
   D. 85%

3. Hospitals established by Dorothea Dix were designed to provide which of the following?

   A. Asylum
   B. Confinement
   C. Therapeutic milieu
   D. Public safety

4. Hildegard Peplau is best known for her writing about which of the following?
   A. Community-based care
   B. Humane treatment
   C. Psychopharmacology
   D. Therapeutic nurse–client relationship

5. How many adults in the United States who need mental health services actually receive care?
   A. 1 in 2
   B. 1 in 3
   C. 1 in 4
   D. 1 in 5

FILL-IN-THE-BLANK QUESTIONS

Indicate what type of information is recorded for each axis of the DSM-IV.

_____ Axis I

_____ Axis II

_____ Axis III

_____ Axis IV

_____ Axis V

SHORT-ANSWER QUESTIONS

1. Explain how the standards of practice developed by the American Nurses Association are used.

2. Discuss three trends of mental health care in the United States.

3. Provide three different concerns nursing students might have as they begin psychiatric nursing clinical experiences.

Neurobiologic Theories and Psychopharmacology

Key Terms

- akathisia
- anticholinergic side effects
- antidepressant drugs
- antipsychotic drugs
- anxiolytic drugs
- black box warning
- computed tomography (CT)
- depot injection
- dopamine
- dystonia
- efficacy
- epinephrine
- extrapyramidal symptoms (EPS)
- half-life
- kindling process
- limbic system
- magnetic resonance imaging (MRI)
- mood-stabilizing drugs
- neuroleptic malignant syndrome (NMS)
- neurotransmitter
- norepinephrine
- off-label use
- positron emission tomography (PET)
- potency
- pseudoparkinsonism
- psychoimmunology
- psychopharmacology
- psychotropic drugs
- rebound
- serotonin
- serotonin syndrome
- single photon emission computed tomography (SPECT)
- stimulant drugs
- tardive dyskinesia
- withdrawal

Learning Objectives

After reading this chapter, you should be able to

1. Discuss the structures, processes, and functions of the brain.

2. Describe the current neurobiologic research and theories that are the basis for current psychopharmacologic treatment of mental disorders.

3. Discuss the nurse's role in educating clients and families about current neurobiologic theories and medication management.

4. Identify pertinent teaching for clients and families about brain imaging techniques.

5. Discuss the categories of drugs used to treat mental illness and their mechanisms of action, side effects, and special nursing considerations.

6. Identify client responses that indicate treatment effectiveness.

7. Discuss common barriers to maintaining the medication regimen.

8. Develop a teaching plan for clients and families for implementation of the prescribed therapeutic regimen.

Visit thePoint. http://thePoint.lww.com for NCLEX-style questions, journal articles, and more!

Although much remains unknown about what causes mental illness, science in the past 20 years has made great strides in helping us understand how the brain works and in presenting possible causes of why some brains work differently from others. Such advances in neurobiologic research are continually expanding the knowledge base in the field of psychiatry and are greatly influencing clinical practice. The psychiatric-mental health nurse must have a basic understanding of how the brain functions and of the current theories regarding mental illness. This chapter includes an overview of the major anatomic structures of the nervous system and how they work—the neurotransmission process. It presents the major current neurobiologic theories regarding what causes mental illness, including genetics and heredity, stress and the immune system, and infectious agents.

The use of medications to treat mental illness (**psychopharmacology**) is related to these neurobiologic theories. These medications directly affect the central nervous system (CNS) and, subsequently, behavior, perceptions, thinking, and emotions. This chapter discusses five categories of drugs used to treat mental illness, including their mechanisms of action, their side effects, and the roles of the nurse in administration and client teaching. Although pharmacologic interventions are the most effective treatment for many psychiatric disorders, adjunctive therapies, such as cognitive and behavioral therapies, family therapy, and psychotherapy, greatly enhance the success of treatment and the client's outcome. Chapter 3 discusses these psychosocial modalities.

THE NERVOUS SYSTEM AND HOW IT WORKS

Central Nervous System

The CNS is composed of the brain, the spinal cord, and associated nerves that control voluntary acts. Structurally, the brain is divided into the cerebrum, cerebellum, brain stem, and limbic system. Figures 2.1 and 2.2 show the locations of brain structures.

CEREBRUM

The cerebrum is divided into two hemispheres; all lobes and structures are found in both halves except for the pineal body, or gland, which is located between the hemispheres. The pineal body is an endocrine gland that influences the activities of the pituitary gland, islets of Langerhans, parathyroids, adrenals, and gonads. The corpus callosum is a pathway connecting the two hemispheres and coordinating their functions. The left hemisphere controls the right side of the body and is the center for logical reasoning and analytic functions such as reading, writing, and mathematical tasks. The right hemisphere controls the left side of the body and is the center for creative thinking, intuition, and artistic abilities.

The cerebral hemispheres are divided into four lobes: frontal, parietal, temporal, and occipital. Some functions of the lobes are distinct; others are integrated. The frontal lobes control the organization of thought, body movement, memories, emotions, and moral behavior. The integration of all this information regulates arousal, focuses attention, and enables problem solving and decision making. Abnormalities in the frontal lobes are associated with schizophrenia, attention deficit hyperactivity disorder (ADHD), and dementia. The parietal lobes interpret sensations of taste and touch and assist in spatial orientation. The temporal lobes are centers for the senses of smell and hearing and for memory and emotional expression. The occipital lobes assist in coordinating language generation and visual interpretation, such as depth perception.

CEREBELLUM

The cerebellum is located below the cerebrum and is the center for coordination of movements and postural adjust-

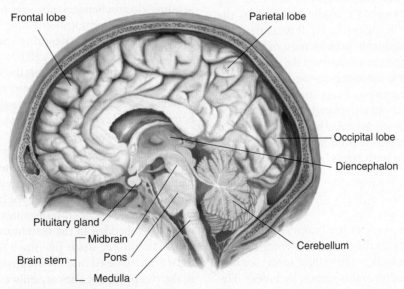

Figure 2.1. Anatomy of the brain.

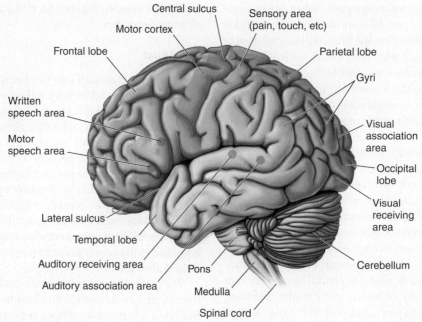

Figure 2.2. The brain and its structures.

ments. The cerebellum receives and integrates information from all areas of the body, such as the muscles, joints, organs, and other components of the CNS. Research has shown that inhibited transmission of dopamine, a neurotransmitter, in this area is associated with the lack of smooth coordinated movements in diseases such as Parkinson's disease and dementia.

BRAIN STEM

The brain stem includes the midbrain, pons, and medulla oblongata and the nuclei for cranial nerves III through XII. The medulla, located at the top of the spinal cord, contains vital centers for respiration and cardiovascular functions. Above the medulla and in front of the cerebrum, the pons bridges the gap both structurally and functionally, serving as a primary motor pathway. The midbrain connects the pons and cerebellum with the cerebrum. It measures only 0.8 inches (2 cm) in length and includes most of the reticular activating system and the extrapyramidal system. The reticular activating system influences motor activity, sleep, consciousness, and awareness. The extrapyramidal system relays information about movement and coordination from the brain to the spinal nerves. The locus ceruleus, a small group of norepinephrine-producing neurons in the brain stem, is associated with stress, anxiety, and impulsive behavior.

LIMBIC SYSTEM

The **limbic system** is an area of the brain located above the brain stem that includes the thalamus, hypothalamus, hippocampus, and amygdala (although some sources differ regarding the structures this system includes). The thalamus regulates activity, sensation, and emotion. The

hypothalamus is involved in temperature regulation, appetite control, endocrine function, sexual drive, and impulsive behavior associated with feelings of anger, rage, or excitement. The hippocampus and amygdala are involved in emotional arousal and memory. Disturbances in the limbic system have been implicated in a variety of mental illnesses, such as the memory loss that accompanies dementia and the poorly controlled emotions and impulses seen with psychotic or manic behavior.

Neurotransmitters

Approximately 100 billion brain cells form groups of neurons, or nerve cells, that are arranged in networks. These neurons communicate information with one another by sending electrochemical messages from neuron to neuron, a process called *neurotransmission*. These electrochemical messages pass from the dendrites (projections from the cell body), through the soma or cell body, down the axon (long extended structures), and across the synapses (gaps between cells) to the dendrites of the next neuron. In the nervous system, the electrochemical messages cross the synapses between neural cells by way of special chemical messengers called neurotransmitters.

Neurotransmitters are the chemical substances manufactured in the neuron that aid in the transmission of information throughout the body. They either excite or stimulate an action in the cells (excitatory) or inhibit or stop an action (inhibitory). These neurotransmitters fit into specific receptor cells embedded in the membrane of the dendrite, just like a certain key shape fits into a lock. After neurotransmitters are released into the synapse and relay the message to the receptor cells, they are either transported back from the synapse to the axon to be stored for later use (reuptake)

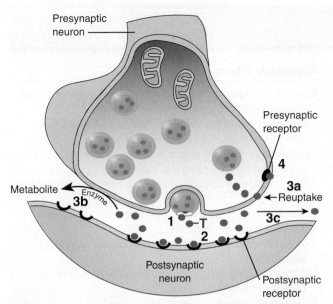

Figure 2.3. Schematic illustration of (1) neurotransmitter (T) release; (2) binding of transmitter to postsynaptic receptor; termination of transmitter action by (3a) reuptake of transmitter into the presynaptic terminal, (3b) enzymatic degradation, or (3c) diffusion away from the synapse; and (4) binding of transmitter to presynaptic receptors for feedback regulation of transmitter release.

or are metabolized and inactivated by enzymes, primarily monoamine oxidase (MAO) (Figure 2.3).

These neurotransmitters are necessary in just the right proportions to relay messages across the synapses. Studies are beginning to show differences in the amount of some neurotransmitters available in the brains of people with certain mental disorders compared with people who have no signs of mental illness (Figure 2.4).

Major neurotransmitters have been found to play a role in psychiatric illnesses as well as in the actions and side effects of psychotropic drugs. Table 2.1 lists the major neurotransmitters and their actions and effects. Dopamine and serotonin have received the most attention in terms of the study and treatment of psychiatric disorders (Tecott & Smart, 2005). The following is a discussion of the major neurotransmitters associated with mental disorders.

DOPAMINE

Dopamine, a neurotransmitter located primarily in the brain stem, has been found to be involved in the control of complex movements, motivation, cognition, and regulation of emotional responses. Dopamine is generally excitatory and is synthesized from tyrosine, a dietary amino acid. Dopamine is implicated in schizophrenia and other psychoses as well as in movement disorders such as Parkinson's disease. Antipsychotic medications work by blocking dopamine receptors and reducing dopamine activity.

NOREPINEPHRINE AND EPINEPHRINE

Norepinephrine, the most prevalent neurotransmitter in the nervous system, is located primarily in the brain stem and plays a role in changes in attention, learning and memory, sleep and wakefulness, and mood regulation. Norepinephrine and its derivative, **epinephrine,** also are known as noradrenaline and adrenaline, respectively. Excess norepinephrine has been implicated in several anxiety disorders; deficits may contribute to memory loss, social withdrawal, and depression. Some antidepressants block the reuptake of norepinephrine, whereas others inhibit MAO from metabolizing it. Epinephrine has limited distribution in the brain but controls the fight-or-flight response in the peripheral nervous system.

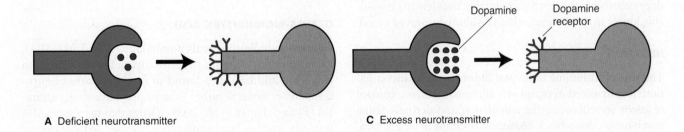

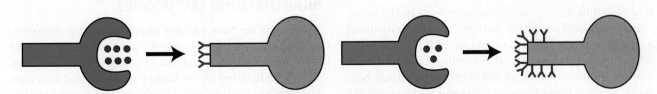

Figure 2.4. Abnormal neurotransmission causing some mental disorders because of excess transmission or excess responsiveness of receptors.

Table 2.1 MAJOR NEUROTRANSMITTERS

Type	Mechanism of Action	Physiologic Effects
Dopamine	Excitatory	Controls complex movements, motivation, cognition; regulates emotional response
Norepinephrine (noradrenaline)	Excitatory	Causes changes in attention, learning and memory, sleep and wakefulness, mood
Epinephrine (adrenaline)	Excitatory	Controls fight-or-flight response
Serotonin	Inhibitory	Controls food intake, sleep and wakefulness, temperature regulation, pain control, sexual behaviors, regulation of emotions
Histamine	Neuromodulator	Controls alertness, gastric secretions, cardiac stimulation, peripheral allergic responses
Acetylcholine	Excitatory or inhibitory	Controls sleep and wakefulness cycle; signals muscles to become alert
Neuropeptides	Neuromodulators	Enhance, prolong, inhibit, or limit the effects of principal neurotransmitters
Glutamate	Excitatory	Results in neurotoxicity if levels are too high
Gamma-aminobutyric acid (GABA)	Inhibitory	Modulates other neurotransmitters

SEROTONIN

Serotonin, a neurotransmitter found only in the brain, is derived from tryptophan, a dietary amino acid. The function of serotonin is mostly inhibitory, and it is involved in the control of food intake, sleep and wakefulness, temperature regulation, pain control, sexual behavior, and regulation of emotions. Serotonin plays an important role in anxiety and mood disorders and schizophrenia. It has been found to contribute to the delusions, hallucinations, and withdrawn behavior seen in schizophrenia. Some antidepressants block serotonin reuptake, thus leaving it available longer in the synapse, which results in improved mood.

HISTAMINE

The role of histamine in mental illness is under investigation. It is involved in peripheral allergic responses, control of gastric secretions, cardiac stimulation, and alertness. Some psychotropic drugs block histamine, resulting in weight gain, sedation, and hypotension.

ACETYLCHOLINE

Acetylcholine is a neurotransmitter found in the brain, spinal cord, and peripheral nervous system, particularly at the neuromuscular junction of skeletal muscle. It can be excitatory or inhibitory. It is synthesized from dietary choline found in red meat and vegetables and has been found to affect the sleep–wake cycle and to signal muscles to become active. Studies have shown that people with Alzheimer's disease have decreased acetylcholine-secreting neurons, and people with myasthenia gravis (a muscular disorder in which impulses fail to pass the myoneural junction, which causes muscle weakness) have reduced acetylcholine receptors.

GLUTAMATE

Glutamate is an excitatory amino acid that at high levels can have major neurotoxic effects. Glutamate has been implicated in the brain damage caused by stroke, hypoglycemia, sustained hypoxia or ischemia, and some degenerative diseases such as Huntington's or Alzheimer's.

GAMMA-AMINOBUTYRIC ACID

Gamma-aminobutyric acid (γ-aminobutyric acid, or GABA), an amino acid, is the major inhibitory neurotransmitter in the brain and has been found to modulate other neurotransmitter systems rather than to provide a direct stimulus (Plata-Salaman et al., 2005). Drugs that increase GABA function, such as benzodiazepines, are used to treat anxiety and to induce sleep.

BRAIN IMAGING TECHNIQUES

At one time, the brain could be studied only through surgery or autopsy. During the past 25 years, however, several brain imaging techniques have been developed that now allow visualization of the brain's structure and function. These techniques are useful for diagnosing some disorders of the brain and have helped to correlate certain areas of the brain with specific functions. Brain imaging techniques also are useful in research to find the causes of mental disorders.

Table 2.2	BRAIN IMAGING TECHNOLOGY		
Procedure	**Imaging Method**	**Results**	**Duration**
Computed tomography (CT)	Serial x-rays of brain	Structural image	20–40 min
Magnetic resonance imaging (MRI)	Radio waves from brain detected from magnet	Structural image	45 min
Positron emission tomography (PET)	Radioactive tracer injected into bloodstream and monitored as client performs activities	Functional	2–3 h
Single photon emission computed tomography (SPECT)	Same as PET	Functional	1–2 h

Table 2.2 describes and compares several of these diagnostic techniques.

Types of Brain Imaging Techniques

Computed tomography (CT), also called computed axial tomography (CAT), is a procedure in which a precise x-ray beam takes cross-sectional images (slices) layer by layer. A computer reconstructs the images on a monitor and also stores the images on magnetic tape or film. CT can visualize the brain's soft tissues, so CT is used to diagnose primary tumors, metastases, and effusions and to determine the size of the ventricles of the brain. Some people with schizophrenia have been shown to have enlarged ventricles; this finding is associated with a poorer prognosis and marked negative symptoms (Figure 2.5; see Chapter 14). The person undergoing a CT must lie motionless on a stretcher-like table for about 20 to 40 minutes as the stretcher passes through a "ring" while the serial x-rays are taken.

In **magnetic resonance imaging (MRI)**, a type of body scan, an energy field is created with a huge magnet and radio waves. The energy field is converted to a visual image or scan. MRI produces more tissue detail and contrast than CT and can show blood flow patterns and tissue changes such as edema. It also can be used to measure the size and thickness of brain structures; persons with schizophrenia can have as much as a 7% reduction in cortical thickness. The person undergoing an MRI must lie in a small, closed chamber and remain motionless during the procedure, which takes about 45 minutes. Those who feel claustrophobic or have increased anxiety may require sedation before the procedure. Clients with pacemakers or metal implants, such as heart valves or orthopedic devices, cannot undergo MRI.

More advanced imaging techniques, such as **positron emission tomography (PET)** and **single photon emission computed tomography (SPECT)**, are used to examine the function of the brain. Radioactive substances are injected into the blood; the flow of those substances in the brain is monitored as the client performs cognitive activities as instructed by the operator. PET uses two photons simultaneously; SPECT uses a single photon. PET provides better resolution with sharper and clearer pictures. PET takes

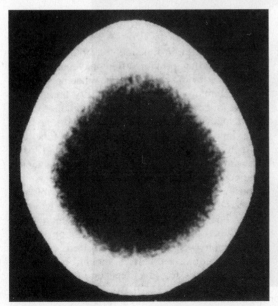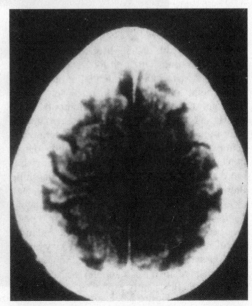

Figure 2.5. Example of computed tomography of the brain of a patient with schizophrenia (*right*) compared with a normal control (*left*).

about 2 to 3 hours; SPECT takes 1 to 2 hours. PET and SPECT are used primarily for research, not for the diagnosis and treatment of clients with mental disorders (Fujita et al., 2005; Vythilingam et al., 2005) (Figure 2.6). A recent breakthrough is the use of the chemical marker FDDNP with PET to identify the amyloid plaques and tangles of Alzheimer's disease in living clients; these conditions previously could be diagnosed only through autopsy. These scans have shown that clients with Alzheimer's disease have decreased glucose metabolism in the brain and decreased cerebral blood flow. Some persons with schizophrenia also demonstrate decreased cerebral blood flow.

Limitations of Brain Imaging Techniques

Although imaging techniques such as PET and SPECT have helped bring about tremendous advances in the study of brain diseases, they have some limitations:

- The use of radioactive substances in PET and SPECT limits the number of times a person can undergo these tests. There is the risk that the client will have an allergic reaction to the substances. Some clients may find receiving intravenous doses of radioactive material frightening or unacceptable.
- Imaging equipment is expensive to purchase and maintain, so availability can be limited. A PET camera costs about $2.5 million; a SPECT camera costs about $500,000.
- Some persons cannot tolerate these procedures because of fear or claustrophobia.

- Researchers are finding that many of the changes in disorders such as schizophrenia are at the molecular and chemical levels and cannot be detected with current imaging techniques (Fujita et al., 2005; Vythilingam et al., 2005).

NEUROBIOLOGIC CAUSES OF MENTAL ILLNESS

Genetics and Heredity

Unlike many physical illnesses that have been found to be hereditary, such as cystic fibrosis, Huntington's disease, and Duchenne's muscular dystrophy, the origins of mental disorders do not seem to be that simple. Current theories and studies indicate that several mental disorders may be linked to a specific gene or combination of genes but that the source is not solely genetic; nongenetic factors also play important roles.

To date, one of the most promising discoveries is the identification in 2007 of variations in the gene *SORL1* that may be a factor in late-onset Alzheimer's disease. Research is continuing in an attempt to find genetic links to other diseases such as schizophrenia and mood disorders. This is the focus of ongoing research in the Human Genome Project, funded by the National Institutes of Health (NIH) and the U.S. Department of Energy. This international research project, started in 1988, is the largest of its kind. It has identified all human DNA and continues with research

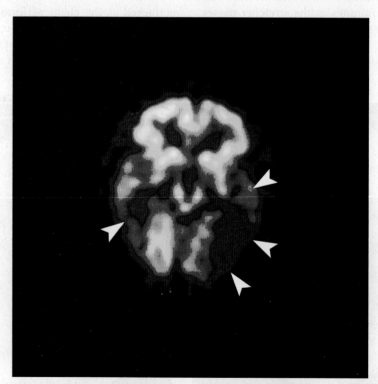

Figure 2.6. Example of axial (horizontal) positron emission tomography of a male patient with Alzheimer's disease, showing defects (*arrowheads*) in metabolism in the regions of the cerebral cortex of brain.

to discover the human characteristics and diseases each gene is related to (encoding). In addition, the project also addresses the ethical, legal, and social implications of human genetics research. This program (known as ELSI) focuses on privacy and fairness in the use and interpretation of genetic information, clinical integration of new genetic technologies, issues surrounding genetics research, and professional and public education (NIH, 2007). The researchers publish their results in the journal *Science;* further information can be obtained at www.genome.gov.

Three types of studies are commonly conducted to investigate the genetic basis of mental illness:

1. *Twin studies* are used to compare the rates of certain mental illnesses or traits in monozygotic (identical) twins, who have an identical genetic makeup, and dizygotic (fraternal) twins, who have a different genetic makeup. Fraternal twins have the same genetic similarities and differences as nontwin siblings.
2. *Adoption studies* are used to determine a trait among biologic versus adoptive family members.
3. *Family studies* are used to compare whether a trait is more common among first-degree relatives (parents, siblings, children) than among more distant relatives or the general population.

Although some genetic links have been found in certain mental disorders, studies have not shown that these illnesses are solely genetically linked. Investigation continues about the influence of inherited traits versus the influence of the environment—the "nature versus nurture" debate. The influence of environmental or psychosocial factors is discussed in Chapter 3.

Stress and the Immune System (Psychoimmunology)

Researchers are following many avenues to discover possible causes of mental illness. **Psychoimmunology**, a relatively new field of study, examines the effect of psychosocial stressors on the body's immune system. A compromised immune system could contribute to the development of a variety of illnesses, particularly in populations already genetically at risk. So far, efforts to link a specific stressor with a specific disease have been unsuccessful.

Infection as a Possible Cause

Some researchers are focusing on infection as a cause of mental illness. Most studies involving viral theories have focused on schizophrenia, but so far none has provided specific or conclusive evidence. Theories that are being developed and tested include the existence of a virus that has an affinity for tissues of the CNS, the possibility that a virus may actually alter human genes, and maternal exposure to a virus during critical fetal development of the nervous system.

Swedo and colleagues (2004) studied the relation of streptococcal bacteria and obsessive-compulsive disorder (OCD) and tics. They found enlarged basal ganglia, indicating a possible autoimmune response to streptococcal infection. When blood plasma (high in streptococcal antibodies) was replaced by transfusion with healthy donor plasma, the incidence of tics decreased by 50%, and other OCD symptoms were reduced by 60%. Studies such as this are promising in discovering a link between infection and mental illness.

THE NURSE'S ROLE IN RESEARCH AND EDUCATION

Amid all the reports of research in these areas of neurobiology, genetics, and heredity, the implications for clients and their families are still not clear or specific. Often, reports in the media regarding new research and studies are confusing, contradictory, or difficult for clients and their families to understand. The nurse must ensure that clients and families are well informed about progress in these areas and must also help them to distinguish between facts and hypotheses. The nurse can explain if or how new research may affect a client's treatment or prognosis. The nurse is a good resource for providing information and answering questions.

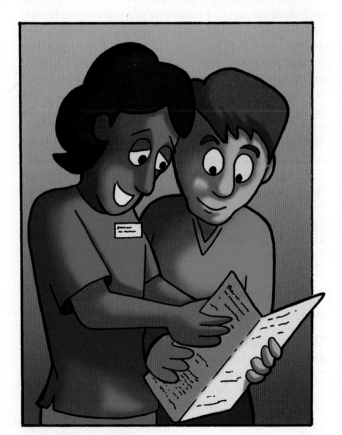

Keeping clients informed

PSYCHOPHARMACOLOGY

Medication management is a crucial issue that greatly influences the outcomes of treatment for many clients with mental disorders. The following sections discuss several categories of drugs used to treat mental disorders (**psychotropic drugs**): antipsychotics, antidepressants, mood stabilizers, anxiolytics, and stimulants. Nurses should understand how these drugs work; their side effects, contraindications, and interactions; and the nursing interventions required to help clients manage medication regimens.

Several terms used in discussions of drugs and drug therapy are important for nurses to know. **Efficacy** refers to the maximal therapeutic effect that a drug can achieve. **Potency** describes the amount of the drug needed to achieve that maximum effect; low-potency drugs require higher dosages to achieve efficacy, whereas high-potency drugs achieve efficacy at lower dosages. **Half-life** is the time it takes for half of the drug to be removed from the bloodstream. Drugs with a shorter half-life may need to be given three or four times a day, but drugs with a longer half-life may be given once a day. The time that a drug needs to leave the body completely after it has been discontinued is about five times its half-life.

The U.S. Food and Drug Administration (FDA) is responsible for supervising the testing and marketing of medications for public safety. These activities include clinical drug trials for new drugs and monitoring the effectiveness and side effects of medications. The FDA approves each drug for use in a particular population and for specific diseases. At times, a drug will prove effective for a disease that differs from the one involved in original testing and FDA approval. This is called **off-label use**. An example is some anticonvulsant drugs (approved to prevent seizures) that are prescribed for their effects in stabilizing the moods of clients with bipolar disorder (off-label use). The FDA also monitors the occurrence and severity of drug side effects. When a drug is found to have serious or life-threatening side effects, even if such side effects are rare, the FDA may issue a **black box warning**. This means that package inserts must have a highlighted box, separate from the text, which contains a warning about the serious or life-threatening side effects. Several psychotropic medications discussed later in this chapter have black box warnings.

Principles That Guide Pharmacologic Treatment

The following are several principles that guide the use of medications to treat psychiatric disorders:

- A medication is selected based on its effect on the client's target symptoms such as delusional thinking, panic attacks, or hallucinations. The medication's effectiveness is evaluated largely by its ability to diminish or eliminate the target symptoms.
- Many psychotropic drugs must be given in adequate dosages for some time before their full effect is realized. For example, tricyclic antidepressants can require 4 to 6 weeks before the client experiences optimal therapeutic benefit.
- The dosage of medication often is adjusted to the lowest effective dosage for the client. Sometimes a client may need higher dosages to stabilize his or her target symptoms, whereas lower dosages can be used to sustain those effects over time.
- As a rule, older adults require lower dosages of medications than do younger clients to experience therapeutic effects. It also may take longer for a drug to achieve its full therapeutic effect in older adults.
- Psychotropic medications often are decreased gradually (tapering) rather than abruptly. This is because of potential problems with **rebound** (temporary return of symptoms), recurrence of the original symptoms, or **withdrawal** (new symptoms resulting from discontinuation of the drug).
- Follow-up care is essential to ensure compliance with the medication regimen, to make needed adjustments in dosage, and to manage side effects.
- Compliance with the medication regimen often is enhanced when the regimen is as simple as possible in terms of both the number of medications prescribed and the number of daily doses.

Antipsychotic Drugs

Antipsychotic drugs, also known as *neuroleptics*, are used to treat the symptoms of psychosis, such as the delusions and hallucinations seen in schizophrenia, schizoaffective disorder, and the manic phase of bipolar disorder. Off-label uses of antipsychotics include treatment of anxiety and insomnia; aggressive behavior; and delusions, hallucinations, and other disruptive behaviors that sometimes accompany Alzheimer's disease. Antipsychotic drugs work by blocking receptors of the neurotransmitter dopamine. They have been in clinical use since the 1950s. They are the primary medical treatment for schizophrenia and also are used in psychotic episodes of acute mania, psychotic depression, and drug-induced psychosis. Clients with dementia who have psychotic symptoms sometimes respond to low dosages of conventional antipsychotics. Atypical antipsychotics can cause increased mortality rate in elderly clients with dementia-related psychosis. Short-term therapy with antipsychotics may be useful for transient psychotic symptoms such as those seen in some clients with borderline personality disorder.

Table 2.3 lists available dosage forms, usual daily oral dosages, and extreme dosage ranges for conventional and atypical antipsychotic drugs. The low end of the extreme range typically is used with older adults or children with psychoses, aggression, or extreme behavior management problems.

Table 2.3 ANTIPSYCHOTIC DRUGS

Generic (Trade) Name	Forms	Daily Dosage*	Extreme Dosage Ranges*
Conventional Antipsychotics			
Phenothiazines			
Chlorpromazine (Thorazine)	T, L, INJ	200–1,600	25–2,000
Perphenazine (Trilafon)	T, L, INJ	16–32	4–64
Fluphenazine (Prolixin)	T, L, INJ	2.5–20	1–60
Thioridazine (Mellaril)	T, L	200–600	40–800
Mesoridazine (Serentil)	T, L, INJ	75–300	30–400
Trifluoperazine (Stelazine)	T, L, INJ	6–50	2–80
Thioxanthene			
Thiothixene (Navane)	C, L, INJ	6–30	6–60
Butyrophenones			
Haloperidol (Haldol)	T, L, INJ	2–20	1–100
Droperidol (Inapsine)	INJ	2.5	
Dibenzazepine			
Loxapine (Loxitane)	C, L, INJ	60–100	30–250
Dihydroindolone			
Molindone (Moban)	T, L	50–100	15–250
Atypical Antipsychotics			
Clozapine (Clozaril)	T	150–500	75–700
Fazclo (clozapine)	DT	150–500	75–700
Risperidone (Risperdal)	T, L, DT	2–8	1–16
Olanzapine (Zyprexa)	T	5–15	5–20
Quetiapine (Seroquel)	T	300–600	200–750
Ziprasidone (Geodon)	C, INJ	40–160	20–200
Paliparidone (Invega)	T	6	3–12
New Generation Antipsychotic			
Aripiprazole (Abilify)	T	15–30	10–40

*Values are mg/day for oral doses only.

T, tablet; C, capsule; L, liquid for oral use; INJ, injection for IM (usually PRN) use; DT, orally disintegrating tablet.

MECHANISM OF ACTION

The major action of all antipsychotics in the nervous system is to block receptors for the neurotransmitter dopamine; however, the therapeutic mechanism of action is only partially understood. Dopamine receptors are classified into subcategories (D1, D2, D3, D4, and D5), and D2, D3, and D4 have been associated with mental illness. The typical antipsychotic drugs are potent antagonists (blockers) of D2, D3, and D4. This makes them effective in treating target symptoms but also produces many extrapyramidal side effects (discussion to follow) because of the blocking of the D2 receptors. Newer, atypical antipsychotic drugs such as clozapine (Clozaril) are relatively weak blockers of D2, which may account for the lower incidence of extrapyramidal side effects. In addition, atypical antipsychotics inhibit the reuptake of serotonin, as do some of the antidepressants, increasing their effectiveness in treating the depressive aspects of schizophrenia. Paliperidone (Invega) is the newest atypical antipsychotic, gaining approval for distribution in the United States in January, 2007. It is chemically similar to risperidone (Risperdal); however, it is an extended release preparation. This means the client can take one daily dose in most cases, which may be a factor in increased compliance.

A new generation of antipsychotics, called dopamine system stabilizers, is being developed. These drugs are thought to stabilize dopamine output; that is, they preserve or enhance dopaminergic transmission when it is too low and reduce it when it is too high. This results in control of symptoms without some of the side effects of other antipsychotic medications. Aripiprazole (Abilify), the first drug of this type, was approved for use in November 2002. In clinical trials, the most common side effects were headache, anxiety, and nausea.

Three antipsychotics are available in **depot injection**, a time-release form of medication for maintenance therapy. Two conventional antipsychotics use sesame oil as the vehicle for these injections, so the medication is absorbed slowly over time; thus, less frequent administration is needed to maintain the desired therapeutic effects. Prolixin (decanoate fluphenazine) has a duration of 7 to 28 days, and Haldol (decanoate haloperidol) has a duration of 4 weeks.

After the client's condition is stabilized with oral doses of these medications, administration by depot injection is required every 2 to 4 weeks to maintain the therapeutic effect. Risperidone (Risperdal Consta), an atypical antipsychotic, encapsulates active medication into polymer-based microspheres that degrade slowly in the body, gradually releasing the drug at a controlled rate. Risperdal Consta, 25 mg, is given every 2 weeks (Kane et al., 2003).

WARNING ⬤

> Elderly patients with dementia-related psychosis treated with atypical antipsychotic drugs are at an increased risk for death. Causes of death were varied, but most of the deaths appeared to be either cardiovascular or infectious in nature.

SIDE EFFECTS

Extrapyramidal Side Effects. **Extrapyramidal symptoms (EPS)**, serious neurologic symptoms, are the major side effects of antipsychotic drugs. They include acute dystonia, pseudoparkinsonism, and akathisia. Although often collectively referred to as EPS, each of these reactions has distinct features. One client can experience all the reactions in the same course of therapy, which makes distinguishing among them difficult. Blockade of D2 receptors in the midbrain region of the brain stem is responsible for the development of EPS. Conventional antipsychotic drugs cause a greater incidence of EPS than do atypical antipsychotic drugs, with ziprasidone (Geodon) rarely causing EPS (Daniel et al., 2006).

WARNING ⬤ Geodon

> Contraindicated in patients with a known history of QT prolongation, recent myocardial infarction, or uncompensated heart failure, it should not be used with other QT-prolonging drugs.

Therapies for acute dystonia, pseudoparkinsonism, and akathisia are similar and include lowering the dosage of the antipsychotic, changing to a different antipsychotic, or administering anticholinergic medication (discussion to follow). Whereas anticholinergic drugs also produce side effects, atypical antipsychotic medications are often prescribed because the incidence of EPS side effects associated with them is decreased.

Acute **dystonia** includes acute muscular rigidity and cramping, a stiff or thick tongue with difficulty swallowing, and, in severe cases, laryngospasm and respiratory difficulties. Dystonia is most likely to occur in the first week of treatment, in clients younger than 40 years, in males, and in those receiving high-potency drugs such as haloperidol and thiothixene. Spasms or stiffness in muscle groups can produce *torticollis* (twisted head and neck), *opisthotonus* (tightness in the entire body with the head back and an arched neck), or *oculogyric crisis* (eyes rolled back in a locked position). Acute dystonic reactions can be painful and frightening for the client. Immediate treatment with anticholinergic drugs, such as intramuscular benztropine mesylate (Cogentin) or intramuscular or intravenous diphenhydramine (Benadryl), usually brings rapid relief.

Table 2.4 lists the drugs, and their routes and dosages, used to treat EPS. The addition of a regularly scheduled oral anticholinergic such as benztropine may allow the client to continue taking the antipsychotic drug with no further dystonia. Recurrent dystonic reactions would necessitate a lower dosage or a change in the antipsychotic drug. Assessment of EPS using the Simpson-Angus rating scale is discussed further in Chapter 14.

Drug-induced parkinsonism, or **pseudoparkinsonism**, is often referred to by the generic label of EPS. Symptoms resemble those of Parkinson's disease and include a stiff, stooped posture; mask-like facies; decreased arm swing; a shuffling, festinating gait (with small steps); cogwheel rigidity (ratchet-like movements of joints); drooling; tremor; bradycardia; and coarse pill-rolling movements of the thumb and fingers while at rest. Parkinsonism is treated by changing

Table 2.4   DRUGS USED TO TREAT EXTRAPYRAMIDAL SIDE EFFECTS

Generic (Trade) Name	Oral Dosages (mg)	IM/IV Doses (mg)	Drug Class
Amantadine (Symmetrel)	100 bid or tid	—	Dopaminergic agonist
Benztropine (Cogentin)	1–3 bid	1–2	Anticholinergic
Biperiden (Akineton)	2 tid–qid	2	Anticholinergic
Diazepam (Valium)	5 tid	5–10	Benzodiazepine
Diphenhydramine (Benadryl)	25–50 tid or qid	25–50	Antihistamine
Lorazepam (Ativan)	1–2 tid	—	Benzodiazepine
Procyclidine (Kemadrin)	2.5–5 tid	—	Anticholinergic
Propranolol (Inderal)	10–20 tid; up to 40 qid	—	Beta-blocker
Trihexyphenidyl (Artane)	2–5 tid	—	Anticholinergic

to an antipsychotic medication that has a lower incidence of EPS or by adding an oral anticholinergic agent or amantadine, which is a dopamine agonist that increases transmission of dopamine blocked by the antipsychotic drug.

Akathisia is reported by the client as an intense need to move about. The client appears restless or anxious and agitated, often with a rigid posture or gait and a lack of spontaneous gestures. This feeling of internal restlessness and the inability to sit still or rest often leads clients to discontinue their antipsychotic medication. Akathisia can be treated by a change in antipsychotic medication or by the addition of an oral agent such as a beta-blocker, anticholinergic, or benzodiazepine.

Neuroleptic Malignant Syndrome. **Neuroleptic malignant syndrome (NMS)** is a potentially fatal idiosyncratic reaction to an antipsychotic (or neuroleptic) drug. Although the *Diagnostic and Statistical Manual of Mental Disorders, 4th edition, Text Revision* (American Psychiatric Association, 2000) notes that the death rate from this syndrome has been reported at 10% to 20%, those figures may have resulted from biased reporting; the reported rates are now decreasing. The major symptoms of NMS are rigidity; high fever; autonomic instability such as unstable blood pressure, diaphoresis, and pallor; delirium; and elevated levels of enzymes, particularly creatine phosphokinase. Clients with NMS usually are confused and often mute; they may fluctuate from agitation to stupor. All antipsychotics seem to have the potential to cause NMS, but high dosages of high-potency drugs increase the risk. NMS most often occurs in the first 2 weeks of therapy or after an increase in dosage, but it can occur at any time.

Dehydration, poor nutrition, and concurrent medical illness all increase the risk for NMS. Treatment includes immediate discontinuance of all antipsychotic medications and the institution of supportive medical care to treat dehydration and hyperthermia until the client's physical condition stabilizes. After NMS, the decision to treat the client with other antipsychotic drugs requires full discussion between the client and the physician to weigh the relative risks against the potential benefits of therapy.

Tardive Dyskinesia. **Tardive dyskinesia (TD),** a syndrome of permanent involuntary movements, is most commonly caused by the long-term use of conventional antipsychotic drugs. The pathophysiology is still not understood, and no effective treatment is available (Chouinard, 2004b). At least 20% of those treated with neuroleptics in the long term develop TD. The symptoms of TD include involuntary movements of the tongue, facial and neck muscles, upper and lower extremities, and truncal musculature. Tongue thrusting and protruding, lip smacking, blinking, grimacing, and other excessive unnecessary facial movements are characteristic. After it has developed, TD is irreversible, although decreasing or discontinuing antipsychotic medications can arrest its progression. Unfortunately, antipsychotic medications can mask the beginning symptoms of TD, that is, increased dosages of the antipsychotic medication cause the initial symptoms to disappear temporarily. As the symptoms of TD worsen, however, they "break through" the effect of the antipsychotic drug.

Preventing TD is one goal when administering antipsychotics. This can be done by keeping maintenance dosages as low as possible, changing medications, and monitoring the client periodically for initial signs of TD using a standardized assessment tool such as the Abnormal Involuntary Movement Scale (see Chapter 14). Clients who have already developed signs of TD but still need to take an antipsychotic medication often are given one of the atypical antipsychotic drugs that have not yet been found to cause or, therefore, worsen TD.

Anticholinergic Side Effects. **Anticholinergic side effects** often occur with the use of antipsychotics and include orthostatic hypotension, dry mouth, constipation, urinary hesitance or retention, blurred near vision, dry eyes, photophobia, nasal congestion, and decreased memory. These side effects usually decrease within 3 to 4 weeks but do not entirely remit. The client who is taking anticholinergic agents for EPS may have increased problems with anticholinergic side effects. Using calorie-free beverages or hard candy may alleviate dry mouth; stool softeners, adequate

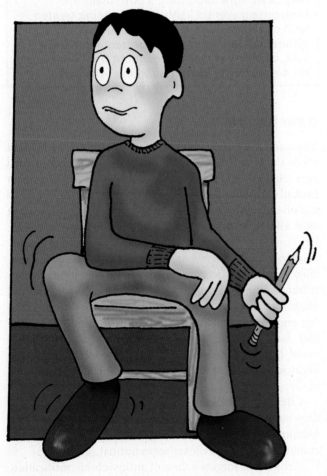

Akathisia

fluid intake, and the inclusion of grains and fruit in the diet may prevent constipation.

Other Side Effects. Antipsychotic drugs also increase blood prolactin levels. Elevated prolactin may cause breast enlargement and tenderness in men and women; diminished libido, erectile and orgasmic dysfunction, and menstrual irregularities; and increased risk for breast cancer and may contribute to weight gain.

Weight gain can accompany most antipsychotic medications, but it is most likely with the atypical antipsychotic drugs, with ziprasidone (Geodon) being the exception. Weight increases are most significant with clozapine (Clozaril) and olanzapine (Zyprexa). In 2004, the FDA informed drug manufacturers that atypical antipsychotics must carry a warning of the increased risk for hyperglycemia and diabetes. Though the exact mechanism of this weight gain is unknown, it is associated with increased appetite, binge eating, carbohydrate craving, food preference changes, and decreased satiety in some clients. In addition, clients with a genetic predisposition for weight gain are at greater risk (Muller & Kennedy, 2006). Prolactin elevation may stimulate feeding centers, histamine antagonism stimulates appetite, and there may be an as yet undetermined interplay of multiple neurotransmitter and receptor interactions with resultant changes in appetite, energy intake, and feeding behavior. Obesity is common in clients with schizophrenia, further increasing the risk for type 2 diabetes mellitus and cardiovascular disease (Newcomer & Haupt, 2006). In addition, clients with schizophrenia are less likely to exercise or eat low-fat nutritionally balanced diets; this pattern decreases the likelihood that they can minimize potential weight gain or lose excess weight. It is recommended that clients taking antipsychotics be involved in an educational program to control weight and decrease body mass index.

Most antipsychotic drugs cause relatively minor cardiovascular adverse effects such as postural hypotension, palpitations, and tachycardia. Certain antipsychotic drugs such as thioridazine (Mellaril), droperidol (Inapsine), and mesoridazine (Serentil) also can cause a lengthening of the QT interval. A QT interval that is longer than 500 ms is considered dangerous and is associated with life-threatening dysrhythmias and sudden death. Though rare, the lengthened QT interval can cause torsade de pointes, a rapid heart rhythm of 150 to 250 beats per minute, causing a "twisted" appearance on the electrocardiogram, giving rise to the name (Glassman, 2005). Thioridazine and mesoridazine are used to treat psychosis; droperidol is most often used as an adjunct to anesthesia or to produce sedation. Sertindole (Serlect) was never approved in the United States to treat psychosis but was used in Europe and subsequently withdrawn from the market because of the number of cardiac dysrhythmias and deaths that it caused.

Clozapine produces fewer traditional side effects than do most antipsychotic drugs, but it has the potentially fatal side effect of agranulocytosis. This develops suddenly and

WARNING ● Droperidol, Thioridazine, Mesoridazine

> May lengthen the QT interval, leading to potentially life-threatening cardiac dysrhythmias or cardiac arrest

is characterized by fever, malaise, ulcerative sore throat, and leukopenia. This side effect may not be manifested immediately and can occur up to 24 weeks after the initiation of therapy. Initially, clients needed to have a weekly white blood cell count (WBC) above 3500/mm^3 to obtain the next week's supply of clozapine. Currently, all clients must have weekly WBCs drawn for the first six months. If the WBC is 3500/mm^3 and the absolute neutrophil count (ANC) is 2000/mm^3, the client may have these labs monitored every 2 weeks for 6 months, and then every 4 weeks. This decreased monitoring is dependent on continuous therapy with clozapine. Any interruption in therapy requires a return to more frequent monitoring for a specified period of time. After clozapine has been discontinued, weekly monitoring of the WBC and ANC is required for 4 weeks.

WARNING ● Clozapine

> May cause agranulocytosis, a potentially life-threatening event. Clients who are being treated with clozapine must have a baseline WBC count and differential before initiation of treatment and a WBC count every week throughout treatment and for 4 weeks after discontinuation of clozapine.

CLIENT TEACHING

The nurse informs clients taking antipsychotic medication about the types of side effects that may occur and encourages clients to report such problems to the physician instead of discontinuing the medication. The nurse teaches the client methods of managing or avoiding unpleasant side effects and maintaining the medication regimen. Drinking sugar-free fluids and eating sugar-free hard candy ease dry mouth. The client should avoid calorie-laden beverages and candy because they promote dental caries, contribute to weight gain, and do little to relieve dry mouth. Methods to prevent or relieve constipation include exercising and increasing water and bulk-forming foods in the diet. Stool softeners are permissible, but the client should avoid laxatives. The use of sunscreen is recommended because photosensitivity can cause the client to sunburn easily.

Clients should monitor the amount of sleepiness or drowsiness they feel. They should avoid driving and performing other potentially dangerous activities until their response times and reflexes seem normal.

If the client forgets a dose of antipsychotic medication, he or she can take the missed dose if it is only 3 or 4 hours late. If the dose is more than 4 hours overdue or the next dose is due, the client can omit the forgotten dose. The nurse encourages clients who have difficulty remembering to take their medication to use a chart and to record doses when taken or to use a pillbox that can be prefilled with accurate doses for the day or week.

Antidepressant Drugs

Antidepressant drugs are primarily used in the treatment of major depressive illness, anxiety disorders, the depressed phase of bipolar disorder, and psychotic depression. Off-label uses of antidepressants include the treatment of chronic pain, migraine headaches, peripheral and diabetic neuropathies, sleep apnea, dermatologic disorders, panic disorder, and eating disorders. Although the mechanism of action is not completely understood, antidepressants somehow interact with the two neurotransmitters, norepinephrine and serotonin, that regulate mood, arousal, attention, sensory processing, and appetite.

Antidepressants are divided into four groups:

1. Tricyclic and the related cyclic antidepressants
2. Selective serotonin reuptake inhibitors (SSRIs)
3. MAO inhibitors (MAOIs)
4. Other antidepressants such as venlafaxine (Effexor), bupropion (Wellbutrin), duloxetine (Cymbalta), trazodone (Desyrel), and nefazodone (Serzone)

Table 2.5 lists the dosage forms, usual daily dosages, and extreme dosage ranges.

The cyclic compounds became available in the 1950s and for years were the first choice of drugs to treat depression even though they cause varying degrees of sedation, orthostatic hypotension (drop in blood pressure on rising), and anticholinergic side effects. In addition, cyclic antidepressants are potentially lethal if taken in an overdose.

Table 2.5 ANTIDEPRESSANT DRUGS

Generic (Trade) Name	Forms	Usual Daily Dosages*	Extreme Dosage Ranges*
Selective Serotonin Reuptake Inhibitors			
Fluoxetine (Prozac)	C, L	20–60	10–80
Fluvoxamine (Luvox)	T	150–200	50–300
Paroxetine (Paxil)	T	20–40	10–50
Sertraline (Zoloft)	T	100–150	50–200
Citalopram (Celexa)	T, L	20–40	20–60
Escitalopram (Lexapro)	T	10–20	5–30
Cyclic Compounds			
Imipramine (Tofranil)	T, C, INJ	150–200	50–300
Desipramine (Norpramin)	T, C	150–200	50–300
Amitriptyline (Elavil)	T, INJ	150–200	50–300
Nortriptyline (Pamelor)	C, L	75–100	25–150
Doxepin (Sinequan)	C, L	150–200	25–300
Trimipramine (Surmontil)	C	150–200	50–300
Protriptyline (Vivactil)	T	15–40	10–60
Maprotiline (Ludiomil)	T	100–150	50–200
Mirtazapine (Remeron)	T	15–45	15–60
Amoxapine (Asendin)	T	150–200	50–250
Clomipramine (Anafranil)	C, INJ	150–200	50–250
Other Compounds			
Bupropion (Wellbutrin)	T	200–300	100–450
Venlafaxine (Effexor)	T, C	75–225	75–375
Trazodone (Desyrel)	T	200–300	100–600
Nefazodone (Serzone)	T	300–600	100–600
Duloxetine (Cymbalta)	C	60	30–90
Monoamine Oxidase Inhibitors			
Phenelzine (Nardil)	T	45–60	15–90
Tranylcypromine (Parnate)	T	30–50	10–90
Isocarboxazid (Marplan)	T	20–40	10–60

*Values are mg/day for oral doses only.

C, capsule; T, tablet; L, liquid; INJ, injection for IM use.

During that same period, the MAOIs were discovered to have a positive effect on people with depression. Although the MAOIs have a low incidence of sedation and anticholinergic effects, they must be used with extreme caution for several reasons:

- A life-threatening side effect, hypertensive crisis, may occur if the client ingests foods containing tyramine (an amino acid) while taking MAOIs.
- Because of the risk for potentially fatal drug interactions, MAOIs cannot be given in combination with other MAOIs, tricyclic antidepressants, meperidine (Demerol), CNS depressants, many antihypertensives, or general anesthetics.
- MAOIs are potentially lethal in overdose and pose a potential risk in clients with depression who may be considering suicide.

The SSRIs, first available in 1987 with the release of fluoxetine (Prozac), have replaced the cyclic drugs as the first choice in treating depression because they are equal in efficacy and produce fewer troublesome side effects. The SSRIs and clomipramine are effective in the treatment of OCD as well. Prozac Weekly is the first and only medication that can be given once a week as maintenance therapy for depression after the client has been stabilized on fluoxetine. It contains 90 mg of fluoxetine with an enteric coating that delays release into the bloodstream.

PREFERRED DRUGS FOR CLIENTS AT HIGH RISK FOR SUICIDE

Suicide is always a primary consideration when treating clients with depression. SSRIs, venlafaxine, nefazodone, and bupropion are often better choices for those who are potentially suicidal or highly impulsive because they carry no risk of lethal overdose, in contrast to the cyclic compounds and the MAOIs. However, SSRIs are only effective for mild and moderate depression. Evaluation of the risk for suicide must continue even after treatment with antidepressants is initiated. The client may feel more energized but still have suicidal thoughts, which increases the likelihood of a suicide attempt. Also, because it often takes weeks before the medications have a full therapeutic effect, clients may become discouraged and tire of waiting to feel better, which can result in suicidal behavior. There is an FDA-required warning for SSRIs and increased suicidal risk in children and adolescents.

MECHANISM OF ACTION

The precise mechanism by which antidepressants produce their therapeutic effects is not known, but much is known about their action on the CNS. The major interaction is with the monoamine neurotransmitter systems in the brain, particularly norepinephrine and serotonin. Both of these neurotransmitters are released throughout the brain and help to regulate arousal, vigilance, attention, mood, sensory processing, and appetite. Norepinephrine, serotonin, and dopamine are removed from the synapses after release by reuptake into presynaptic neurons. After reuptake, these three neurotransmitters are reloaded for subsequent release or metabolized by the enzyme MAO. The SSRIs block the reuptake of serotonin; the cyclic antidepressants and venlafaxine block the reuptake of norepinephrine primarily and block serotonin to some degree; and the MAOIs interfere with enzyme metabolism. This is not the complete explanation, however; the blockade of serotonin and norepinephrine reuptake and the inhibition of MAO occur in a matter of hours, whereas antidepressants are rarely effective until taken for several weeks. The cyclic compounds may take 4 to 6 weeks to be effective; MAOIs need 2 to 4 weeks for effectiveness; and SSRIs may be effective in 2 to 3 weeks. Researchers believe that the actions of these drugs are an "initiating event" and that eventual therapeutic effectiveness results when neurons respond more slowly, making serotonin available at the synapses (Lehne, 2006).

SIDE EFFECTS OF SELECTIVE SEROTONIN REUPTAKE INHIBITORS

SSRIs have fewer side effects compared with the cyclic compounds. Enhanced serotonin transmission can lead to several common side effects such as anxiety, agitation, akathisia (motor restlessness), nausea, insomnia, and sexual dysfunction, specifically diminished sexual drive or difficulty achieving an erection or orgasm. In addition, weight gain is both an initial and ongoing problem during antidepressant therapy, although SSRIs cause less weight gain than other antidepressants. Taking medications with food usually can minimize nausea. Akathisia usually is treated with a beta-blocker such as propranolol (Inderal) or a benzodiazepine. Insomnia may continue to be a problem even if the client takes the medication in the morning; a sedative-hypnotic or low-dosage trazodone may be needed.

Less common side effects include sedation (particularly with paroxetine [Paxil]), sweating, diarrhea, hand tremor, and headaches. Diarrhea and headaches usually can be managed with symptomatic treatment. Sweating and continued sedation most likely indicate the need for a change to another antidepressant.

SIDE EFFECTS OF CYCLIC ANTIDEPRESSANTS

Cyclic compounds have more side effects than do SSRIs and the newer miscellaneous compounds. The individual medications in this category vary in terms of the intensity of side effects, but generally side effects fall into the same categories. The cyclic antidepressants block cholinergic receptors, resulting in anticholinergic effects such as dry mouth, constipation, urinary hesitancy or retention, dry nasal passages, and blurred near vision. More severe anticholinergic effects such as agitation, delirium, and ileus may occur, particularly in older adults. Other common side effects include orthostatic hypotension, sedation, weight gain, and tachycardia. Clients may develop tolerance to anticholinergic effects, but these side effects are common reasons that clients discontinue drug therapy. Clients taking cyclic compounds frequently report sexual dysfunction similar to problems experienced with SSRIs. Both weight gain and sexual dysfunction are cited as common reasons for noncompliance (Hitt, 2003).

SIDE EFFECTS OF MONOAMINE OXIDASE INHIBITORS

The most common side effects of MAOIs include daytime sedation, insomnia, weight gain, dry mouth, orthostatic hypotension, and sexual dysfunction. The sedation and insomnia are difficult to treat and may necessitate a change in medication. Of particular concern with MAOIs is the potential for a life-threatening hypertensive crisis if the client ingests food that contains tyramine or takes sympathomimetic drugs. Because the enzyme MAO is necessary to break down the tyramine in certain foods, its inhibition results in increased serum tyramine levels, causing severe hypertension, hyperpyrexia, tachycardia, diaphoresis, tremulousness, and cardiac dysrhythmias. Drugs that may cause potentially fatal interactions with MAOIs include SSRIs, certain cyclic compounds, buspirone (BuSpar), dextromethorphan, and opiate derivatives such as meperidine. The client must be able to follow a tyramine-free diet; Box 2.1 lists the foods to avoid. Studies are currently underway to determine whether a selegiline transdermal patch would be effective in treating depression without the risks of dietary tyramine and orally ingested MAOIs.

SIDE EFFECTS OF OTHER ANTIDEPRESSANTS

Of the other or novel antidepressant medications, nefazodone, trazodone, and mirtazapine (Remeron) commonly cause sedation. Both nefazodone and trazodone commonly cause headaches. Nefazodone also can cause dry mouth and nausea. Bupropion and venlafaxine may cause loss of appetite, nausea, agitation, and insomnia. Venlafaxine also may cause dizziness, sweating, or sedation. Sexual dysfunction is much less common with the novel antidepressants, with one notable exception: Trazodone can cause priapism (a sustained and painful erection that necessitates immediate treatment and discontinuation of the drug). Priapism also may result in impotence.

WARNING ● Nefazodone

> May cause rare but potentially life-threatening liver damage, which could lead to liver failure

WARNING ● Bupropion

> Can cause seizures at a rate four times that of other antidepressants. The risk for seizures increases when doses exceed 450 mg/day (400 mg SR); dose increases are sudden or in large increments; the client has a history of seizures, cranial trauma, excessive use of or withdrawal from alcohol, or addiction to opiates, cocaine, or stimulants; the client uses OTC stimulants or anorectics; or the client has diabetes being treated with oral hypoglycemics or insulin.

DRUG INTERACTIONS

An uncommon but potentially serious drug interaction, called **serotonin** or serotonergic **syndrome**, can result from taking an MAOI and an SSRI at the same time. It also can occur if the client takes one of these drugs too close to the end of therapy with the other. In other words, one drug must clear the person's system before initiation of ther-

---

Box 2.1   FOODS (CONTAINING TYRAMINE) TO AVOID WHEN TAKING MAOIs

- Mature or aged cheeses or dishes made with cheese, such as lasagna or pizza. All cheese is considered aged except cottage cheese, cream cheese, ricotta cheese, and processed cheese slices.
- Aged meats such as pepperoni, salami, mortadella, summer sausage, beef logs, meat extracts, and similar products. Make sure meat and chicken are fresh and have been properly refrigerated.

- Italian broad beans (fava), bean curd (tofu), banana peel, over ripe fruit, avocado
- All tap beers and microbrewery beer. Drink no more than two cans or bottles of beer (including nonalcoholic beer) or 4 ounces of wine per day.
- Sauerkraut, soy sauce or soybean condiments, or marmite (concentrated yeast)
- Yogurt, sour cream, peanuts, Brewer's yeast, MSG

Adapted from University of North Carolina Clinical Research Center. (2004).

apy with the other. Symptoms include agitation, sweating, fever, tachycardia, hypotension, rigidity, hyperreflexia, and, in extreme reactions, even coma and death (Krishnan, 2006). These symptoms are similar to those seen with an SSRI overdose.

CLIENT TEACHING

Clients should take SSRIs first thing in the morning unless sedation is a problem; generally paroxetine most often causes sedation. If the client forgets a dose of an SSRI, he or she can take it up to 8 hours after the missed dose. To minimize side effects, clients generally should take cyclic compounds at night in a single daily dose when possible. If the client forgets a dose of a cyclic compound, he or she should take it within 3 hours of the missed dose or omit the dose for that day. Clients should exercise caution when driving or performing activities requiring sharp, alert reflexes until sedative effects can be determined.

Clients taking MAOIs need to be aware that a life-threatening hyperadrenergic crisis can occur if they do not observe certain dietary restrictions. They should receive a written list of foods to avoid while taking MAOIs. The nurse should make clients aware of the risk for serious or even fatal drug interactions when taking MAOIs and instruct them not to take any additional medication, including over-the-counter preparations, without checking with the physician or pharmacist.

Mood-Stabilizing Drugs

Mood-stabilizing drugs are used to treat bipolar disorder by stabilizing the client's mood, preventing or minimizing the highs and lows that characterize bipolar illness, and treating acute episodes of mania. Lithium is the most established mood stabilizer; some anticonvulsant drugs, particularly carbamazepine (Tegretol) and valproic acid (Depakote, Depakene), are effective mood stabilizers. Other anticonvulsants, such as gabapentin (Neurontin), topiramate (Topamax), oxcarbazepine (Trileptal), and lamotrigine (Lamictal), are also used for mood stabilization. Occasionally, clonazepam (Klonopin) also is used to treat acute mania. Clonazepam is included in the discussion of anti-anxiety agents.

MECHANISM OF ACTION

Although lithium has many neurobiologic effects, its mechanism of action in bipolar illness is poorly understood. Lithium normalizes the reuptake of certain neurotransmitters such as serotonin, norepinephrine, acetylcholine, and dopamine. It also reduces the release of norepinephrine through competition with calcium. Lithium produces its effects intracellularly rather than within neuronal synapses; it acts directly on G proteins and certain enzyme subsystems such as cyclic adenosine monophosphates and phosphatidylinositol. Lithium is considered a first-line

agent in the treatment of bipolar disorder (Bauer & Mitchner, 2004).

The mechanism of action for anticonvulsants is not clear as it relates to their off-label use as mood stabilizers. Valproic acid and topiramate are known to increase levels of the inhibitory neurotransmitter GABA. Both valproic acid and carbamazepine are thought to stabilize mood by inhibiting the **kindling process**. This can be described as the snowball-like effect seen when minor seizure activity seems to build up into more frequent and severe seizures. In seizure management, anticonvulsants raise the level of the threshold to prevent these minor seizures. It is suspected that this same kindling process also may occur in the development of full-blown mania with stimulation by more frequent, minor episodes. This may explain why anticonvulsants are effective in the treatment and prevention of mania as well (Plata-Salaman et al., 2005).

DOSAGE

Lithium is available in tablets, capsules, liquid, and a sustained-released form; no parenteral forms are available. The effective dosage of lithium is determined by monitoring serum lithium levels and assessing the client's clinical response to the drug. Daily dosages generally range from 900 to 3,600 mg; more importantly, the serum lithium level should be about 1.0 mEq/L. Serum lithium levels of less than 0.5 mEq/L are rarely therapeutic, and levels of more than 1.5 mEq/L are usually considered toxic. The lithium level should be monitored every 2 to 3 days while the therapeutic dosage is being determined; then, it should be monitored weekly. When the client's condition is stable, the level may need to be checked once a month or less frequently.

WARNING ● Lithium

> Toxicity is closely related to serum lithium levels and can occur at therapeutic doses. Facilities for serum lithium determinations are required to monitor therapy.

Carbamazepine is available in liquid, tablet, and chewable tablet forms. Dosages usually range from 800 to 1,200 mg/day; the extreme dosage range is 200 to 2,000 mg/day. Valproic acid is available in liquid, tablet, and capsule forms and as sprinkles with dosages ranging from 1,000 to 1,500 mg/day; the extreme dosage range is 750 to 3,000 mg/day. Serum drug levels, obtained 12 hours after the last dose of the medication, are monitored for therapeutic levels of both these anticonvulsants.

SIDE EFFECTS

Common side effects of lithium therapy include mild nausea or diarrhea, anorexia, fine hand tremor, polydipsia, polyuria, a metallic taste in the mouth, and fatigue or lethargy. Weight gain and acne are side effects that occur later in lithium therapy; both are distressing for clients. Taking the medication with food may help with nausea, and the use of propranolol often improves the fine tremor. Lethargy and weight gain are difficult to manage or minimize and frequently lead to noncompliance.

Toxic effects of lithium are severe diarrhea, vomiting, drowsiness, muscle weakness, and lack of coordination. Untreated, these symptoms worsen and can lead to renal failure, coma, and death. When toxic signs occur, the drug should be discontinued immediately. If lithium levels exceed 3.0 mEq/L, dialysis may be indicated.

Side effects of carbamazepine and valproic acid include drowsiness, sedation, dry mouth, and blurred vision. In addition, carbamazepine may cause rashes and orthostatic hypotension, and valproic acid may cause weight gain, alopecia, and hand tremor. Topiramate causes dizziness, sedation, weight loss (rather than gain), and increased incidence of renal calculi (Bauer & Mitchner, 2004).

WARNING ⬤ Valproic Acid and Its Derivatives

> Can cause hepatic failure, resulting in fatality. Liver function tests should be performed before therapy and at frequent intervals thereafter, especially for the first 6 months. Can produce teratogenic effects such as neural tube defects (e.g., spina bifida). Can cause life-threatening pancreatitis in both children and adults. Can occur shortly after initiation or after years of therapy.

WARNING ⬤ Carbamazepine

> Can cause aplastic anemia and agranulocytosis at a rate five to eight times greater than the general population. Pretreatment hematologic baseline data should be obtained and monitored periodically throughout therapy to discover lowered WBC or platelet counts.

WARNING ⬤ Lamotrigine

> Can cause serious rashes requiring hospitalization, including Stevens-Johnson syndrome, and, rarely, life-threatening toxic epidermal necrolysis. The risk for serious rashes is greater in children younger than 16 years.

CLIENT TEACHING

For clients taking lithium and the anticonvulsants, monitoring blood levels periodically is important. The time of the last dose must be accurate so that plasma levels can be checked 12 hours after the last dose has been taken. Taking these medications with meals minimizes nausea. The client should not attempt to drive until dizziness, lethargy, fatigue, or blurred vision has subsided.

Antianxiety Drugs (Anxiolytics)

Antianxiety drugs, or **anxiolytic drugs**, are used to treat anxiety and anxiety disorders, insomnia, OCD, depression, posttraumatic stress disorder, and alcohol withdrawal. Antianxiety drugs are among the most widely prescribed medications today. A wide variety of drugs from different classifications have been used in the treatment of anxiety and insomnia. Benzodiazepines have proved to be the most effective in relieving anxiety and are the drugs most frequently prescribed. Benzodiazepines also may be prescribed for their anticonvulsant and muscle relaxant effects. Buspirone is a nonbenzodiazepine often used for the relief of anxiety and therefore is included in this section. Other drugs such as propranolol, clonidine (Catapres), and hydroxyzine (Vistaril) that may be used to relieve anxiety are much less effective and are not included in this discussion.

MECHANISM OF ACTION

Benzodiazepines mediate the actions of the amino acid GABA, the major inhibitory neurotransmitter in the brain. Because GABA receptor channels selectively admit the anion

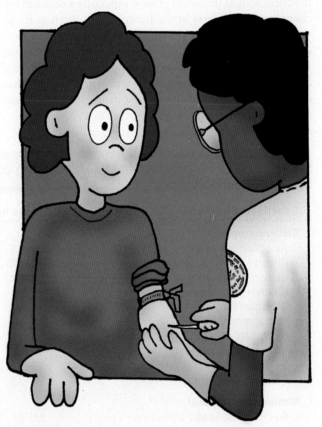

Periodic blood levels

chloride into neurons, activation of GABA receptors hyper-polarizes neurons and thus is inhibitory. Benzodiazepines produce their effects by binding to a specific site on the GABA receptor. Buspirone is believed to exert its anxiolytic effect by acting as a partial agonist at serotonin receptors, which decreases serotonin turnover (Chouinard, 2004a).

The benzodiazepines vary in terms of their half-lives, the means by which they are metabolized, and their effectiveness in treating anxiety and insomnia. Table 2.6 lists dosages, half-lives, and speed of onset after a single dose. Drugs with a longer half-life require less frequent dosing and produce fewer rebound effects between doses; however, they can accumulate in the body and produce "next-day sedation" effects. Conversely, drugs with a shorter half-life do not accumulate in the body or cause next-day sedation, but they do have rebound effects and require more frequent dosing.

Temazepam (Restoril), triazolam (Halcion), and flurazepam (Dalmane) are most often prescribed for sleep rather than for relief of anxiety. Diazepam (Valium), chlordiazepoxide (Librium), and clonazepam often are used to manage alcohol withdrawal as well as to relieve anxiety.

SIDE EFFECTS

Although not a side effect in the true sense, one chief problem encountered with the use of benzodiazepines is their tendency to cause physical dependence. Significant discontinuation symptoms occur when the drug is stopped; these symptoms often resemble the original symptoms for which the client sought treatment. This is especially a problem for clients with long-term benzodiazepine use, such as those with panic disorder or generalized anxiety disorder. Psychological dependence on benzodiazepines is common: Clients fear the return of anxiety symptoms or believe they are incapable of handling anxiety without the drugs. This can lead to overuse or abuse of these drugs. Buspirone does not cause this type of physical dependence.

The side effects most commonly reported with benzodiazepines are those associated with CNS depression, such as drowsiness, sedation, poor coordination, and impaired memory or clouded sensorium. When used for sleep, clients may complain of next-day sedation or a hangover effect. Clients often develop a tolerance to these symptoms, and they generally decrease in intensity. Common side effects from buspirone include dizziness, sedation, nausea, and headache (Chouinard, 2004a).

Elderly clients may have more difficulty managing the effects of CNS depression. They may be more prone to falls from the effects on coordination and sedation. They also may have more pronounced memory deficits and may have problems with urinary incontinence, particularly at night.

CLIENT TEACHING

Clients need to know that antianxiety agents are aimed at relieving symptoms such as anxiety or insomnia but do not treat the underlying problems that cause the anxiety. Benzodiazepines strongly potentiate the effects of alcohol: One drink may have the effect of three drinks. Therefore, clients should not drink alcohol while taking benzodiazepines. Clients should be aware of decreased response time, slower reflexes, and possible sedative effects of these drugs when attempting activities such as driving or going to work.

Benzodiazepine withdrawal can be fatal. After the client has started a course of therapy, he or she should never discontinue benzodiazepines abruptly or without the supervision of the physician (Lehne, 2006).

Stimulants

Stimulant drugs, specifically amphetamines, were first used to treat psychiatric disorders in the 1930s for their pronounced effects of CNS stimulation. In the past, they were used to treat depression and obesity, but those uses are

Table 2.6 ANTIANXIETY (ANXIOLYTIC) DRUGS

Generic (Trade) Name	Daily Dosage Range	Half-Life (h)	Speed of Onset
Benzodiazepines			
Alprazolam (Xanax)	0.75–1.5	12–15	Intermediate
Chlordiazepoxide (Librium)	15–100	50–100	Intermediate
Clonazepam (Klonopin)	1.5–20	18–50	Intermediate
Chlorazepate (Tranxene)	15–60	30–200	Fast
Diazepam (Valium)	4–40	30–100	Very fast
Flurazepam (Dalmane)	15–30	47–100	Fast
Lorazepam (Ativan)	2–8	10–20	Moderately slow
Oxazepam (Serax)	30–120	3–21	Moderately slow
Temazepam (Restoril)	15–30	9.5–20	Moderately fast
Triazolam (Halcion)	0.25–0.5	2–4	Fast
Nonbenzodiazepine			
Buspirone (BuSpar)	15–30	3–11	Very slow

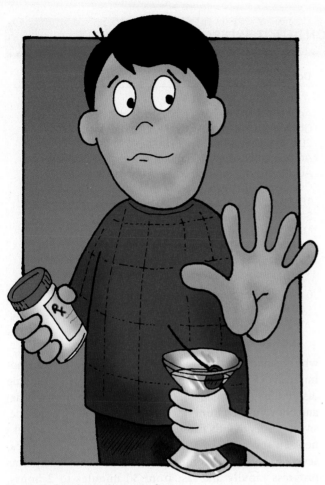

No alcohol with psychotropic drugs

uncommon in current practice. Dextroamphetamine (Dexedrine) has been widely abused to produce a high or to remain awake for long periods. Today, the primary use of stimulants is for ADHD in children and adolescents, residual attention deficit disorder in adults, and narcolepsy (attacks of unwanted but irresistible daytime sleepiness that disrupt the person's life).

The primary stimulant drugs used to treat ADHD are methylphenidate (Ritalin), amphetamine (Adderall), and dextroamphetamine (Dexedrine). Pemoline (Cylert) is infrequently used for ADHD because of the potential for liver problems. Of these drugs, methylphenidate accounts for 90% of the stimulant medication given to children for ADHD (Maxmen & Ward, 2002). About 10% to 30% of clients with ADHD who do not respond adequately to the stimulant medications have been treated with antidepressants. In 2003, atomoxetine (Strattera), a selective norepinephrine reuptake inhibitor, was approved for the treatment of ADHD, becoming the first nonstimulant medication specifically designed and tested for ADHD.

MECHANISM OF ACTION

Amphetamines and methylphenidate are often termed *indirectly acting amines* because they act by causing release of

the neurotransmitters (norepinephrine, dopamine, and serotonin) from presynaptic nerve terminals as opposed to having direct agonist effects on the postsynaptic receptors. They also block the reuptake of these neurotransmitters. Methylphenidate produces milder CNS stimulation than amphetamines; pemoline primarily affects dopamine and therefore has less effect on the sympathetic nervous system. It was originally thought that the use of methylphenidate and pemoline to treat ADHD in children produced the reverse effect of most stimulants—a calming or slowing of activity in the brain. However, this is not the case; the inhibitory centers in the brain are stimulated, so the child has greater abilities to filter out distractions and manage his or her own behavior. Atomoxetine helps to block the reuptake of norepinephrine into neurons, thereby leaving more of the neurotransmitter in the synapse to help convey electrical impulses in the brain.

WARNING ● Amphetamines

Potential for abuse is high. Administration for prolonged periods may lead to drug dependence.

DOSAGE

For the treatment of narcolepsy in adults, both dextroamphetamine and methylphenidate are given in divided doses totaling 20 to 200 mg/day. The higher dosages may be needed because adults with narcolepsy develop tolerance to the stimulants and so require more medication to sustain improvement. Stimulant medications are also available in sustained-release preparations so that once-a-day dosing is possible. Tolerance is not seen in persons with ADHD.

WARNING ● Methylphenidate

Use with caution in emotionally unstable clients such as those with alcohol or drug dependence because they may increase the dosage on their own. Chronic abuse can lead to marked tolerance and psychic dependence.

The dosages used to treat ADHD in children vary widely depending on the physician; the age, weight, and behavior of the child; and the tolerance of the family for the child's behavior. Table 2.7 lists the usual dosage ranges for these stimulants. Arrangements must be made for the school nurse or another authorized adult to administer the stimulants to the child at school. Sustained-released preparations eliminate the need for additional dosing at school.

SIDE EFFECTS

The most common side effects of stimulants are anorexia, weight loss, nausea, and irritability. The client should avoid

| Table 2.7 | DRUGS USED TO TREAT ATTENTION DEFICIT HYPERACTIVITY DISORDER |

Generic (Trade) Name	Dosage
Stimulants	
Methylphenidate (Ritalin)	Adults: 20–200 mg/day, orally, in divided doses
	Children: 10–60 mg/day, orally, in 2–4 divided doses
Sustained release (Ritalin-SR, Concerta, Metadate-CD)	20–60 mg/day, orally, single dose
Transdermal patch (Daytrana)	Adults and Children: 15mg patch worn for 9 hours per day
Dextroamphetamine (Dexedrine)	Adults: 20–200 mg/day, orally, in divided doses
	Children: 5–40 mg/day, orally, in 2 or 3 divided doses
Sustained release (Dexedrine-SR)	10–30 mg/day, orally, single dose
Amphetamine (Adderall)	5–40 mg/day, orally, in divided doses
Sustained release (Adderall-SR)	10–30 mg/day, orally, single dose
Pemoline (Cylert)	Children: 37.5–112.5 mg/day, orally, single dose in the morning
Selective Norepinephrine Reuptake Inhibitor	
Atomoxetine (Strattera)	0.5–1.5 mg/kg/day, orally, single dose

caffeine, sugar, and chocolate, which may worsen these symptoms. Less common side effects include dizziness, dry mouth, blurred vision, and palpitations. The most common long-term problem with stimulants is the growth and weight suppression that occurs in some children. This can usually be prevented by taking "drug holidays" on weekends and holidays or during summer vacation, which helps to restore normal eating and growth patterns. Atomoxetine can cause decreased appetite, nausea, vomiting, fatigue, or upset stomach.

WARNING ● Pemoline

Can cause life-threatening liver failure, which can result in death or require liver transplantation in 4 weeks from the onset of symptoms. The physician should obtain written consent before the initiation of this drug.

CLIENT TEACHING

The potential for abuse exists with stimulants, but this is seldom a problem in children. Taking doses of stimulants after meals may minimize anorexia and nausea. Caffeine-free beverages are suggested; clients should avoid chocolate and excessive sugar. Most important is to keep the medication out of the child's reach because as little as a 10-day supply can be fatal.

Disulfiram (Antabuse)

Disulfiram is a sensitizing agent that causes an adverse reaction when mixed with alcohol in the body. This agent's only use is as a deterrent to drinking alcohol in persons receiving treatment for alcoholism. It is useful for persons who are motivated to abstain from drinking and who are not impulsive. Five to 10 minutes after someone who is taking disulfiram ingests alcohol, symptoms begin to appear: facial and body flushing from vasodilation, a throbbing headache, sweating, dry mouth, nausea, vomiting, dizziness, and weakness. In severe cases, there may be chest pain, dyspnea, severe hypotension, confusion, and even death. Symptoms progress rapidly and last from 30 minutes to 2 hours. Because the liver metabolizes disulfiram, it is most effective in persons whose liver enzyme levels are within or close to normal range.

Disulfiram inhibits the enzyme aldehyde dehydrogenase, which is involved in the metabolism of ethanol. Acetaldehyde levels are then increased from 5 to 10 times higher than normal, resulting in the disulfiram–alcohol reaction. This reaction is potentiated by decreased levels of epinephrine and norepinephrine in the sympathetic nervous system caused by inhibition of dopamine beta-hydroxylase (dopamine β-hydroxylase) (Cornish et al., 2006).

Education is extremely important for the client taking disulfiram. Many common products such as shaving cream, aftershave lotion, cologne, and deodorant and over-the-counter medications such as cough preparations contain alcohol; when used by the client taking disulfiram, these products can produce the same reaction as drinking alcohol. The client must read product labels carefully and select items that are alcohol-free.

WARNING ● Disulfiram

Never give to a client in a state of alcohol intoxication or without the client's full knowledge. Instruct the client's relatives accordingly.

Other side effects reported by persons taking disulfiram include fatigue, drowsiness, halitosis, tremor, and impotence. Disulfiram also can interfere with the metabolism of other drugs the client is taking, such as phenytoin (Dilantin), isoniazid, warfarin (Coumadin), barbiturates, and long-acting benzodiazepines such as diazepam and chlordiazepoxide.

Acamprosate (Campral) was approved in 2004 for persons in recovery from alcohol abuse or dependence. It helps reduce the physical and emotional discomfort encountered during the first weeks or months of sobriety, such as sweating, anxiety, and sleep disturbances. The dosage is two tablets (333 mg each) three times a day. Persons with renal impairments cannot take this drug. Side effects are reported as mild and include diarrhea, nausea, flatulence, and pruritus.

CULTURAL CONSIDERATIONS

Studies have shown that people from different ethnic backgrounds respond differently to certain drugs used to treat mental disorders. The nurse should be familiar with these cultural differences.

Studies have shown that African Americans respond more rapidly to antipsychotic medications and tricyclic antidepressants than do whites. Also, African Americans have a greater risk for developing side effects from both these classes of drugs than do whites. Asians metabolize antipsychotics and tricyclic antidepressants more slowly than do whites and therefore require lower dosages to achieve the same effects. Hispanics also require lower dosages of antidepressants than do whites to achieve the desired results (Woods et al., 2003).

Asians respond therapeutically to lower dosages of lithium than do whites. African Americans have higher blood levels of lithium than whites when given the same dosage, and they also experience more side effects. This suggests that African Americans require lower dosages of lithium than do whites to produce desired effects (Chen et al., 2002).

Herbal medicines have been used for hundreds of years in many countries and are now being used with increasing frequency in the United States. St. John's wort is used to treat depression and is the second most commonly purchased herbal product in the United States (Malaty, 2005). Kava is used to treat anxiety and can potentiate the effects of alcohol, benzodiazepines, and other sedative-hypnotic agents. Valerian helps produce sleep and is sometimes used to relieve stress and anxiety. Ginkgo biloba is primarily used to improve memory but is also taken for fatigue, anxiety, and depression.

It is essential for the nurse to ask clients specifically if they use any herbal preparations. Clients may not consider these products as "medicine" or may be reluctant to admit their use for fear of censure by health professionals. Herbal medicines are often chemically complex and are not standardized or regulated for use in treating illnesses. Combining herbal preparations with other medicines can lead to unwanted interactions, so it essential to assess the clients' use of these products.

SELF-AWARENESS ISSUES

Nurses must examine their own beliefs and feelings about mental disorders as illnesses and the role of drugs in treating mental disorders. Some nurses may be skeptical about some mental disorders and may believe that clients could gain control of their lives if they would just put forth enough effort. Nurses who work with clients with mental disorders come to understand that many disorders are similar to chronic physical illnesses such as asthma or diabetes, which require lifelong medication to maintain health. Without proper medication management, clients with certain mental disorders, such as schizophrenia or bipolar affective disorder, cannot survive in and cope with the world around them. The nurse must explain to the client and family that this is an illness that requires continuous medication management and follow-up, just like a chronic physical illness.

It is also important for the nurse to know about current biologic theories and treatments. Many clients and their families will have questions about reports in the news about research or discoveries. The nurse can help them distinguish between what is factual and what is experimental. Also, it is important to keep discoveries and theories in perspective.

Clients and families need more than factual information to deal with mental illness and its effect on their lives. Many clients do not understand the nature of their illness and ask, "Why is this happening to me?" They need simple but thorough explanations about the nature of the illness and how they can manage it. The nurse must learn to give out enough information about the illness while providing the care and support needed by all those confronting mental illness.

Points to Consider When Working on Self-Awareness

- Chronic mental illness has periods of remission and exacerbation just like chronic physical illness. A recurrence of symptoms is not the client's fault, nor is it a failure of treatment or nursing care.
- Research regarding the neurobiologic causes of mental disorders is still in its infancy. Do not dismiss new ideas just because they may not yet help in the treatment of these illnesses.
- Often, when clients stop taking medication or take medication improperly, it is not because they intend to; rather, it is the result of faulty thinking and reasoning, which is part of the illness.

Critical Thinking Questions

1. It is possible to identify a gene associated with increased risk for the late onset of Alzheimer's disease. Should this test be available to anyone who requests it? Why or why not? What dilemmas might arise from having such knowledge?

2. What are the implications for nursing if it becomes possible to predict certain illnesses such as schizophrenia through the identification of genes responsible for or linked to the disease? Should this influence whether people who carry such genes should have children? Who should make that decision, given that many people with chronic mental illness depend on government programs for financial support?

3. Drug companies research and develop new drugs. Much more money and effort are expended to produce new drugs for common disorders rather than drugs (often called "orphan drugs") needed to treat rare disorders such as Tourette's syndrome. What are the ethical and financial dilemmas associated with research designed to produce new drugs?

KEY POINTS

- Neurobiologic research is constantly expanding our knowledge in the field of psychiatry and is significantly affecting clinical practice.
- The cerebrum is the center for coordination and integration of all information needed to interpret and respond to the environment.
- The cerebellum is the center for coordination of movements and postural adjustments.
- The brain stem contains centers that control cardiovascular and respiratory functions, sleep, consciousness, and impulses.
- The limbic system regulates body temperature, appetite, sensations, memory, and emotional arousal.
- Neurotransmitters are the chemical substances manufactured in the neuron that aid in the transmission of infor-

mation from the brain throughout the body. Several important neurotransmitters including dopamine, norepinephrine, serotonin, histamine, acetylcholine, GABA, and glutamate have been found to play a role in mental disorders and are targets of pharmacologic treatment.

- Researchers continue to examine the roles of genetics, heredity, and viruses in the development of mental illness.
- Pharmacologic treatment is based on the ability of medications to eliminate or minimize identified target symptoms.
- The following factors must be considered in the selection of medications to treat mental disorders: the efficacy, potency, and half-life of the drug; the age and race of the client; other medications the client is taking; and the side effects of the drugs.
- Antipsychotic drugs are the primary treatment for psychotic disorders such as schizophrenia, but they produce a host of side effects that also may require pharmacologic intervention. Neurologic side effects, which can be treated with anticholinergic medications, are called EPS and include acute dystonia, akathisia, and pseudoparkinsonism. Some of the more serious neurologic side effects include tardive dyskinesia (permanent involuntary movements) and neuroleptic malignant syndrome, which can be fatal.
- Because of the serious side effects of antipsychotic medications, clients must be well educated regarding their medications, medication compliance, and side effects. Health care professionals must closely supervise the regimen.
- Antidepressant medications include cyclic compounds, SSRIs, MAOIs, and a group of newer drugs.
- The nurse must carefully instruct clients receiving MAOIs to avoid foods containing tyramine because the combination produces a hypertensive crisis that can become life threatening.
- The risk for suicide may increase as clients begin taking antidepressants. Although suicidal thoughts are still present, the medication may increase the client's energy, which may allow the client to carry out a suicide plan.
- Lithium and selected anticonvulsants are used to stabilize mood, particularly in bipolar affective disorder.
- The nurse must monitor serum lithium levels regularly to ensure the level is in the therapeutic range and to avoid lithium toxicity. Symptoms of toxicity include

INTERNET RESOURCES

RESOURCE	INTERNET ADDRESS
Clinical Pharmacology Online	http://www.cponline.gsm.som
Research Project Relating to DNA, Genetics, and Mental Disorders	http://www.nhgri.gov
U.S. Food and Drug Administration	http://www.fda.gov

severe diarrhea and vomiting, drowsiness, muscle weakness, and loss of coordination. Untreated, lithium toxicity leads to coma and death.

- Benzodiazepines are used to treat a wide variety of problems related to anxiety and insomnia. Clients taking them should avoid alcohol, which increases the effects of the benzodiazepines.

- The primary use of stimulants such as methylphenidate (Ritalin) is the treatment of children with ADHD. Methylphenidate has been proved successful in allowing these children to slow down their activity and focus on the tasks at hand and their schoolwork. Its exact mechanism of action is unknown.

- Clients from various cultures may metabolize medications at different rates and therefore require alterations in standard dosages.

- Assessing use of herbal preparations is essential for all clients.

REFERENCES

American Psychiatric Association. (2000). *Diagnostic and statistical manual of mental disorders* (4th ed., text revision). Washington, DC: American Psychiatric Association.

Bauer, M. S., & Mitchner, L. (2004). What is a "mood stabilizer"? An evidence-based response. *American Journal of Psychiatry, 161*(1), 3–18.

Chen, J. P., Barron, C., Lin, K. M., et al. (2002). Prescribing medication for Asians with mental disorders. *Western Journal of Medicine, 176*(4), 271–275.

Chouinard, G. (2004a). Issues in the clinical use of benzodiazepines: Potency, withdrawal, and rebound. *Journal of Clinical Psychiatry, 65*(Suppl. 5), 7–12.

Chouinard, G. (2004b). New nomenclature for drug-induced movement disorders including tardive dyskinesia. *Journal of Clinical Psychiatry, 65*(Suppl. 9), 9–15.

Cornish, J. W., McNicholas, L. F., & O'Brien, C. P. (2006). Treatment of substance-related disorders. In A. F. Schatzberg & C. B. Nemeroff (Eds.), *Essentials of clinical pharmacology* (2nd ed., pp. 647–667). Washington, DC: American Psychiatric Publishing.

Daniel, D. G., Copeland, L. F., & Tamminga, C. (2006). Ziprasidone. In A. F. Schatzberg & C. B. Nemeroff (Eds.), *Essentials of clinical pharmacology,* (2nd ed., pp. 297–305). Washington, DC: American Psychiatric Publishing.

Fujita, M., Kugaya, A., & Innis, R. B. (2005). Radiotracer imaging: Basic principles and exemplary findings in neuropsychiatric disorders. In B. J. Sadock & V. A. Sadock (Eds.), *Comprehensive textbook of psychiatry* (Vol. 1, 8th ed., pp. 222–236). Philadelphia: Lippincott Williams & Wilkins.

Glassman, A. H. (2005). Schizophrenia, antipsychotic drugs, and cardiovascular disease. *Journal of Clinical Psychiatry, 66*(Suppl 6), 5–10.

Hitt, E. (2003). Managing weight gain as a side effect of antidepressant therapy. *Cleveland Clinical Journal, 70,* 614–623.

Kane, J. M., Eerdekens, M., Lindenmayer, J., et al. (2003). Long-acting injectable risperidone: Efficacy and safety for the first long-acting atypical antipsychotic. *American Journal of Psychiatry, 160*(6), 1125–1132.

Krishnan, K. R. R. (2006). Monoamine oxidase inhibitors. In A. F. Schatzberg & C. B. Nemeroff (Eds.), *Essentials of clinical pharmacology* (2nd ed., pp. 113–125). Washington, DC: American Psychiatric Publishing.

Lehne, R. A. (2006). *Pharmacology for nursing care* (6th ed.). Philadelphia: W. B. Saunders.

Malaty, W. (2005). St. John's wort for depression. *American Family Physician, 71*(7), 1375–1376.

Muller, D. J., & Kennedy, J. L. (2006). Genetics of antipsychotic treatment emergent weight gain in schizophrenia. *Pharmacogenomics, 7*(6), 863–887.

National Institutes of Health. (2007). About ELSI. Retrieved February 3, 2002, from http://www.nhgri.nhi.gov/ELSI.

Newcomer, J. N., & Haupt, D. W. (2006). The metabolic effects of antipsychotic medications. *Canadian Journal of Psychiatry 51*(8): 480–491.

Plata-Salaman, C. R., Shank, R. P., & Smith-Swintosky, V. L. (2005). Amino acid neurotransmitters. In B. J. Sadock & V. A. Sadock (Eds.), *Comprehensive textbook of psychiatry* (Vol. 1, 8th ed., pp. 60–72). Philadelphia: Lippincott Williams & Wilkins.

Swedo, S. E., Leonard, H. L., & Rapoport, J. L. (2004). The pediatric autoimmune neuropsychiatric disorders associated with streptococcal infection (PANDAS) subgroup: Separating fact from fiction. *Pediatrics, 113*(4), 907–911.

Tecott, L. H., & Smart, S. L. (2005). Monoamine transmitters. In B. J. Sadock & V. A. Sadock (Eds.), *Comprehensive textbook of psychiatry* (Vol. 1, 8th ed., pp. 49–60). Philadelphia: Lippincott Williams & Wilkins.

Vythilingam, M., Shen, J., Drevets, W. C., et al. (2005). Nuclear magnetic resonance imaging: Basic principles and recent findings in neuropsychiatric disorders. In B. J. Sadock & V. A. Sadock (Eds.), *Comprehensive textbook of psychiatry* (Vol. 1, 8th ed., pp. 201–222). Philadelphia: Lippincott Williams & Wilkins.

Woods, S. W., Sullivan, M. C., Neuse, E. C., et al. (2003). Racial and ethnic effects on antipsychotic prescribing practices in a community mental health center. *Psychiatric Services, 54*(2), 177–179.

ADDITIONAL READINGS

Janicak, P. G., & Beedle, D. (2005). Medication-induced movement disorders. In B. J. Sadock & V. A. Sadock (Eds.), *Comprehensive textbook of psychiatry* (Vol. 2, 8th ed., pp. 2712–2718). Philadelphia: Lippincott Williams & Wilkins.

Mathews, C. A., & Friemer, N. B. (2005). Genetic linkage analysis of the psychiatric disorders. In B. J. Sadock & V. A. Sadock (Eds.), *Comprehensive textbook of psychiatry* (Vol. 1, 8th ed., pp. 252–272). Philadelphia: Lippincott Williams & Wilkins.

Chapter Study Guide

MULTIPLE-CHOICE QUESTIONS

Select the best answer for each of the following questions.

1. The nurse is teaching a client taking an MAOI about foods with tyramine that he or she should avoid. Which of the following statements indicates that the client needs further teaching?
   A. "I'm so glad I can have pizza as long as I don't order pepperoni."
   B. "I will be able to eat cottage cheese without worrying."
   C. "I will have to avoid drinking nonalcoholic beer."
   D. "I can eat green beans on this diet."

2. A client who has been depressed and suicidal started taking a tricyclic antidepressant 2 weeks ago and is now ready to leave the hospital to go home. Which of the following is a concern for the nurse as discharge plans are finalized?
   A. The client may need a prescription for diphenhydramine (Benadryl) to use for side effects.
   B. The nurse will evaluate the risk for suicide by overdose of the tricyclic antidepressant.
   C. The nurse will need to include teaching regarding the signs of neuroleptic malignant syndrome.
   D. The client will need regular laboratory work to monitor therapeutic drug levels.

3. The signs of lithium toxicity include which of the following?
   A. Sedation, fever, restlessness
   B. Psychomotor agitation, insomnia, increased thirst
   C. Elevated white blood cell count, sweating, confusion
   D. Severe vomiting, diarrhea, weakness

4. Which of the following is a concern for children taking stimulants for ADHD for several years?
   A. Dependence on the drug
   B. Insomnia
   C. Growth suppression
   D. Weight gain

5. The nurse is caring for a client with schizophrenia who is taking haloperidol (Haldol). The client complains of restlessness, cannot sit still, and has muscle stiffness. Of the following PRN medications, which would the nurse administer?
   A. Haloperidol (Haldol), 5 mg PO
   B. Benztropine (Cogentin), 2 mg PO
   C. Propranolol (Inderal), 20 mg PO
   D. Trazodone, 50 mg PO

6. Client teaching for lamotrigine (Lamictal) should include which of the following?
   A. Eat a well-balanced diet to avoid weight gain.
   B. Report any rashes to your doctor immediately.
   C. Take each dose with food to avoid nausea.
   D. This drug may cause psychological dependence.

7. Which of the following physician orders would the nurse question for a client who has stated "I'm allergic to phenothiazines"?
   A. Haldol, 5 mg PO bid
   B. Navane, 10 mg PO bid
   C. Prolixin, 5 mg PO tid
   D. Risperdal, 2 mg bid

8. Clients taking which of the following types of psychotropic medications need close monitoring of their cardiac status?
   A. Antidepressants
   B. Antipsychotics
   C. Mood stabilizers
   D. Stimulants

FILL-IN-THE-BLANK QUESTIONS

Identify the drug classification for each of the following medications.

_____ 1. Clozapine (Clozaril)

_____ 2. Fluoxetine (Prozac)

_____   3. Amitriptyline (Elavil)

_____   4. Benztropine (Cogentin)

_____   5. Methylphenidate (Ritalin)

_____   6. Carbamazepine (Tegretol)

_____   7. Clonazepam (Klonopin)

_____   8. Quetiapine (Seroquel)

SHORT-ANSWER QUESTIONS

1. Explain the rationale for tapering psychotropic medication doses before the client discontinues the drug.

2. Describe the teaching needed for a client who is scheduled for PET.

3. Explain the kindling process as it relates to the manic episodes of bipolar affective disorder.

Psychosocial Theories and Therapy

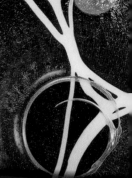

Key Terms

- alternative medicine
- behavior modification
- behaviorism
- client-centered therapy
- closed group
- cognitive therapy
- complementary medicine
- countertransference
- crisis
- crisis intervention
- dream analysis
- education group
- ego
- ego defense mechanisms
- family therapy
- free association
- group therapy
- hierarchy of needs
- humanism
- id
- individual psychotherapy
- integrative medicine
- milieu therapy
- negative reinforcement
- open group
- operant conditioning

- parataxic mode
- participant observer
- positive reinforcement
- prototaxic mode
- psychiatric rehabilitation
- psychoanalysis
- psychosocial interventions
- psychotherapy
- psychotherapy group
- self-actualization

- self-help group
- subconscious
- superego
- support group
- syntaxic mode
- systematic desensitization
- therapeutic community or milieu
- therapeutic nurse–patient relationship
- transference

Learning Objectives

After reading this chapter, you should be able to

1. Explain the basic beliefs and approaches of the following psychosocial theories: psychoanalytic, developmental, interpersonal, humanistic, behavioral, existential, and crisis intervention.

2. Describe the following psychosocial treatment modalities: individual psychotherapy, group psychotherapy, family therapy, behavior modification, systematic desensitization, token economy, self-help groups, support groups, education groups, cognitive therapy, milieu therapy, and psychiatric rehabilitation.

3. Identify the psychosocial theory on which each treatment strategy is based.

4. Identify how several of the theoretical perspectives have influenced current nursing practice.

Visit the Point http://thePoint.lww.com for NCLEX-style questions, journal articles, and more!

Today's mental health treatment has an eclectic approach, meaning one that incorporates concepts and strategies from a variety of sources. This chapter presents an overview of major psychosocial theories, highlights the ideas and concepts in current practice, and explains the various psychosocial treatment modalities. The psychosocial theories have produced many models currently used in individual and group therapy and various treatment settings. The medical model of treatment is based on the neurobiologic theories discussed in Chapter 2.

PSYCHOSOCIAL THEORIES

Many theories attempt to explain human behavior, health, and mental illness. Each theory suggests how normal development occurs based on the theorist's beliefs, assumptions, and view of the world. These theories suggest strategies that the clinician can use to work with clients. Many theories discussed in this chapter were not based on empirical or research evidence; rather, they evolved from individual experiences and might more appropriately be called conceptual models or frameworks.

This chapter discusses the following types of psychosocial theories:

- Psychoanalytic
- Developmental
- Interpersonal
- Humanistic
- Behavioral
- Existential

Psychoanalytic Theories

SIGMUND FREUD: THE FATHER OF PSYCHOANALYSIS

Sigmund Freud (1856–1939; Figure 3.1) developed psychoanalytic theory in the late 19th and early 20th centuries in Vienna, where he spent most of his life. Several other noted psychoanalysts and theorists have contributed to this body of knowledge, but Freud is its undisputed founder. Many clinicians and theorists did not agree with much of Freud's psychoanalytic theory and later developed their own theories and styles of treatment.

Psychoanalytic theory supports the notion that all human behavior is caused and can be explained (deterministic theory). Freud believed that *repressed* (driven from conscious awareness) sexual impulses and desires motivate much human behavior. He developed his initial ideas and explanations of human behavior from his experiences with a few clients, all of them women who displayed unusual behaviors such as disturbances of sight and speech, inability to eat, and paralysis of limbs. These symptoms had no physiologic basis, so Freud considered them to be the "hysterical" or neurotic behavior of women. After several years of working with these women, Freud concluded that many of their problems resulted from childhood trauma or fail-

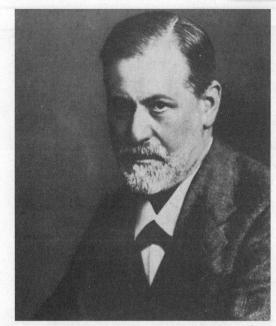

Figure 3.1. Sigmund Freud: the father of psychoanalysis.

ure to complete tasks of psychosexual development. These women repressed their unmet needs and sexual feelings as well as traumatic events. The "hysterical" or neurotic behaviors resulted from these unresolved conflicts.

Personality Components: Id, Ego, and Superego. Freud conceptualized personality structure as having three components: id, ego, and superego (Freud, 1923/1962). The **id** is the part of one's nature that reflects basic or innate desires such as pleasure-seeking behavior, aggression, and sexual impulses. The id seeks instant gratification, causes impulsive unthinking behavior, and has no regard for rules or social convention. The **superego** is the part of a person's nature that reflects moral and ethical concepts, values, and parental and social expectations; therefore, it is in direct opposition to the id. The third component, the **ego**, is the balancing or mediating force between the id and the superego. The ego represents mature and adaptive behavior that allows a person to function successfully in the world. Freud believed that anxiety resulted from the ego's attempts to balance the impulsive instincts of the id with the stringent rules of the superego. The accompanying drawing demonstrates the relationship of these personality structures.

Behavior Motivated by Subconscious Thoughts and Feelings. Freud believed that the human personality functions at three levels of awareness: conscious, preconscious, and unconscious (Freud, 1923/1962). *Conscious* refers to the perceptions, thoughts, and emotions that exist in the person's awareness, such as being aware of happy feelings or thinking about a loved one. *Preconscious* thoughts and emotions are not currently in the person's awareness, but he or she can recall them with some effort—for example, an adult remembering what he or she did, thought, or felt as a child. The *unconscious* is the realm of thoughts and feelings that motivate a person even though he or she is

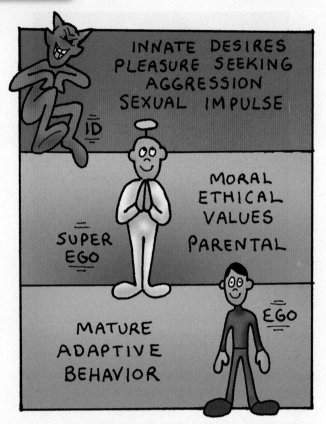

Freud's components of personality

totally unaware of them. This realm includes most defense mechanisms (see discussion to follow) and some instinctual drives or motivations. According to Freud's theories, the person represses into the unconscious the memory of traumatic events that are too painful to remember.

Freud believed that much of what we do and say is motivated by our **subconscious** thoughts or feelings (those in the preconscious or unconscious level of awareness). A "Freudian slip" is a term we commonly use to describe slips of the tongue—for example, saying "You look portly today" to an overweight friend instead of "You look pretty today." Freud believed these slips are not accidents or coincidences but rather are indications of subconscious feelings or thoughts that accidentally emerge in casual day-to-day conversation.

Freud's Dream Analysis. Freud believed that a person's dreams reflect his or her subconscious and have significant meaning, although sometimes the meaning is hidden or symbolic (Loden, 2002). **Dream analysis,** a primary method used in psychoanalysis, involves discussing a client's dreams to discover their true meaning and significance. For example, a client might report having recurrent frightening dreams about snakes chasing her. Freud's interpretation might be that the woman fears intimacy with men; he would view the snake as a phallic symbol, representing the penis.

Another method used to gain access to subconscious thoughts and feelings is **free association,** in which the therapist tries to uncover the client's true thoughts and feelings

by saying a word and asking the client to respond quickly with the first thing that comes to mind. Freud believed that such quick responses would be likely to uncover subconscious or repressed thoughts or feelings.

Ego Defense Mechanisms. Freud believed the self, or ego, uses **ego defense mechanisms,** which are methods of attempting to protect the self and cope with basic drives or emotionally painful thoughts, feelings, or events. Defense mechanisms are explained in Table 3.1. For example, a person who has been diagnosed with cancer and told he has 6 months to live but refuses to talk about his illness is using the defense mechanism of denial, or refusal to accept the reality of the situation. If a person dying of cancer exhibits continuously cheerful behavior, he could be using the defense mechanism of reaction formation to protect his emotions. Most defense mechanisms operate at the unconscious level of awareness, so people are not aware of what they are doing and often need help to see the reality.

Five Stages of Psychosexual Development. Freud based his theory of childhood development on the belief that sexual energy, termed *libido,* was the driving force of human behavior. He proposed that children progress through five stages of psychosexual development: oral (birth to 18 months), anal (18 to 36 months), phallic/oedipal (3 to 5 years), latency (5 to 11 or 13 years), and genital (11 to 13 years). Table 3.2 describes these stages and the accompanying developmental tasks. Psychopathology results when a person has difficulty making the transition from one stage to the next or when a person remains stalled at a particular stage or regresses to an earlier stage. Freud's open discussion of sexual impulses, particularly in children, was considered shocking for his time (Freud, 1923/1962).

Transference and Countertransference. Freud developed the concepts of transference and countertransference. **Transference** occurs when the client displaces onto the therapist attitudes and feelings that the client originally experienced in other relationships (Freud, 1923/1962). Transference patterns are automatic and unconscious in the therapeutic relationship. For example, an adolescent female client working with a nurse who is about the same age as the teen's parents might react to the nurse like she reacts to her parents. She might experience intense feelings of rebellion or make sarcastic remarks; these reactions are actually based on her experiences with her parents, not the nurse.

Countertransference occurs when the therapist displaces onto the client attitudes or feelings from his or her past. For example, a female nurse who has teenage children and who is experiencing extreme frustration with an adolescent client may respond by adopting a parental or chastising tone. The nurse is countertransfering her own attitudes and feelings toward her children onto the client. Nurses can deal with countertransference by examining their own feelings and responses, using self-awareness, and talking with colleagues.

CURRENT PSYCHOANALYTIC PRACTICE

Psychoanalysis focuses on discovering the causes of the client's unconscious and repressed thoughts, feelings, and

Table 3.1   EGO DEFENSE MECHANISMS

Compensation	Overachievement in one area to offset real or perceived deficiencies in another area • Napoleon complex: diminutive man becoming emperor • Nurse with low self-esteem works double shifts so her supervisor will like her.
Conversion	Expression of an emotional conflict through the development of a physical symptom, usually senso-rimotor in nature • Teenager forbidden to see X-rated movies is tempted to do so by friends and develops blindness, and the teenager is unconcerned about the loss of sight.
Denial	Failure to acknowledge an unbearable condition; failure to admit the reality of a situation or how one enables the problem to continue • Diabetic person eating chocolate candy • Spending money freely when broke • Waiting 3 days to seek help for severe abdominal pain
Displacement	Ventilation of intense feelings toward persons less threatening than the one who aroused those feelings • Person who is mad at the boss yells at his or her spouse. • Child who is harassed by a bully at school mistreats a younger sibling.
Dissociation	Dealing with emotional conflict by a temporary alteration in consciousness or identity • Amnesia that prevents recall of yesterday's auto accident • Adult remembers nothing of childhood sexual abuse.
Fixation	Immobilization of a portion of the personality resulting from unsuccessful completion of tasks in a developmental stage • Never learning to delay gratification • Lack of a clear sense of identity as an adult
Identification	Modeling actions and opinions of influential others while searching for identity, or aspiring to reach a personal, social, or occupational goal • Nursing student becoming a critical care nurse because this is the specialty of an instructor she admires
Intellectualization	Separation of the emotions of a painful event or situation from the facts involved; acknowledging the facts but not the emotions • Person shows no emotional expression when discussing serious car accident.
Introjection	Accepting another person's attitudes, beliefs, and values as one's own • Person who dislikes guns becomes an avid hunter, just like a best friend.
Projection	Unconscious blaming of unacceptable inclinations or thoughts on an external object • Man who has thought about same-gender sexual relationship, but never had one, beats a man who is gay. • Person with many prejudices loudly identifies others as bigots.
Rationalization	Excusing own behavior to avoid guilt, responsibility, conflict, anxiety, or loss of self-respect • Student blames failure on teacher being mean. • Man says he beats his wife because she doesn't listen to him.
Reaction formation	Acting the opposite of what one thinks or feels • Woman who never wanted to have children becomes a super-mom. • Person who despises the boss tells everyone what a great boss she is.
Regression	Moving back to a previous developmental stage to feel safe or have needs met • Five-year-old asks for a bottle when new baby brother is being fed. • Man pouts like a 4-year-old if he is not the center of his girlfriend's attention.
Repression	Excluding emotionally painful or anxiety-provoking thoughts and feelings from conscious awareness • Woman has no memory of the mugging she suffered yesterday. • Woman has no memory before age 7, when she was removed from abusive parents.
Resistance	Overt or covert antagonism toward remembering or processing anxiety-producing information • Nurse is too busy with tasks to spend time talking to a dying patient. • Person attends court-ordered treatment for alcoholism but refuses to participate.
Sublimation	Substituting a socially acceptable activity for an impulse that is unacceptable • Person who has quit smoking sucks on hard candy when the urge to smoke arises. • Person goes for a 15-minute walk when tempted to eat junk food.

Table 3.1	EGO DEFENSE MECHANISMS (Continued)
Substitution	Replacing the desired gratification with one that is more readily available • Woman who would like to have her own children opens a day care center.
Suppression	Conscious exclusion of unacceptable thoughts and feelings from conscious awareness • Student decides not to think about a parent's illness to study for a test. • Woman tells a friend she cannot think about her son's death right now.
Undoing	Exhibiting acceptable behavior to make up for or negate unacceptable behavior • Person who cheats on a spouse brings the spouse a bouquet of roses. • Man who is ruthless in business donates large amounts of money to charity.

conflicts believed to cause anxiety and on helping the client to gain insight into and resolve these conflicts and anxieties. The analytic therapist uses the techniques of free association, dream analysis, and interpretation of behavior.

Psychoanalysis is still practiced today but on a very limited basis. Analysis is lengthy, with weekly or more frequent sessions for several years. It is costly and not covered by conventional health insurance programs; thus, it has become known as "therapy for the wealthy."

Developmental Theories

ERIK ERIKSON AND PSYCHOSOCIAL STAGES OF DEVELOPMENT

Erik Erikson (1902–1994) was a German-born psychoanalyst who extended Freud's work on personality development across the life span while focusing on social and psychological development in the life stages. In 1950, Erikson published *Childhood and Society,* in which he described eight psychosocial stages of development. In each stage, the person must complete a life task that is essential to his or her well-being and mental health. These tasks allow the person to achieve life's virtues: hope, purpose, fidelity, love, caring, and wisdom. The stages, life tasks, and virtues are described in Table 3.3.

Erikson's eight psychosocial stages of development are still used in a variety of disciplines. In his view, psychosocial growth occurs in sequential phases, and each stage is dependent on completion of the previous stage and life task. For example, in the infant stage (birth to 18 months), trust versus mistrust, the infant must learn to develop basic

Table 3.2	FREUD'S DEVELOPMENTAL STAGES	
Phase	**Age**	**Focus**
Oral	Birth to 18 months	Major site of tension and gratification is the mouth, lips, and tongue; includes biting and sucking activities. Id present at birth Ego develops gradually from rudimentary structure present at birth.
Anal	18–36 months	Anus and surrounding area are major source of interest. Acquisition of voluntary sphincter control (toilet training)
Phallic/oedipal	3–5 years	Genital focus of interest, stimulation, and excitement Penis is organ of interest for both sexes. Masturbation is common. Penis envy (wish to possess penis) seen in girls; oedipal complex (wish to marry opposite-sex parent and be rid of same-sex parent) seen in boys and girls.
Latency	5–11 or 13 years	Resolution of oedipal complex Sexual drive channeled into socially appropriate activities such as school work and sports Formation of the superego Final stage of psychosexual development
Genital	11–13 years	Begins with puberty and the biologic capacity for orgasm; involves the capacity for true intimacy

Adapted from Freud, S. (1962). *The ego and the id (The standard edition of the complete psychological works of Sigmund Freud;* J. Strachey, Trans.). New York: W. W. Norton & Company.

Table 3.3	ERIKSON'S STAGES OF PSYCHOSOCIAL DEVELOPMENT	
Stage	**Virtue**	**Task**
Trust vs. mistrust (infant)	Hope	Viewing the world as safe and reliable; relationships as nurturing, stable, and dependable
Autonomy vs. shame and doubt (toddler)	Will	Achieving a sense of control and free will
Initiative vs. guilt (preschool)	Purpose	Beginning development of a conscience; learning to manage conflict and anxiety
Industry vs. inferiority (school age)	Competence	Emerging confidence in own abilities; taking pleasure in accomplishments
Identity vs. role confusion (adolescence)	Fidelity	Formulating a sense of self and belonging
Intimacy vs. isolation (young adult)	Love	Forming adult, loving relationships and meaningful attachments to others
Generativity vs. stagnation (middle adult)	Care	Being creative and productive; establishing the next generation
Ego integrity vs. despair (maturity)	Wisdom	Accepting responsibility for one's self and life

trust (the positive outcome) such as that he or she will be fed and taken care of. The formation of trust is essential: mistrust, the negative outcome of this stage, will impair the person's development throughout his or her life.

JEAN PIAGET AND COGNITIVE STAGES OF DEVELOPMENT

Jean Piaget (1896–1980) explored how intelligence and cognitive functioning develop in children. He believed that human intelligence progresses through a series of stages based on age, with the child at each successive stage demonstrating a higher level of functioning than at previous stages. In his schema, Piaget strongly believed that biologic changes and maturation were responsible for cognitive development.

Piaget's four stages of cognitive development are as follows:

1. Sensorimotor—birth to 2 years: The child develops a sense of self as separate from the environment and the concept of object permanence; that is, tangible objects do not cease to exist just because they are out of sight. He or she begins to form mental images.
2. Preoperational—2 to 6 years: The child develops the ability to express self with language, understands the meaning of symbolic gestures, and begins to classify objects.
3. Concrete operations—6 to 12 years: The child begins to apply logic to thinking, understands spatiality and reversibility, and is increasingly social and able to apply rules; however, thinking is still concrete.
4. Formal operations—12 to 15 years and beyond: The child learns to think and reason in abstract terms, further develops logical thinking and reasoning, and achieves cognitive maturity.

Piaget's theory suggests that individuals reach cognitive maturity by middle to late adolescence. Some critics of Piaget believe that cognitive development is less rigid and more individualized than his theory suggests. Piaget's theory is useful when working with children. The nurse may better understand what the child means if the nurse is aware of his or her level of cognitive development. Also, teaching for children is often structured with their cognitive development in mind.

Interpersonal Theories

HARRY STACK SULLIVAN: INTERPERSONAL RELATIONSHIPS AND MILIEU THERAPY

Harry Stack Sullivan (1892–1949) was an American psychiatrist who extended the theory of personality development to include the significance of interpersonal relationships. Sullivan believed that one's personality involves more than individual characteristics, particularly how one interacts with others. He thought that inadequate or nonsatisfying relationships produce anxiety, which he saw as the basis for all emotional problems (Sullivan, 1953). The importance and significance of interpersonal relationships in one's life is probably Sullivan's greatest contribution to the field of mental health.

Five Life Stages. Sullivan established five life stages of development—infancy, childhood, juvenile, preadolescence, and adolescence, each focusing on various interpersonal relationships (Table 3.4). Sullivan also described three developmental cognitive modes of experience and believed that mental disorders are related to the persistence of one of the early modes. The **prototaxic mode**, characteristic of infancy and childhood, involves brief, unconnected experiences that have no relationship to one another. Adults with schizophrenia exhibit persistent prototaxic experiences. The **parataxic mode** begins in early childhood as the

Table 3.4 SULLIVAN'S LIFE STAGES

Stage	Ages	Focus
Infancy	Birth to onset of language	Primary need for bodily contact and tenderness Prototaxic mode dominates (no relation between experiences). Primary zones are oral and anal. If needs are met, infant has sense of well-being; unmet needs lead to dread and anxiety.
Childhood	Language to 5 years	Parents viewed as source of praise and acceptance. Shift to parataxic mode (experiences are connected in sequence to each other) Primary zone is anal. Gratification leads to positive self-esteem. Moderate anxiety leads to uncertainty and insecurity; severe anxiety results in self-defeating patterns of behavior.
Juvenile	5–8 years	Shift to the syntaxic mode begins (thinking about self and others based on analysis of experiences in a variety of situations). Opportunities for approval and acceptance of others Learn to negotiate own needs Severe anxiety may result in a need to control or in restrictive, prejudicial attitudes.
Preadolescence	8–12 years	Move to genuine intimacy with friend of the same sex Move away from family as source of satisfaction in relationships Major shift to syntaxic mode Capacity for attachment, love, and collaboration emerges or fails to develop.
Adolescence	Puberty to adulthood	Lust is added to interpersonal equation. Need for special sharing relationship shifts to the opposite sex. New opportunities for social experimentation lead to the consolidation of self-esteem or self-ridicule. If the self-system is intact, areas of concern expand to include values, ideals, career decisions, and social concerns.

Adapted from Sullivan, H. S. (1953). *The interpersonal theory of psychiatry*. New York: W. W. Norton & Company.

child begins to connect experiences in sequence. The child may not make logical sense of the experiences and may see them as coincidence or chance events. The child seeks to relieve anxiety by repeating familiar experiences, although he or she may not understand what he or she is doing. Sullivan explained paranoid ideas and slips of the tongue as a person operating in the parataxic mode. In the **syntaxic mode**, which begins to appear in school-aged children and becomes more predominant in preadolescence, the person begins to perceive him or herself and the world within the context of the environment and can analyze experiences in a variety of settings. Maturity may be defined as predominance of the syntaxic mode (Sullivan, 1953).

Therapeutic Community or Milieu. Sullivan envisioned the goal of treatment as the establishment of satisfying interpersonal relationships. The therapist provides a corrective interpersonal relationship for the client. Sullivan coined the term **participant observer** for the therapist's role, meaning that the therapist both participates in and observes the progress of the relationship.

Sullivan is also credited with developing the first **therapeutic community or milieu** with young men with schizophrenia in 1929 (although the term *therapeutic community*

was not used extensively until Maxwell Jones published *The Therapeutic Community* in 1953). In the concept of therapeutic community or milieu, the interaction among clients is seen as beneficial, and treatment emphasizes the role of this client-to-client interaction. Until this time, it was believed that the interaction between the client and the psychiatrist was the one essential component to the client's treatment. Sullivan and later Jones observed that interactions among clients in a safe, therapeutic setting provided great benefits to clients. The concept of **milieu therapy**, originally developed by Sullivan, involved clients' interactions with one another, including practicing interpersonal relationship skills, giving one another feedback about behavior, and working cooperatively as a group to solve day-to-day problems.

Milieu therapy was one of the primary modes of treatment in the acute hospital setting. In today's health care environment, however, inpatient hospital stays are often too short for clients to develop meaningful relationships with one another. Therefore, the concept of milieu therapy receives little attention. Management of the milieu, or environment, is still a primary role for the nurse in terms of providing safety and protection for all clients and promoting social interaction.

HILDEGARD PEPLAU: THERAPEUTIC NURSE–PATIENT RELATIONSHIP

Hildegard Peplau (1909–1999; Figure 3.2) was a nursing theorist and clinician who built on Sullivan's interpersonal theories and also saw the role of the nurse as a participant observer. Peplau developed the concept of the **therapeutic nurse–patient relationship**, which includes four phases: orientation, identification, exploitation, and resolution (Table 3.5).

During these phases, the client accomplishes certain tasks and makes relationship changes that help the healing process (Peplau, 1952).

1. The *orientation phase* is directed by the nurse and involves engaging the client in treatment, providing explanations and information, and answering questions.
2. The *identification phase* begins when the client works interdependently with the nurse, expresses feelings, and begins to feel stronger.
3. In the *exploitation phase,* the client makes full use of the services offered.
4. In the *resolution phase,* the client no longer needs professional services and gives up dependent behavior. The relationship ends.

Peplau's concept of the nurse–client relationship, with tasks and behaviors characteristic of each stage, has been modified but remains in use today (see Chapter 5).

Roles of the Nurse in the Therapeutic Relationship. Peplau also wrote about the roles of the nurse in the therapeutic relationship and how these roles help meet the client's needs. The primary roles she identified are as follows:

- *Stranger:* offering the client the same acceptance and courtesy that the nurse would to any stranger
- *Resource person:* providing specific answers to questions within a larger context
- *Teacher:* helping the client to learn formally or informally
- *Leader:* offering direction to the client or group
- *Surrogate:* serving as a substitute for another such as a parent or sibling
- *Counselor:* promoting experiences leading to health for the client such as expression of feelings

Peplau also believed that the nurse could take on many other roles, including consultant, tutor, safety agent, mediator, administrator, observer, and researcher. These were not defined in detail but were "left to the intelligence and imagination of the readers" (Peplau, 1952, p. 70).

Four Levels of Anxiety. Peplau defined anxiety as the initial response to a psychic threat. She described four levels of anxiety: mild, moderate, severe, and panic (Table 3.6). These serve as the foundation for working with clients with anxiety in a variety of contexts (see Chapter 13).

1. *Mild anxiety* is a positive state of heightened awareness and sharpened senses, allowing the person to learn new behaviors and solve problems. The person can take in all available stimuli (perceptual field).
2. *Moderate anxiety* involves a decreased perceptual field (focus on immediate task only); the person can learn new behavior or solve problems only with assistance. Another person can redirect the person to the task.
3. *Severe anxiety* involves feelings of dread or terror. The person cannot be redirected to a task; he or she focuses only on scattered details and has physiologic symptoms of tachycardia, diaphoresis, and chest pain. A person with severe anxiety may go to an emergency department, believing he or she is having a heart attack.
4. *Panic anxiety* can involve loss of rational thought, delusions, hallucinations, and complete physical immobility and muteness. The person may bolt and run aimlessly, often exposing himself or herself to injury.

Humanistic Theories

Humanism represents a significant shift away from the psychoanalytic view of the individual as a neurotic, impulse-driven person with repressed psychic problems and away from the focus on and examination of the client's past experiences. **Humanism** focuses on a person's positive qualities, his or her capacity to change (human potential), and the promotion of self-esteem. Humanists do consider the person's past experiences, but they direct more attention toward the present and future.

ABRAHAM MASLOW: HIERARCHY OF NEEDS

Abraham Maslow (1921–1970) was an American psychologist who studied the needs or motivations of the individual. He differed from previous theorists in that he focused on the total person, not just on one facet of the person, and emphasized health instead of simply illness and problems.

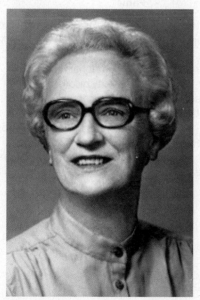

Figure 3.2. Hildegard Peplau, who developed the phases of the nurse–client therapeutic relationship, which has made great contributions to the foundation of nursing practice today.

Table 3.5   PEPLAU'S STAGES AND TASKS OF RELATIONSHIPS

Stage	Tasks
Orientation	Clarification of patient's problems and needs
	Patient asks questions.
	Explanation of hospital routines and expectations
	Patient harnesses energy toward meeting problems.
	Patient's full participation is elicited.
Identification	Patient responds to persons he or she perceives as helpful.
	Patient feels stronger.
	Expression of feelings
	Interdependent work with the nurse
	Clarification of roles of both patient and nurse
Exploitation	Patient makes full use of available services.
	Goals such as going home and returning to work emerge.
	Patient's behaviors fluctuate between dependence and independence.
Resolution	Patient gives up dependent behavior.
	Services are no longer needed by patient.
	Patient assumes power to meet own needs, set new goals, and so forth.

Adapted from Peplau, H. (1952). *Interpersonal relations in nursing.* New York: G. P. Putnam's Sons.

Maslow (1954) formulated the **hierarchy of needs**, in which he used a pyramid to arrange and illustrate the basic drives or needs that motivate people. The most basic needs—the physiologic needs of food, water, sleep, shelter, sexual expression, and freedom from pain—must be met first. The second level involves safety and security needs, which include protection, security, and freedom from harm or threatened deprivation. The third level is love and belonging needs, which include enduring intimacy, friendship, and acceptance. The fourth level involves esteem

Table 3.6   ANXIETY LEVELS

Mild	Moderate	Severe	Panic
Sharpened senses	Selectively attentive	Perceptual field reduced to one detail or scattered details	Perceptual field reduced to focus on self
Increased motivation	Perceptual field limited to the immediate task	Cannot complete tasks	Cannot process environmental stimuli
Alert	Can be redirected	Cannot solve problems or learn effectively	Distorted perceptions
Enlarged perceptual field	Cannot connect thoughts or events independently	Behavior geared toward anxiety relief and is usually ineffective	Loss of rational thought
Can solve problems	Muscle tension	Feels awe, dread, horror	Personality disorganization
Learning is effective	Diaphoresis	Doesn't respond to redirection	Doesn't recognize danger
Restless	Pounding pulse	Severe headache	Possibly suicidal
Gastrointestinal "butterflies"	Headache	Nausea, vomiting, diarrhea	Delusions or hallucination possible
Sleepless	Dry mouth	Trembling	Can't communicate verbally
Irritable	Higher voice pitch	Rigid stance	Either cannot sit (may bolt and run) or
Hypersensitive to noise	Increased rate of speech	Vertigo	is totally mute and immobile
	Gastrointestinal upset	Pale	
	Frequent urination	Tachycardia	
	Increased automatisms (nervous mannerisms)	Chest pain	
		Crying	
		Ritualistic (purposeless, repetitive) behavior	

Adapted from Peplau, H. (1952). *Interpersonal relations in nursing.* New York: G. P. Putnam's Sons.

needs, which include the need for self-respect and esteem from others. The highest level is self-actualization, the need for beauty, truth, and justice.

Maslow hypothesized that the basic needs at the bottom of the pyramid would dominate the person's behavior until those needs were met, at which time the next level of needs would become dominant. For example, if needs for food and shelter are not met, they become the overriding concern in life: the hungry person risks danger and social ostracism to find food.

Maslow used the term **self-actualization** to describe a person who has achieved all the needs of the hierarchy and has developed his or her fullest potential in life. Few people ever become fully self-actualized.

Maslow's theory explains individual differences in terms of a person's motivation, which is not necessarily stable throughout life. Traumatic life circumstances or compromised health can cause a person to regress to a lower level of motivation. For example, if a 35-year-old woman who is functioning at the "love and belonging" level discovers she has cancer, she may regress to the "safety" level to undergo treatment for the cancer and preserve her own health. This theory helps nurses understand how clients' motivations and behaviors change during life crises (see Chapter 7).

CARL ROGERS: CLIENT-CENTERED THERAPY

Carl Rogers (1902–1987) was a humanistic American psychologist who focused on the therapeutic relationship and developed a new method of client-centered therapy. Rogers

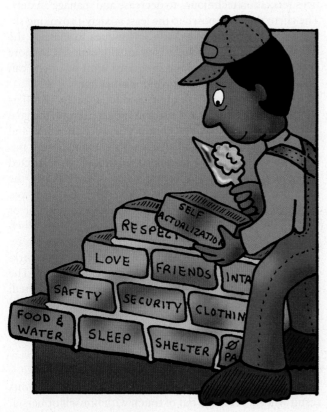

Maslow's hierarchy of needs

was one of the first to use the term *client* rather than *patient*. **Client-centered therapy** focuses on the role of the client, rather than the therapist, as the key to the healing process. Rogers believed that each person experiences the world differently and knows his or her own experience best (Rogers, 1961). According to Rogers, clients do "the work of healing," and within a supportive and nurturing client–therapist relationship, clients can cure themselves. Clients are in the best position to know their own experiences and make sense of them, to regain their self-esteem, and to progress toward self-actualization.

The therapist takes a person-centered approach, a supportive role, rather than a directive or expert role, because Rogers viewed the client as the expert on his or her life. The therapist must promote the client's self-esteem as much as possible through three central concepts:

- *Unconditional positive regard*—a nonjudgmental caring for the client that is not dependent on the client's behavior
- *Genuineness*—realness or congruence between what the therapist feels and what he or she says to the client
- *Empathetic understanding*—in which the therapist senses the feelings and personal meaning from the client and communicates this understanding to the client

Unconditional positive regard promotes the client's self-esteem and decreases his or her need for defensive behavior. As the client's self-acceptance grows, the natural self-actualization process can continue.

Rogers also believed that the basic nature of humans is to become self-actualized, or to move toward self-improvement and constructive change. We are all born with a positive self-regard and a natural inclination to become self-actualized. If relationships with others are supportive and nurturing, the person retains feelings of self-worth and progresses toward self-actualization, which is healthy. If the person encounters repeated conflicts with others or is in nonsupportive relationships, he or she loses self-esteem, becomes defensive, and is no longer inclined toward self-actualization; this is not healthy.

Behavioral Theories

Behaviorism grew out of a reaction to introspection models that focused on the contents and operations of the mind. **Behaviorism** is a school of psychology that focuses on observable behaviors and what one can do externally to bring about behavior changes. It does not attempt to explain how the mind works.

Behaviorists believe that behavior can be changed through a system of rewards and punishments. For adults, receiving a regular paycheck is a constant positive reinforcer that motivates people to continue to go to work every day and to try to do a good job. It helps motivate positive behavior in the workplace. If someone stops receiving a paycheck, he or she is most likely to stop working.

If a motorist consistently speeds (negative behavior) and does not get caught, he or she is likely to continue to speed. If the driver receives a speeding ticket (a negative reinforcer), he or she is likely to slow down. However, if the motorist does not get caught for speeding for the next 4 weeks (negative reinforcer is removed), he or she is likely to resume speeding.

IVAN PAVLOV: CLASSICAL CONDITIONING

Laboratory experiments with dogs provided the basis for the development of Ivan Pavlov's theory of classical conditioning: Behavior can be changed through conditioning with external or environmental conditions or stimuli. His experiment with dogs involved his observation that dogs naturally began to salivate (response) when they saw or smelled food (stimulus). Pavlov (1849–1936) set out to change this salivating response or behavior through conditioning. He would ring a bell (new stimulus), then produce the food, and the dogs would salivate (the desired response). Pavlov repeated this ringing of the bell along with the presentation of food many times. Eventually he could ring the bell and the dogs would salivate without seeing or smelling food. The dogs had been "conditioned," or had learned a new response—to salivate when they heard the bell. Their behavior had been modified through classical conditioning, or a conditioned response.

B. F. SKINNER: OPERANT CONDITIONING

One of the most influential behaviorists was B. F. Skinner (1904–1990), an American psychologist. He developed the theory of **operant conditioning**, which says people learn their behavior from their history or past experiences, particularly those experiences that were repeatedly reinforced. Although some criticize his theories for not considering the role that thoughts, feelings, or needs play in motivating behavior, his work has provided several important principles still used today. Skinner did not deny the existence of feelings and needs in motivation; however, he viewed behavior as only that which could be observed, studied, and learned or unlearned. He maintained that if the behavior could be changed, then so too could the accompanying thoughts or feelings. Changing the behavior was what was important.

The following principles of operant conditioning described by Skinner (1974) form the basis for behavior techniques in use today:

1. All behavior is learned.
2. Consequences result from behavior—broadly speaking, reward and punishment.
3. Behavior that is rewarded with reinforcers tends to recur.
4. Positive reinforcers that follow a behavior increase the likelihood that the behavior will recur.
5. Negative reinforcers that are removed after a behavior increase the likelihood that the behavior will recur.
6. Continuous reinforcement (a reward every time the behavior occurs) is the fastest way to increase that behavior, but the behavior will not last long after the reward ceases.
7. Random intermittent reinforcement (an occasional reward for the desired behavior) is slower to produce an increase in behavior, but the behavior continues after the reward ceases.

These behavioral principles of rewarding or reinforcing behaviors are used to help people change their behaviors in a therapy known as behavior modification. **Behavior modification** is a method of attempting to strengthen a desired behavior or response by reinforcement, either positive or negative. For example, if the desired behavior is assertiveness, whenever the client uses assertiveness skills in a communication group, the group leader provides **positive reinforcement** by giving the client attention and positive feedback. **Negative reinforcement** involves removing a stimulus immediately after a behavior occurs so that the behavior is more likely to occur again. For example, if a client becomes anxious when waiting to talk in a group, he or she may volunteer to speak first to avoid the anxiety.

In a group home setting, operant principles may come into play in a token economy, a way to involve residents in performing activities of daily living. A chart of desired behaviors, such as getting up on time, taking a shower, and getting dressed, is kept for each resident. Each day the chart is marked when the desired behavior occurs. At the end of the day or week, the resident gets a reward or token for each time each of the desired behaviors occurred. The resident can redeem the tokens for items such as snacks, TV time, or a relaxed curfew.

Conditioned responses, such as fears or phobias, can be treated with behavioral techniques. **Systematic desensitization** can be used to help clients overcome irrational fears and anxiety associated with phobias. The client is asked to make a list of situations involving the phobic object, from the least to the most anxiety-provoking. The client learns and practices relaxation techniques to decrease and manage anxiety. The client then is exposed to the least anxiety-provoking situation and uses the relaxation techniques to manage the resulting anxiety. The client is gradually exposed to more and more anxiety-provoking situations until he or she can manage the most anxiety-provoking situation.

Behavioral techniques can be used for a variety of different problems. In the treatment of anorexia nervosa, the goal is weight gain. A behavioral contract between the client and therapist or physician is initiated when treatment begins. Initially, the client has little unsupervised time and is restricted to the hospital unit. The contract may specify that if the client gains a certain amount of weight, such as 0.2 kg/day, in return he or she will get increased unsupervised time or time off the unit as long as the weight gain progresses. When working with children with attention deficit hyperactivity disorder, goals include task completion for homework, hygiene tasks, turn-taking when talking, and so forth. The child is given a "star" or sticker when tasks are completed. Upon reaching a specified numbers of stars, the child receives a reward.

Existential Theories

Existential theorists believe that behavioral deviations result when a person is out of touch with himself or herself or the environment. The person who is self-alienated is lonely and sad and feels helpless. Lack of self-awareness, coupled with harsh self-criticism, prevents the person from participating in satisfying relationships. The person is not free to choose from all possible alternatives because of self-imposed restrictions. Existential theorists believe that the person is avoiding personal responsibility and giving in to the wishes or demands of others.

All existential therapies have the goal of helping the person discover an authentic sense of self. They emphasize personal responsibility for one's self, feelings, behaviors, and choices. These therapies encourage the person to live fully in the present and to look forward to the future. Carl Rogers is sometimes grouped with existential therapists. Table 3.7 summarizes existential therapies.

COGNITIVE THERAPY

Many existential therapists use **cognitive therapy**, which focuses on immediate thought processing—how a person perceives or interprets his or her experience and determines how he or she feels and behaves. For example, if a person interprets a situation as dangerous, he or she experiences anxiety and tries to escape. Basic emotions of sadness, elation, anxiety, and anger are reactions to perceptions of loss, gain, danger, and wrongdoing by others (Beck & Rush, 1995). Aaron Beck is credited with pioneering cognitive therapy in persons with depression.

RATIONAL EMOTIVE THERAPY

Albert Ellis, founder of rational emotive therapy, identified 11 "irrational beliefs" that people use to make themselves unhappy. An example of an irrational belief is "If I love someone, he or she must love me back just as much." Ellis claimed that continuing to believe this patently untrue statement will make the person utterly unhappy, but he or she will blame it on the person who does not return his or her love. Ellis also believes that people have "automatic thoughts" that cause them unhappiness in certain situations. He used the ABC technique to help people identify these automatic thoughts: A is the activating stimulus or event, C is the excessive inappropriate response, and B is the blank in the person's mind that he or she must fill in by identifying the automatic thought.

VIKTOR FRANKL AND LOGOTHERAPY

Viktor Frankl based his beliefs on his observations of people in Nazi concentration camps during World War II. His curiosity about why some survived and others did not led him to conclude that survivors were able to find meaning in their lives even under miserable conditions. Hence, the search for meaning (*logos*) is the central theme in logotherapy. Counselors and therapists who work with clients in spirituality and grief counseling often use the concepts that Frankl developed.

GESTALT THERAPY

Gestalt therapy, founded by Frederick "Fritz" Perls, emphasizes identifying the person's feelings and thoughts in the here and now. Perls believed that self-awareness leads to self-acceptance and responsibility for one's own thoughts and feelings. Therapists often use gestalt therapy to increase clients' self-awareness by having them write and read letters, keep journals, and perform other activities designed to put the past to rest and focus on the present.

REALITY THERAPY

William Glasser devised an approach called reality therapy that focuses on the person's behavior and how that behavior keeps him or her from achieving life goals. He developed this approach while working with persons with delinquent behavior, unsuccessful school performance, and emotional problems. He believed that persons who were unsuccessful often blamed their problems on other people, the system, or society. He believed they needed to find their own identities through responsible behavior. Reality therapy challenges clients to examine the ways in which their own behavior thwarts their attempts to achieve life goals.

Table 3.7   EXISTENTIAL THERAPIES

Therapy	Therapist	Therapeutic Process
Rational emotive therapy	Albert Ellis	A cognitive therapy using confrontation of "irrational beliefs" that prevent the individual from accepting responsibility for self and behavior
Logotherapy	Viktor E. Frankl	A therapy designed to help individuals assume personal responsibility. The search for meaning (*logos*) in life is a central theme.
Gestalt therapy	Frederick S. Perls	A therapy focusing on the identification of feelings in the here and now, which leads to self-acceptance
Reality therapy	William Glasser	Therapeutic focus is need for identity through responsible behavior. Individuals are challenged to examine ways in which their behavior thwarts their attempts to achieve life goals.

Crisis Intervention

A **crisis** is a turning point in an individual's life that produces an overwhelming emotional response. Individuals experience a crisis when they confront some life circumstance or stressor that they cannot effectively manage through use of their customary coping skills. Caplan (1964) identified the stages of crisis: (1) the person is exposed to a stressor, experiences anxiety, and tries to cope in a customary fashion; (2) anxiety increases when customary coping skills are ineffective; (3) the person makes all possible efforts to deal with the stressor, including attempts at new methods of coping; and (4) when coping attempts fail, the person experiences disequilibrium and significant distress.

Crises occur in response to a variety of life situations and events and fall into three categories:

- *Maturational crises*, sometimes called *developmental crises*, are predictable events in the normal course of life, such as leaving home for the first time, getting married, having a baby, and beginning a career.
- *Situational crises* are unanticipated or sudden events that threaten the individual's integrity, such as the death of a loved one, loss of a job, and physical or emotional illness in the individual or family member.
- *Adventitious crises*, sometimes called social crises, include natural disasters like floods, earthquakes, or hurricanes; war; terrorist attacks; riots; and violent crimes such as rape or murder.

Note that not all events that result in crisis are "negative" in nature. Events like marriage, retirement, and childbirth are often desirable for the individual but may still present overwhelming challenges. Aguilera (1998) identified three factors that influence whether or not an individual experiences a crisis: the individual's perception of the event, the availability of emotional supports, and the availability of adequate coping mechanisms. When the person in crisis seeks assistance, these three factors represent a guide for effective intervention. The person can be assisted to view the event or issue from a different perspective, for example, as an opportunity for growth or change rather than as a threat. Assisting the person to use existing supports or helping the individual find new sources of support can decrease the feelings of being alone or overwhelmed. Finally, assisting the person to learn new methods of coping will help to resolve the current crisis and give him or her new coping skills to use in the future.

Crisis is described as self-limiting; that is, the crisis does not last indefinitely but usually exists for 4 to 6 weeks. At the end of that time, the crisis is resolved in one of three ways. In the first two, the person either returns to his or her pre-crisis level of functioning or begins to function at a higher level; both are positive outcomes for the individual. The third resolution is that the person's functioning stabilizes at a level lower than pre-crisis functioning, which is a negative outcome for the individual. Positive outcomes are more likely when the problem (crisis response and precipitating event or issue) is clearly and thoroughly defined. Likewise, early intervention is associated with better outcomes.

Persons experiencing a crisis usually are distressed and likely to seek help for their distress. They are ready to learn and even eager to try new coping skills as a way to relieve their distress. This is an ideal time for intervention that is likely to be successful. **Crisis intervention** includes a variety of techniques based on the assessment of the individual. *Directive interventions* are designed to assess the person's health status and promote problem-solving, such as offering the person new information, knowledge, or meaning; raising the person's self-awareness by providing feedback about behavior; and directing the person's behavior by offering suggestions or courses of action. *Supportive interventions* aim at dealing with the person's needs for empathetic understanding, such as encouraging the person to identify and discuss feelings, serving as a sounding board for the person, and affirming the person's self-worth. Techniques and strategies that include a balance of these different types of intervention are the most effective.

CULTURAL CONSIDERATIONS

The major psychosocial theorists were white and born in Europe or the United States, as were many of the people whom they treated. What they considered normal or typical may not apply equally well to people with different racial, ethnic, or cultural backgrounds. For example, Erikson's developmental stages focus on autonomy and independence for toddlers, but this focus may not be appropriate for people from other cultures in which early individual independence is not a developmental milestone. Therefore, it is important that the nurse avoids reaching faulty conclusions when working with clients and families from other cultures. Chapter 7 discusses cultural factors in depth.

TREATMENT MODALITIES

Benefits of Community Mental Health Treatment

Recent changes in health care and reimbursement have affected mental health treatment, as they have all areas of medicine, nursing, and related health disciplines (see Chapter 4). Inpatient treatment is often the last, rather than the first, mode of treatment for mental illness. Current treatment reflects the belief that it is more beneficial and certainly more cost-effective for clients to remain in the community and receive outpatient treatment whenever possible. The client can often continue to work and can stay connected to family, friends, and other support systems while participating in therapy. Outpatient therapy also takes into account that a person's personality or behavior patterns, such as coping skills, styles of communication, and level of self-esteem, gradually develop over the course of a lifetime and cannot be changed in a relatively short inpatient course of treatment. Hospital admission is indicated when the person is severely depressed and suicidal, severely psychotic, experiencing alcohol or drug withdrawal, or exhibiting behaviors that require close supervision in a safe, supportive environment. This section briefly describes the treatment modalities currently used in both inpatient and outpatient settings.

Individual Psychotherapy

Individual psychotherapy is a method of bringing about change in a person by exploring his or her feelings, attitudes, thinking, and behavior. It involves a one-to-one relationship between the therapist and the client. People generally seek this kind of therapy based on their desire to understand themselves and their behavior, to make personal changes, to improve interpersonal relationships, or to get relief from emotional pain or unhappiness. The relationship between the client and the therapist proceeds through stages similar to those of the nurse–client relationship: introduction, working, and termination. Cost-containment measures mandated by health maintenance organizations and other insurers may necessitate moving into the working phase rapidly so the client can get the maximum benefit possible from therapy.

The therapist–client relationship is key to the success of this type of therapy. The client and the therapist must be compatible for therapy to be effective. Therapists vary in their formal credentials, experience, and model of practice. Selecting a therapist is extremely important in terms of successful outcomes for the client. The client must select a therapist whose theoretical beliefs and style of therapy are congruent with the client's needs and expectations of therapy. The client also may have to try different therapists to find a good match.

A therapist's theoretical beliefs strongly influence his or her style of therapy (discussed earlier in this chapter). For example, a therapist grounded in interpersonal theory emphasizes relationships, whereas an existential therapist focuses on the client's self-responsibility.

The nurse or other health care provider who is familiar with the client may be in a position to recommend a therapist or a choice of therapists. He or she also may help the client understand what different therapists have to offer.

The client should select a therapist carefully and should ask about the therapist's treatment approach and area of specialization. State laws regulate the practice and licensing of therapists; thus, from state to state, the qualifications to practice psychotherapy, the requirements for licensure, or even the need for a license can vary. A few therapists have little or no formal education, credentials, or experience but still practice entirely within the legal limits of their states. A client can verify a therapist's legal credentials with the state licensing board; state government listings are in the local phone book. The Better Business Bureau can inform consumers if a particular therapist has been reported to them for investigation. Calling the local mental health services agency or contacting the primary care provider is another way for a client to check a therapist's credentials and ethical practices.

Groups

A group is a number of persons who gather in a face-to-face setting to accomplish tasks that require cooperation, collaboration, or working together. Each person in a group is in a position to influence and to be influenced by other group members. Group content refers to what is said in the context of the group, including educational material, feelings and emotions, or discussions of the project to be completed. Group process refers to the behavior of the group and its individual members, including seating arrangements, tone of voice, who speaks to whom, who is quiet, and so forth. Content and process occur continuously throughout the life of the group.

STAGES OF GROUP DEVELOPMENT

A group may be established to serve a particular purpose in a specified period such as a work group to complete an assigned project or a therapy group that meets with the same members to explore ways to deal with depression. These groups develop in observable stages. In the pregroup stages, members are selected, the purpose or work of the group is identified, and group structure is addressed. Group structure includes where and how often the group will meet, identification of a group leader, and the rules of the group—for example, whether individuals can join the group after it begins, how to handle absences, and expectations for group members.

The beginning stage of group development, or the initial stage, commences as soon as the group begins to meet. Members introduce themselves, a leader can be selected (if not done previously), the group purpose is discussed, and rules and expectations for group participation are reviewed. Group members begin to "check out" one another and the leader as they determine their levels of comfort in the group setting.

The working stage of group development begins as members begin to focus their attention on the purpose or task the group is trying to accomplish. This may happen relatively quickly in a work group with a specific assigned project but may take two or three sessions in a therapy group because members must develop some level of trust before sharing personal feelings or difficult situations. During this phase, several group characteristics may be seen. Group cohesiveness is the degree to which members work together cooperatively to accomplish the purpose. Cohesiveness is a desirable group characteristic and is associated with positive group outcomes. Cohesiveness is evidenced when members value one another's contributions to the group; members think of themselves as "we" and share responsibility for the work of the group. When a group is cohesive, members feel free to express all opinions, positive and negative, with little fear of rejection or retribution. If a group is "overly cohesive," in that uniformity and agreement become the group's implicit goals, there may be a negative effect on the group outcome. In a therapy group, members do not give one another needed feedback if the group is overly cohesive. In a work group, critical thinking and creative problem-solving are unlikely, which may make the work of the group less meaningful.

Some groups exhibit competition, or rivalry, among group members. This may positively affect the outcome of the group if the competition leads to compromise, improved group performance, and growth for individual members. Many times, however, competition can be destructive for the group; when conflicts are not resolved, members become hostile, or the group's energy is diverted from accomplishing its purpose to bickering and power struggles.

The final stage, or termination, of the group occurs before the group disbands. The work of the group is reviewed, with the focus on group accomplishments, growth of group members, or both, depending on the purpose of the group.

Observing the stages of group development in groups that are ongoing is difficult with members joining and leaving the group at various times. Rather, the group involvement of new members as they join the group evolves as they feel accepted by the group, take a more active role, and join in the work of the group. An example of this type of group would be Alcoholics Anonymous, a self-help group with stated purposes. Members may attend Alcoholics Anonymous meetings as often or infrequently as they choose; group cohesiveness or competition can still be observed in ongoing groups.

GROUP LEADERSHIP

Groups often have an identified or formal leader—someone designated to lead the group. In therapy groups and education groups, a formal leader is usually identified based on his or her education, qualifications, and experience. Some work groups have formal leaders appointed in advance, whereas other work groups select a leader at the initial meeting. Support groups and self-help groups usually do not have identified formal leaders; all members are seen as equals. An informal leader may emerge from a "leaderless" group or from a group that has an identified formal leader. Informal leaders are generally members recognized by others as having the knowledge, experience, or characteristics that members admire and value.

Effective group leaders focus on group process as well as on group content. Tasks of the group leader include giving feedback and suggestions; encouraging participation from all members (eliciting responses from quiet members, placing limits on members who may monopolize the group's time); clarifying thoughts, feelings, and ideas; summarizing progress and accomplishments; and facilitating progress through the stages of group development.

GROUP ROLES

Roles are the parts that members play within the group. Not all members are aware of their "role behavior," and changes in members' behavior may be a topic that the group will need to address. Some roles facilitate the work of the group, whereas other roles can negatively affect the process or outcome of the group. Growth-producing roles include the information-seeker, opinion-seeker, information-giver, energizer, coordinator, harmonizer, encourager, and elaborator. Growth-inhibiting roles include the monopolizer, aggressor, dominator, critic, recognition-seeker, and passive follower.

GROUP THERAPY

In **group therapy**, clients participate in sessions with a group of people. The members share a common purpose and are expected to contribute to the group to benefit others and receive benefit from others in return. Group rules are established that all members must observe. These rules vary according to the type of group. Being a member of a group allows the client to learn new ways of looking at a problem or ways of coping with or solving problems and also helps him or her to learn important interpersonal skills. For example, by interacting with other members, clients often receive feedback on how others perceive and react to them and their behavior. This is extremely important information for many clients with mental disorders, who often have difficulty with interpersonal skills.

The therapeutic results of group therapy (Yalom, 1995) include the following:
* Gaining new information, or learning
* Gaining inspiration or hope
* Interacting with others
* Feeling acceptance and belonging
* Becoming aware that one is not alone and that others share the same problems
* Gaining insight into one's problems and behaviors and how they affect others
* Giving of oneself for the benefit of others (altruism)

Therapy groups vary with different purposes, degrees of formality, and structures. Our discussion includes psychotherapy groups, family therapy, family education, education groups, support groups, and self-help groups.

Psychotherapy Groups. The goal of a **psychotherapy group** is for members to learn about their behavior and to make positive changes in their behavior by interacting and communicating with others as a member of a group. Groups may be organized around a specific medical diagnosis, such as depression, or a particular issue, such as improving interpersonal skills or managing anxiety. Group techniques and processes are used to help group members learn about their behavior with other people and how it relates to core personality traits. Members also learn they have responsibilities to others and can help other members achieve their goals.

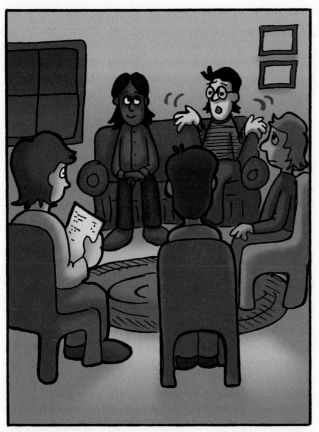

Group therapy

Psychotherapy groups are often formal in structure, with one or two therapists as the group leaders. One task of the group leader or the entire group is to establish the rules for the group. These rules deal with confidentiality, punctuality, attendance, and social contact between members outside of group time.

There are two types of groups: open groups and closed groups. **Open groups** are ongoing and run indefinitely, allowing members to join or leave the group as they need to. **Closed groups** are structured to keep the same members in the group for a specified number of sessions. If the group is closed, the members decide how to handle members who wish to leave the group and the possible addition of new group members (Yalom, 1995).

Family Therapy. **Family therapy** is a form of group therapy in which the client and his or her family members participate. The goals include understanding how family dynamics contribute to the client's psychopathology, mobilizing the family's inherent strengths and functional resources, restructuring maladaptive family behavioral styles, and strengthening family problem-solving behaviors (Sadock & Sadock, 2004). Family therapy can be used both to assess and treat various psychiatric disorders. Although one family member usually is identified initially as the one who has problems and needs help, it often becomes evident through the therapeutic process that other family members also have emotional problems and difficulties.

Family Education. The National Alliance for the Mentally Ill (NAMI) developed a unique 12-week Family to Family Education course taught by trained family members. The curriculum focuses on schizophrenia, bipolar disorder, clinical depression, panic disorder, and obsessive-compulsive disorder. The course discusses the clinical treatment of these illnesses and teaches the knowledge and skills that family members need to cope more effectively. The specific features of this education program include emphasis on emotional understanding and healing in the personal realm and on power and action in the social realm. NAMI also conducts Provider Education programs taught by two consumers, two family members, and a mental health professional who is also a family member or consumer. This course is designed to help providers realize the hardships that families and consumers endure and to appreciate the courage and persistence it takes to reconstruct lives that must be lived, through no fault of the consumer or family, "on the verge" (NAMI, 2004, p. 1).

Education Groups. The goal of an **education group** is to provide information to members on a specific issue—for instance, stress management, medication management, or assertiveness training. The group leader has expertise in the subject area and may be a nurse, therapist, or other health professional. Education groups usually are scheduled for a specific number of sessions and retain the same members for the duration of the group. Typically, the leader presents the information and then members can ask questions or practice new techniques.

In a medication management group, the leader may discuss medication regimens and possible side effects, screen clients for side effects, and in some instances actually administer the medication (e.g., depot injections of haloperidol [Haldol] decanoate or fluphenazine [Prolixin] decanoate).

Support Groups. **Support groups** are organized to help members who share a common problem to cope with it. The group leader explores members' thoughts and feelings and creates an atmosphere of acceptance so that members feel comfortable expressing themselves. Support groups often provide a safe place for group members to express their feelings of frustration, boredom, or unhappiness and also to discuss common problems and potential solutions. Rules for support groups differ from those in psychotherapy in that members are allowed—in fact, encouraged—to contact one another and socialize outside the sessions. Confidentiality may be a rule for some groups; the members decide this. Support groups tend to be open groups in which members can join or leave as their needs dictate.

Common support groups include those for cancer or stroke victims, persons with AIDS, and family members of someone who has committed suicide. One national support group, Mothers Against Drunk Driving (MADD), is for family members of someone killed in a car accident caused by a drunk driver.

Self-Help Groups. In a **self-help group**, members share a common experience, but the group is not a formal or structured therapy group. Although professionals organize some self-help groups, many are run by members and do not have a formally identified leader. Various self-help groups are available. Some are locally organized and announce their meetings in local newspapers. Others are nationally organized, such as Alcoholics Anonymous, Parents Without Partners, Gamblers Anonymous, and Al-Anon (a group for spouses and partners of alcoholics), and have national headquarters and Internet Web sites (see Internet Resources).

Most self-help groups have a rule of confidentiality: whoever is seen at and whatever is said at the meetings cannot be divulged to others or discussed outside the group. In many 12-step programs, such as Alcoholics Anonymous and Gamblers Anonymous, people use only their first names so their identities are not divulged (although in some settings, group members do know one another's names).

Complementary and Alternative Therapies

The National Center for Complementary and Alternative Medicine (NCCAM) is a federal government agency for scientific research on complementary and alternative medicine (CAM). This agency is part of the National Institutes of Health in the Department of Health and Human Services. **Complementary medicine** includes therapies *used with* conventional medicine practices (the medical model). **Alternative medicine** includes therapies *used in place of* conventional treatment. NCCAM conducts clinical research to help determine the safety and efficacy of these practices (NCCAM, 2006). Studying the use of St. John's wort to treat depression (instead of using antidepressant medication) would be an example of researching alternative medicine. Conducting research on the use of chiropractic massage and antidepressant medication to treat depression is an example of complementary medicine research. **Integrative medicine** combines conventional medical therapy and CAM therapies that have scientific evidence supporting their safety and effectiveness.

NCCAM studies a wide variety of complementary and alternative therapies:

- *Alternative medical systems* include homeopathic medicine and naturopathic medicine in Western cultures, and traditional Chinese medicine, which includes herbal and nutritional therapy, restorative physical exercises (yoga, Tai chi), meditation, acupuncture, and remedial massage.
- *Mind–body interventions* include meditation, prayer, mental healing, and creative therapies that use art, music, or dance.
- *Biologically based therapies* use substances found in nature, such as herbs, food, and vitamins. Dietary supplements, herbal products, medicinal teas, aromatherapy, and a variety of diets are included.
- *Manipulative and body-based therapies* are based on manipulation or movement of one or more parts of the body, such as therapeutic massage and chiropractic or osteopathic manipulation.
- *Energy therapies* include two types of therapy: biofield therapies, intended to affect energy fields that are believed to surround and penetrate the body, such as therapeutic touch, qi gong, and Reiki; and bioelectric-based therapies involving the unconventional use of electromagnetic fields, such as pulsed fields, magnetic fields, and AC or DC fields. Qi gong is part of Chinese medicine that combines movement, meditation, and regulated breathing to enhance the flow of vital energy and promote healing. Reiki (Japanese meaning universal life energy) is based on the belief that when spiritual energy is channeled through a Reiki practitioner, the patient's spirit and body are healed.

Clients may be reluctant to tell the psychiatrist or primary care provider about the use of CAM. Therefore, it is important that the nurse ask clients specifically about use of herbs, vitamins, or other health practices in a nonjudgmental way.

Psychiatric Rehabilitation

Psychiatric rehabilitation involves providing services to people with severe and persistent mental illness to help them to live in the community. These programs are often called *community support services* or *community support programs.* Psychiatric rehabilitation focuses on the client's strengths, not just on his or her illness. The client actively participates in program planning. The programs are designed to help the client manage the illness and symptoms, gain access to needed services, and live successfully in the community.

These programs assist clients with activities of daily living such as transportation, shopping, food preparation, money management, and hygiene. Social support and interpersonal relationships are recognized as a primary need for successful community living. Psychiatric rehabilitation programs provide opportunities for socialization, such as drop-in centers and places where clients can go to be with others in a safe, supportive environment. Vocational referral, training, job coaching, and support are available for clients who want to seek and maintain employment. Community support programs also provide education about the client's illness and treatment and help the client to obtain health care when needed.

Lecomte, Wallace, Perreault, and Caron (2005) emphasize the importance of including the client in identifying rehabilitation goals. There is often a disparity between what health care professionals view as the client's needs and what the client perceives as valuable. Offering services that meet each client's most important goals can significantly improve his or her quality of life and promote recovery and well-being.

THE NURSE AND PSYCHOSOCIAL INTERVENTIONS

Intervention is a crucial component of the nursing process. **Psychosocial interventions** are nursing activities that enhance the client's social and psychological functioning and improve social skills, interpersonal relationships, and communication. Nurses often use psychosocial interventions to help meet clients' needs and achieve outcomes in all practice settings, not just mental health. For example, a medical-surgical nurse might need to use interventions that incorporate behavioral principles such as setting limits with manipulative behavior or giving positive feedback.

For example, a client with diabetes tells the nurse,

"I promise to have just one bite of cake. Please! It's my grandson's birthday cake" (manipulative behavior).

The nurse might use behavioral limit-setting by saying,

"I can't give you permission to eat the cake. Your blood glucose level will go up if you do, and your insulin can't be adjusted properly."

When a client first attempts to change a colostomy bag but needs some assistance, the nurse might say,

"You gave it a good effort. You were able to complete the task with a little assistance" (giving positive feedback).

Understanding the theories and treatment modalities presented in this chapter can help the nurse select appropriate and effective intervention strategies. In later chapters that present particular mental disorders or problems, specific psychosocial interventions that the nurse might use are described.

SELF-AWARENESS ISSUES

The nurse must examine his or her beliefs about the theories of psychosocial development and realize that many treatment approaches are available. Different treatments may work for different clients: no one approach works for everyone. Sometimes the nurse's personal opinions may not agree with those of the client, but the nurse must make sure that those beliefs do not inadvertently affect the therapeutic process. For example, an overweight client may be working on accepting herself as being overweight rather than trying to lose weight, but the nurse believes the client really just needs to lose weight. The nurse's responsibility is to support the client's needs and goals, not to promote the nurse's own ideas about what the client should do. Hence, the nurse must support the client's decision to work on self-acceptance. For the nurse who believes that being overweight is simply a lack of will power, it might be difficult to support a client's participation in a self-help weight-loss group, such as Overeaters Anonymous, that emphasizes overeating as a disease and accepting oneself.

Points to Consider When Working on Self-Awareness

Points to consider regarding psychosocial theories and treatment:

- No one theory explains all human behavior. No one approach will work with all clients.
- Becoming familiar with the variety of psychosocial approaches for working with clients will increase the nurse's effectiveness in promoting the client's health and well-being.
- The client's feelings and perceptions about his or her situation are the most influential factors in determining his or her response to therapeutic interventions, rather than what the nurse believes the client should do.

Critical Thinking Questions

1. Can sound parenting and nurturing in a loving environment overcome a genetic or biologic predisposition to mental illness?
2. Can children raised in a hostile environment without parental love, support, and consistency avoid mental health problems as adults? If so, how, or what factors could help a person overcome a neglectful or traumatic childhood?

KEY POINTS

- Psychosocial theories help to explain human behavior—both mental health and mental illness. There are several types of psychosocial theories, including psychoanalytic theories, interpersonal theories, humanistic theories, behavioral theories, and existential theories.
- Freud believed that human behavior is motivated by repressed sexual impulses and desires and that childhood development is based on sexual energy (libido) as the driving force.
- Erik Erikson's theories focused on both social and psychological development across the life span. He proposed eight stages of psychosocial development; each stage includes a developmental task and a virtue to be achieved (hope, will, purpose, fidelity, love, caring, and wisdom). Erikson's theories remain in wide use today.
- Jean Piaget described four stages of cognitive development: sensorimotor, preoperational, concrete operations, and formal operations.
- Harry Stack Sullivan's theories focused on development in terms of interpersonal relationships. He viewed the therapist's role (termed *participant observer*) as key to the client's treatment.
- Hildegard Peplau is a nursing theorist whose theories formed much of the foundation of modern nursing practice, including the therapeutic nurse–patient relationship, the role of the nurse in the relationship, and the four anxiety levels.
- Abraham Maslow developed a hierarchy of needs stating that people are motivated by progressive levels of needs;

INTERNET RESOURCES

RESOURCE	INTERNET ADDRESS
• Albert Ellis Institute (Rational Emotive Behavior Therapy)	http://www.rebt.org
• Alcoholics Anonymous	http://www.alcoholics-anonymous.org
• American Group Psychotherapy Association	http://www.agpa.org
• Beck Institute for Cognitive Therapy and Research	http://www.beckinstitute.org
• Gamblers Anonymous	http://www.gamblersanonymous.org
• NAMI Family to Family Education Program	http://www.nami.org/family
• National Association of Cognitive-Behavioral Therapists	http://www.nacbt.org

each level must be satisfied before the person can progress to the next level. The levels begin with physiologic needs and then proceed to safety and security needs, belonging needs, esteem needs, and finally self-actualization needs.

• Carl Rogers developed client-centered therapy in which the therapist plays a supportive role, demonstrating unconditional positive regard, genuineness, and empathetic understanding to the client.

• Behaviorism focuses on the client's observable performance and behaviors and external influences that can bring about behavior changes rather than on feelings and thoughts.

• Systematic desensitization is an example of conditioning in which a person who has an excessive fear of something, such as frogs or snakes, learns to manage his or her anxiety response through being exposed to the feared object.

• B. F. Skinner was a behaviorist who developed the theory of operant conditioning in which people are motivated to learn or change behavior with a system of rewards or reinforcement.

• Existential theorists believe that problems result when the person is out of touch with the self or the environment. The person has self-imposed restrictions, criticizes himself or herself harshly, and does not participate in satisfying interpersonal relationships.

• Founders of existentialism include Albert Ellis (rational emotive therapy), Viktor Frankl (logotherapy), Frederick Perls (gestalt therapy), and William Glasser (reality therapy).

• All existential therapies have the goal of returning the person to an authentic sense of self through emphasizing personal responsibility for oneself and one's feelings, behavior, and choices.

• A crisis is a turning point in an individual's life that produces an overwhelming response. Crises may be maturational, situational, or adventitious. Effective crisis intervention includes assessment of the person in crisis, promotion of problem-solving, and provision of empathetic understanding.

• Cognitive therapy is based on the premise that how a person thinks about or interprets life experiences determines how he or she will feel or behave. It seeks to help the person change how he or she thinks about things to bring about an improvement in mood and behavior.

• Treatment of mental disorders and emotional problems can include one or more of the following: individual psychotherapy, group psychotherapy, family therapy, family education, psychiatric rehabilitation, self-help groups, support groups, education groups, and other psychosocial interventions such as setting limits or giving positive feedback.

• An understanding of psychosocial theories and treatment modalities can help the nurse select appropriate and effective intervention strategies to use with clients.

REFERENCES

Aguilera, D. C. (1998). *Crisis intervention: Theory and methodology* (7th ed.). St. Louis: Mosby.

Beck, A. T., & Rush, A. J. (1995). Cognitive therapy. In H. I. Kaplan & B. J. Sadock (Eds.), *Comprehensive textbook of psychiatry, Vol. 2* (6th ed., pp. 1847–1856). Philadelphia: J. B. Lippincott.

Caplan, G. (1964). *Principles of preventive psychiatry.* New York: Basic Books.

Erikson, E. H. (1963). *Childhood and society* (2nd ed.). New York: Norton.

Freud, S. (1962). *The ego and the id (The standard edition of the complete psychological works of Sigmund Freud;* J. Strachey, Trans.). New York: W. W. Norton & Company. (Original work published 1923.)

Lecomte, T., Wallace, C. J., Perreault, M., & Caron, J. (2005). Consumer's goals in psychiatric rehabilitation and their concordance with existing services. *Psychiatric Services, 56*(2), 209–211.

Loden, S. (2002). The fate of the dream in contemporary psychoanalysis. *Journal of the American Psychoanalytic Association, 5*(1), 43–70.

Maslow, A. H. (1954). *Motivation and personality.* New York: Harper & Row.

National Alliance for the Mentally Ill (NAMI). (2004). Family to Family Education Program. Available: http://www.nami.org/family.

National Center for Complementary and Alternative Medicine. (2006). What is complementary and alternative medicine? Available: http://nccam.nih.gov/health.

Peplau, H. (1952). *Interpersonal relations in nursing.* New York: G. P. Putnam's Sons.

Rogers, C. R. (1961). *On becoming a person: A therapist's view of psychotherapy*. Boston: Houghton Mifflin.

Sadock, B. J., & Sadock, V. A. (2004). *Concise textbook of clinical psychiatry* (3rd ed.). Philadelphia: Lippincott Williams & Wilkins.

Skinner, B. F. (1974). *About behaviorism*. New York: Alfred A. Knopf, Inc.

Sullivan, H. S. (1953). *The interpersonal theory of psychiatry*. New York: Norton.

Yalom, I. D. (1995). *The theory and practice of group psychotherapy*. New York: Basic Books.

ADDITIONAL READINGS

Beck, A. T. (1976). *Cognitive therapy and the emotional disorders*. New York: New American Library, Inc.

Berne, E. (1964). *Games people play*. New York: Grove Press.

Caplan, G. (1964). *Principles of preventive psychiatry*. New York: Basic Books.

Crain, W. C. (1980). *Theories of development: Concepts and application*. Englewood Cliffs, NJ: Prentice Hall, Inc.

Frankl, V. E. (1959). *Man's search for meaning: An introduction to logotherapy*. New York: Beacon Press.

Glasser, W. (1965). *Reality therapy: A new approach to psychiatry*. New York: Harper & Row.

Hendrick, S. S. (2004). Close relationships research: A resource for couple and family therapists. *Journal of Marital and Family Therapy, 30*(1), 13–27.

Miller, P. H. (1983). *Theories of developmental psychology*. San Francisco: W. H. Freeman & Co.

Millon, T. (Ed.). (1967). *Theories of psychopathology*. Philadelphia: W. B. Saunders.

Perls, F. S., Hefferline, R. F., & Goodman, P. (1951). *Gestalt therapy: Excitement and growth in the human personality*. New York: Dell Publishing Co., Inc.

Sugarman, L. (1986). *Life-span development: Concepts, theories and interventions*. London: Methuen & Co., Ltd.

Szasz, T. (1961). *The myth of mental illness*. New York: Hoeber-Harper.

Viscott, D. (1996). *Emotional resilience: Simple truths for dealing with the unfinished business of your past*. New York: Harmony Books.

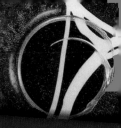

Chapter Study Guide

MULTIPLE-CHOICE QUESTIONS

Select the best answer for each of the following questions.

1. Which of the following theorists believed that a corrective interpersonal relationship with the therapist was the primary mode of treatment?
   A. Sigmund Freud
   B. William Glasser
   C. Hildegard Peplau
   D. Harry Stack Sullivan

2. Dream analysis and free association are techniques in which of the following?
   A. Client-centered therapy
   B. Gestalt therapy
   C. Logotherapy
   D. Psychoanalysis

3. Four levels of anxiety were described by
   A. Erik Erikson
   B. Sigmund Freud
   C. Hildegard Peplau
   D. Carl Rogers

4. Correcting how one thinks about the world and oneself is the focus of
   A. Behaviorism
   B. Cognitive therapy
   C. Psychoanalysis
   D. Reality therapy

5. The personality structures of id, ego, and superego were described by
   A. Sigmund Freud
   B. Hildegard Peplau
   C. Frederick Perls
   D. Harry Stack Sullivan

6. The nursing role that involves being a substitute for another, such as a parent, is called
   A. Counselor
   B. Resource person
   C. Surrogate
   D. Teacher

7. Psychiatric rehabilitation focuses on
   A. Client's strengths
   B. Medication compliance
   C. Social skills deficits
   D. Symptom reduction

8. When a nurse develops feelings toward a client that are based on the nurse's past experience, it is called
   A. Countertransference
   B. Role reversal
   C. Transference
   D. Unconditional regard

9. A group that was designed to meet weekly for 10 sessions to deal with feelings of depression would be a(n)
   A. Closed group
   B. Educational group
   C. Open group
   D. Support group

FILL-IN-THE-BLANK QUESTIONS

Write the name of the appropriate theorist beside the statement or theory. Names may be used more than once.

1. The client is the key to his or her own healing. _____

2. Social and psychological factors influence development. _____

3. Behavior change occurs through conditioning with environmental stimuli. _____

4. People make themselves unhappy by clinging to irrational beliefs. _____

5. Behavior is learned from past experience that is reinforcing. _____

6. Client-centered therapy _____

7. Gestalt therapy _____

8. Hierarchy of needs _____

9. Logotherapy _____

10. Rational emotive therapy _____

11. Reality therapy _____

SHORT-ANSWER QUESTIONS

Describe each of the following types of groups, and give an example.

1. Group psychotherapy

2. Education group

3. Support group

4. Self-help group

Treatment Settings and Therapeutic Programs

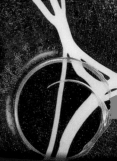

Key Terms

- **Access to Community Care and Effective Services and Support (ACCESS) Demonstration Project**
- **assertive community treatment (ACT)**
- **case management**
- **clubhouse model**
- **criminalization of mental illness**
- **day treatment**
- **evolving consumer household**
- **interdisciplinary (multidisciplinary) team**
- **partial hospitalization program (PHP)**
- **residential treatment settings**

Learning Objectives

After reading this chapter, you should be able to

1. Discuss traditional treatment settings.

2. Describe different types of residential treatment settings and the services they provide.

3. Describe community treatment programs that provide services to people with mental illness.

4. Identify barriers to effective treatment for homeless people with mental illness.

5. Discuss the issues related to people with mental illness in the criminal justice system.

6. Describe the roles of different members of a multidisciplinary mental health care team.

7. Identify the different roles of the nurse in varied treatment settings and programs.

Visit the Point http://thePoint.lww.com for NCLEX-style questions, journal articles, and more!

Mental health care has undergone profound changes in the past 50 years. Before the 1950s, humane treatment in large state facilities was the best available strategy for people with chronic and persistent mental illness, many of whom stayed in such facilities for months or years. The introduction of psychotropic medications in the 1950s offered the first hope of successfully treating the symptoms of mental illness in a meaningful way. By the 1970s, focus on client rights and changes in commitment laws led to deinstitutionalization and a new era of treatment. Institutions could no longer hold clients with mental illness indefinitely, and treatment in the "least restrictive environment" became a guiding principle and right. Large state hospitals emptied. Treatment in the community was intended to replace much of state hospital inpatient care. Adequate funding, however, has not kept pace with the need for community programs and treatment (see Chapter 1).

Today, people with mental illness receive treatment in a variety of settings. This chapter describes the range of treatment settings available for those with mental illness and the psychiatric rehabilitation programs that have been developed to meet their needs. Both of these sections discuss the challenges of integrating people with mental illness into the community. The chapter also addresses two populations who are receiving inadequate treatment because they are not connected with needed services: homeless clients and clients who are in jail. In addition, the chapter describes the multidisciplinary team, including the role of the nurse as a member. Finally, it briefly discusses psychosocial nursing in public health and home care.

TREATMENT SETTINGS

Inpatient Hospital Treatment

In the 1980s, inpatient psychiatric care was still a primary mode of treatment for people with mental illness. A typical psychiatric unit emphasized *talk therapy,* or one-on-one interactions between residents and staff, and *milieu therapy,* meaning the total environment and its effect on the client's treatment. Individual and group interactions focused on trust, self-disclosure by clients to staff and one another, and active participation in groups. Effective milieu therapy required long lengths of stay because clients with more stable conditions helped to provide structure and support for newly admitted clients with more acute conditions.

By the 1990s, the economics of health care began to change dramatically, and the lengths of stay in hospitals decreased to just a few days. Today, most Americans are insured under some form of managed care. Managed care exerts cost-control measures such as recertification of admissions, utilization review, and case management—all of which have altered inpatient treatment significantly. The growth of managed care has been associated with declining admissions, shorter lengths of stay, reduced reimbursement, and increased acuity of inpatients. Therefore, clients are sicker when they are admitted and do not stay as long in the hospital.

Today, inpatient units must provide rapid assessment, stabilization of symptoms, and discharge planning, and they must accomplish goals quickly. A client-centered multidisciplinary approach to a brief stay is essential. Clinicians help clients recognize symptoms, identify coping skills, and choose discharge supports. When the client is safe and stable, the clinicians and the client identify long-term issues for the client to pursue in outpatient therapy.

Some inpatient units have a locked entrance door, requiring staff with keys to let persons in or out of the unit. This situation has both advantages and disadvantages (Haglund, von Knorring, & von Essen, 2006). Nurses identify the advantages of providing protection against the "outside world" in a safe and secure environment as well as the primary disadvantages of making clients feel confined or dependent, and emphasizing the staff members' power over them.

SCHEDULED INPATIENT STAYS

Tucker, Moore, and Luedtke (2000) studied brief inpatient hospital stays for clients with anxiety and mood disorders. Clients participated in the program for an average of 7 days. Three months after the hospital stay, clients had maintained the gains achieved during the program and had few readmissions to the hospital.

The Department of Veterans Affairs (VA) hospital system has piloted a variety of alternatives to inpatient hospital admission that occurs when the client's condition has worsened or a crisis has developed. Scheduled, intermittent hospital stays did not lessen veterans' days in the hospital, but did improve their self-esteem and feelings of self-control. Another alternative available to veterans, the Short-Term Acute Residential Treatment (START) program (Hawthorne et al., 2005), is based in San Diego and is available at six facilities, all of which are non–hospital-based residential treatment centers. Over a 2-year period, veterans treated in the START program had the same improvement in symptoms and functioning as those treated at a VA hospital, but were significantly more satisfied with the services. The cost of treatment in a START program was 65% lower than treatment in the hospital.

LONG-STAY CLIENTS

Long-stay clients are people with severe and persistent mental illness who continue to require acute care services despite the current emphasis on decreased hospital stays. This population includes clients who were hospitalized before deinstitutionalization and remain hospitalized despite efforts at community placement. It also includes clients who have been hospitalized consistently for long periods despite efforts to minimize their hospital stays. Community placement of clients with problematic behaviors still meets resistance from the public, creating a barrier to successful placement in community settings.

One approach to working with long-stay clients is a "hospital hostel," a unit within a hospital that is designed to be more home-like and less institutional. In Great Britain, several hospital hostel projects have been established that provide access to community facilities and focus on "normal expectations," such as cooking, cleaning, and doing housework. A study of one such program found that clients had improved functioning and fewer aggressive episodes, and were more satisfied with their care. Some clients remained in the hostel setting, whereas others were eventually resettled in the community (King, Singh, & Sheperd, 2000).

The concept of a "crisis hostel" has been successful in a rural community–based program in Colorado (Knight, 2004). The only criterion for using the service is the client's perception of being in crisis and needing a more structured environment. Knight believed that if the client does not have to exhibit any certain "symptoms" to gain access to the hostel, he or she is more likely to perceive his or her situation more accurately, feel better about asking for help, and avoid rehospitalization.

Lunsky and colleagues (2006) studied more than 12,000 long-stay clients in the tertiary mental health care system in Ontario. They found that 1 in 8 clients had a dual diagnosis of a major mental illness and mental retardation. These clients required, but did not often receive, a higher level of care with more intensive services and supervision than clients with a mental illness and normal intellectual functioning. As a group, the clients with a dual diagnosis had more severe symptoms, more instances of aggressive behavior, and a greater lack of financial and health care resources. The authors suggested that reform in the tertiary mental health care system should address the needs of clients with a dual diagnosis, which often exceed current available services.

CASE MANAGEMENT

Case management, or management of care on a case-by-case basis, is an important concept in both inpatient and community settings. Inpatient case managers are usually nurses or social workers who follow the client from admission to discharge and serve as liaisons between the client and community resources, home care, and third-party payers. In the community, the case manager works with clients on a broad range of issues, from accessing needed medical and psychiatric services to carrying out tasks of daily living such as using public transportation, managing money, and buying groceries.

DISCHARGE PLANNING

An important concept in any inpatient treatment setting is discharge planning. Environmental supports, such as housing and transportation, and access to community resources and services are crucial to successful discharge planning. In fact, the adequacy of discharge plans is a better predictor of how long the person could remain in the community than are clinical indicators such as psychiatric diagnoses.

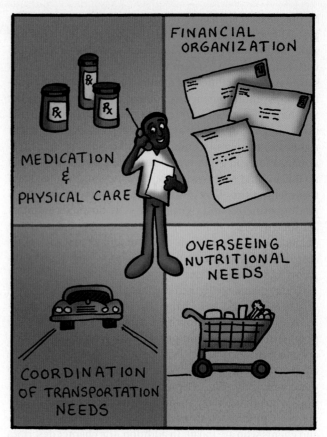

Case manager

Impediments to successful discharge planning include alcohol and drug abuse, criminal or violent behavior, noncompliance with medication regimens, and suicidal ideation. For example, optimal housing often is not available to people with a recent history of drug or alcohol abuse or criminal behavior. Also, clients who have suicidal ideas or a history of noncompliance with medication regimens may be ineligible for some treatment programs or services. Therefore, clients with these impediments to successful discharge planning may have a marginal discharge plan in place because optimal services or plans are not available to them. Consequently, people discharged with marginal plans are readmitted more quickly and more frequently than those who have better discharge plans.

However, discharge plans cannot be successful if clients do not follow through with the established plan. Clients do not keep follow-up appointments or referrals if they don't feel connected to the outpatient services or if these services aren't perceived as helpful or valuable. Attention to psychosocial factors that address the client's well-being, his or her preference for follow-up services, inclusion of the family, and familiarity with outpatient providers is critical to the success of a discharge plan (Williams, 2004).

Prince (2006) found that three types of intervention are significant in preventing rehospitalization for individuals with four or more prior inpatient stays. These interventions are symptom education, service continuity, and establishment of daily structure. Clients who can recognize signs of impending relapse and seek help, participate in out-patient appointments and services, and have a daily plan of activities and responsibilities are least likely to require rehospitalization.

Creating successful discharge plans that offer optimal services and housing is essential if people with mental illness are to be integrated into the community. A holistic approach to reintegrating persons into the community is the best way to prevent repeated hospital admissions and improve quality of life for clients. Community programs after discharge from the hospital should include social services, day treatment, and housing programs, all geared toward survival in the community, compliance with treatment recommendations, rehabilitation, and independent living. **Assertive community treatment (ACT)** programs provide many of the services that are necessary to stop the revolving door of repeated hospital admissions punctuated by unsuccessful attempts at community living. ACT programs are discussed in detail later in this chapter.

Partial Hospitalization Programs

Partial hospitalization programs (PHPs) are designed to help clients make a gradual transition from being inpatients to living independently and to prevent repeat admissions. In **day treatment** programs, clients return home at night; evening programs are just the reverse. The services that different PHPs offer vary, but most programs include groups for building communication and social skills, solving problems, monitoring medications, and learning coping strategies and skills for daily living. Individual sessions are available in some PHPs, as are vocational assistance and occupational and recreation therapies.

Each client has an individualized treatment plan and goals, which the client develops with the case manager and other members of the treatment team. Eight broad categories of goals usually addressed in PHPs are summarized in Box 4.1.

Clients in PHPs may complete the program after an inpatient hospital stay, which is usually too short to address anything other than stabilization of symptoms and medication effectiveness. Other clients may come to a PHP to treat problems before they really start, thus avoiding a costly and unwanted hospital stay. Others may make the transition from a PHP to longer-term outpatient therapy. Bateman and Fonagy (2003) reported that completion of a day treatment program was effective in stabilizing symptoms and improving daily functioning, and it encouraged poorly functioning clients with personality disorders to participate in outpatient therapy. Day treatment has also been successful with depressed clients, who reported a significant reduction in symptoms as well as improvements in social adaptation and overall functioning (Mazza et al., 2004).

Residential Settings

Persons with mental illness may live in community **residential treatment settings** that vary according to structure, level of supervision, and services provided (Box 4.2). Some settings are designed as transitional housing with the expectation that residents will progress to more independent living. Other residential programs serve clients for as long as the need exists, sometimes years. Board and care homes often provide a room, bathroom, laundry facilities, and one common meal each day. Adult foster homes may care for one to three clients in a family-like atmosphere, including meals and social activities with the family. Halfway houses usually serve as temporary placements that provide support as the clients prepare for independence. Group homes house 6 to 10 residents, who take turns cooking meals and sharing household chores under the supervision of one or two staff persons. Independent living programs are often housed in apartment complexes, where clients share apartments. Staff members are available for crisis intervention, transportation, assistance with daily living tasks, and, sometimes, drug monitoring. In addition to on-site staff, many residential settings provide case management services for clients and put them in touch with other programs (e.g., vocational rehabilitation; medical, dental, and psychiatric care; psychosocial rehabilitation programs or services) as needed.

Box 4.1 PARTIAL HOSPITALIZATION PROGRAM GOALS

- Stabilizing psychiatric symptoms
- Monitoring drug effectiveness
- Stabilizing living environment
- Improving activities of daily living
- Learning to structure time
- Developing social skills
- Obtaining meaningful work, paid employment, or a volunteer position
- Providing follow-up of any health concerns

Box 4.2 RESIDENTIAL SETTINGS

Group homes
Supervised apartments
Board and care homes
Adult foster care
Respite/crisis housing

Some agencies provide respite housing, or crisis housing services, for clients in need of short-term temporary shelter. These clients may live in group homes or independently most of the time but have a need for "respite" from their usual residences. This usually occurs when clients experience a crisis, feel overwhelmed, or cannot cope with problems or emotions. Respite services often provide increased emotional support and assistance with problem solving in a setting away from the source of the clients' distress.

A client's living environment affects his or her level of functioning, rate of reinstitutionalization, and duration of remaining in the community setting. In fact, the living environment is often more predictive of the client's success than the characteristics of his or her illness. A client with a poor living environment often leaves the community or is readmitted to the hospital. Finding quality living situations for clients is a difficult task. Many clients live in crime-ridden or commercial, rather than residential, areas (Segal & Riley, 2003).

Frequently, residents oppose plans to establish a group home or residential facility in their neighborhood. They argue that having a group home will decrease their property values, and they may believe that people with mental illness are violent, will act bizarrely in public, or will be a menace to their children. These people have strongly ingrained stereotypes and a great deal of misinformation. Local residents must be given the facts so that safe, affordable, and desirable housing can be established for persons needing residential care. Nurses are in a position to advocate for clients by providing education to members of the community.

Evolving Consumer Households

The **evolving consumer household** is a group-living situation in which the residents make the transition from a traditional group home to a residence where they fulfill their own responsibilities and function without on-site supervision from paid staff. This concept was developed as part of the Boston McKinney Research Demonstration Project in the early 1990s, which is sponsored by the National Institute of Mental Health. One of the problems with housing for people with mental illness is that they may have to move many times, from one type of setting to another, as their independence increases. This continual moving necessitates readjustment in each setting, making it difficult for clients to sustain their gains in independence. Because the evolving consumer household is a permanent living arrangement, it eliminates the problem of relocation.

During the demonstration project, it was found that poverty among people with mental illness was a significant barrier to maintaining housing, which psychiatric rehabilitation seldom addressed. Residents often rely on government entitlements, such as Social Security Insurance or Social Security Disability Insurance, for their income, which averages $400 to $450 per month. Although many clients express the desire to work, many cannot do so consistently. Even

with vocational services, the jobs available tend to be unskilled and part-time, resulting in income that is inadequate to maintain independent living. In addition, the Social Security Insurance system is often a disincentive to making the transition to paid employment: the client would have to trade a reliable source of income and much-needed health insurance for a poorly paying, relatively insecure job that is unlikely to include fringe benefits. Both psychiatric rehabilitation programs and society must address poverty among people with mental illness to remove this barrier to independent living and self-sufficiency.

PSYCHIATRIC REHABILITATION PROGRAMS

Psychiatric rehabilitation, sometimes called *psychosocial rehabilitation,* refers to services designed to promote the recovery process for clients with mental illness (Box 4.3). This recovery goes beyond symptom control and medication management to include personal growth, reintegration into the community, empowerment, increased independence, and improved quality of life (Palmer & Wegener, 2003). Community support programs and services provide psychiatric rehabilitation to varying degrees, often depending on the resources and funding available. Some programs focus primarily on reducing hospital readmissions through symptom control and medication management, whereas others include social and recreation services. There are not enough programs available nationwide to meet the needs of people with mental illnesses.

Hughes (1999) stated that the likelihood of achieving even minimal treatment goals is low without a broad array of psychosocial, vocational, and housing services, even though these services are typically not included under the "medically necessary" services funded under managed care. He identified 10 reasons (listed in Box 4.4) why comprehensive

Box 4.3   GOALS OF PSYCHIATRIC REHABILITATION

- Recovery from mental illness
- Personal growth
- Quality of life
- Community reintegration
- Empowerment
- Increased independence
- Decreased hospital admissions
- Improved social functioning
- Improved vocational functioning
- Continuous treatment
- Increased involvement in treatment decisions
- Improved physical health
- Recovered sense of self

services for people with mental illness should include community support.

Psychiatric rehabilitation has improved client outcomes by providing community support services to decrease hospital readmission rates and increase community integration. At the same time, managed care has reduced the "medically necessary" services that are funded. For example, because skills training was found to be successful in assisting clients in the community, managed care organizations defined psychiatric rehabilitation as only skills training and did not fund other aspects of rehabilitation such as socialization or environmental supports. Clients and providers identified poverty, lack of jobs, and inadequate vocational skills as barriers to community integration, but because these barriers were not included in the "medically necessary" definition of psychiatric rehabilitation by managed care, services to overcome these barriers were not funded.

Clubhouse Model

In 1948, Fountain House pioneered the **clubhouse model** of community-based rehabilitation in New York City. Cur-

rently, more than 400 such clubhouses have been established in 27 countries throughout the world (Ferguson, 2004). Fountain House is an "intentional community" based on the belief that men and women with serious and persistent psychiatric disabilities can and will achieve normal life goals when given the opportunity, time, support, and fellowship. The essence of membership in the clubhouse is based on the four guaranteed rights of members:

- A place to come to
- Meaningful work
- Meaningful relationships
- A place to return to (lifetime membership)

The clubhouse model provides members with many opportunities, including daytime work activities focused on the care, maintenance, and productivity of the clubhouse; evening, weekend, and holiday leisure activities; transitional and independent employment support and efforts; and housing options. Members are encouraged and assisted to use psychiatric services, which are usually local clinics or private practitioners.

The clubhouse model recognizes the physician–client relationship as a key to successful treatment and rehabili-

---

Box 4.4   TEN REASONS TO INCLUDE COMMUNITY SUPPORT IN EVERY BEHAVIORAL HEALTH PLAN

1. Decreased hospitalization. This facilitates lower cost of care. Clients who have access to more intensive support are less likely to decompensate to a point where they require inpatient hospitalization.
2. Normalization. Clients respond favorably to community interactions that are more "normal" and not directly treatment-related such as pursuing a hobby or joining the YMCA or YWCA with the help of their community support workers.
3. Linkage to resources. Community support workers can identify and access resources for the client when he or she may be unable to do so.
4. Effective advocacy. Community support workers can confront individuals or institutions in a professional manner to resolve any attempts to prevent a client from reaching goals.
5. Improved quality of life. Because clients often survive on Social Security Insurance benefits, they need assistance to access such services as food pantries, energy grants, and weatherization programs to help make ends meet.
6. Respite for natural caregivers. Community support workers can arrange doctors' appointments and lab work, pick up drugs, and monitor compliance with medications

to alleviate the stress of these tasks on the client's caregiver. They also can provide direct support and information to caregivers to make their tasks easier.
7. Consolidated funding. Services in the community are often provided and funded by a variety of programs and agencies. Community support workers can advocate for the enhancement of community support services and improved, adequate funding of these services.
8. Equalization of a two-tiered system. Private sector mental health care is often limited when the illness is persistent and severe. Consequently, clients revert to care provided through public funds. All payers, public or private, could benefit from community support programs to promote wellness and manage crises or serious mental illness.
9. Flexibility. Community support employs a variety of persons at different skill levels to provide assistance with everything from daily activities to psychiatric care, depending on the needs of the client.
10. Continuum of care. Community support provides the opportunity for clients to move along a continuum of services without repeated transfers to different programs with unfamiliar staff.

Hughes, W. C. (1999). Managed care, meet community support. Health & Social Work, 24(2), 103–110.

tation while acknowledging that brief encounters that focus on symptom management are not sufficient to promote rehabilitation efforts. The "rehabilitation alliance" refers to the network of relationships that must develop over time to support people with psychiatric disabilities and includes the client, family, friends, clinicians, and even landlords, employers, and neighbors. The rehabilitation alliance needs community support, opportunities for success, coordination of service providers, and member involvement to maintain a positive focus on life goals, strengths, creativity, and hope as the members pursue recovery. The clubhouse model exists to promote the rehabilitation alliance as a positive force in the members' lives.

The clubhouse focus is on health, not illness. Taking prescribed drugs, for example, is not a condition of participation in the clubhouse. Members, not staff, must ultimately make decisions about treatment, such as whether or not they need hospital admission. Clubhouse staff supports members, helps them to obtain needed assistance, and most of all allows them to make the decisions that ultimately affect all aspects of their lives. This approach to psychiatric rehabilitation is the cornerstone and the strength of the clubhouse model.

Assertive Community Treatment (1973)

One of the most effective approaches to community-based treatment for people with mental illness is ACT (Box 4.5). Marx, Test, and Stein (1973) conceived this idea in 1973 in Madison, Wisconsin, while working at Mendota State Hospital. They believed that skills training, support, and teaching should be done in the community where it was needed rather than in the hospital. Their program was first known as the Madison model, then "training in community living," and, finally, ACT, or the program for assertive treatment. The mobile outreach and continuous treatment programs of today all have their roots in the Madison model.

An ACT program has a problem-solving orientation: Staff members attend to specific life issues, no matter how mundane. ACT programs provide most services directly rather than relying on referrals to other programs or agencies, and they implement the services in the clients' homes or communities, not in offices. The ACT services are also intense; three or more face-to-face contacts with clients are tailored to meet clients' needs. The team approach allows all staff to be equally familiar with all clients, so clients do not have to wait for an assigned person. ACT programs also make a long-term commitment to clients, providing services for as long as the need persists and with no time constraints (Redko et al., 2004).

ACT programs were developed and flourished in urban settings. ACT programs have also been effective in rural areas, where traditional psychiatric services are more limited, fragmented, and difficult to obtain than in cities. Rural areas have less money to fund services, and social stigma about mental illness is greater in rural areas, as are negative

---

Box 4.5 COMPONENTS OF AN ACT PROGRAM

- Having a multidisciplinary team that includes a psychiatrist, psychiatric mental health nurse, vocational rehabilitation specialist, and social worker for each 100 clients (low staff-to-client ratio)
- Identifying a fixed point of responsibility for clients with a primary provider of services
- Ameliorating or eliminating the debilitating symptoms of mental illness
- Improving client functioning in adult social and employment roles and activities
- Decreasing the family's burden of care by providing opportunities for clients to learn skills in real-life situations
- Implementing an individualized, ongoing treatment program defined by clients' needs
- Involving all needed support systems for holistic treatment of clients
- Promoting mental health through the use of a vast array of resources and treatment modalities
- Emphasizing and promoting client independence
- Using daily team meetings to discuss strategies to improve the care of clients
- Providing services 24 hours a day that would include respite care to deflect unnecessary hospitalization and crisis intervention to prevent destabilization with unnecessary emergency department visits
- Measuring client outcomes on the following aspects: symptomatology; social, psychological, and familial functioning; gainful employment; client independence; client empowerment; use of ancillary services; client, family, and societal satisfaction; hospital use; agency use; rehospitalization; quality of life; and costs

---

attitudes about public service programs. Rural ACT programs have resulted in fewer hospital admissions, greater housing stability, improved quality of life, and improved psychiatric symptoms. This success occurred even though certain modifications of traditional ACT programs were required, such as two-person teams, fewer and shorter contacts with clients, and minimal participation from some disciplines.

ACT programs have also been successful in Canada and Australia (Latimer, 2005; Udechuku et al., 2005) in decreasing hospital admissions and fostering community integration for persons with mental illness. In New York, ACT services have been modified to include services designed to prevent arrest and incarceration of adults with severe mental illness who have been involved in the criminal justice system (Lamberti, Weisman, & Faden, 2004). This special population is discussed later in the chapter.

SPECIAL POPULATIONS OF CLIENTS WITH MENTAL ILLNESS

Homeless Population

Homeless people with mental illness have been the focus of recent studies. For this population, shelters, rehabilitation programs, and prisons may serve as makeshift alternatives to inpatient care or supportive housing. Frequent shifts between the street, programs, and institutions worsen the marginal existence of this population. Compared with homeless people without mental illness, mentally ill homeless people are homeless longer, spend more time in shelters, have fewer contacts with family, spend more time in jail, and face greater barriers to employment (National Resource and Training Center on Homelessness and Mental Illness, 2006). For this population, professionals supersede families as the primary source of help.

Providing housing alone does not significantly alter the prognosis of homelessness for persons with mental illness. In a study conducted in Philadelphia, Min, Wong, and Rothbard (2004) found that psychosocial rehabilitation services, peer support, vocational training, and daily living skill training were effective in decreasing the number of days the clients stayed at shelters. In the early 1990s, the Federal government authorized a grant program to address the needs of people who are homeless and have mental illness. The program, Projects for Assistance in Transition from Homelessness (PATH), funds community-based outreach, mental health, substance abuse, case management, and other support services. Some limited housing services are available, but PATH works primarily with existing housing services in the given community (Substance Abuse and Mental Health Services Administration, 2006).

The Center for Mental Health Services initiated the **Access to Community Care and Effective Services and Support (ACCESS) Demonstration Project** in 1994 to assess whether more integrated systems of service delivery enhance the quality of life of homeless people with serious mental disabilities through the use of services and outreach. ACCESS was a 5-year demonstration program located within 15 U.S cities in nine states that represented most geographic areas of the continental United States. Each site provided outreach and intensive case management to 100 homeless people with severe mental illnesses every year.

Participants in the first 2 years of the ACCESS demonstration project were surveyed to determine whether they had formed a relationship with their assigned case managers and what, if any, differences they experienced in terms of homelessness, symptom management, and use of substances. A total of 2,798 participants completed the survey process. Only 48% reported having relationships or personal connections with their case managers, underscoring the difficulty in establishing therapeutic relationships with homeless mentally ill clients. Clients reporting such relationships described more social support, received more public support and education, were less psychotic, were homeless fewer days, and were intoxicated fewer days than participants who reported having no relationship with their assigned case managers. Although engaging this population in therapeutic relationships is difficult, results are positive when those relationships are established.

The most recent report from the ACCESS project found that participants reported multiple factors that influence their quality of life; managing psychiatric symptoms and receiving social support were most important. The data from this report suggest that focusing treatment on the multiple independent domains of psychiatric illness, social support networks, work and income, housing, and increased service use is necessary to maximally improve clients' self-assessed quality of life and decrease the number of homeless days. These positive outcomes were maintained after termination of the intervention (Rothbard et al., 2004). Desai and Rosenheck (2005) studied persons in the ACCESS project in terms of unmet physical health needs. They found that collaborative case management played an important role in improving the physical health of participants by linking them to appropriate medical services.

Prisoners

McCoy and colleagues (2004) reported that 16% of people in jails, in state prisons, and on probation have experienced a mental illness or psychiatric hospitalization. The rate of mental illness in the jailed population is 13%, compared with 2% in the general population. Offenders generally have acute and chronic mental illness and poor functioning, and many are homeless. Factors cited as reasons that mentally ill people are placed in the criminal justice system include deinstitutionalization, more rigid criteria for civil commitment, lack of adequate community support, economizing on treatment for mental illness, and the attitudes of police and society (Konrad, 2002). **Criminalization of mental illness** refers to the practice of arresting and prosecuting mentally ill offenders, even for misdemeanors, at a rate four times that of the general population in an effort to contain them in some type of institution where they might receive needed treatment. However, if offenders with mental illness had obtained needed treatment, some might not have engaged in criminal activity.

The public concern about the potential danger of people with mental illness is fueled by the media attention that surrounds any violent criminal act committed by a mentally ill person. Although it is true that people with major mental illnesses who do not take prescribed medication are at increased risk for being violent, most people with mental illness do not represent a significant danger to others. This fact, however, does not keep citizens from clinging to stereotypes of the mentally ill as people to be feared, avoided, and institutionalized. If such people cannot be confined in mental hospitals for any period, there seems to be public support for arresting and incarcerating them instead.

People with mental illness who are in the criminal justice system face several barriers to successful community reintegration (McCoy et al., 2004):

- Poverty
- Homelessness
- Substance use
- Violence
- Victimization, rape, and trauma
- Self-harm

Some communities have mobile crisis services linked to their police departments. These professionals are called to the scene (after the situation is stabilized) when police officers believe mental health issues are involved. Frequently, the mentally ill individual can be diverted to crisis counseling services or to the hospital, if needed, instead of being arrested and going to jail. Often, these same professionals provide education to police to help them recognize mental illness and perhaps change their attitude about mentally ill offenders.

Steadman and associates (2005) piloted the Brief Jail Mental Health Screen (BJMHS) at Cook County jail in Chicago. This is an eight-item questionnaire that can be administered in 2.5 minutes. Each detainee was given the questionnaire to see if further evaluation or referral for mental health services was indicated. The BJMHS correctly classified 73.5% of males, but only 61.6% of females. This led the authors to suggest that this brief screening tool would increase effective identification and referral of male detainees and, therefore, could be useful as a standard part of jail admission.

INTERDISCIPLINARY TEAM

Regardless of the treatment setting, rehabilitation program, or population, an **interdisciplinary (multidisciplinary) team** approach is most useful in dealing with the multifaceted problems of clients with mental illness. Different members of the team have expertise in specific areas. By collaborating, they can meet clients' needs more effectively. Members of the interdisciplinary team include the pharmacist, psychiatrist, psychologist, psychiatric nurse, psychiatric social worker, occupational therapist, recreation therapist, and vocational rehabilitation specialist. Their primary roles are described in Box 4.6. Not all settings have a full-time member from each discipline on their team; the programs and services that the team offers determine its composition in any setting.

Functioning as an effective team member requires the development and practice of several core skill areas (White & Brooker, 2001):

- Interpersonal skills, such as tolerance, patience, and understanding
- Humanity, such as warmth, acceptance, empathy, genuineness, and nonjudgmental attitude
- Knowledge base about mental disorders, symptoms, and behavior

- Communication skills
- Personal qualities, such as consistency, assertiveness, and problem-solving abilities
- Teamwork skills, such as collaborating, sharing, and integrating
- Risk assessment and risk management skills

The role of the case manager has become increasingly important with the proliferation of managed care and the variety of services that clients need. No standard formal educational program to become a case manager exists, however, and people from many different backgrounds may fill this role. In some settings, a social worker or psychiatric nurse may be the case manager. In other settings, people who work in psychosocial rehabilitation settings may take on the role of case manager with a baccalaureate degree in a related field, such as psychology, or by virtue of their experience and demonstrated skills. Liberman and coworkers (2001) identified three distinct sets of competencies necessary for effective case managers: clinical skills, relationship skills, and liaison and advocacy skills. Clinical skills include treatment planning, symptom and functional assessment, and skills training. Relationship skills include the ability to establish and maintain collaborative, respectful, and therapeutic alliances with a wide variety of clients. Liaison and advocacy skills are necessary to develop and maintain effective interagency contacts for housing, financial entitlements, and vocational rehabilitation.

As clients' needs become more varied and complex, the psychiatric nurse is in an ideal position to fulfill the role of case manager. In 1994, the American Nurses Association stated that the psychiatric nurse can assess, monitor, and refer clients for general medical problems as well as psychiatric problems; administer drugs; monitor for drug side effects; provide drug and client and family health education; and monitor for general medical disorders that have psychological and physiologic components. Registered nurses bring unique nursing knowledge and skills to the multidisciplinary team.

PSYCHOSOCIAL NURSING IN PUBLIC HEALTH AND HOME CARE

Psychosocial nursing is an important area of public health nursing practice and home care. Public health nurses working in the community provide mental health prevention services to reduce risks to the mental health of persons, families, and communities. Examples include primary prevention, such as stress management education; secondary prevention, such as early identification of potential mental health problems; and tertiary prevention, such as monitoring and coordinating rehabilitation services for the mentally ill.

The clinical practice of public health and home care nurses includes caring for clients and families with issues such as substance abuse, domestic violence, child abuse, grief, and depression. In addition, public health nurses care

---

Box 4.6 INTERDISCIPLINARY TEAM PRIMARY ROLES

- **Pharmacist:** The registered pharmacist is a member of the interdisciplinary team when medications, management of side effects, and/or interactions with nonpsychiatric medications are complex. Clients with refractory symptoms may also benefit from the pharmacist's knowledge of chemical structure and actions of medications.

- **Psychiatrist:** The psychiatrist is a physician certified in psychiatry by the American Board of Psychiatry and Neurology, which requires a 3-year residency, 2 years of clinical practice, and completion of an examination. The primary function of the psychiatrist is diagnosis of mental disorders and prescription of medical treatments.

- **Psychologist:** The clinical psychologist has a doctorate (Ph.D.) in clinical psychology and is prepared to practice therapy, conduct research, and interpret psychological tests. Psychologists may also participate in the design of therapy programs for groups of individuals.

- **Psychiatric nurse:** The registered nurse gains experience in working with clients with psychiatric disorders after graduation from an accredited program of nursing and completion of the licensure examination. The nurse has a solid foundation in health promotion, illness prevention, and rehabilitation in all areas, allowing him or her to view the client holistically. The nurse is also an essential team member in evaluating the effectiveness of medical treatment, particularly medications. Registered nurses who obtain master's degrees in mental health may be certified as clinical specialists or licensed as advanced practitioners, depending on individual state nurse practice acts.

- Advanced practice nurses are certified to prescribe drugs in many states.

- **Psychiatric social worker:** Most psychiatric social workers are prepared at the master's level, and they are licensed in some states. Social workers may practice therapy and often have the primary responsibility for working with families, community support, and referral.

- **Occupational therapist:** Occupational therapists may have an associate degree (certified occupational therapy assistant) or a baccalaureate degree (certified occupational therapist). Occupational therapy focuses on the functional abilities of the client and ways to improve client functioning, such as working with arts and crafts and focusing on psychomotor skills.

- **Recreation therapist:** Many recreation therapists complete a baccalaureate degree, but in some instances persons with experience fulfill these roles. The recreation therapist helps the client to achieve a balance of work and play in his or her life and provides activities that promote constructive use of leisure or unstructured time.

- **Vocational rehabilitation specialist:** Vocational rehabilitation includes determining clients' interests and abilities and matching them with vocational choices. Clients are also assisted in job-seeking and job-retention skills as well as in pursuit of further education, if that is needed and desired. Vocational rehabilitation specialists can be prepared at the baccalaureate or master's level and may have different levels of autonomy and program supervision based on their education.

---

for children in schools and teach health-related subjects to community groups and agencies. Mental health services that public health and home care nurses provide can reduce the suffering that many people experience as a result of physical disease, mental disorders, social and emotional disadvantages, and other vulnerabilities.

SELF-AWARENESS ISSUES

Psychiatric-mental health nursing is evolving as changes continue in health care. The focus is shifting from traditional hospital-based goals of symptom and medication management to more client-centered goals, which include improved quality of life and recovery from mental illness. Therefore, the nurse also must expand his or her repertoire of skills and abilities to assist clients in their efforts. These challenges may overwhelm the nurse at times, and he or she may feel underprepared or ill-equipped to meet them.

Mental health services are moving into some nontraditional settings such as jails and homeless shelters. As nursing roles expand in these alternative settings, the nurse does not have the array of backup services found in hospitals or clinics, such as on-site physicians and colleagues, medical services, and so forth. This requires the nurse to practice in a more autonomous and independent manner, which can be unsettling.

Empowering clients to make their own decisions about treatment is an essential part of full recovery. This differs from the model of the psychiatrist or treatment team as the authority on what is the best course for the client to follow. It is a challenge for the nurse to be supportive of the client when the nurse believes the client has made choices that are less than ideal.

The nurse may experience frustration when working with mentally ill adults who are homeless, incarcerated, or both. Typically, these clients are difficult to engage in therapeutic relationships and may present great challenges to the nurse. The nurse may feel rejected by clients who do not engage readily in a relationship, or the nurse may feel inadequate in attempts to engage these clients.

Points to Consider When Working in Community-Based Settings

- The client can make mistakes, survive them, and learn from them. Mistakes are a part of normal life for everyone, and it is not the nurse's role to protect clients from such experiences.
- The nurse will not always have the answer to solve a client's problems or resolve a difficult situation.
- As clients move toward recovery, they need support to make decisions and follow a course of action, even if the nurse thinks the client is making decisions that are unlikely to be successful.
- Working with clients in community settings is a more collaborative relationship than the traditional role of caring for the client. The nurse may be more familiar and comfortable with the latter.

Critical Thinking Questions

1. Discuss the role of the nurse in advocating for social or legislative policy changes needed to provide psychiatric rehabilitation services for clients in all settings.
2. When are programs for special populations, such as mentally ill adults who are offenders or homeless, considered successful?
3. How can the nurse reconcile the trend for short-term inpatient hospitalization with the long-term needs of some clients with severe and persistent mental illness?

KEY POINTS

- People with mental illness are treated in a variety of settings, and some are not in touch with needed services at all.
- Shortened inpatient hospital stays necessitate changes in the ways hospitals deliver services to clients.
- Adequate discharge planning is a good indicator of how successful the client's community placement will be.
- Impediments to successful discharge planning include alcohol and drug abuse, criminal or violent behavior, noncompliance with medications, and suicidal ideation.
- PHPs usually address the client's psychiatric symptoms, medication use, living environment, activities of daily living, leisure time, social skills, work, and health concerns.
- Community residential settings vary in terms of structure, level of supervision, and services provided. Some

residential settings are transitional, with the expectation that clients will progress to independent living; others serve the client for as long as he or she needs.

- Types of residential settings include board and care homes, adult foster homes, halfway houses, group homes, and independent living programs.
- A client's ability to remain in the community is closely related to the quality and adequacy of his or her living environment.
- Poverty among persons with mental illness is a significant barrier to maintaining housing in the community and is seldom addressed in psychiatric rehabilitation.
- Psychiatric rehabilitation refers to services designed to promote the recovery process for clients with mental illness. This recovery goes beyond symptom control and medication management to include personal growth, reintegration into the community, empowerment, increased independence, and improved quality of life.
- The clubhouse model of psychosocial rehabilitation is an intentional community based on the belief that men and women with mental illness can and will achieve normal life goals when provided time, opportunity, support, and fellowship.
- ACT is one of the most effective approaches to community-based treatment. It includes 24-hour-a-day services, low staff-to-client ratios, in-home or community services, intense and frequent contact, and unlimited length of service.
- Psychiatric rehabilitation services such as ACT must be provided along with stable housing to produce positive outcomes for mentally ill adults who are homeless.
- Adults with mental illness may be placed in the criminal justice system more frequently because of deinstitutionalization, rigid criteria for civil commitment, lack of adequate community support, economizing on treatment for mental illness, and the attitudes of police and society.
- Barriers to community reintegration for mentally ill persons who have been incarcerated include poverty, homelessness, substance abuse, violence, victimization, rape, trauma, and self-harm.
- The multidisciplinary team includes the psychiatrist, psychologist, psychiatric nurse, psychiatric social worker, occupational therapist, recreation therapist, vocational rehabilitation specialist, and sometimes pharmacist.
- The psychiatric nurse is in an ideal position to fulfill the role of case manager. The nurse can assess, monitor, and refer clients for general medical and psychiatric problems; administer drugs; monitor for drug side effects; provide drug and patient and family health education; and monitor for general medical disorders that have psychological and physiologic components.
- Empowering clients to pursue full recovery requires collaborative working relationships with clients rather than the traditional approach of caring for clients.

INTERNET RESOURCES

RESOURCE	INTERNET ADDRESS
• Fountain House (clubhouse model)	http://www.fountainhouse.org
• National Association for Home Care and Hospice	http://www.nahc.org
• National Law Center on Homelessness and Poverty	http://www.nlchp.org
• National Mental Health Association	http://www.nmha.org
• National Mental Health Information Center	http://www.mentalhealth.org
• National Rehabilitation Information Center	http://www.naric.com

REFERENCES

Bateman, A., & Fonagy, P. (2003). Health service utilization costs for borderline personality disorder patients treated with psychoanalytically oriented partial hospitalization versus general psychiatric care. *American Journal of Psychiatry, 160*(1), 169–171.

Desai, M. M., & Rosenheck, R. A. (2005). Unmet need for medical care among homeless adults with serious mental illness. *General Hospital Psychiatry, 27*(6), 418–425.

Ferguson, A. (2004). Clubhouse: The recovery model. *Mental Health Practice, 7*(9), 22–23.

Haglund, K, von Knorring, L., & von Essen, L. (2006). Psychiatric wards with locked doors: Advantages and disadvantages according to nurses and mental health assistants. *Journal of Clinical Nursing, 15*(4), 387–394.

Hawthorne, W. B., Green, E. E., Gilmer, T., et al. (2005). A randomized trial of short-term acute residential treatment for veterans. *Psychiatric Services, 56*(11), 1379–1386.

Hughes, W. C. (1999). Managed care, meet community support: Ten reasons to include direct support services in every behavioral health plan. *Health & Social Work, 24*(2), 103–110.

King, C., Singh, K., & Sheperd, G. (2000). An analysis of process and outcomes for new long-stay patients in a "ward-in-a-house." *Journal of Mental Health, 9*(2), 179–191.

Knight, E. L. (2004). Exemplary rural mental health services delivery. *Behavioral Healthcare Tomorrow, 13*(3), 20–24.

Konrad, N. (2002). Prisons as new asylums. *Current Opinions in Psychiatry, 15*(6), 583–587.

Lamberti, J. S., Weisman, R., & Faden, D. I. (2004). Forensic assertive community treatment: Preventing incarceration of adults with severe mental illness. *Psychiatric Services, 55*(11), 1285–1293.

Latimer, E. (2005). Economic considerations associated with assertive community treatment and supported employment for people with severe mental illness. *Journal of Psychiatry & Neuroscience, 30*(5), 355–359.

Liberman, R. P., Hilty, D. M., Drake, R. E., et al. (2001). Requirements for multidisciplinary teamwork in psychiatric rehabilitation. *Psychiatric Services, 52*(10), 1331–1342.

Lunsky, Y., Bradley, E., Durbin, J., et al. (2006). The clinical profile and service needs of hospitalized adults with mental retardation and a psychiatric diagnosis. *Psychiatric Services, 57*(1), 77–83.

Marx, A. J., Test, M. A., & Stein, L. I. (1973). Extrohospital management of severe mental illness: Feasibility and effects of social functioning. *Archives of General Psychiatry, 29*(4), 505–511.

Mazza, M., Barbarinoe, E., Capitani, S., et al. (2004). Day treatment for mood disorders. *Psychiatric Services, 55*(4), 436–438.

McCoy, M. L., Roberts, D. L., Hanrahan, P., et al. (2004). Jail linkage assertive community treatment services for individuals with mental illnesses. *Psychiatric Rehabilitation Journal, 27*(3), 243–250.

Min, S., Wong, Y. L. I., & Rothbard, A. B. (2004). Outcomes of shelter use among homeless persons with serious mental illness. *Psychiatric Services, 55*(3), 284–289.

National Resource and Training Center on Homelessness and Mental Illness. (2006). Why are so many people with mental illness homeless? Available: http://www.nrchmi.sanhsa.gov/facts.

Palmer, S., & Wegener, S. T. (2003). Rehabilitation psychology: Overview and key concepts. *Maryland Medicine, 4*(4), 20–22.

Prince, J. D. (2006). Practices preventing rehospitalization of individuals with schizophrenia. *Journal of Nervous and Mental Disease, 194*(6), 397–403.

Redko, C., Durbin, J., Waysylenki, D., et al. (2004). Participant perspectives on satisfaction with assertive community treatment. *Psychiatric Rehabilitation Journal, 27*(3), 283–286.

Rothbard, A. B., Min, S. Y., Kuno, E., & Wong, Y. L. (2004). Long-term effectiveness of the ACCESS program in linking community mental health services to homeless persons with serious mental illness. *Journal of Behavioral Health Services & Research, 31*(4), 441–449.

Segal, S. P., & Riley, S. (2003). Caring for persons with serious mental illness: Policy and practice suggestions. *Social Work in Mental Health, 1*(3), 1–17.

Steadman, H. J., Scott, J. E., Osher, F., et al. (2005). Validation of the brief jail mental health screen. *Psychiatric Services, 56*(7), 816–822.

Substance Abuse and Mental Health Services Administration (SAMHSA). (2006). PATH: Overview of the program. Available: http://pathprogram.samhsa.gov/about/overview.asp.

Tucker, S., Moore, W., & Luedtke, C. (2000). Outcomes of a brief inpatient program for mood and anxiety disorders. *Outcomes Management for Nursing Practice, 4*(3), 117–123.

Udechuku, A., Oliver, J., Hallam, K., et al. (2005). Assertive community treatment of the mentally ill: Service model and effectiveness. *Australasian Psychiatry, 13*(2), 129–134.

White, L., & Brooker, C. (2001). Working with a multidisciplinary team in a secure psychiatric environment. *Journal of Psychosocial Nursing, 39*(9), 26–31.

Williams, C. C. (2004). Discharge planning process on a general psychiatry unit. *Social Work in Mental Health, 2*(1), 17–31.

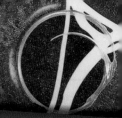

Chapter Study Guide

MULTIPLE-CHOICE QUESTIONS

Select the best answer for each of the following questions.

1. All the following are characteristics of ACT except
   A. Services are provided in the home or community.
   B. Services are provided by the client's case manager.
   C. There are no time limitations on ACT services.
   D. All needed support systems are involved in ACT.

2. Research shows that scheduled intermittent hospital admissions result in which of the following?
   A. Fewer inpatient hospital stays
   B. Increased sense of control for the client
   C. Feelings of failure when hospitalized
   D. Shorter hospital stays

3. Inpatient psychiatric care focuses on all the following except
   A. Brief interventions
   B. Discharge planning
   C. Independent living skills
   D. Symptom management

4. How many persons in the state prison population have severe mental illness?
   A. Less than 9%
   B. 16%
   C. 33%
   D. More than 45%

5. Which of the following interventions is an example of primary prevention implemented by a public health nurse?
   A. Reporting suspected child abuse
   B. Monitoring compliance with medications for a client with schizophrenia
   C. Teaching effective problem-solving skills to high school students
   D. Helping a client to apply for disability benefits

6. The primary purpose of psychiatric rehabilitation is to
   A. Control psychiatric symptoms
   B. Manage clients' medications
   C. Promote the recovery process
   D. Reduce hospital readmissions

7. Managed care provides funding for psychiatric rehabilitation programs to
   A. Develop vocational skills
   B. Improve medication compliance
   C. Provide community skills training
   D. Teach social skills

8. The mentally ill homeless population benefits most from
   A. Case management services
   B. Outpatient psychiatric care to manage psychiatric symptoms
   C. Stable housing in a residential neighborhood
   D. A combination of housing, rehabilitation services, and community support

FILL-IN-THE-BLANK QUESTIONS

Identify the interdisciplinary team member responsible for the functions listed below.

_____ Works with families, community supports, and referrals

_____ Focuses on functional abilities and work using arts and crafts

_____ Makes diagnoses and prescribes treatment

_____ Emphasizes job-seeking and job-retention skills

SHORT-ANSWER QUESTIONS

1. Identify three barriers to community reintegration faced by mentally ill offenders.

2. Discuss the concept of evolving consumer households.

3. List factors that have caused an increased number of persons with mental illness to be detained in jails.

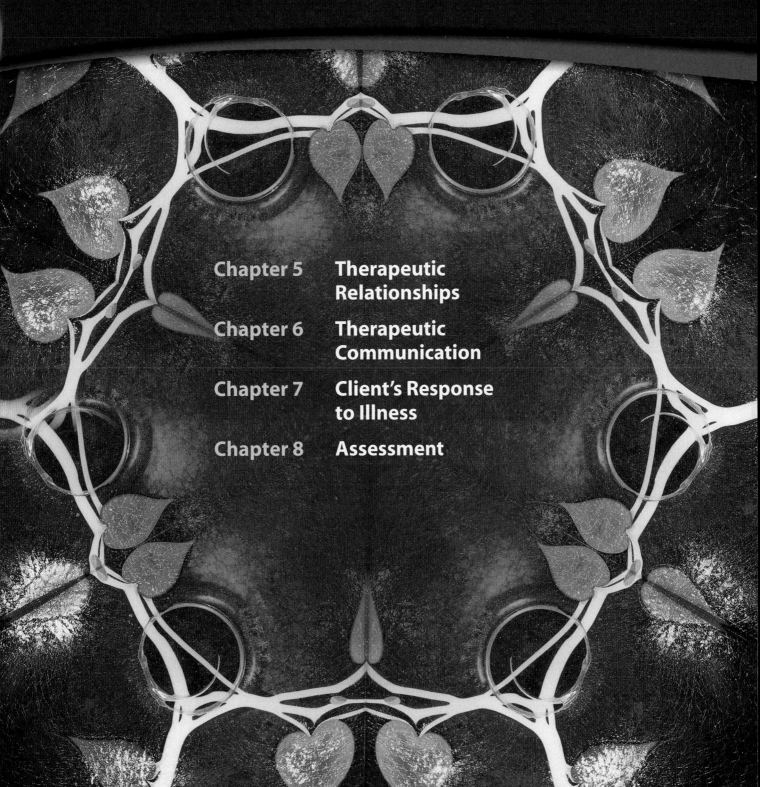

Unit 2

Building the Nurse–Client Relationship

Unit 2

Building the
Nurse–Client Relationship

Chapter 5   Therapeutic Relationships

Chapter 6   Therapeutic Communication

Chapter 7   Client's Response to Illness

Chapter 8   Assessment

Chapter 5

Therapeutic Relationships

Key Terms

- acceptance
- advocacy
- attitudes
- beliefs
- confidentiality
- congruence
- countertransference
- duty to warn
- empathy
- exploitation
- genuine interest
- intimate relationship
- orientation phase
- patterns of knowing
- positive regard
- preconceptions
- problem identification
- self-awareness
- self-disclosure
- social relationship
- termination or resolution phase
- therapeutic relationship
- therapeutic use of self
- transference
- unknowing
- values
- working phase

Learning Objectives

After reading this chapter, you should be able to

1. Describe how the nurse uses the necessary components involved in building and enhancing the nurse–client relationship (trust, genuine interest, empathy, acceptance, and positive regard).

2. Explain the importance of values, beliefs, and attitudes in the development of the nurse–client relationship.

3. Describe the importance of self-awareness and therapeutic use of self in the nurse–client relationship.

4. Identify self-awareness issues that can enhance or hinder the nurse–client relationship.

5. Define Carper's four patterns of knowing and give examples of each.

6. Describe the differences between social, intimate, and therapeutic relationships.

7. Describe and implement the phases of the nurse–client relationship as outlined by Hildegard Peplau.

8. Explain the negative behaviors that can hinder or diminish the nurse–client relationship.

9. Explain the various possible roles of the nurse (teacher, caregiver, advocate, and parent surrogate) in the nurse–client relationship.

The ability to establish therapeutic relationships with clients is one of the most important skills a nurse can develop. Although important in all nursing specialties, the therapeutic relationship is especially crucial to the success of interventions with clients requiring psychiatric care because the therapeutic relationship and the communication within it serve as the underpinning for treatment and success.

This chapter examines the crucial components involved in establishing appropriate therapeutic nurse–client relationships: trust, genuine interest, acceptance, positive regard, self-awareness, and therapeutic use of self. It explores the tasks that should be accomplished in each phase of the nurse–client relationship and the techniques the nurse can use to help do so. It also discusses each of the therapeutic roles of the nurse: teacher, caregiver, advocate, and parent surrogate.

COMPONENTS OF A THERAPEUTIC RELATIONSHIP

Many factors can enhance the nurse–client relationship, and it is the nurse's responsibility to develop them. These factors promote communication and enhance relationships in all aspects of the nurse's life.

Trust

The nurse–client relationship requires trust. Trust builds when the client is confident in the nurse and when the nurse's presence conveys integrity and reliability. Trust develops when the client believes that the nurse will be consistent in his or her words and actions and can be relied on to do what he or she says. Some behaviors the nurse can exhibit to help build the client's trust include being friendly, caring, interested, understanding, and consistent; keeping promises; and listening to and being honest with the client (Box 5.1).

Congruence occurs when words and actions match. For example, the nurse says to the client, "I have to leave now to go to a clinical conference, but I will be back at 2 PM" and indeed returns at 2 PM to see the client. The nurse needs to exhibit congruent behaviors to build trust with the client.

Trust erodes when a client sees inconsistency between what the nurse says and does. Inconsistent or incongruent behaviors include making verbal commitments and not following through on them. For example, the nurse tells the client she will work with him every Tuesday at 10 AM, but the very next week she has a conflict with her conference schedule and does not show up. Another example of incongruent behavior is when the nurse's voice or body language is inconsistent with the words he or she speaks. For example, an angry client confronts a nurse and accuses her of not liking her. The nurse responds by saying, "Of course I like you, Nancy! I am here to help you." But as she says these words, the nurse backs away from Nancy and looks over her shoulder: the verbal and nonverbal components of the message do not match.

Box 5.1 TRUSTING BEHAVIORS

Trust is built in the nurse–client relationship when the nurse exhibits the following behaviors:

- Friendliness
- Caring
- Interest
- Understanding
- Consistency
- Treating the client as a human being
- Suggesting without telling
- Approachability
- Listening
- Keeping promises
- Providing schedules of activities
- Honesty

When working with a client with psychiatric problems, some of the symptoms of the disorder, such as paranoia, low self-esteem, and anxiety, may make trust difficult to establish. For example, a client with depression has little psychic energy to listen to or to comprehend what the nurse is saying. Likewise, a client with panic disorder may be too anxious to focus on the nurse's communication. Although clients with mental disorders frequently give incongruent messages because of their illness, the nurse must continue to provide consistent congruent messages. Examining one's own behavior and doing one's best to make messages clear, simple, and congruent help to facilitate trust between the nurse and the client.

Genuine Interest

When the nurse is comfortable with himself or herself, aware of his or her strengths and limitations, and clearly focused, the client perceives a genuine person showing **genuine interest**. A client with mental illness can detect when someone is exhibiting dishonest or artificial behavior such as asking a question and then not waiting for the answer, talking over him or her, or assuring him or her everything will be all right. The nurse should be open and honest and display congruent behavior. Sometimes, however, responding with truth and honesty alone does not provide the best professional response. In such cases, the nurse may choose to disclose to the client a personal experience related to the client's current concerns. Doing so helps to develop trust and allows the client to see the nurse as a real person with perhaps similar problems. The client then may choose to reveal more information to the nurse. This self-disclosure, revealing personal information (e.g., biographical data, ideas, thoughts,

CLINICAL VIGNETTE: THERAPEUTIC RELATIONSHIPS

Twelve nursing students have arrived for their first day on the psychiatric unit. They are apprehensive, uncertain what to expect, and standing in a row just inside the locked doors. They are not at all sure how to react to these clients and are fearful of what to say at the first meeting. Suddenly they hear one of the clients shout, "Oh look, the students are here.

Now we can have some fun!" Another client replies, "Not me, I just want to be left alone." A third client says, "I want to talk to the good-looking one." And so, these students' nurse–client relationships have just begun—not quite in the best or text-book circumstances.

feelings), can enhance openness and honesty. Nevertheless, the nurse must not shift emphasis to his or her own problems rather than the client's.

Empathy

Empathy is the ability of the nurse to perceive the meanings and feelings of the client and to communicate that understanding to the client. It is considered one of the essential skills a nurse must develop. Being able to put himself or herself in the client's shoes does not mean that the nurse has had the same exact experiences as the client. Nevertheless, by listening and sensing the importance of the situation to the client, the nurse can imagine the client's feelings about the experience. Both the client and the nurse give a "gift of self" when empathy occurs—the client by feeling safe enough to share feelings and the nurse by listening closely enough to understand. Empathy has been shown to positively influence client outcomes. Clients tend to feel better about themselves and more understood when the nurse is empathetic (Welch, 2005).

Several therapeutic communication techniques, such as reflection, restatement, and clarification, help the nurse to send empathetic messages to the client. For example, a client says,

"I'm so confused! My son just visited and wants to know where the safety deposit box key is."

Using reflection, the nurse responds,

"You're confused because your son asked for the safety deposit key?"

The nurse, using clarification, responds,

"Are you confused about the purpose of your son's visit?"

From these empathetic moments, a bond can be established to serve as the foundation for the nurse–client relationship. More examples of therapeutic communication techniques are found in Chapter 6.

The nurse must understand the difference between empathy and *sympathy* (feelings of concern or compassion one shows for another). By expressing sympathy, the nurse may project his or her personal concerns onto the client, thus inhibiting the client's expression of feelings. In the above example, the nurse using sympathy would have responded, "I know how confusing sons can be. My son confuses me, too, and I know how bad that makes you feel." The nurse's feelings of sadness or even pity could influence the relationship and hinder the nurse's abilities to focus on the client's needs. Sympathy often shifts the emphasis to the nurse's feelings, hindering the nurse's ability to view the client's needs objectively.

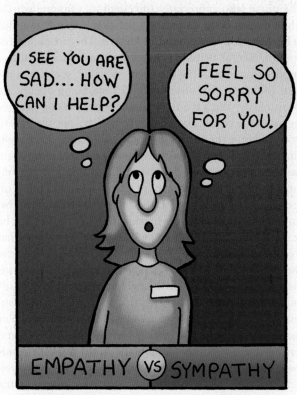

Empathy vs. sympathy

Acceptance

The nurse who does not become upset or respond negatively to a client's outbursts, anger, or acting out conveys **acceptance** to the client. Avoiding judgments of the person, no matter what the behavior, is acceptance. This does not mean acceptance of inappropriate behavior but acceptance of the person as worthy. The nurse must set boundaries for behavior in the nurse–client relationship. By being clear and firm without anger or judgment, the nurse allows the client to feel intact while still conveying that certain behavior is unacceptable. For example, a client puts his arm around the nurse's waist. An appropriate response would be for the nurse to remove his hand and say,

> *"John, do not place your hand on me. We are working on your relationship with your girlfriend and that does not require you to touch me. Now, let's continue."*

An inappropriate response would be,

> *"John, stop that! What's gotten into you? I am leaving, and maybe I'll return tomorrow."*

Leaving and threatening not to return punish the client while failing to clearly address the inappropriate behavior.

Positive Regard

The nurse who appreciates the client as a unique worthwhile human being can respect the client regardless of his or her behavior, background, or lifestyle. This unconditional nonjudgmental attitude is known as **positive regard** and implies respect. Calling the client by name, spending time with the client, and listening and responding openly are measures by which the nurse conveys respect and positive regard to the client. The nurse also conveys positive regard by considering the client's ideas and preferences when planning care. Doing so shows that the nurse believes the client has the ability to make positive and meaningful contributions to his or her own plan of care. The nurse relies on presence, or *attending,* which is using nonverbal and verbal communication techniques to make the client aware that he or she is receiving full attention. Nonverbal techniques that create an atmosphere of presence include leaning toward the client, maintaining eye contact, being relaxed, having arms resting at the sides, and having an interested but neutral attitude. Verbally attending means that the nurse avoids communicating value judgments about the client's behavior. For example, the client may say, "I was so mad, I yelled and screamed at my mother for an hour." If the nurse responds with "Well, that didn't help, did it?" or "I can't believe you did that," the nurse is communicating a value judgment that the client was "wrong" or "bad." A better response would be

"What happened then?" or "You must have been really upset." The nurse maintains attention on the client and avoids communicating negative opinions or value judgments about the client's behavior.

Self-Awareness and Therapeutic Use of Self

Before he or she can begin to understand clients, the nurse must first know himself or herself. **Self-awareness** is the process of developing an understanding of one's own values, beliefs, thoughts, feelings, attitudes, motivations, prejudices, strengths, and limitations and how these qualities affect others. Self-awareness allows the nurse to observe, pay attention to, and understand the subtle responses and reactions of clients when interacting with them.

Values are abstract standards that give a person a sense of right and wrong and establish a code of conduct for living. Sample values include hard work, honesty, sincerity, cleanliness, and orderliness. To gain insight into oneself and personal values, the values clarification process is helpful.

The values clarification process has three steps: choosing, prizing, and acting. *Choosing* is when the person considers a range of possibilities and freely chooses the value that feels right. *Prizing* is when the person considers the value, cherishes it, and publicly attaches it to himself or herself. *Acting* is when the person puts the value into action. For example, a clean and orderly student has been assigned to live with another student who leaves clothes and food all over their room. At first the orderly student is unsure why she hesitates to return to the room and feels tense around her roommate. As she examines the situation, she realizes that they view the use of personal space differently (choosing). Next she discusses her conflict and choices with her adviser and friends (prizing). Finally, she decides to negotiate with her roommate for a compromise (acting).

Beliefs are ideas that one holds to be true, for example, "All old people are hard of hearing," "If the sun is shining, it will be a good day," or "Peas should be planted on St. Patrick's Day." Some beliefs have objective evidence to substantiate them. For example, people who believe in evolution have accepted the evidence that supports this explanation for the origins of life. Other beliefs are irrational and may persist, despite these beliefs having no supportive evidence or the existence of contradictory empirical evidence. For example, many people harbor irrational beliefs about cultures different from their own that they developed simply from others' comments or fear of the unknown, not from any evidence to support such beliefs.

Attitudes are general feelings or a frame of reference around which a person organizes knowledge about the world. Attitudes, such as hopeful, optimistic, pessimistic, positive, and negative, color how we look at the world and people. A positive mental attitude occurs when a person chooses to put a positive spin on an experience, comment, or judgment. For example, in a crowded grocery line, the person at the front pays with change, slowly counting it

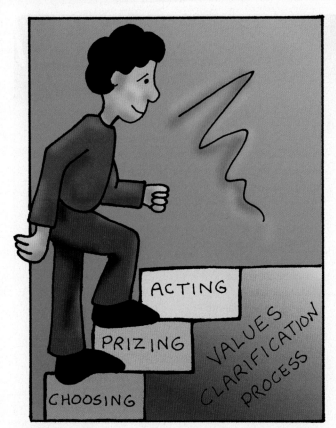

Values clarification process

Box 5.2   CULTURAL AWARENESS QUESTIONS

ACKNOWLEDGING YOUR CULTURAL HERITAGE

- To what ethnic group, socioeconomic class, religion, age group, and community do you belong?
- What experiences have you had with people from ethnic groups, socioeconomic classes, religions, age groups, or communities different from your own?
- What were those experiences like? How did you feel about them?
- When you were growing up, what did your parents and significant others say about people who were different from your family?
- What about your ethnic group, socioeconomic class, religion, age, or community do you find embarrassing or wish you could change? Why?
- What sociocultural factors in your background might contribute to being rejected by members of other cultures?
- What personal qualities do you have that will help you establish interpersonal relationships with people from other cultural groups? What personal qualities may be detrimental?

out. The person waiting in line who has a positive attitude would be thankful for the extra minutes and would begin to use them to do deep-breathing exercises and to relax. A negative attitude also colors how one views the world and other people. For example, a person who has had an unpleasant experience with a rude waiter may develop a negative attitude toward all waiters. Such a negative attitude might cause the person to behave impolitely and unpleasantly with every waiter he or she encounters.

The nurse should re-evaluate and readjust beliefs and attitudes periodically as he or she gains experience and wisdom. Ongoing self-awareness allows the nurse to accept values, attitudes, and beliefs of others that may differ from his or her own. Box 5.2 lists questions designed to increase the nurse's cultural awareness. A person who does not assess personal attitudes and beliefs may hold a prejudice (hostile attitude) toward a group of people because of preconceived ideas or stereotypical images of that group. For example, a nursing student comes from a white, Protestant, middle-class environment; until beginning nursing school in a multicultural urban environment, she had little experience with cultures other than her own. She came with an ethnocentric attitude of believing that her culture was superior to all others. Once she became friends with students from Mexico and Kenya, she began to realize that each culture has its own beauty and style and each is as important as the other. By letting her new experiences and friends become part of her view of the world, the student

has revised her beliefs and attitudes and expanded her understanding of people and the world. Box 5.3 provides an example of a values clarification exercise that can assist nurses to become aware of their own beliefs and thoughts about other cultures.

THERAPEUTIC USE OF SELF

By developing self-awareness and beginning to understand his or her attitudes, the nurse can begin to use aspects of his or her personality, experiences, values, feelings, intelligence, needs, coping skills, and perceptions to establish relationships with clients. This is called **therapeutic use of self.** Nurses use themselves as a therapeutic tool to establish therapeutic relationships with clients and to help clients grow, change, and heal. Peplau (1952), who described this therapeutic use of self in the nurse–client relationship, believed that nurses must clearly understand themselves to promote their clients' growth and to avoid limiting clients' choices to those that nurses value.

The nurse's personal actions arise from conscious and unconscious responses that are formed by life experiences and educational, spiritual, and cultural values. Nurses (and all people) tend to use many automatic responses or behaviors just because they are familiar. They need to examine such accepted ways of responding or behaving and evaluate how they help or hinder the therapeutic relationship.

Box 5.3 VALUES CLARIFICATION EXERCISE

VALUES CLARIFICATION

Your values are your ideas about what is most important to you in your life—what you want to live by and live for. They are the silent forces behind many of your actions and decisions. The goal of "values clarification" is for their influence to become fully conscious, for you to explore and honestly acknowledge what you truly value at this time. You can be more self-directed and effective when you know which values you really choose to keep and live by as an adult and which ones will get priority over others. Identify your values first, and then rank your top three or five.

- ☐ Being with people
- ☐ Being loved
- ☐ Being married
- ☐ Having a special partner
- ☐ Having companionship
- ☐ Loving someone
- ☐ Taking care of others
- ☐ Having someone's help
- ☐ Having a close family
- ☐ Having good friends
- ☐ Being liked
- ☐ Being popular
- ☐ Getting someone's approval
- ☐ Being appreciated
- ☐ Being treated fairly
- ☐ Being admired

- ☐ Being independent
- ☐ Being courageous
- ☐ Having things in control
- ☐ Having self-control
- ☐ Being emotionally stable
- ☐ Having self-acceptance
- ☐ Having pride or dignity
- ☐ Being well organized
- ☐ Being competent
- ☐ Learning and knowing a lot
- ☐ Achieving highly
- ☐ Being productively busy
- ☐ Having enjoyable work
- ☐ Having an important position
- ☐ Making money

- ☐ Striving for perfection
- ☐ Making a contribution to the world
- ☐ Fighting injustice
- ☐ Living ethically
- ☐ Being a good parent (or child)
- ☐ Being a spiritual person
- ☐ Having a relationship with God
- ☐ Having peace and quiet
- ☐ Making a home
- ☐ Preserving your roots
- ☐ Having financial security
- ☐ Holding on to what you have
- ☐ Being safe physically
- ☐ Being free from pain

- ☐ Not getting taken advantage of
- ☐ Having it easy
- ☐ Being comfortable
- ☐ Avoiding boredom
- ☐ Having fun
- ☐ Enjoying sensual pleasures
- ☐ Looking good
- ☐ Being physically fit
- ☐ Being healthy
- ☐ Having prized possessions
- ☐ Being a creative person
- ☐ Having deep feelings
- ☐ Growing as a person
- ☐ Living fully
- ☐ "Smelling the flowers"
- ☐ Having a purpose

By Joyce Sichel. From Bernard, M. E., & Wolfe, J. L. (Eds.) (2000). The RET resource book for practitioners. *New York: Albert Ellis Institute.*

One tool that is useful in learning more about oneself is the Johari window (Luft, 1970), which creates a "word portrait" of a person in four areas and indicates how well that person knows himself or herself and communicates with others. The four areas evaluated are as follows:

- Quadrant 1: Open/public self—qualities one knows about oneself and others also know
- Quadrant 2: Blind/unaware self—qualities known only to others
- Quadrant 3: Hidden/private self—qualities known only to oneself
- Quadrant 4: Unknown—an empty quadrant to symbolize qualities as yet undiscovered by oneself or others

In creating a Johari window, the first step is for the nurse to appraise his or her own qualities by creating a list of them: values, attitudes, feelings, strengths, behaviors, accomplishments, needs, desires, and thoughts. The second step is to find out the perceptions of others by interviewing them and asking them to identify qualities, both positive and negative, they see in the nurse. To learn from this exercise, the opinions given must be honest; there must be no sanctions taken against those who list negative qualities. The third step is to compare lists and to assign qualities to the appropriate quadrant.

If quadrant 1 is the longest list, this indicates that the nurse is open to others; a smaller quadrant 1 means that the nurse shares little about himself or herself with others. If quadrants 1 and 3 are both small, the person demonstrates little insight. Any change in one quadrant is reflected by changes in other quadrants. The goal is to work toward moving qualities from quadrants 2, 3, and 4 into quadrant 1 (qualities known to self and others). Doing so indicates that the nurse is gaining self-knowledge and awareness. See the accompanying figure for an example of a Johari window.

PATTERNS OF KNOWING

Nurse theorist Hildegard Peplau (1952) identified **preconceptions,** or ways one person expects another to behave or speak, as a roadblock to the formation of an authentic rela-

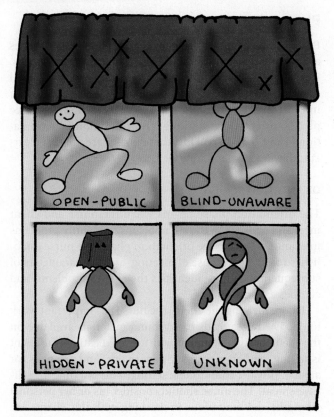

Johari window

tionship. Preconceptions often prevent people from getting to know one another. Preconceptions and different or conflicting personal beliefs and values may prevent the nurse from developing a therapeutic relationship with a client. Here is an example of preconceptions that interfere with a therapeutic relationship: Mr. Lopez, a client, has the preconceived stereotypical idea that all male nurses are homosexual and refuses to have Samuel, a male nurse, take care of him. Samuel has a preconceived stereotypical notion that all Hispanics use switchblades, so he is relieved that Mr. Lopez has refused to work with him. Both men are miss-

ing the opportunity to do some important work together because of incorrect preconceptions.

Carper (1978) identified four **patterns of knowing** in nursing: empirical knowing (derived from the science of nursing), personal knowing (derived from life experiences), ethical knowing (derived from moral knowledge of nursing), and aesthetic knowing (derived from the art of nursing). These patterns provide the nurse with a clear method of observing and understanding every client interaction. Understanding where knowledge comes from and how it affects behavior helps the nurse become more self-aware (Table 5.1). Munhall (1993) added another pattern that she called **unknowing**: For the nurse to admit she or he does not know the client or the client's subjective world opens the way for a truly authentic encounter. The nurse in a state of unknowing is open to seeing and hearing the client's views without imposing any of his or her values or viewpoints. In psychiatric nursing, negative preconceptions on the nurse's part can adversely affect the therapeutic relationship; thus, it is especially important for the nurse to work on developing this openness and acceptance toward the client.

TYPES OF RELATIONSHIPS

Each relationship is unique because of the various combinations of traits and characteristics of and circumstances related to the people involved. Although every relationship is different, all relationships may be categorized into three major types: social, intimate, and therapeutic.

Social Relationship

A **social relationship** is primarily initiated for the purpose of friendship, socialization, companionship, or accomplishment of a task. Communication, which may be superficial, usually focuses on sharing ideas, feelings, and experiences and meets the basic need for people to interact. Advice is often given. Roles may shift during social interactions. Out-

Table 5.1	CARPER'S PATTERNS OF NURSING KNOWLEDGE
Pattern	**Example**
Empirical knowing (obtained from the science of nursing)	Client with panic disorder begins to have an attack. Panic attack will raise pulse rate.
Personal knowing (obtained from life experience)	Client's face shows the panic.
Ethical knowing (obtained from the moral knowledge of nursing)	Although the nurse's shift has ended, she remains with the client.
Aesthetic knowing (obtained from the art of nursing)	Although the client shows outward signals now, the nurse has sensed previously the client's jumpiness and subtle differences in the client's demeanor and behavior.

Adapted from Carper, B. (1978). Fundamental patterns of knowing in nursing. *Advances in Nursing Sciences, 1*(1), 13–23.

comes of this kind of relationship are rarely assessed. When a nurse greets a client and chats about the weather or a sports event or engages in small talk or socializing, this is a social interaction. This is acceptable in nursing, but for the nurse–client relationship to accomplish the goals that have been decided on, social interaction must be limited. If the relationship becomes more social than therapeutic, serious work that moves the client forward will not be done.

Intimate Relationship

A healthy **intimate relationship** involves two people who are emotionally committed to each other. Both parties are concerned about having their individual needs met and helping each other to meet needs as well. The relationship may include sexual or emotional intimacy as well as sharing of mutual goals. Evaluation of the interaction may be ongoing or not. The intimate relationship has no place in the nurse–client interaction.

Therapeutic Relationship

The **therapeutic relationship** differs from the social or intimate relationship in many ways because it focuses on the needs, experiences, feelings, and ideas of the client only. The nurse and client agree about the areas to work on and evaluate the outcomes. The nurse uses communication skills, personal strengths, and understanding of human behavior to interact with the client. In the therapeutic relationship the parameters are clear: the focus is the client's needs, not the nurse's. The nurse should not be concerned about whether or not the client likes him or her or is grateful. Such concern is a signal that the nurse is focusing on a personal need to be liked or needed. The nurse must guard against allowing the therapeutic relationship to slip into a more social relationship. The nurse must constantly focus on the client's needs, not his or her own.

The nurse's level of self-awareness can either benefit or hamper the therapeutic relationship. For example, if the nurse is nervous around the client, the relationship is more apt to stay social because superficiality is safer. If the nurse is aware of his or her fears, he or she can discuss them with the instructor, paving the way for a more therapeutic relationship to develop.

ESTABLISHING THE THERAPEUTIC RELATIONSHIP

The nurse who has self-confidence rooted in self-awareness is ready to establish appropriate therapeutic relationships with clients. Because personal growth is ongoing over one's lifetime, the nurse cannot expect to have complete self-knowledge. Awareness of his or her strengths and limitations at any particular moment, however, is a good start.

Phases

Peplau studied and wrote about the interpersonal processes and the phases of the nurse–client relationship for 35 years. Her work provides the nursing profession with a model that can be used to understand and document progress with interpersonal interactions. Peplau's model (1952) has three phases: orientation, working, and resolution or termination (Table 5.2). In real life, these phases are not that clear-cut; they overlap and interlock.

ORIENTATION

The **orientation phase** begins when the nurse and client meet and ends when the client begins to identify problems to examine. During the orientation phase, the nurse establishes roles, the purpose of meeting, and the parameters of subsequent meetings; identifies the client's problems; and clarifies expectations.

Before meeting the client, the nurse has important work to do. The nurse reads background materials available on the client, becomes familiar with any medications the client is taking, gathers necessary paperwork, and arranges for a quiet, private, comfortable setting. This is a time for self-assessment. The nurse should consider his or her personal strengths and limitations in working with this client. Are there any areas that might signal difficulty because of past experiences? For example, if this client is a spouse batterer and the nurse's father was also, the nurse needs to consider the situation: How does it make him or her feel? What memories does it prompt, and can he or she work with the client without these memories interfering? The nurse must examine preconceptions about the client and ensure that he or she can put them aside and get to know the real person. The nurse must come to each client without preconceptions or prejudices. It may be useful for the nurse to discuss all potential problem areas with the instructor.

During the orientation phase, the nurse begins to build trust with the client. It is the nurse's responsibility to establish a therapeutic environment that fosters trust and understanding (Table 5.3). The nurse should share appropriate information about himself or herself at this time, including name, reason for being on the unit, and level of schooling: For example, "Hello, James. My name is Miss Ames and I will be your nurse for the next six Tuesdays. I am a senior nursing student at the University of Mississippi."

The nurse needs to listen closely to the client's history, perceptions, and misconceptions. He or she needs to convey empathy and understanding (Forchuk, 2002). If the relationship gets off to a positive start, it is more likely to succeed and to meet established goals.

At the first meeting, the client may be distrustful if previous relationships with nurses have been unsatisfactory. The client may use rambling speech, act out, or exaggerate episodes as ploys to avoid discussing the real problems. It may take several sessions until the client believes that he or she can trust the nurse.

Table 5.2 PHASES OF THE NURSE–CLIENT RELATIONSHIP

Orientation	Working		Termination
	Identification	Exploitation	
Client			
• Seeks assistance	• Participates in identifying problems	• Makes full use of services	• Abandons old needs
• Conveys needs	• Begins to be aware of time	• Identifies new goals	• Aspires to new goals
• Asks questions	• Responds to help	• Attempts to attain new goals	• Becomes independent of helping person
• Shares preconceptions and expectations of nurse based on past experience	• Identifies with nurse	• Rapid shifts in behavior: dependent, independent	• Applies new problem-solving skills
	• Recognizes nurse as a person	• Exploitative behavior	• Maintains changes in style of communication and interaction
	• Explores feelings	• Self-directing	
	• Fluctuates dependence, independence, and inter-dependence in relationship with nurse	• Develops skill in inter-personal relationships and problem solving	• Shows positive changes in view of self
	• Increases focal attention	• Displays changes in manner of communication (more open, flexible)	• Integrates illness
	• Changes appearance (for better or worse)		• Exhibits ability to stand alone
	• Understands continuity between sessions (process and content)		
	• Testing maneuvers decrease		
Nurse			
• Responds to client	• Maintains separate identity	• Continues assessment	• Sustains relationship as long as client feels necessary
• Gives parameters of meetings	• Exhibits ability to edit speech or control focal attention	• Meets needs as they emerge	• Promotes family inter-action to assist with goal planning
• Explains roles	• Shows unconditional acceptance	• Understands reason for shifts in behavior	• Teaches preventive measures
• Gathers data	• Helps express needs, feelings	• Initiates rehabilitative plans	• Uses community agencies
• Helps client identify problem	• Assesses and adjusts to needs	• Reduces anxiety	• Teaches self-care
• Helps client plan use of community resources and services	• Provides information	• Identifies positive factors	• Terminates nurse–client relationship
• Reduces anxiety and tension	• Provides experiences that diminish feelings of helplessness	• Helps plan for total needs	
• Practices active listening	• Does not allow anxiety to overwhelm client	• Facilitates forward move-ment of personality	
• Focuses client's energies	• Helps client focus on cues	• Deals with therapeutic impasse	
• Clarifies preconceptions and expectations of nurse	• Helps client develop responses to cues		
	• Uses word stimuli		

Adapted from Forchuck, C., & Brown, B. (1989). Establishing a nurse–client relationship. *Journal of Psychosocial Nursing, 27*(2), 30–34.

Nurse–Client Contracts. Although many clients have had prior experiences in the mental health system, the nurse must once again outline the responsibilities of the nurse and client. At the outset, both nurse and client should agree on these responsibilities in an informal or verbal contract. In some instances, a formal or written contract may be appropriate;

examples include if a written contract has been necessary in the past with the client or if the client "forgets" the agreed-on verbal contract.

The contract should state the following:
- Time, place, and length of sessions
- When sessions will terminate

Table 5.3	COMMUNICATION DURING THE PHASES OF THE NURSE–CLIENT RELATIONSHIP	
Phase of Relationship	**Sample Conversation**	**Communication Skill**
Orientation	**Nurse**: "Hello, Mr. O'Hare. I am Sally Fourth, a nursing student from Orange County Community College. I will be coming to the hospital for the next 6 Mondays. I would like to meet with you each time I am here to help support you as you work on your treatment goals."	Establishing trust; placing boundaries on the relationship and first mention of termination in 6 weeks
Orientation	**Nurse**: "Mr. O'Hare, we will meet every Monday from June 1 to July 15 at 11 am in conference room 2. We can use that time to work on your feelings of loss since the death of your twin sister."	Establishing specifics of the relationship time, date, place, and duration of meetings (can be written as a formal contract or stated as an informal contract)
Orientation	**Nurse**: "Mr. O'Hare, it is important that I tell you I will be sharing some of what we talk about with my instructor, peers, and staff at clinical conference. I will not be sharing any information with your wife or children without your permission. If I feel a piece of information may be helpful, I will ask you first if I may share it with your wife."	Establishing confidentiality
Working	**Client**: "Nurse, I miss my sister Eileen so much." **Nurse**: "Mr. O'Hare, how long have you been without your sister?"	Gathering data
Working	**Client**: "Without my twin, I am not half the person I was." **Nurse**: "Mr. O'Hare, let's look at the strengths you have."	Promoting self-esteem
Working	**Client**: "Oh, why talk about me. I'm nothing without my twin." **Nurse**: "Mr. O'Hare, you are a person in your own right. I believe working together we can identify strengths you have. Will you try with me?"	Overcoming resistance
Termination	**Nurse**: "Well, Mr. O'Hare, as you know I only have 1 week left to meet with you." **Client**: "I am going to miss you. I feel better when you are here." **Nurse**: "I will miss you also, Mr. O'Hare."	Sharing of the termination experience with the client demonstrates the partnership and the caring of the relationship

• Who will be involved in the treatment plan (family members, health team members)
• Client responsibilities (arrive on time, end on time)
• Nurse's responsibilities (arrive on time, end on time, maintain confidentiality at all times, evaluate progress with client, document sessions)

Confidentiality. **Confidentiality** means respecting the client's right to keep private any information about his or her mental and physical health and related care. Confidentiality means allowing only those dealing with the client's care to have access to the information that the client divulges. Only under precisely defined conditions can third parties have access to this information; for example, many states require that staff report suspected child and elder abuse.

Adult clients can decide which family members, if any, may be involved in treatment and may have access to clinical information. Ideally, the people close to the client and responsible for his or her care are involved. The client must decide, however, who will be included. For the client to feel safe, boundaries must be clear. The nurse must clearly state information about who will have access to client assessment data and progress evaluations. He or she should tell the client that members of the mental health team share appropriate information among themselves to provide consistent care and that only with the client's permission will they include a family member. If the client has an appointed guardian, that person can review client information and make treatment decisions that are in the client's best interest. For a child, the parent or appointed guardian is allowed access to information and can make treatment decisions as outlined by the health care team.

The nurse must be alert if a client asks him or her to keep a secret because this information may relate to the client's harming himself or herself or others. The nurse must avoid any promises to keep secrets. If the nurse has promised not to tell before hearing the message, he or she could be jeopardizing the client's trust. In most cases, even when the nurse refuses to agree to keep information secret, the client continues to relate issues anyway. The following is an example of a good response to a client who is suicidal but requests secrecy:

Client: *"I am going to jump off the 14th floor of my apartment building tonight, but please don't tell anyone."*

Nurse: *"I cannot keep such a promise, especially if it involves your safety. I sense you are feeling frightened. The staff and I will help you stay safe."*

The *Tarasoff vs. Regents of the University of California* (1976) decision releases professionals from privileged communication with their clients should a client make a homicidal threat. The decision requires the nurse to notify intended victims and police of such a threat. In this circumstance, the nurse must report the homicidal threat to the nursing supervisor and attending physician so that both the police and intended victim can be notified. This is called a **duty to warn** and is discussed more fully in Chapter 9.

The nurse documents the client's problems with planned interventions. The client must understand that the nurse will collect data about him or her that helps in making a diagnosis, planning health care (including medications), and protecting the client's civil rights. The client needs to know the limits of confidentiality in nurse–client interactions and how the nurse will use and share this information with professionals involved in client care.

Self-Disclosure. **Self-disclosure** means revealing personal information such as biographical information and personal ideas, thoughts, and feelings about oneself to clients. Traditionally, conventional wisdom held that nurses should share only their name, marital status, and number of children and perhaps should give a general idea about their residence, such as "I live in Ocean County." Now, however, it is believed that more self-disclosure can improve rapport between the nurse and client. The nurse can use self-disclosure to convey support, educate clients, demonstrate that a client's anxiety is normal, and even facilitate emotional healing (Ashmore & Banks, 2003a).

Nurses should remember these therapeutic goals of self-disclosure and use disclosure to help the client feel more comfortable and more willing to share thoughts and feelings. Sharing may help the client gain insight about his or her situation or encourage him or her to resolve concerns. The nurse should not use self-disclosure to meet personal needs.

When using self-disclosure, the nurse must consider cultural factors. For example, if the client is from a culture that is stoic and noncommunicative, he or she may deem self-disclosure inappropriate. The nurse should keep self-disclosure brief and comfortable, respect the client's privacy by making sure the discussion takes place away from others, and understand that each experience is different. The nurse must monitor his or her own comfort level. If the nurse has unresolved feelings about the issue, he or she should not share personal experiences.

Disclosing personal information can be harmful and inappropriate for a client, so the nurse must give it careful thought. For example, when working with a client whose parents are getting a divorce, the nurse says, "My parents got a divorce when I was 12 and it was a horrible time for me." The nurse has shifted the focus away from the client and has given the client the idea that this experience will be horrible for the client. Although the nurse may have meant to communicate empathy, the result can be quite the opposite. If the client does not seem ready to deal with the issue or if the conversation is purely social, it is not a good time to disclose information about oneself (Ashmore & Banks, 2003b).

WORKING

The **working phase** of the nurse–client relationship is usually divided into two subphases: During **problem identification**, the client identifies the issues or concerns causing problems. During **exploitation**, the nurse guides the client to examine feelings and responses and to develop better coping skills and a more positive self-image; this encourages behavior change and develops independence. (Note that Peplau's use of the word *exploitation* had a very different meaning than current usage, which involves unfairly

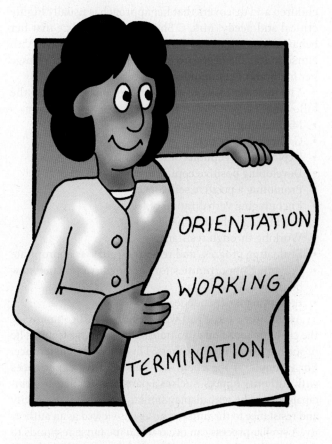

Phases of nurse–client relationship

using or taking advantage of a person or situation. For that reason, this phase is better conceptualized as intense exploration and elaboration on earlier themes that the client discussed.) The trust established between nurse and client at this point allows them to examine the problems and to work on them within the security of the relationship. The client must believe that the nurse will not turn away or be upset when the client reveals experiences, issues, behaviors, and problems. Sometimes the client will use outrageous stories or acting-out behaviors to test the nurse. Testing behavior challenges the nurse to stay focused and not to react or to be distracted. Often when the client becomes uncomfortable because he or she is getting too close to the truth, he or she will use testing behaviors to avoid the subject. The nurse may respond by saying, "It seems as if we have hit an uncomfortable spot for you. Would you like to let it go for now?" This statement focuses on the issue at hand and diverts attention from the testing behavior.

The nurse must remember that it is the client who examines and explores problem situations and relationships. The nurse must be nonjudgmental and refrain from giving advice; the nurse should allow the client to analyze situations. The nurse can guide the client to observe patterns of behavior and whether or not the expected response occurs. For example, Mrs. O'Shea suffers from depression. She continues to complain to the nurse about the lack of concern her children show her. With Nurse Jones' assistance, Mrs. O'Shea explores how she communicates with her children and discovers that her approach is usually highly critical and needy. Mrs. O'Shea begins to realize that her behavior contributes to driving her children away. With Nurse Jones, she begins to explore how she might change her methods of communication.

The specific tasks of the working phase include the following:

- Maintaining the relationship
- Gathering more data
- Exploring perceptions of reality
- Developing positive coping mechanisms
- Promoting a positive self-concept
- Encouraging verbalization of feelings
- Facilitating behavior change
- Working through resistance
- Evaluating progress and redefining goals as appropriate
- Providing opportunities for the client to practice new behaviors
- Promoting independence

As the nurse and client work together, it is common for the client unconsciously to transfer to the nurse feelings he or she has for significant others. This is called **transference**. For example, if the client has had negative experiences with authority figures, such as a parent or teachers or principals, he or she may display similar reactions of negativity and resistance to the nurse, who also is viewed as an authority. A similar process can occur when the nurse responds to the client based on personal unconscious needs and con-

flicts; this is called **countertransference**. For example, if the nurse is the youngest in her family and often felt as if no one listened to her when she was a child, she may respond with anger to a client who does not listen or resists her help. Again, self-awareness is important so that the nurse can identify when transference and countertransference might occur. By being aware of such "hot spots," the nurse has a better chance of responding appropriately rather than letting old unresolved conflicts interfere with the relationship.

TERMINATION

The **termination or resolution phase** is the final stage in the nurse–client relationship. It begins when the problems are resolved, and it ends when the relationship is ended. Both nurse and client usually have feelings about ending the relationship; the client especially may feel the termination as an impending loss. Often clients try to avoid termination by acting angry or as if the problem has not been resolved. The nurse can acknowledge the client's angry feelings and assure the client that this response is normal to ending a relationship. If the client tries to reopen and discuss old resolved issues, the nurse must avoid feeling as if the sessions were unsuccessful; instead, he or she should identify the client's stalling maneuvers and refocus the client on newly learned behaviors and skills to handle the problem. It is appropriate to tell the client that the nurse enjoyed the time spent with the client and will remember him or her, but it is inappropriate for the nurse to agree to see the client outside the therapeutic relationship.

Nurse Jones comes to see Mrs. O'Shea for the last time. Mrs. O'Shea is weeping quietly.

Mrs. O'Shea: *"Oh, Ms. Jones, you have been so helpful to me. I just know I will go back to my old self without you here to help me."*

Nurse Jones: *"Mrs. O'Shea, I think we've had a very productive time together. You have learned so many new ways to have better relationships with your children, and I know you will go home and be able to use those skills. When you come back for your follow-up visit, I will want to hear all about how things have changed at home."*

AVOIDING BEHAVIORS THAT DIMINISH THE THERAPEUTIC RELATIONSHIP

The nurse has power over the client by virtue of his or her professional role. That power can be abused if excessive familiarity or an intimate relationship occurs or if confidentiality is breached.

Inappropriate Boundaries

All staff members, both new and veteran, are at risk for allowing a therapeutic relationship to expand into an inappropriate relationship. Self-awareness is extremely important: The nurse who is in touch with his or her feelings and aware of his or her influence over others can help maintain the boundaries of the professional relationship. The nurse must maintain professional boundaries to ensure the best therapeutic outcomes. It is the nurse's responsibility to define the boundaries of the relationship clearly in the orientation phase and to ensure those boundaries are maintained throughout the relationship. The nurse must act warmly and empathetically but must not try to be friends with the client. Social interactions that continue beyond the first few minutes of a meeting contribute to the conversation staying on the surface. This lack of focus on the problems that have been agreed on for discussion erodes the professional relationship.

If a client is attracted to a nurse or vice versa, it is up to the nurse to maintain professional boundaries. Accepting gifts or giving a client one's home address or phone number would be considered a breach of ethical conduct. Nurses must continually assess themselves and ensure they keep their feelings in check and focus on the clients' interests and needs. Nurses can assess their behavior by using the Nursing Boundary Index in Table 5.4. A full discussion of ethical dilemmas encountered in relationships is found in Chapter 9.

Feelings of Sympathy and Encouraging Client Dependency

The nurse must not let feelings of empathy turn into sympathy for the client. Unlike the therapeutic use of empathy, the nurse who feels sorry for the client often tries to compensate by trying to please him or her. When the nurse's behavior is rooted in sympathy, the client finds it easier to manipulate the nurse's feelings. This discourages the client from exploring his or her problems, thoughts, and feelings; discourages client growth; and often leads to client dependency.

The client may make increased requests of the nurse for help and assistance or may regress and act as if he or she cannot carry out tasks previously done. These can be signals that the nurse has been "overdoing" for the client and may be contributing to the client's dependency. Clients often test the nurse to see how much the nurse is willing to do. If the client cooperates only when the nurse is in attendance and does not carry out agreed-on behavior in the nurse's absence, the client has become too dependent. In any of these instances, the nurse needs to reassess his or her professional behavior and refocus on the client's needs and therapeutic goals.

Table 5.4	NURSING BOUNDARY INDEX			
Please rate yourself according to the frequency that the following statements reflect your behavior, thoughts, or feelings within the past 2 years while providing patient care.				
1. Have you ever received any feedback about your behavior for being overly intrusive with patients or their families?	Never	Rarely	Sometimes	Often
2. Do you ever have difficulty setting limits with patients?	Never	Rarely	Sometimes	Often
3. Do you arrive early or stay late to be with your patient for a longer period of time?	Never	Rarely	Sometimes	Often
4. Do you ever find yourself relating to patients or peers as you might a family member?	Never	Rarely	Sometimes	Often
5. Have you ever acted on sexual feelings you have for a patient?	Never	Rarely	Sometimes	Often
6. Do you feel that you are the only one who understands the patient?	Never	Rarely	Sometimes	Often
7. Have you ever received feedback that you get "too involved" with patients or families?	Never	Rarely	Sometimes	Often
8. Do you derive conscious satisfaction from patients' praise, appreciation, or affection?	Never	Rarely	Sometimes	Often
9. Do you ever feel that other staff members are too critical of "your" patient?	Never	Rarely	Sometimes	Often
10. Do you ever feel that other staff members are jealous of your relationship with a patient?	Never	Rarely	Sometimes	Often
11. Have you ever tried to "match-make" a patient with one of your friends?	Never	Rarely	Sometimes	Often
12. Do you find it difficult to handle patients' unreasonable requests for assistance, verbal abuse, or sexual language?	Never	Rarely	Sometimes	Often
Any item that is responded to with a "sometimes" or "often" should alert the nurse to a possible area of vulnerability. If the item is responded to with a "rarely," the nurse should determine whether it was an isolated event or a possible pattern of behavior.				

Pilette, P., Berck, C., & Achber, L. (1995). Therapeutic management. *Journal of Psychosocial Nursing, 33*(1), 45.

Nonacceptance and Avoidance

The nurse–client relationship can be jeopardized if the nurse finds the client's behavior unacceptable or distasteful and allows those feelings to show by avoiding the client or making verbal responses or facial expressions of annoyance or turning away from the client. The nurse should be aware of the client's behavior and background before beginning the relationship; if the nurse believes there may be conflict, he or she must explore this possibility with a colleague. If the nurse is aware of a prejudice that would place the client in an unfavorable light, he or she must explore this issue as well. Sometimes by talking about and confronting these feelings, the nurse can accept the client and not let a prejudice hinder the relationship. If the nurse cannot resolve such negative feelings, however, he or she should consider requesting another assignment. It is the nurse's responsibility to treat each client with acceptance and positive regard, regardless of the client's history. Part of the nurse's responsibility is to continue to become more self-aware and to confront and resolve any prejudices that threaten to hinder the nurse–client relationship (Box 5.4).

ROLES OF THE NURSE IN A THERAPEUTIC RELATIONSHIP

As when working with clients in any other nursing setting, the psychiatric nurse uses various roles to provide needed care to the client. The nurse understands the importance of assuming the appropriate role for the work that he or she is doing with the client.

Teacher

The teacher role is inherent in most aspects of client care. During the working phase of the nurse–client relationship, the nurse may teach the client new methods of coping and solving problems. He or she may instruct about the medication regimen and available community resources. To be a good teacher, the nurse must feel confident about the knowledge he or she has and must know the limitations of that knowledge base. The nurse should be familiar with the resources in the health care setting and community and on the Internet, which can provide needed information for clients. The nurse must be honest about what information he or she can provide and when and where to refer clients for further information. This behavior and honesty build trust in clients.

Caregiver

The primary caregiving role in mental health settings is the implementation of the therapeutic relationship to build trust, explore feelings, assist the client in problem solving, and help the client meet psychosocial needs. If the client also requires physical nursing care, the nurse may need to explain to the client the need for touch while performing physical care. Some clients may confuse physical care with intimacy and sexual interest, which can erode the therapeutic relationship. The nurse must consider the relationship boundaries and parameters that have been established and must repeat the goals that were established together at the beginning of the relationship.

Advocate

In the advocate role, the nurse informs the client and then supports him or her in whatever decision he or she makes (Edd, Fox, & Burns, 2005). In psychiatric-mental health nursing, advocacy is a bit different from medical-surgical settings because of the nature of the client's illness. For example, the nurse cannot support a client's decision to hurt himself or herself or another person. **Advocacy** is the process of acting on the client's behalf when he or she cannot do so. This includes ensuring privacy and dignity, promoting informed consent, preventing unnecessary examinations and procedures, accessing needed services and benefits, and ensuring safety from abuse and exploitation by a health professional or authority figure. For example, if a physician begins to examine a client without closing the curtains and the nurse steps in and properly drapes the client and closes the curtains, the nurse has just acted as the client's advocate.

Box 5.4   POSSIBLE WARNINGS OR SIGNALS OF ABUSE OF THE NURSE–CLIENT RELATIONSHIP

- Secrets, reluctance to talk to others about the work being done with clients
- Sudden increase in phone calls between nurse and client or calls outside clinical hours
- Nurse making more exceptions for client than normal
- Inappropriate gift-giving between client and nurse
- Loaning, trading, or selling goods or possessions

- Nurse disclosure of personal issues or information
- Inappropriate touching, comforting, or physical contact
- Overdoing, overprotecting, or overidentifying with client
- Change in nurse's body language, dress, or appearance (with no other satisfactory explanation)
- Extended one-on-one sessions or home visits

Being an advocate has risks. In the previous example, the physician may be embarrassed and angry and make a comment to the nurse. The nurse needs to stay focused on the appropriateness of his or her behavior and not be intimidated.

The role of advocate also requires the nurse to be observant of other health care professionals. At times, staff members may be reluctant to see what is happening or become involved when a colleague violates the boundaries of a professional relationship. Nurses must take action by talking to the colleague or a supervisor when they observe boundary violations. State nurse practice acts include the nurse's legal responsibility to report boundary violations and unethical conduct on the part of other health care providers. There is a full discussion of ethical conduct in Chapter 9.

There is debate about the role of nurse as advocate. There are times when the nurse does not advocate for the client's autonomy or right to self-determination, such as by supporting involuntary hospitalization for a suicidal client. At these times, acting in the client's best interest (keeping the client safe) is in direct opposition to the client's wishes. Some critics view this as paternalism and interference with the true role of advocacy. In addition, they do not see advocacy as a role exclusive to nursing but also relevant to the domains of physicians, social workers, and other health care professionals.

Parent Surrogate

When a client exhibits child-like behavior or when a nurse is required to provide personal care such as feeding or bathing, the nurse may be tempted to assume the parental role as evidenced in choice of words and nonverbal communication. The nurse may begin to sound authoritative with an attitude of "I know what's best for you." Often, the client responds by acting more child-like and stubborn.

Neither party realizes they have fallen from adult–adult communication to parent–child communication. It is easy for the client to view the nurse in such circumstances as a parent surrogate. In such situations, the nurse must be clear and firm and set limits or reiterate the previously set limits. By retaining an open, easygoing, nonjudgmental attitude, the nurse can continue to nurture the client while establishing boundaries. The nurse must ensure the relationship remains therapeutic and does not become social or intimate (Box 5.5).

SELF-AWARENESS ISSUES

Self-awareness is crucial in establishing therapeutic nurse–client relationships. For example, a nurse who is prejudiced against people from a certain culture or religion but is not consciously aware of it may have difficulty relating to a client from that culture or religion. If the nurse is aware of, acknowledges, and is open to reassessing the prejudice, the relationship has a better chance of being authentic. If the nurse has certain beliefs and attitudes that he or she will not change, it may be best for another nurse to care for the client. Examining personal strengths and weaknesses helps one gain a strong sense of self. Understanding oneself helps one understand and accept others who may have different ideas and values. The nurse must continue on a path of self-discovery to become more self-aware and more effective in caring for clients.

Nurses also need to learn to "care for themselves." This means balancing work with leisure time, building satisfying personal relationships with friends, and taking time to relax and pamper oneself. Nurses who are overly committed to work become burned out, never find time to relax or see friends, and sacrifice their own personal lives in the process. When this happens, the nurse is more prone to

---

Box 5.5   **METHODS TO AVOID INAPPROPRIATE RELATIONSHIPS BETWEEN NURSES AND CLIENTS**

- Realize that all staff members, whether male or female, junior or senior, or from any discipline, are at risk for over-involvement and loss of boundaries.
- Assume that boundary violations will occur. Supervisors should recognize potential "problem" clients and regularly raise the issue of sexual feelings or boundary loss with staff members.
- Provide opportunities for staff members to discuss their dilemmas and effective ways of dealing with them.
- Develop orientation programs to include how to set limits, how to recognize clues that the relationship is losing boundaries, what the institution expects of the professional, clearly

- defined consequences, case studies, how to develop skills to maintain boundaries, and recommended reading.
- Provide resources for confidential and nonjudgmental assistance.
- Hold regular meetings to discuss inappropriate relationships and feelings toward clients.
- Provide senior staff to lead groups and model effective therapeutic interventions with difficult clients.
- Use clinical vignettes for training.
- Use situations that reflect not only sexual dilemmas but also other boundary violations, including problems with abuse of authority and power.

INTERNET RESOURCES

RESOURCE	INTERNET ADDRESS
• American Psychological Association Brochure About Sexual Relationships in Therapy	http://www.apa.org/pi/therapy.htm
• Countertransference and the Therapeutic Relationship	http:/psychematters.com/papers/hinshelwood.htm
• Managing Countertransference	http://www.hafmc.org/hr/recommendations.htm
• Summary of the Work of Hildegard Peplau	http://www.enursescribe.com/Peplau.htm

boundary violations with clients (e.g., sharing frustrations, responding to the client's personal interest in the nurse). In addition, the nurse who is stressed or overwhelmed tends to lose the objectivity that comes with self-awareness and personal growth activities. In the end, nurses who fail to take good care of themselves also cannot take good care of clients and families.

Points to Consider When Building Therapeutic Relationships

- Attend workshops about values clarification, beliefs, and attitudes to help you assess and learn about yourself.
- Keep a journal of thoughts, feelings, and lessons learned to provide self-insight.
- Listen to feedback from colleagues about your relationships with clients.
- Participate in group discussions on self-growth at the local library or health center to aid self-understanding.
- Develop a continually changing care plan for self-growth.
- Read books on topics that support the strengths you have identified and help to develop your areas of weakness.

Critical Thinking Questions

1. When is it appropriate to accept a gift from a client? What types of gifts are acceptable? Under what circumstances should the nurse accept a gift from a client?
2. What relationship-building behaviors would the nurse use with a client who is very distrustful of the health care system?
3. What preconceptions do you have about mental health clients?

KEY POINTS

- Factors that enhance the nurse–client relationship include trust and congruence, genuine interest, empathy, acceptance, and positive regard.

- Self-awareness is crucial in the therapeutic relationship. The nurse's values, beliefs, and attitudes all come into play as he or she forms a relationship with a client.
- Carper identified four patterns of knowing: empirical, aesthetic, personal, and ethical.
- Munhall established the pattern of unknowing as an openness that the nurse brings to the relationship that prevents preconceptions from clouding his or her view of the client.
- The three types of relationships are social, intimate, and therapeutic. The nurse–client relationship should be therapeutic, not social or intimate.
- Nurse theorist Hildegard Peplau developed the phases of the nurse–client relationship: orientation, working (with subphases of problem identification and exploitation), and termination, or resolution. These phases are ongoing and overlapping.
- The orientation phase begins when the nurse and client meet and ends when the client begins to identify problems to examine.
- Tasks of the working phase include maintaining the relationship, gathering more data, exploring perceptions of reality, developing positive coping mechanisms, promoting a positive self-concept, encouraging verbalization of feelings that facilitate behavior change, working through resistance, evaluating progress and redefining goals as appropriate, providing opportunities for the client to practice new behaviors, and promoting independence.
- Termination begins when the problems are resolved and ends when the relationship is ended.
- Factors that diminish the nurse–client relationship include loss of or unclear boundaries, intimacy, and abuse of power.
- Therapeutic roles of the nurse in the nurse–client relationship include teacher, caregiver, advocate, and parent surrogate.

REFERENCES

Ashmore, R., & Banks, D. (2003a). Mental health nursing students' rationales for self-disclosure. 1. *British Journal of Nursing, 12*(20), 1220–1227.
Ashmore, R., & Banks, D. (2003b). Mental health nursing students' rationales for self-disclosure. 2. *British Journal of Nursing, 12*(21), 1274–1280.
Carper, B. (1978). Fundamental patterns of knowing in nursing. *Advances in Nursing Science, 1*(1), 13–23.

Edd, J. R., Fox, P. G., & Burns, K. (2005). Advocating for the rights of the mentally ill: A global issue. *International Journal of Psychiatric Nursing Research, 11*(1), 1211–1217.

Forchuk, C. (2002). People with enduring mental health problems described the importance of communication, continuity of care, and stigma. *Evidence-Based Nursing, 5*(3), 93–99.

Luft, J. (1970). *Group processes: An introduction in group dynamics.* Palo Alto, CA: National Press Books.

Munhall, P. (1993). Unknowing: Toward another pattern of knowing in nursing. *Nursing Outlook, 41*(3), 125–128.

Peplau, H. E. (1952). *Interpersonal relations in nursing.* New York: G. P. Putnam's Sons.

Welch, M. (2005). Pivotal moments in the therapeutic relationship. *International Journal of Mental Health Nursing, 14*(3), 161–165.

ADDITIONAL READINGS

Beeber, L. S. (2000). Hildahood: Taking the interpersonal theory of nursing to the neighborhood. *Journal of the American Psychiatric Nurses Association, 6*(2), 49–55.

Hanson, B., & Taylor, M. F. (2000). Being-with, doing-with: A model of the nurse-client relationship in mental health nursing. *Journal of Psychiatric and Mental Health Nursing, 7,* 417–423.

Mead, N., & Bower, P. (2000). Patient-centredness: A conceptual framework and review of the empirical literature. *Social Science & Medicine, 51,* 1087–1110.

O'Brien, L. (2000). Nurse-client relationships: The experience of community psychiatric nurses. *Australian and New Zealand Journal of Mental Health Nursing, 9,* 184–194.

Chapter Study Guide

MULTIPLE-CHOICE QUESTIONS

Select the best answer for each of the following questions.

1. Building trust is important in
   A. The orientation phase of the relationship
   B. The problem identification subphase of the relationship
   C. All phases of the relationship
   D. The exploitation subphase of the relationship

2. Abstract standards that provide a person with his or her code of conduct are
   A. Values
   B. Attitudes
   C. Beliefs
   D. Personal philosophy

3. Ideas that one holds as true are
   A. Values
   B. Attitudes
   C. Beliefs
   D. Personal philosophy

4. The emotional frame of reference by which one sees the world is created by
   A. Values
   B. Attitudes
   C. Beliefs
   D. Personal philosophy

FILL-IN-THE-BLANK QUESTIONS

Identify the pattern of knowing as described by Carper.

_____ The nurse reviews the client's medication regimen.

_____ The nurse notices that the client is in a dark cluttered room. Knowing the importance of environment, the nurse begins to open the drapes.

_____ The nurse's grandmother also suffered from dementia, so the client's behavior does not surprise her.

_____ As report is given, the nurse realizes client confidentiality has been breached.

SHORT-ANSWER QUESTIONS

1. Give a dialogue example of each of the following:

   Congruence

   Positive regard

   Acceptance

2. For each of the following client statements, write a response the nurse might make and the rationale for each.

   Client: "I don't believe my doctor really went to medical school."

   Client: "I thought you said you were going to be here for 8 weeks, not 6!"

CLINICAL EXAMPLE

Mr. V., 56 years of age, immigrated to the United States 25 years ago. He has seen many groups of student nurses come and go on his unit. He looks over the newest group and points at one nurse. "I'll take the cute little thing over there," he announces to the instructor and students. He sidles up to the chosen student and puts his arm around her. You are the nurse he has chosen. Create a dialogue that indicates an orientation phase with evidence of trust-building and relationship-enhancing behaviors for working with this client.

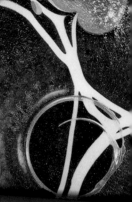

Chapter

6

Therapeutic Communication

Key Terms

- abstract messages
- active listening
- active observation
- body language
- circumstantiality
- cliché
- closed body positions
- communication
- concrete messages
- congruent message
- content
- context
- contract
- cues (overt and covert)
- culture
- directive role
- distance zones
- eye contact
- incongruent message
- intimate zone
- metaphor
- nondirective role
- nonverbal communication
- personal zone
- process
- proverbs

- proxemics
- public zone
- religion
- social zone

- spirituality
- therapeutic communication
- verbal communication

Learning Objectives

After reading this chapter, you should be able to

1. Describe the goals of therapeutic communication.

2. Identify therapeutic and nontherapeutic verbal communication skills.

3. Discuss nonverbal communication skills such as facial expression, body language, vocal cues, eye contact, and understanding of levels of meaning and context.

4. Discuss boundaries in therapeutic communication with respect to distance and use of touch.

5. Distinguish between concrete and abstract messages.

6. Given a hypothetical situation, select an effective therapeutic response to the client.

Visit thePoint http://thePoint.lww.com for NCLEX-style questions, journal articles, and more!

Communication is the process that people use to exchange information. Messages are simultaneously sent and received on two levels: verbally through the use of words and nonverbally by behaviors that accompany the words (DeVito, 2004).

Verbal communication consists of the words a person uses to speak to one or more listeners. Words represent the objects and concepts being discussed. Placement of words into phrases and sentences that are understandable to both speaker and listeners gives an order and a meaning to these symbols. In verbal communication, **content** is the literal words that a person speaks. **Context** is the environment in which communication occurs and can include the time and the physical, social, emotional, and cultural environments. Context includes the circumstances or parts that clarify the meaning of the content of the message (Greene & Burleson, 2003). It is discussed in more detail throughout this chapter.

Nonverbal communication is the behavior that accompanies verbal content such as body language, eye contact, facial expression, tone of voice, speed and hesitations in speech, grunts and groans, and distance from the listeners. Nonverbal communication can indicate the speaker's thoughts, feelings, needs, and values that he or she acts out mostly unconsciously.

Process denotes all nonverbal messages that the speaker uses to give meaning and context to the message. The process component of communication requires the listeners to observe the behaviors and sounds that accent the words and to interpret the speaker's nonverbal behaviors to assess whether they agree or disagree with the verbal content. A **congruent message** is when content and process agree. For example, a client says, "I know I haven't been myself. I need help." She has a sad facial expression and a genuine and sincere voice tone. The process validates the content as being true. But when the content and process disagree—when what the speaker says and what he or she does do not agree—the speaker is giving an **incongruent message**. For example, if the client says, "I'm here to get help," but has a rigid posture, clenched fists, an agitated and frowning facial expression, and snarls the words through clenched teeth, the message is incongruent. The process or observed behavior invalidates what the speaker says (content).

Nonverbal process represents a more accurate message than does verbal content. "I'm sorry I yelled and screamed at you" is readily believable when the speaker has a slumped posture, a resigned voice tone, downcast eyes, and a shameful facial expression because the content and process are congruent. The same sentence said in a loud voice and with raised eyebrows, a piercing gaze, an insulted facial expression, hands on hips, and outraged body language invalidates the words (incongruent message). The message conveyed is "I'm apologizing because I think I have to. I'm not really sorry."

WHAT IS THERAPEUTIC COMMUNICATION?

Therapeutic communication is an interpersonal interaction between the nurse and client during which the nurse focuses on the client's specific needs to promote an effective exchange of information. Skilled use of therapeutic communication techniques helps the nurse understand and empathize with the client's experience. All nurses need skills in therapeutic communication to effectively apply the nursing process and to meet standards of care for their clients.

Therapeutic communication can help nurses to accomplish many goals:

- Establish a therapeutic nurse–client relationship.
- Identify the most important client concern at that moment (the client-centered goal).
- Assess the client's perception of the problem as it unfolds. This includes detailed actions (behaviors and messages) of the people involved and the client's thoughts and feelings about the situation, others, and self.
- Facilitate the client's expression of emotions.
- Teach the client and family necessary self-care skills.
- Recognize the client's needs.
- Implement interventions designed to address the client's needs.
- Guide the client toward identifying a plan of action to a satisfying and socially acceptable resolution.

Establishing a therapeutic relationship is one of the most important responsibilities of the nurse when working with clients. Communication is the means by which a therapeutic relationship is initiated, maintained, and terminated. The therapeutic relationship is discussed in depth in Chapter 5, including confidentiality, self-disclosure, and therapeutic use of self. To have effective therapeutic communication, the nurse also must consider privacy and respect of boundaries, use of touch, and active listening and observation.

Privacy and Respecting Boundaries

Privacy is desirable but not always possible in therapeutic communication. An interview or conference room is optimal if the nurse believes this setting is not too isolative for the interaction. The nurse also can talk with the client at the end of the hall or in a quiet corner of the day room or lobby, depending on the physical layout of the setting. The nurse needs to evaluate whether interacting in the client's room is therapeutic. For example, if the client has difficulty maintaining boundaries or has been making sexual comments, then the client's room is not the best setting. A more formal setting would be desirable.

Proxemics is the study of distance zones between people during communication. People feel more comfortable with smaller distances when communicating with someone they know rather than with strangers (DeVito, 2004).

People from the United States, Canada, and many Eastern European nations generally observe four **distance zones**:

- **Intimate zone** (0 to 18 inches between people): This amount of space is comfortable for parents with young children, people who mutually desire personal contact, or people whispering. Invasion of this intimate zone by anyone else is threatening and produces anxiety.
- **Personal zone** (18 to 36 inches): This distance is comfortable between family and friends who are talking.
- **Social zone** (4 to 12 feet): This distance is acceptable for communication in social, work, and business settings.
- **Public zone** (12 to 25 feet): This is an acceptable distance between a speaker and an audience, small groups, and other informal functions (Hall, 1963).

People from some cultures (e.g., Hispanic, Mediterranean, East Indian, Asian, Middle Eastern) are more comfortable with less than 4 to 12 feet of space between them while talking. The nurse of European American or African American heritage may feel uncomfortable if clients from these cultures stand close when talking. Conversely, clients from these backgrounds may perceive the nurse as remote and indifferent (Andrews & Boyle, 2003).

Both the client and the nurse can feel threatened if one invades the other's personal or intimate zone, which can result in tension, irritability, fidgeting, or even flight. When the nurse must invade the intimate or personal zone, he or she always should ask the client's permission. For example, if a nurse performing an assessment in a community setting needs to take the client's blood pressure, he or she should say, "Mr. Smith, to take your blood pressure I will wrap this cuff around your arm and listen with my stethoscope. Is this acceptable to you?" He or she should ask permission in a yes/no format so the client's response is clear. This is one of the times when yes/no questions are appropriate.

The therapeutic communication interaction is most comfortable when the nurse and client are 3 to 6 feet apart. If a client invades the nurse's intimate space (0 to 18 inches), the nurse should set limits gradually, depending on how often the client has invaded the nurse's space and the safety of the situation.

Touch

As intimacy increases, the need for distance decreases. Knapp (1980) identified five types of touch:

- *Functional-professional* touch is used in examinations or procedures such as when the nurse touches a client to assess skin turgor or a masseuse performs a massage.
- *Social-polite* touch is used in greeting, such as a handshake and the "air kisses" some women use to greet acquaintances, or when a gentle hand guides someone in the correct direction.
- *Friendship-warmth* touch involves a hug in greeting, an arm thrown around the shoulder of a good friend, or the back slapping some men use to greet friends and relatives.
- *Love-intimacy* touch involves tight hugs and kisses between lovers or close relatives.
- *Sexual-arousal* touch is used by lovers.

Touching a client can be comforting and supportive when it is welcome and permitted. The nurse should observe the client for cues that show whether touch is desired or indicated. For example, holding the hand of a sobbing mother whose child is ill is appropriate and therapeutic. If the mother pulls her hand away, however, she signals to the

---

CLINICAL VIGNETTE: PERSONAL BOUNDARIES BETWEEN NURSE AND CLIENT

Saying he wanted to discuss his wife's condition, a man accompanied the nurse down the narrow hallway of his house but did not move away when they reached the parlor. He was 12 inches from the nurse. The nurse was uncomfortable with his closeness, but she did not perceive any physical threat from him. Because this was the first visit to this home, the nurse indicated two easy chairs and said, "Let's sit over here, Mr. Barrett" (offering collaboration). If sitting down were not an option and Mr. Barrett moved in to compensate for the nurse's backing up, the nurse could neutrally say, "I feel uncomfortable when anyone invades my personal space, Mr. Barrett. Please back up at least 12 inches" (setting limits). In this message, the nurse has taken the blame instead of shaming the other person and has gently given an order for a specific distance between herself and Mr. Barrett. If Mr. Barrett were to move closer to the nurse again, the nurse would note

the behavior and ask the client about it—for example, "You have moved in again very close to me, Mr. Barrett. What is that about?" (encouraging evaluation). The use of an open-ended question provides an opportunity for the client to address his behavior. He may have difficulty hearing the nurse, want to keep this discussion confidential so his wife will not hear it, come from a culture in which 12 inches is an appropriate distance for a conversation, or be using his closeness as a manipulative behavior (ensure attention, threat, or sexual invitation). After discussing Mr. Barrett's response and understanding that he can hear adequately, the nurse can add, "We can speak just fine from 2 or 3 feet apart, Mr. Barrett. Otherwise, I will leave or we can continue this discussion in your wife's room" (setting limits). If Mr. Barrett again moves closer, the nurse will leave or move to the wife's room to continue the interview.

nurse that she feels uncomfortable being touched. The nurse also can ask the client about touching (e.g., "Would it help you to squeeze my hand?").

Although touch can be comforting and therapeutic, it is an invasion of intimate and personal space. Some clients with mental illness have difficulty understanding the concept of personal boundaries or knowing when touch is or is not appropriate. Consequently, most psychiatric inpatient, outpatient, and ambulatory care units have policies against clients touching one another or staff. Unless they need to get close to a client to perform some nursing care, staff members should serve as role models and refrain from invading clients' personal and intimate space. When a staff member is going to touch a client while performing nursing care, he or she must verbally prepare the client before starting the procedure. A client with paranoia may interpret being touched as a threat and may attempt to protect himself or herself by striking the staff person.

Active Listening and Observation

To receive the sender's simultaneous messages, the nurse must use active listening and active observation. **Active listening** means refraining from other internal mental activities and concentrating exclusively on what the client says. **Active observation** means watching the speaker's nonverbal actions as he or she communicates.

Peplau (1952) used observation as the first step in the therapeutic interaction. The nurse observes the client's behavior and guides him or her in giving detailed descrip-

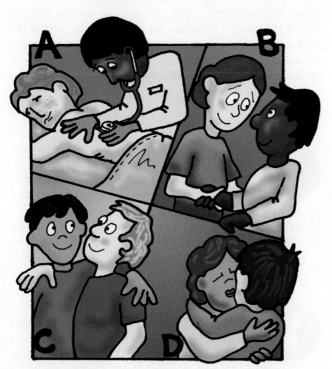

Four types of touch: **A,** Functional-professional touch;
B, Social-polite touch; **C,** Friendship-warmth touch;
D, Love-intimacy touch

tions of that behavior. The nurse also documents these details. To help the client develop insight into his or her interpersonal skills, the nurse analyzes the information obtained, determines the underlying needs that relate to the behavior, and connects pieces of information (makes links between various sections of the conversation).

A common misconception by students learning the art of therapeutic communication is that they always must be ready with questions the instant the client has finished speaking. Hence, they are constantly thinking ahead regarding the next question rather than actively listening to what the client is saying. The result can be that the nurse does not understand the client's concerns, and the conversation is vague, superficial, and frustrating to both participants. When a superficial conversation occurs, the nurse may complain that the client is not cooperating, is repeating things, or is not taking responsibility for getting better. Superficiality, however, can be the result of the nurse's failure to listen to cues in the client's responses and repeatedly asking the same question. The nurse does not get details and works from his or her assumptions rather than from the client's true situation.

While listening to a client's story, it is almost impossible for the nurse not to make assumptions. A person's life experiences, knowledge base, values, and prejudices often color the interpretation of a message. In therapeutic communication, the nurse must ask specific questions to get the entire story from the client's perspective, to clarify assumptions, and to develop empathy with the client. Empathy is the ability to place oneself into the experience of another for a moment in time. Nurses develop empathy by gathering as much information about an issue as possible directly from the client to avoid interjecting their personal experiences and interpretations of the situation. The nurse asks as many questions as needed to gain a clear understanding of the client's perceptions of an event or issue.

Active listening and observation help the nurse to

- Recognize the issue that is most important to the client at this time.
- Know what further questions to ask the client.
- Use additional therapeutic communication techniques to guide the client to describe his or her perceptions fully.
- Understand the client's perceptions of the issue instead of jumping to conclusions.
- Interpret and respond to the message objectively.

VERBAL COMMUNICATION SKILLS

Using Concrete Messages

The nurse should use words that are as clear as possible when speaking to the client so that the client can understand the message. Anxious people lose cognitive processing skills—the higher the anxiety, the less ability to process concepts—so **concrete messages** are important for accurate information exchange. In a concrete message, the words are explicit and need no interpretation; the speaker uses nouns instead of pronouns—for example, "What health symptoms caused you to come to the hospital today?" or "When was the last time you took your antidepressant medications?" Concrete questions are clear, direct, and easy to understand. They elicit more accurate responses and avoid the need to go back and rephrase unclear questions, which interrupts the flow of a therapeutic interaction.

Abstract messages, in contrast, are unclear patterns of words that often contain figures of speech that are difficult to interpret. They require the listener to interpret what the speaker is asking. For example, a nurse who wants to know why a client was admitted to the unit asks, "How did you get here?" This is an abstract message: the terms *how* and *here* are vague. An anxious client might not be aware of where he or she is and reply, "Where am I?" or might interpret this as a question about how he or she was conveyed to the hospital and respond, "The ambulance brought me." Clients who are anxious, from different cultures, cognitively impaired, or suffering from some mental disorders often function at a concrete level of comprehension and have difficulty answering abstract questions. The nurse must be sure that statements and questions are clear and concrete.

The following are examples of abstract and concrete messages:

Abstract (unclear): *"Get the stuff from him."*
Concrete (clear): *"John will be home today at 5 PM, and you can pick up your clothes at that time."*
Abstract (unclear): *"Your clinical performance has to improve."*
Concrete (clear): *"To administer medications tomorrow, you'll have to be able to calculate dosages correctly by the end of today's class."*

Using Therapeutic Communication Techniques

The nurse can use many therapeutic communication techniques to interact with clients. The choice of technique depends on the intent of the interaction and the client's ability to communicate verbally. Overall, the nurse selects techniques that facilitate the interaction and enhance communication between client and nurse. Table 6.1 lists these techniques and gives examples. Techniques such as exploring, focusing, restating, and reflecting encourage the client to discuss his or her feelings or concerns in more depth. Other techniques help focus or clarify what is being said. The nurse may give the client feedback using techniques such as making an observation or presenting reality.

Avoiding Nontherapeutic Communication

In contrast, there are many nontherapeutic techniques that nurses should avoid (Table 6.2). These responses cut off communication and make it more difficult for the interaction to continue. Responses such as "Everything will work out" or "Maybe tomorrow will be a better day" may be intended to comfort the client, but instead may impede the communication process. Asking "Why" questions (in an effort to gain information) may be perceived as criticism by the client, conveying a negative judgment from the nurse. Many of these responses are common in social interaction. Therefore, it takes practice for the nurse to avoid making these types of comments.

Interpreting Signals or Cues

To understand what a client means, the nurse watches and listens carefully for cues. **Cues** are verbal or nonverbal messages that signal key words or issues for the client. Finding cues is a function of active listening. Cues can be buried in what a client says or can be acted out in the process of communication. Often, cue words introduced by the client can help the nurse to know what to ask next or how to respond to the client. The nurse builds his or her responses on these cue words or concepts. Understanding this can relieve pressure on students who are worried and anxious about what question to ask next. The following example illustrates questions the nurse might ask when responding to a client's cue:

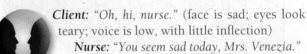

Client: *"I had a boyfriend when I was younger."*
Nurse: *"You had a boyfriend?"* (reflecting)
"Tell me about you and your boyfriend." (encouraging description)
"How old were you when you had this boyfriend?" (placing events in time or sequence)

If a client has difficulty attending to a conversation and drifts into a rambling discussion or a flight of ideas, the nurse listens carefully for a theme, or a topic around which the client composes his or her words. Using the theme, the nurse can assess the nonverbal behaviors that accompany the client's words and build responses based on these cues. In the following examples, the underlined words are themes and cues to help the nurse formulate further communication.

Theme of sadness:

Client: *"Oh, hi, nurse."* (face is sad; eyes look teary; voice is low, with little inflection)
Nurse: *"You seem sad today, Mrs. Venezia."*
Client: *"Yes, it is the <u>anniversary</u> of my <u>husband's death</u>."*
Nurse: *"<u>How long ago</u> did your husband die?"* (Or the nurse can use the other cue.)
Nurse: *"Tell me about your <u>husband's death,</u> Mrs. Venezia."*

Theme of loss of control:

Client: *"I had a fender bender this morning. I'm okay. I lost my wallet, and I have to go to the bank to cover a check I wrote last night. I can't get in contact with my husband at work. <u>I don't know where to start.</u>"*
Nurse: *"I sense you feel out of control."* (translating into feelings)

Table 6.1	THERAPEUTIC COMMUNICATION TECHNIQUES	

Therapeutic Communication Technique	Examples	Rationale
Accepting—indicating reception	"Yes." "I follow what you said." Nodding	An accepting response indicates the nurse has heard and followed the train of thought. It does not indicate agreement but is nonjudgmental. Facial expression, tone of voice, and so forth also must convey acceptance or the words lose their meaning.
Broad openings—allowing the client to take the initiative in introducing the topic	"Is there something you'd like to talk about?" "Where would you like to begin?"	Broad openings make explicit that the client has the lead in the interaction. For the client who is hesitant about talking, broad openings may stimulate him or her to take the initiative.
Consensual validation—searching for mutual understanding, for accord in the meaning of the words	"Tell me whether my understanding of it agrees with yours." "Are you using this word to convey that . . . ?"	For verbal communication to be meaningful, it is essential that the words being used have the same meaning for both (all) participants. Sometimes, words, phrases, or slang terms have different meanings and can be easily misunderstood.
Encouraging comparison—asking that similarities and differences be noted	"Was it something like . . . ?" "Have you had similar experiences?"	Comparing ideas, experiences, or relationships brings out many recurring themes. The client benefits from making these comparisons because he or she might recall past coping strategies that were effective or remember that he or she has survived a similar situation.
Encouraging description of perceptions—asking the client to verbalize what he or she perceives	"Tell me when you feel anxious." "What is happening?" "What does the voice seem to be saying?"	To understand the client, the nurse must see things from his or her perspective. Encouraging the client to describe ideas fully may relieve the tension the client is feeling, and he or she might be less likely to take action on ideas that are harmful or frightening.
Encouraging expression—asking the client to appraise the quality of his or her experiences	"What are your feelings in regard to . . . ?" "Does this contribute to your distress?"	The nurse asks the client to consider people and events in light of his or her own values. Doing so encourages the client to make his or her own appraisal rather than to accept the opinion of others.
Exploring—delving further into a subject or idea	"Tell me more about that." "Would you describe it more fully?" "What kind of work?"	When clients deal with topics superficially, exploring can help them examine the issue more fully. Any problem or concern can be better understood if explored in depth. If the client expresses an unwillingness to explore a subject, however, the nurse must respect his or her wishes.
Focusing—concentrating on a single point	"This point seems worth looking at more closely." "Of all the concerns you've mentioned, which is most troublesome?"	The nurse encourages the client to concentrate his or her energies on a single point, which may prevent a multitude of factors or problems from overwhelming the client. It is also a useful technique when a client jumps from one topic to another.
Formulating a plan of action—asking the client to consider kinds of behavior likely to be appropriate in future situations	"What could you do to let your anger out harmlessly?" "Next time this comes up, what might you do to handle it?"	It may be helpful for the client to plan in advance what he or she might do in future similar situations. Making definite plans increases the likelihood that the client will cope more effectively in a similar situation.
General leads—giving encouragement to continue	"Go on." "And then?" "Tell me about it."	General leads indicate that the nurse is listening and following what the client is saying without taking away the initiative for the interaction. They also encourage the client to continue if he or she is hesitant or uncomfortable about the topic.
Giving information—making available the facts that the client needs	"My name is . . ." "Visiting hours are . . ." "My purpose in being here is . . ."	Informing the client of facts increases his or her knowledge about a topic or lets the client know what to expect. The nurse is functioning as a resource person. Giving information also builds trust with the client.

(continued)

Table 6.1   THERAPEUTIC COMMUNICATION TECHNIQUES (Continued)

Therapeutic Communication Technique	Examples	Rationale
Giving recognition—acknowledging, indicating awareness	"Good morning, Mr. S. . . ." "You've finished your list of things to do." "I notice that you've combed your hair."	Greeting the client by name, indicating awareness of change, or noting efforts the client has made all show that the nurse recognizes the client as a person, as an individual. Such recognition does not carry the notion of value, that is, of being "good" or "bad."
Making observations—verbalizing what the nurse perceives	"You appear tense." "Are you uncomfortable when . . . ?" "I notice that you're biting your lip."	Sometimes clients cannot verbalize or make themselves understood. Or the client may not be ready to talk.
Offering self—making oneself available	"I'll sit with you awhile." "I'll stay here with you." "I'm interested in what you think."	The nurse can offer his or her presence, interest, and desire to understand. It is important that this offer is unconditional, that is, the client does not have to respond verbally to get the nurse's attention.
Placing event in time or sequence—clarifying the relationship of events in time	"What seemed to lead up to . . . ?" "Was this before or after . . . ?" "When did this happen?"	Putting events in proper sequence helps both the nurse and client to see them in perspective. The client may gain insight into cause-and-effect behavior and consequences, or the client may be able to see that perhaps some things are not related. The nurse may gain information about recurrent patterns or themes in the client's behavior or relationships.
Presenting reality—offering for consideration that which is real	"I see no one else in the room." "That sound was a car backfiring." "Your mother is not here; I am a nurse."	When it is obvious that the client is misinterpreting reality, the nurse can indicate what is real. The nurse does this by calmly and quietly expressing the nurse's perceptions or the facts, not by way of arguing with the client or belittling his or her experience. The intent is to indicate an alternative line of thought for the client to consider, not to "convince" the client that he or she is wrong.
Reflecting—directing client actions, thoughts, and feelings back to client	*Client*: "Do you think I should tell the doctor . . . ?" *Nurse*: "Do you think you should?" *Client*: "My brother spends all my money and then has nerve to ask for more." *Nurse*: "This causes you to feel angry?"	Reflection encourages the client to recognize and accept his or her own feelings. The nurse indicates that the client's point of view has value, and that the client has the right to have opinions, make decisions, and think independently.
Restating—repeating the main idea expressed	*Client*: "I can't sleep. I stay awake all night." *Nurse*: "You have difficulty sleeping." *Client*: "I'm really mad, I'm really upset." *Nurse*: "You're really mad and upset."	The nurse repeats what the client has said in approximately or nearly the same words the client has used. This restatement lets the client know that he or she communicated the idea effectively. This encourages the client to continue. Or if the client has been misunderstood, he or she can clarify his or her thoughts.
Seeking information—seeking to make clear that which is not meaningful or that which is vague	"I'm not sure that I follow." "Have I heard you correctly?"	The nurse should seek clarification throughout interactions with clients. Doing so can help the nurse to avoid making assumptions that understanding has occurred when it has not. It helps the client to articulate thoughts, feelings, and ideas more clearly.

Table 6.1	THERAPEUTIC COMMUNICATION TECHNIQUES *(Continued)*

Therapeutic Communication Technique	Examples	Rationale
Silence—absence of verbal communication, which provides time for the client to put thoughts or feelings into words, to regain composure, or to continue talking	Nurse says nothing but continues to maintain eye contact and conveys interest.	Silence often encourages the client to verbalize, provided that it is interested and expectant. Silence gives the client time to organize thoughts, direct the topic of interaction, or focus on issues that are most important. Much nonverbal behavior takes place during silence, and the nurse needs to be aware of the client and his or her own nonverbal behavior.
Suggesting collaboration—offering to share, to strive, to work with the client for his or her benefit	"Perhaps you and I can discuss and discover the triggers for your anxiety." "Let's go to your room, and I'll help you find what you're looking for."	The nurse seeks to offer a relationship in which the client can identify problems in living with others, grow emotionally, and improve the ability to form satisfactory relationships. The nurse offers to do things with, rather than for, the client.
Summarizing—organizing and summing up that which has gone before	"Have I got this straight?" "You've said that . . ." "During the past hour, you and I have discussed . . ."	Summarization seeks to bring out the important points of the discussion and to increase the awareness and understanding of both participants. It omits the irrelevant and organizes the pertinent aspects of the interaction. It allows both client and nurse to depart with the same ideas and provides a sense of closure at the completion of each discussion.
Translating into feelings—seeking to verbalize client's feelings that he or she expresses only indirectly	*Client*: "I'm dead." *Nurse*: "Are you suggesting that you feel lifeless?" *Client*: "I'm way out in the ocean." *Nurse*: "You seem to feel lonely or deserted."	Often what the client says, when taken literally, seems meaningless or far removed from reality. To understand, the nurse must concentrate on what the client might be feeling to express himself or herself this way.
Verbalizing the implied—voicing what the client has hinted at or suggested	*Client*: "I can't talk to you or anyone. It's a waste of time." *Nurse:* "Do you feel that no one understands?"	Putting into words what the client has implied or said indirectly tends to make the discussion less obscure. The nurse should be as direct as possible without being unfeelingly blunt or obtuse. The client may have difficulty communicating directly. The nurse should take care to express only what is fairly obvious; otherwise, the nurse may be jumping to conclusions or interpreting the client's communication.
Voicing doubt—expressing uncertainty about the reality of the client's perceptions	"Isn't that unusual?" "Really?" "That's hard to believe."	Another means of responding to distortions of reality is to express doubt. Such expression permits the client to become aware that others do not necessarily perceive events in the same way or draw the same conclusions. This does not mean the client will alter his or her point of view, but at least the nurse will encourage the client to reconsider or re-evaluate what has happened. The nurse neither agreed nor disagreed; however, he or she has not let the misperceptions and distortions pass without comment.

Adapted from Hays, J. S., & Larson, K. (1963). *Interactions with patients*. New York: Macmillan Press.

Table 6.2   NONTHERAPEUTIC COMMUNICATION TECHNIQUES

Techniques	Examples	Rationale
Advising—telling the client what to do	"I think you should . . ." "Why don't you . . ."	Giving advice implies that only the nurse knows what is best for the client.
Agreeing—indicating accord with the client	"That's right." "I agree."	Approval indicates the client is "right" rather than "wrong." This gives the client the impression that he or she is "right" because of agreement with the nurse. Opinions and conclusions should be exclusively the client's. When the nurse agrees with the client, there is no opportunity for the client to change his or her mind without being "wrong."
Belittling feelings expressed—misjudging the degree of the client's discomfort	*Client*: "I have nothing to live for . . . I wish I was dead." *Nurse*: "Everybody gets down in the dumps," or "I've felt that way myself."	When the nurse tries to equate the intense and overwhelming feelings the client has expressed to "everybody" or to the nurse's own feelings, the nurse implies that the discomfort is temporary, mild, self-limiting, or not very important. The client is focused on his or her own worries and feelings; hearing the problems or feelings of others is not helpful.
Challenging—demanding proof from the client	"But how can you be president of the United States?" "If you're dead, why is your heart beating?"	Often the nurse believes that if he or she can challenge the client to prove unrealistic ideas, the client will realize there is no "proof" and then will recognize reality. Actually, challenging causes the client to defend the delusions or misperceptions more strongly than before.
Defending—attempting to protect someone or something from verbal attack?	"This hospital has a fine reputation." "I'm sure your doctor has your best interests in mind."	Defending what the client has criticized implies that he or she has no right to express impressions, opinions, or feelings. Telling the client that his or her criticism is unjust or unfounded does not change the client's feelings but only serves to block further communication.
Disagreeing—opposing the client's ideas	"That's wrong." "I definitely disagree with . . ." "I don't believe that."	Disagreeing implies the client is "wrong." Consequently, the client feels defensive about his or her point of view or ideas.
Disapproving—denouncing the client's behavior or ideas	"That's bad." "I'd rather you wouldn't . . ."	Disapproval implies that the nurse has the right to pass judgment on the client's thoughts or actions. It further implies that the client is expected to please the nurse.
Giving approval—sanctioning the client's behavior or ideas	"That's good." "I'm glad that . . ."	Saying what the client thinks or feels is "good" implies that the opposite is "bad." Approval, then, tends to limit the client's freedom to think, speak, or act in a certain way. This can lead to the client's acting in a particular way just to please the nurse.
Giving literal responses—responding to a figurative comment as though it were a statement of fact	*Client*: "They're looking in my head with a television camera." *Nurse*: "Try not to watch television," or "What channel?"	Often the client is at a loss to describe his or her feelings, so such comments are the best he or she can do. Usually, it is helpful for the nurse to focus on the client's feelings in response to such statements.
Indicating the existence of an external source—attributing the source of thoughts, feelings, and behavior to others or to outside influences	"What makes you say that?" "What made you do that?" "Who told you that you were a prophet?"	The nurse can ask, "What happened?" or "What events led you to draw such a conclusion?" But to question, "What made you think that?" implies that the client was made or compelled to think in a certain way. Usually, the nurse does not intend to suggest that the source is external, but that is often what the client thinks.
Interpreting—asking to make conscious that which is unconscious; telling the client the meaning of his or her experience	"What you really mean is . . ." "Unconsciously you're saying . . ."	The client's thoughts and feelings are his or her own, not to be interpreted by the nurse for hidden meaning. Only the client can identify or confirm the presence of feelings.

Table 6.2   NONTHERAPEUTIC COMMUNICATION TECHNIQUES (Continued)

Techniques	Examples	Rationale
Introducing an unrelated topic—changing the subject	*Client*: "I'd like to die." *Nurse*: "Did you have visitors last evening?"	The nurse takes the initiative for the interaction away from the client. This usually happens because the nurse is uncomfortable, doesn't know how to respond, or has a topic he or she would rather discuss.
Making stereotyped comments—offering meaningless clichés or trite comments	"It's for your own good." "Keep your chin up." "Just have a positive attitude and you'll be better in no time."	Social conversation contains many clichés and much meaningless chitchat. Such comments are of no value in the nurse–client relationship. Any automatic responses lack the nurse's consideration or thoughtfulness.
Probing—persistent questioning of the client	"Now tell me about this problem. You know I have to find out." "Tell me your psychiatric history."	Probing tends to make the client feel used or invaded. Clients have the right not to talk about issues or concerns if they choose. Pushing and probing by the nurse will not encourage the client to talk.
Reassuring—indicating there is no reason for anxiety or other feelings of discomfort	"I wouldn't worry about that." "Everything will be all right." "You're coming along just fine."	Attempts to dispel the client's anxiety by implying that there is not sufficient reason for concern completely devalue the client's feelings. Vague reassurances without accompanying facts are meaningless to the client.
Rejecting—refusing to consider or showing contempt for the client's ideas or behaviors	"Let's not discuss . . ." "I don't want to hear about . . ."	When the nurse rejects any topic, he or she closes it off from exploration. In turn, the client may feel personally rejected along with his or her ideas.
Requesting an explanation—asking the client to provide reasons for thoughts, feelings, behaviors, events	"Why do you think that?" "Why do you feel that way?"	There is a difference between asking the client to describe what is occurring or has taken place and asking him to explain why. Usually, a "why" question is intimidating. In addition, the client is unlikely to know "why" and may become defensive trying to explain himself or herself.
Testing—appraising the client's degree of insight	"Do you know what kind of hospital this is?" "Do you still have the idea that . . . ?"	These types of questions force the client to try to recognize his or her problems. The client's acknowledgement that he or she doesn't know these things may meet the nurse's needs but is not helpful for the client.
Using denial—refusing to admit that a problem exists	*Client*: "I'm nothing." *Nurse*: "Of course you're something—everybody's something." *Client*: "I'm dead." *Nurse*: "Don't be silly."	The nurse denies the client's feelings or the seriousness of the situation by dismissing his or her comments without attempting to discover the feelings or meaning behind them.

Adapted from Hays, J. S., & Larson, K. (1963). *Interactions with patients.* New York: Macmillan Press.

Clients may use many word patterns to cue the listener to their intent. **Overt cues** are clear statements of intent, such as "I want to die." The message is clear that the client is thinking of suicide or self-harm. **Covert cues** are vague or hidden messages that need interpretation and exploration—for example, if a client says, "Nothing can help me." The nurse is unsure, but it sounds as if the client might be saying he feels so hopeless and helpless that he plans to commit suicide. The nurse can explore this covert cue to clarify the client's intent and to protect the client. Most suicidal people are ambivalent about whether to live or die and often admit their plan when directly asked about it. When the nurse suspects self-harm or suicide, he or she uses a yes/no question to elicit a clear response.

Theme of hopelessness and suicidal ideation:

Client: "Life is hard. I want it to be done. There is no rest. Sleep, sleep is good . . . forever."
Nurse: "I hear you saying things seem hopeless. I wonder if you are planning to kill yourself."
(verbalizing the implied)

Other word patterns that need further clarification for meaning include metaphors, proverbs, and clichés. When a client uses these figures of speech, the nurse must follow up with questions to clarify what the client is trying to say.

A **metaphor** is a phrase that describes an object or situation by comparing it to something else familiar.

> **Client:** *"My son's bedroom looks like a bomb went off."*
> **Nurse:** *"You're saying your son is not very neat."* (verbalizing the implied)
> **Client:** *"My mind is like mashed potatoes."*
> **Nurse:** *"I sense you find it difficult to put thoughts together."* (translating into feelings)

Proverbs are old accepted sayings with generally accepted meanings.

> **Client:** *"People who live in glass houses shouldn't throw stones."*
> **Nurse:** *"Who do you believe is criticizing you but actually has similar problems?"* (encouraging description of perception)

A **cliché** is an expression that has become trite and generally conveys a stereotype. For example, if a client says "she has more guts than brains," the implication is that the speaker believes the woman to whom he or she refers is not smart, acts before thinking, or has no common sense. The nurse can clarify what the client means by saying, "Give me one example of how you see Mary as having more guts than brains" (focusing).

NONVERBAL COMMUNICATION SKILLS

Nonverbal communication is behavior that a person exhibits while delivering verbal content. It includes facial expression, eye contact, space, time, boundaries, and body movements. Nonverbal communication is as important, if not more so, than verbal communication. It is estimated that one third of meaning is transmitted by words and two thirds is communicated nonverbally. The speaker may verbalize what he or she believes the listener wants to hear, whereas nonverbal communication conveys the speaker's actual meaning. Nonverbal communication involves the unconscious mind acting out emotions related to the verbal content, the situation, the environment, and the relationship between the speaker and the listener.

Knapp and Hall (2002) listed the ways in which nonverbal messages accompany verbal messages:

- Accent: using flashing eyes or hand movements
- Complement: giving quizzical looks, nodding
- Contradict: rolling eyes to demonstrate that the meaning is the opposite of what one is saying
- Regulate: taking a deep breath to demonstrate readiness to speak, using "and uh" to signal the wish to continue speaking
- Repeat: using nonverbal behaviors to augment the verbal message, such as shrugging after saying "Who knows?"

- Substitute: using culturally determined body movements that stand in for words, such as pumping the arm up and down with a closed fist to indicate success

Facial Expression

The human face produces the most visible, complex, and sometimes confusing nonverbal messages. Facial movements connect with words to illustrate meaning; this connection demonstrates the speaker's internal dialogue (Greene & Burleson, 2003). Facial expressions can be categorized into expressive, impassive, and confusing:

- An *expressive* face portrays the person's moment-by-moment thoughts, feelings, and needs. These expressions may be evident even when the person does not want to reveal his or her emotions.
- An *impassive* face is frozen into an emotionless deadpan expression similar to a mask.
- A *confusing* facial expression is one that is the opposite of what the person wants to convey. A person who is verbally expressing sad or angry feelings while smiling is exhibiting a confusing facial expression.

Facial expressions often can affect the listener's response. Strong and emotional facial expressions can persuade the listener to believe the message. For example, by appearing perplexed and confused, a client could manipulate the nurse into staying longer than scheduled. Facial expressions such as happy, sad, embarrassed, or angry usually have the same meaning across cultures, but the nurse should identify the facial expression and ask the client to validate the nurse's interpretation of it—for instance, "You're smiling, but I sense you are very angry" (Sheldon, 2004).

Frowns, smiles, puzzlement, relief, fear, surprise, and anger are common facial communication signals. Looking away, not meeting the speaker's eyes, and yawning indicate that the listener is disinterested, lying, or bored. To ensure the accuracy of information, the nurse identifies the nonverbal communication and checks its congruency with the content (Sheldon, 2004). An example is "Mr. Jones, you said everything is fine today, yet you frowned as you spoke. I sense that everything is not really fine" (verbalizing the implied).

Body Language

Body language (gestures, postures, movements, and body positions) is a nonverbal form of communication. **Closed body positions,** such as crossed legs or arms folded across the chest, indicate that the interaction might threaten the listener who is defensive or not accepting. A better, more accepting body position is to sit facing the client with both feet on the floor, knees parallel, hands at the side of the body, and legs uncrossed or crossed only at the ankle. This open posture demonstrates unconditional positive regard, trust, care, and acceptance. The nurse indicates interest in and acceptance of the client by facing and slightly leaning toward him or her while maintaining nonthreatening eye contact.

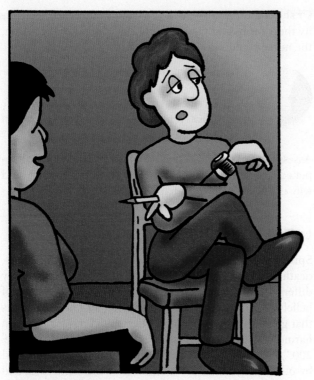

Closed body position

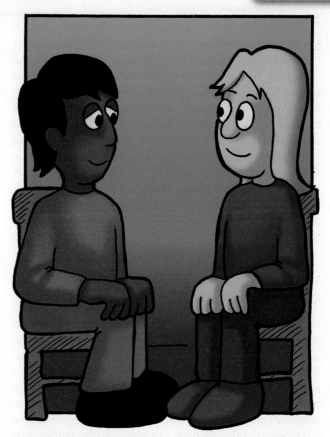

Accepting body position

Hand gestures add meaning to the content. A slight lift of the hand from the arm of a chair can punctuate or strengthen the meaning of words. Holding both hands with palms up while shrugging the shoulders often means "I don't know." Some people use many hand gestures to demonstrate or act out what they are saying, whereas others use very few gestures.

The positioning of the nurse and client in relation to each other is also important. Sitting beside or across from the client can put the client at ease, whereas sitting behind a desk (creating a physical barrier) can increase the formality of the setting and may decrease the client's willingness to open up and communicate freely. The nurse may wish to create a more formal setting with some clients, however, such as those who have difficulty maintaining boundaries.

Vocal Cues

Vocal cues are nonverbal sound signals transmitted along with the content: voice volume, tone, pitch, intensity, emphasis, speed, and pauses augment the sender's message. Volume, the loudness of the voice, can indicate anger, fear, happiness, or deafness. Tone can indicate whether someone is relaxed, agitated, or bored. Pitch varies from shrill and high to low and threatening. Intensity is the power, severity, and strength behind the words, indicating the importance of the message. Emphasis refers to accents on words or phrases that highlight the subject or give insight on the topic. Speed is number of words spoken per

minute. Pauses also contribute to the message, often adding emphasis or feeling.

The high-pitched rapid delivery of a message often indicates anxiety. The use of extraneous words with long tedious descriptions is called **circumstantiality**. Circumstantiality can indicate the client is confused about what is important or is a poor historian. Slow, hesitant responses can indicate that the person is depressed, confused and searching for the correct words, having difficulty finding the right words to describe an incident, or reminiscing. It is important for the nurse to validate these nonverbal indicators rather than to assume that he or she knows what the client is thinking or feeling (e.g., "Mr. Smith, you sound anxious. Is that how you're feeling?").

Eye Contact

The eyes have been called the mirror of the soul because they often reflect our emotions. Messages that the eyes give include humor, interest, puzzlement, hatred, happiness, sadness, horror, warning, and pleading. **Eye contact**, looking into the other person's eyes during communication, is used to assess the other person and the environment and to indicate whose turn it is to speak; it increases during listening but decreases while speaking (DeVito, 2004). Although maintaining good eye contact is usually desirable, it is important that the nurse doesn't "stare" at the client.

Silence

Silence or long pauses in communication may indicate many different things. The client may be depressed and struggling to find the energy to talk. Sometimes pauses indicate the client is thoughtfully considering the question before responding. At times, the client may seem to be "lost in his or her own thoughts" and not paying attention to the nurse. It is important to allow the client sufficient time to respond, even if it seems like a long time. It may confuse the client if the nurse "jumps in" with another question or tries to restate the question differently. Also, in some cultures, verbal communication is slow with many pauses, and the client may believe the nurse is impatient or disrespectful if he or she does not wait for the client's response.

UNDERSTANDING THE MEANING OF COMMUNICATION

Few messages in social and therapeutic communication have only one level of meaning; messages often contain more meaning than just the spoken words (DeVito, 2004). The nurse must try to discover all the meaning in the client's communication. For example, the client with depression might say, "I'm so tired that I just can't go on." If the nurse considers only the literal meaning of the words, he or she might assume the client is experiencing the fatigue that often accompanies depression. However, statements such as the previous example often mean the client wishes to die. The nurse would need to further assess the client's statement to determine whether or not the client is suicidal.

It is sometimes easier for clients to act out their emotions than to organize their thoughts and feelings into words to describe feelings and needs. For example, people who outwardly appear dominating and strong and often manipulate and criticize others in reality may have low self-esteem and feel insecure. They do not verbalize their true feelings but act them out in behavior toward others. Insecurity and low self-esteem often translate into jealousy and mistrust of others and attempts to feel more important and strong by dominating or criticizing them.

UNDERSTANDING CONTEXT

Understanding the context of communication is extremely important in accurately identifying the meaning of a message. Think of the difference in the meaning of "I'm going to kill you!" when stated in two different contexts: anger during an argument and when one friend discovers another is planning a surprise party for him or her. Understanding the context of a situation gives the nurse more information and reduces the risk for assumptions.

To clarify context, the nurse must gather information from verbal and nonverbal sources and validate findings with the client. For example, if a client says, "I collapsed," she may mean she fainted or felt weak and had to sit down.

Or she could mean she was tired and went to bed. To clarify these terms and view them in the context of the action, the nurse could say

"What do you mean collapsed?" (seeking clarification) or
"Describe where you were and what you were doing when you collapsed." (placing events in time and sequence)

Assessment of context focuses on *who* was there, *what* happened, *when* it occurred, *how* the event progressed, and *why* the client believes it happened as it did.

UNDERSTANDING SPIRITUALITY

Spirituality is a client's belief about life, health, illness, death, and one's relationship to the universe. Spirituality differs from **religion**, which is an organized system of beliefs about one or more all-powerful, all-knowing forces that govern the universe and offer guidelines for living in harmony with the universe and others (Andrews & Boyle, 2003). Spiritual and religious beliefs usually are supported by others who share them and follow the same rules and rituals for daily living. Spirituality and religion often provide comfort and hope to people and can greatly affect a person's health and health care practices.

The nurse must first assess his or her own spiritual and religious beliefs. Religion and spirituality are highly subjective and can be vastly different among people. The nurse must remain objective and nonjudgmental regarding the client's beliefs and must not allow them to alter nursing care. The nurse must assess the client's spiritual and religious needs and guard against imposing his or her own on the client. The nurse must ensure that the client is not ignored or ridiculed because his or her beliefs and values differ from those of the staff (Chant et al., 2002).

As the therapeutic relationship develops, the nurse must be aware of and respect the client's religious and spiritual beliefs. Ignoring or being judgmental will quickly erode trust and could stall the relationship. For example, a nurse working with a Native American client could find him looking up at the sky and talking to "Grandmother Moon." If the nurse did not realize that the client's beliefs embody all things with spirit, including the sun, moon, earth, and trees, the nurse might misinterpret the client's actions as inappropriate. Chapter 7 gives a more detailed discussion on spirituality.

CULTURAL CONSIDERATIONS

Culture is all the socially learned behaviors, values, beliefs, and customs transmitted down to each generation. The rules about the way in which to conduct communication vary because they arise from each culture's specific social relationship patterns (Sheldon, 2004). Each culture has its own rules governing verbal and nonverbal communication. For example, in Western cultures, the handshake is a nonverbal greeting used primarily by men often to size up or judge someone they just met. For women, a polite "hello" is an accepted form of greeting. In some Asian cultures, bowing is the accepted form of greeting and departing and a method of designating social status.

Because of these differences, cultural assessment is necessary when establishing a therapeutic relationship. The nurse must assess the client's emotional expression, beliefs, values, and behaviors; modes of emotional expression; and views about mental health and illness.

When caring for people who do not speak English, the services of a qualified translator who is skilled at obtaining accurate data are necessary. He or she should be able to translate technical words into another language while retaining the original intent of the message and not injecting his or her own biases. The nurse is responsible for knowing how to contact a translator, regardless of whether the setting is inpatient, outpatient, or in the community.

The nurse must understand the differences in how various cultures communicate. It helps to see how a person from another culture acts toward and speaks with others. U.S. and many European cultures are individualistic; they value self-reliance and independence and focus on individual goals and achievements. Other cultures, such as Chinese and Korean, are collectivistic, valuing the group and observing obligations that enhance the security of the group. Persons from these cultures are more private and guarded when speaking to members outside the group and sometimes may even ignore outsiders until they are formally introduced to the group. Cultural differences in greetings, personal space, eye contact, touch, and beliefs about health and illness are discussed in-depth in Chapter 7.

THE THERAPEUTIC COMMUNICATION SESSION

Goals

The nurse uses all the therapeutic communication techniques and skills previously described to help achieve the following goals:

- Establish rapport with the client by being empathetic, genuine, caring, and unconditionally accepting of the client regardless of his or her behavior or beliefs.
- Actively listen to the client to identify the issues of concern and to formulate a client-centered goal for the interaction.
- Gain an in-depth understanding of the client's perception of the issue, and foster empathy in the nurse–client relationship.
- Explore the client's thoughts and feelings.
- Facilitate the client's expression of thoughts and feelings.
- Guide the client to develop new skills in problem-solving.
- Promote the client's evaluation of solutions.

Often the nurse can plan the time and setting for therapeutic communication, such as having an in-depth, one-on-one interaction with an assigned client. The nurse has time

to think about where to meet and what to say and will have a general idea of the topic, such as finding out what the client sees as his or her major concern or following up on interaction from a previous encounter. At times, however, a client may approach the nurse saying, "Can I talk to you right now?" Or the nurse may see a client sitting alone, crying, and decide to approach the client for an interaction. In these situations, the nurse may know that he or she will be trying to find out what is happening with the client at that moment in time.

When meeting the client for the first time, introducing oneself and establishing a contract for the relationship is an appropriate start for therapeutic communication. The nurse can ask the client how he or she prefers to be addressed. A **contract** for the relationship includes outlining the care the nurse will give, the times the nurse will be with the client, and acceptance of these conditions by the client.

Nurse: "Hello, Mr. Kirk. My name is Joan, and I'll be your nurse today. I'm here from 7 AM to 3:30 PM. Right now I have a few minutes, and I see you are dressed and ready for the day. I would like to spend some time talking with you if this is convenient." (giving recognition and introducing self, setting limits of contract)

After making the introduction and establishing the contract, the nurse can engage in small talk to break the ice and to help get acquainted with the client if they have not met before. Then the nurse can use a broad opening question to guide the client toward identifying the major topic of concern. Broad opening questions are helpful to begin the therapeutic communication session because they allow the client to focus on what he or she considers important. The following is a good example of how to begin the therapeutic communication:

Nurse: "Hello, Mrs. Nagy. My name is Donna, and I am your nurse today and tomorrow from 7 AM to 3 PM. What do you like to be called?" (introducing self, establishing limits of relationship)

Client: "Hi, Donna. You can call me Peggy."

Nurse: "The rain today has been a welcome relief from the heat of the past few days."

Client: "Really? It's hard to tell what it's doing outside. Still seems hot in here to me."

Nurse: "It does get stuffy here sometimes. So tell me, how are you doing today?" (broad opening)

NONDIRECTIVE ROLE

When beginning therapeutic interaction with a client, it is often the client (not the nurse) who identifies the problem he or she wants to discuss. The nurse uses active listening skills to identify the topic of concern. The client identifies the goal, and information-gathering about this topic focuses on the client. The nurse acts as a guide in this conversation. The therapeutic communication centers on achieving the goal within the time limits of the conversation.

The following are examples of client-centered goals:

- Client will discuss her concerns about her 16-year-old daughter, who is having trouble in school.
- Client will describe difficulty she has with side effects of her medication.
- Client will share his distress about son's drug abuse.
- Client will identify the greatest concerns he has about being a single parent.

The nurse is assuming a **nondirective role** in this type of therapeutic communication, using broad openings and open-ended questions to collect information and help the client to identify and discuss the topic of concern. The client does most of the talking. The nurse guides the client through the interaction, facilitating the client's expression of feelings and identification of issues. The following is an example of the nurse's nondirective role:

Client: "I'm so upset about my family."
    Nurse: "You're so upset?" (reflecting)
    Client: "Yes, I am. I can't sleep. My appetite is poor. I just don't know what to do."
Nurse: "Go on." (using a general lead)
Client: "Well, my husband works long hours and is very tired when he gets home. He barely sees the children before their bedtime."
Nurse: "I see." (accepting)
Client: "I'm busy trying to fix dinner, trying to keep an eye on the children, but I also want to talk to my husband."
Nurse: "How do you feel when all this is happening?" (encouraging expression)
Client: "Like I'm torn in several directions at once. Nothing seems to go right, and I can't straighten everything out."
Nurse: "It sounds like you're feeling overwhelmed." (translating into feelings)
Client: "Yes, I am. I can't do everything at once all by myself. I think we have to make some changes."
Nurse: "Perhaps you and I can discuss some potential changes you'd like to make." (suggesting collaboration)

In some therapeutic interactions, the client wants only to talk to an interested listener and feel like he or she has been heard. Often just sharing a distressing event can allow the client to express thoughts and emotions that he or she has been holding back. It serves as a way to lighten the emotional load and release feelings without a need to alter the situation. Other times, the client may need to reminisce and share pleasant memories of past events. Older adults often find great solace in reminiscing about events in their lives such as what was happening in the world when they were growing up, how they met and when they married their spouses, and so forth. Reminiscence is discussed further in Chapter 21.

DIRECTIVE ROLE

When the client is suicidal, experiencing a crisis, or out of touch with reality, the nurse uses a **directive role**, asking direct yes/no questions and using problem-solving to help the client develop new coping mechanisms to deal with present here-and-now issues. The following is an example of therapeutic communication using a more directive role:

Nurse: "I see you sitting here in the corner of the room away from everyone else." (making observation)
    Client: "Yeah, what's the point?"
    Nurse: "What's the point of what?" (seeking clarification)
Client: "Of anything"
Nurse: "You sound hopeless." (verbalizing the implied) "Are you thinking about suicide?" (seeking information)
Client: "I have been thinking I'd be better off dead."

The nurse uses a very directive role in this example because the client's safety is at issue.

As the nurse–client relationship progresses, the nurse uses therapeutic communication to implement many interventions in the client's plan of care. In Unit 4, specific mental illnesses and disorders are discussed, as are specific therapeutic communication interventions and examples of how to use the techniques effectively.

How to Phrase Questions

The manner in which the nurse phrases questions is important. Open-ended questions elicit more descriptive information; yes/no questions yield just an answer. The nurse asks different types of questions based on the information the nurse wishes to obtain. The nurse uses active listening to build questions based on the cues the client has given in his or her responses.

In English, people frequently substitute the word *feel* for the word *think*. Emotions differ from the cognitive process of thinking, so using the appropriate term is important. For example, "What do you feel about that test?" is a vague question that could elicit several types of answers. A more specific question is, "How well do you think you did on the test?" The nurse should ask, "What did you think about . . . ?" when discussing cognitive issues and "How did you feel about . . . ?" when trying to elicit the client's emotions and feelings. Box 6.1 lists "feeling" words that are commonly used to express or describe emotions. The following are examples of different responses that clients could give to questions using "think" and "feel":

Nurse: "What did you think about your daughter's role in her automobile accident?"
    Client: "I believe she is just not a careful driver. She drives too fast."
Nurse: "How did you feel when you heard about your daughter's automobile accident?"
Client: "Relieved that neither she nor anyone else was injured."

Using active listening skills, asking many open-ended questions, and building on the client's responses help the

Box 6.1   "FEELING" WORDS

Afraid	Hopeless
Alarmed	Horrified
Angry	Impatient
Anxious	Irritated
Ashamed	Jealous
Bewildered	Joyful
Calm	Lonely
Carefree	Pleased
Confused	Powerless
Depressed	Relaxed
Ecstatic	Resentful
Embarrassed	Sad
Enraged	Scared
Envious	Surprised
Excited	Tense
Fearful	Terrified
Frustrated	Threatened
Guilty	Thrilled
Happy	Uptight
Hopeful	

nurse obtain a complete description of an issue or an event and understand the client's experience. Some clients do not have the skill or patience to describe how an event unfolded over time without assistance from the nurse. Clients tend to recount the beginning and the end of a story, leaving out crucial information about their own behavior. The nurse can help the client by using techniques such as clarification and placing an event in time or sequence.

ASKING FOR CLARIFICATION

Nurses often believe they always should be able to understand what the client is saying. This is not always the case: The client's thoughts and communications may be unclear. The nurse never should assume that he or she understands; rather, the nurse should ask for clarification if there is doubt. Asking for clarification to confirm the nurse's understanding of what the client intends to convey is paramount to accurate data collection (Summers, 2002).

If the nurse needs more information or clarification on a previously discussed issue, he or she may need to return to that issue. The nurse also may need to ask questions in some areas to clarify information. The nurse then can use the therapeutic technique of consensual validation, or repeating his or her understanding of the event that the client just described to see whether their perceptions agree. It is important to go back and clarify rather than to work from assumptions.

The following is an example of clarifying and focusing techniques:

> **Client:** *"I saw it coming. No one else had a clue this would happen."*
>
> **Nurse:** *"What was it that you saw coming?"* (seeking information)
>
> **Client:** *"We were doing well, and then the floor dropped out from under us. There was little anyone could do but hope for the best."*
>
> **Nurse:** *"Help me understand by describing what 'doing well' refers to."* (seeking information)
>
> *"Who are the 'we' you refer to?"* (focusing)
>
> *"How did the floor drop out from under you?"* (encouraging description of perceptions)
>
> *"What did you hope would happen when you 'hoped for the best'?"* (seeking information)

CLIENT'S AVOIDANCE OF THE ANXIETY-PRODUCING TOPIC

Sometimes clients begin discussing a topic of minimal importance because it is less threatening than the issue that is increasing the client's anxiety. The client is discussing a topic but seems to be focused elsewhere. Active listening and observing changes in the intensity of the nonverbal process help to give the nurse a sense of what is going on. Many options can help the nurse to determine which topic is more important:

1. Ask the client which issue is more important at this time.
2. Go with the new topic because the client has given nonverbal messages that this is the issue that needs to be discussed.
3. Reflect the client's behavior signaling there is a more important issue to be discussed.
4. Mentally file the other topic away for later exploration.
5. Ignore the new topic because it seems that the client is trying to avoid the original topic.

The following example shows how the nurse can try to identify which issue is most important to the client:

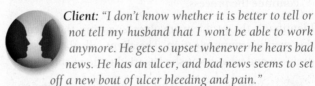

> **Client:** *"I don't know whether it is better to tell or not tell my husband that I won't be able to work anymore. He gets so upset whenever he hears bad news. He has an ulcer, and bad news seems to set off a new bout of ulcer bleeding and pain."*
>
> **Nurse:** *"Which issue is more difficult for you to confront right now: your bad news or your husband's ulcer?"* (encouraging expression)

Guiding the Client in Problem-Solving and Empowering the Client to Change

Many therapeutic situations involve problem-solving. The nurse is not expected to be an expert or to tell the client what to do to fix his or her problem. Rather, the nurse should help the client explore possibilities and find solutions to his or her problem. Often just helping the client to discuss and explore his or her perceptions of a problem stimulates potential solutions in the client's mind (Adkins, 2003). The nurse should introduce the concept of problem-solving and offer himself or herself in this process.

Virginia Satir (1967) explained how important the client's participation is to finding effective and meaningful solutions to problems. If someone else tells the client how to solve his or her problems and does not allow the client to participate and develop problem-solving skills and paths for change, the client may fear growth and change. The nurse who gives advice or directions about the way to fix a problem does not allow the client to play a role in the process and implies that the client is less than competent. This process makes the client feel helpless and not in control and lowers self-esteem. The client may even resist the directives in an attempt to regain a sense of control.

When a client is more involved in the problem-solving process, he or she is more likely to follow through on the solutions. The nurse who guides the client to solve his or her own problems helps the client to develop new coping strategies, maintains or increases the client's self-esteem, and demonstrates the belief that the client is capable of change. These goals encourage the client to expand his or her repertoire of skills and to feel competent; feeling effective and in control is a comfortable state for any client.

Problem-solving is frequently used in crisis intervention but is equally effective for general use. The problem-solving process is used when the client has difficulty finding ways to solve the problem or when working with a group of people whose divergent viewpoints hinder finding solutions. It involves several steps:

1. Identify the problem.
2. Brainstorm all possible solutions.
3. Select the best alternative.
4. Implement the selected alternative.
5. Evaluate the situation.
6. If dissatisfied with results, select another alternative and continue the process.

Identifying the problem involves engaging the client in therapeutic communication. The client tells the nurse the problem and what he or she has tried to do to solve it:

> **Nurse:** *"I see you frowning. What is going on?"* (making observation; broad opening)
> **Client:** *"I've tried to get my husband more involved with the children other than yelling at them when he comes in from work, but I've had little success."*
> **Nurse:** *"What have you tried that has not worked?"* (encouraging expression)
> **Client:** *"Before my surgery, I tried to involve him in their homework. My husband is a math whiz. Then I tried TV time together, but the kids like cartoons and he wants to watch stuff about history, natural science, or travel."*

> **Nurse:** *"How have you involved your husband in this plan for him to get more involved with the children?"* (seeking information)
> **Client:** *"Uh, I haven't. I mean, he always says he wants to spend more quality time with the kids, but he doesn't. Do you mean it would be better for him to decide how he wants to do this—I mean, spend quality time with the kids?"*
> **Nurse:** *"That sounds like a place to start. Perhaps you and your husband could discuss this issue when he comes to visit and decide what would work for both of you."* (formulating a plan of action)

It is important to remember that the nurse is facilitating the client's problem-solving abilities. The nurse may not believe the client is choosing the best or most effective solution, but it is essential that the nurse supports the client's choice and assists him or her to implement the chosen alternative. If the client makes a mistake or the selected alternative isn't successful, the nurse can support the client's efforts and assist the client to try again. Effective problem-solving involves helping the client to resolve his or her own problems as independently as possible.

COMMUNITY-BASED CARE

As community care for people with physical and mental health problems continues to expand, the nurse's role expands as well. The nurse may become the major caregiver and resource person for increasingly high-risk clients treated in the home, and their families and may become more responsible for primary prevention in wellness and health maintenance. Therapeutic communication techniques and skills are essential to successful management of clients in the community.

Caring for older adults in the family unit and in communities today is a major nursing concern and responsibility. It is important to assess the relationships of family members; identifying their areas of agreement and conflict can greatly affect the care of clients. To be responsive to the needs of these clients and their families for support and caring, the nurse must communicate and relate to clients and establish a therapeutic relationship.

When practicing in the community, the nurse needs self-awareness and knowledge about cultural differences. When the nurse enters the home of a client, the nurse is the outsider and must learn to negotiate the cultural context of each family by understanding their beliefs, customs, and practices and not judging them according to his or her own cultural context. Asking the family for help in learning about their culture demonstrates the nurse's unconditional positive regard and genuineness. Families from other cultural backgrounds often respect nurses and health care professionals and are quite patient and forgiving of the cultural mistakes that nurses might make as they learn different customs and behaviors.

Another reason the nurse needs to understand the health care practices of various cultures is to make sure these practices do not hinder or alter the prescribed therapeutic regimens. Some cultural healing practices, remedies, and even dietary practices may alter the client's immune system and may enhance or interfere with prescribed medications.

The nurse in community care is a member of the health care team and must learn to collaborate with the client and family as well as with other health care providers who are involved in the client's care such as physicians, physical therapists, psychologists, and home health aides.

Working with several people at one time rather than just with the client is the standard in community care. Self-awareness and sensitivity to the beliefs, behaviors, and feelings of others are paramount to the successful care of clients in the community setting.

 ## SELF-AWARENESS ISSUES

Therapeutic communication is the primary vehicle that nurses use to apply the nursing process in mental health settings. The nurse's skill in therapeutic communication influences the effectiveness of many interventions. Therefore, the nurse must evaluate and improve his or her communication skills on an ongoing basis. When the nurse examines his or her personal beliefs, attitudes, and values as they relate to communication, he or she is gaining awareness of the factors influencing communication. Gaining awareness of how one communicates is the first step toward improving communication.

The nurse will experience many different emotional reactions to clients, such as sadness, anger, frustration, and discomfort. The nurse must reflect on these experiences to determine how emotional responses affect both verbal and nonverbal communication. When working with clients from different cultural or ethnic backgrounds, the nurse needs to know or find out what communication styles are comfortable for the client in terms of eye contact, touch, proximity, and so forth. The nurse can then adapt his or her communication style in ways that are beneficial to the nurse–client relationship.

Points to Consider When Working on Therapeutic Communication Skills

- Remember that nonverbal communication is just as important as the words you speak. Be mindful of your facial expression, body posture, and other nonverbal aspects of communication as you work with clients.
- Ask colleagues for feedback about your communication style. Ask them how they communicate with clients in difficult or uncomfortable situations.
- Examine your communication by asking questions such as "How do I relate to men? To women? To authority figures? To elderly persons? To people from cultures different from my own?" "What types of clients or situations make me uncomfortable? Sad? Angry? Frustrated?" Use these self-assessment data to improve your communication skills.

Critical Thinking Questions

1. Explain why the nurse's attempt to solve the client's problem is less effective than guiding the client to identify his or her own ways to resolve the issue.
2. The nurse is working with a client whose culture includes honoring one's parents and being obedient, keeping "private" matters within the family only, and not talking with strangers about family matters. Given this client's belief system, how will the nurse use therapeutic communication effectively?

KEY POINTS

- Communication is the process people use to exchange information through verbal and nonverbal messages. It is composed of both the literal words or content and all the nonverbal messages (process), including body language, eye contact, facial expression, tone of voice, rate of speech, context, and hesitations that accompany the words. To communicate effectively, the nurse must be skilled in the analysis of both content and process.
- Therapeutic communication is an interpersonal interaction between the nurse and client during which the nurse focuses on the needs of the client to promote an effective exchange of information between the nurse and client.
- Goals of therapeutic communication include establishing rapport, actively listening, gaining the client's perspective, exploring the client's thoughts and feelings, and guiding the client in problem-solving.
- The crucial components of therapeutic communication are confidentiality, privacy, respect for boundaries, self-disclosure, use of touch, and active listening and observation skills.
- Proxemics is concerned with the distance zones between people when they communicate: intimate, personal, social, and public.
- Active listening involves refraining from other internal mental activities and concentrating exclusively on what the client is saying.
- Verbal messages need to be clear and concrete rather than vague and abstract. Abstract messages requiring the client to make assumptions can be misleading and confusing. The nurse needs to clarify any areas of confusion so that he or she does not make assumptions based on his or her own experiences.
- Nonverbal communication includes facial expressions, body language, eye contact, proxemics (environmental distance), touch, and vocal cues. All are important in understanding the speaker's message.
- Understanding the context is important to the accuracy of the message. Assessment of context focuses on the who, what, when, how, and why of an event.

INTERNET RESOURCES

RESOURCE	INTERNET ADDRESS
• Resources for Listening and Communicating	http://www.allaboutcounseling.com
• Seven Keys to Listening	http://www.stresscure.com/relation/7keys.html
• Team Communication	http://www.yorkteam.com/teamc.htm

- Spirituality and religion can greatly affect a client's health and health care. These beliefs vary widely and are highly subjective. The nurse must be careful not to impose his or her beliefs on the client or to allow differences to erode trust.
- Cultural differences can greatly affect the therapeutic communication process.
- When guiding a client in the problem-solving process, it is important that the client (not the nurse) chooses and implements solutions.
- Therapeutic communication techniques and skills are essential to successful management of clients in the community.
- The greater the nurse's understanding of his or her own feelings and responses, the better the nurse can communicate and understand others.

REFERENCES

Adkins, E. (2003). The first day of the rest of their lives. *Journal of Psychosocial Nursing and Mental Services, 41*(7), 28–32.

Andrews, M., & Boyle, J. (2003). *Transcultural concepts in nursing care* (4th ed.). Philadelphia: Lippincott Williams & Wilkins.

Chant, S., Jenkinson, T., Randle, J., et al. (2002). Communication skills: Some problems in nursing education and practice. *Journal of Clinical Nursing, 11*(1), 12–21.

DeVito, J. A. (2004). *The interpersonal communication handbook* (10th ed.). Boston: Pearson Education.

Greene, J. O., & Burleson, B. R. (Eds.). (2003). *Handbook of communication and social interaction skills.* Mahwah, NJ: Erlbaum Associates.

Hall, E. (1963). Proxemics: The study of man's spatial relationships. In J. Gladstone (Ed.), *Man's image in medicine and anthropology* (pp. 109–120). Philadelphia: Mosby.

Knapp, M. L. (1980). *Essentials of nonverbal communication.* New York: Holt, Rinehart & Winston.

Knapp, M. L., & Hall, J. (2002). *Nonverbal behavior in human interaction* (5th ed.). New York: Wadsworth.

Peplau, H. (1952). *Interpersonal relations in nursing.* New York: G. P. Putnam.

Satir, V. (1967). *Conjoint family therapy: A guide to theory and technique* (rev. ed.). Palo Alto, CA: Science and Behavior Books, Inc.

Sheldon, L. K. (2004). *Communication for nurses: Talking with patients.* Thorofare, NJ: SLACK, Inc.

Summers, L. C. (2002). Mutual timing: An essential component of provider/patient communication. *Journal of the American Academy of Nurse Practitioners, 14*(1), 19–25.

ADDITIONAL READINGS

Castledine, G. (2002). Nurses' bedside manner: Is it deteriorating? *British Journal of Nursing, 11*(10), 723.

Crouch, R. (2002). Communication is the key. *Emergency Nurse, 10*(3), 3–5.

Dineen, K. (2002). Gift of presence. *Nursing 02, 32*(6), 76.

Fox, V. (2000). Empathy: The wonder quality of mental health treatment. *Psychiatric Rehabilitation Journal, 23*(3), 292–293.

Kuehn, A. (2002). Communication and the nursing shortage. *American Nurse, 34*(3), 6–7.

Puentas, W. J. (2000). Using social reminiscence to teach therapeutic communication skills. *Geriatric Nursing, 21*(6), 315–318.

Wallace, L. (2002). More than good manners. *Nursing 02, 33*(7), 32.

Chapter Study Guide

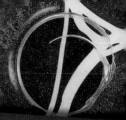

MULTIPLE-CHOICE QUESTIONS

Select the best answer for each of the following questions.

1. Client: "I had an accident."

   Nurse: "Tell me about your accident."

   This is an example of which therapeutic communication technique?
   A. Making observations
   B. Offering self
   C. General lead
   D. Reflection

2. "Earlier today you said you were concerned that your son was still upset with you. When I stopped by your room about an hour ago, you and your son seemed relaxed and smiling as you spoke to each other. How did things go between the two of you?"

   This is an example of which therapeutic communication technique?
   A. Consensual validation
   B. Encouraging comparison
   C. Accepting
   D. General lead

3. "Why do you always complain about the night nurse? She is a nice woman and a fine nurse and has five kids to support. You're wrong when you say she is noisy and uncaring."

   This example reflects which nontherapeutic technique?
   A. Requesting an explanation
   B. Defending
   C. Disagreeing
   D. Advising

4. "How does Jerry make you upset?" is a nontherapeutic communication technique because it
   A. Gives a literal response
   B. Indicates an external source of the emotion
   C. Interprets what the client is saying
   D. Is just another stereotyped comment

5. Client: "I was so upset about my sister ignoring my pain when I broke my leg."

   Nurse: "When are you going to your next diabetes education program?"

   This is a nontherapeutic response because the nurse has
   A. Used testing to evaluate the client's insight
   B. Changed the topic
   C. Exhibited an egocentric focus
   D. Advised the client what to do

6. When the client says, "I met Joe at the dance last week," what is the best way for the nurse to ask the client to describe her relationship with Joe?
   A. "Joe who?"
   B. "Tell me about Joe."
   C. "Tell me about you and Joe."
   D. "Joe, you mean that blond guy with the dark blue eyes?"

7. Which of the following is a concrete message?
   A. "Help me put this pile of books on Marsha's desk."
   B. "Get this out of here."
   C. "When is she coming home?"
   D. "They said it is too early to get in."

SHORT-ANSWER QUESTIONS

Define the following.

1. Culture

2. Proxemics

3. Incongruent message

4. Spirituality

5. Nonverbal communication

6. Cliché

7. Metaphor

8. Therapeutic use of self

In the following client statements, underline the cues (words, phrases, or issues) that should be followed up with therapeutic communication interventions. Then, write a therapeutic response.

1. "I feel good."

2. "I can't take it anymore."

3. "I have two children, one from my wife and one from my girlfriend."

4. "We were standing on the corner."

5. "My son is never going to understand the way his wife is ruining them."

Client's Response to Illness

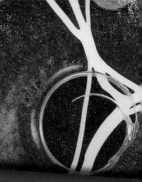

Key Terms

- culturally competent
- culture
- environmental control
- ethnicity
- hardiness
- race
- resilience
- resourcefulness
- self-efficacy
- sense of belonging
- social network
- social organization
- social support
- socioeconomic status
- spirituality
- time orientation

Learning Objectives

After reading this chapter, you should be able to

1. Discuss the influences of age, growth, and development on a client's response to illness.

2. Identify the roles that physical health and biologic makeup play in a client's emotional responses.

3. Explain the importance of personal characteristics, such as self-efficacy, hardiness, resilience, resourcefulness, and spirituality, in a client's response to stressors.

4. Explain the influence of interpersonal factors, such as sense of belonging, social networks, and family support, on the client's response to illness.

5. Describe various cultural beliefs and practices that can affect mental health or illness.

6. Explain the cultural factors that the nurse must assess and consider when working with clients of different cultural backgrounds.

7. Explain the nurse's role in assessing and working with clients of different cultural backgrounds.

Visit the **Point** http://thePoint.lww.com for NCLEX-style questions, journal articles, and more!

Nursing philosophies often describe the person or individual as a biopsychosocial being who possesses unique characteristics and responds to others and the world in various and diverse ways. This view of the individual as unique requires nurses to assess each person and his or her responses to plan and provide nursing care that is personally meaningful. This uniqueness of response may partially explain why some people become ill and others do not. Understanding why two people raised in a stressful environment (e.g., one with neglect or abuse) turn out differently is difficult: one person becomes reasonably successful and maintains a satisfying marriage and family, whereas the other feels isolated, depressed, and lonely; is divorced; and abuses alcohol. Although we do not know exactly what makes the difference, studies have begun to show that certain personal, interpersonal, and cultural factors influence a person's response.

Culture is all the socially learned behaviors, values, beliefs, customs, and ways of thinking of a population that guide its members' views of themselves and the world. This view affects all aspects of the person's being, including health, illness, and treatment. Cultural diversity refers to the vast array of differences that exist among populations.

This chapter examines some of the personal, interpersonal, and cultural factors that create the unique individual response to both illness and treatment. In determining how a person copes with illness, we cannot single out one or two factors. Rather, we must consider each person as a combination of all these overlapping and interacting factors.

INDIVIDUAL FACTORS

Age, Growth, and Development

A person's age seems to affect how he or she copes with illness. For instance, the age at onset of schizophrenia is a strong predictor of the prognosis of the disease (Buchanan & Carpenter, 2005). People with a younger age at onset have poorer outcomes, such as more negative signs (apathy, social isolation, lack of volition) and less effective coping skills, than do people with a later age at onset. A possible reason for this difference is that younger clients have not had experiences of successful independent living or the opportunity to work and be self-sufficient and have a less well-developed sense of personal identity than older clients.

A client's age also can influence how he or she expresses illness. A young child with attention deficit hyperactivity disorder may lack the understanding and ability to describe his or her feelings, which may make management of the disorder more challenging. Nurses must be aware of the child's level of language and work to understand the experience as he or she describes it.

Erik Erikson described psychosocial development across the life span in terms of developmental tasks to accomplish at each stage (Table 7.1). Each stage of development depends on the successful completion of the previous stage. In each stage, the person must complete a critical life task that is essential to well-being and mental health. Failure to complete the critical task results in a negative outcome for that stage of development and impedes completion of future tasks. For example, the infancy stage (birth to 18 months) is the stage of "trust versus mistrust," when infants must learn to develop basic trust that their parents or guardians will take care of them, feed them, change their diapers, love them, and keep them safe. If the infant does not develop trust in this stage, he or she may be unable to love and trust others later in life because the ability to trust others is essential to establishing good relationships. Specific developmental tasks for adults are summarized in Table 7.2.

According to Erikson's theory, people may get "stuck" at any stage of development. For example, a person who

Table 7.1	ERIKSON'S STAGES OF PSYCHOSOCIAL DEVELOPMENT
Stage	**Tasks**
Trust vs. mistrust (infant)	Viewing the world as safe and reliable
	Viewing relationships as nurturing, stable, and dependable
Autonomy vs. shame and doubt (toddler)	Achieving a sense of control and free will
Initiative vs. guilt (preschool)	Beginning to develop a conscience
	Learning to manage conflict and anxiety
Industry vs. inferiority (school age)	Building confidence in own abilities
	Taking pleasure in accomplishments
Identity vs. role diffusion (adolescence)	Formulating a sense of self and belonging
Intimacy vs. isolation (young adult)	Forming adult, loving relationships and meaningful attachment to others
	Being creative and productive
Generativity vs. stagnation (middle adult)	Establishing the next generation
Ego integrity vs. despair (maturity)	Accepting responsibility for one's self and life

Table 7.2   ADULT GROWTH AND DEVELOPMENT TASKS

Stage	Tasks
Young adult (25–45 years of age)	Accept self.
	Stabilize self-image.
	Establish independence from parental home and financial independence.
	Establish a career or vocation.
	Form an intimate bond with another person.
	Build a congenial social and friendship group.
	Become an involved citizen.
	Establish and maintain a home.
Middle adult (45–65 years of age)	Express love through more than sexual contacts.
	Maintain healthy life patterns.
	Develop sense of unity with mate.
	Help growing and grown children to be responsible adults.
	Relinquish central role in lives of grown children.
	Accept children's mates and friends.
	Create a comfortable home.
	Be proud of accomplishments of self and mate/spouse.
	Reverse roles with aging parents.
	Achieve mature civic and social responsibility.
	Adjust to physical changes of middle age.
	Use leisure time creatively.
	Cherish old friends and make new ones.
Older adult (65 years of age and older)	Prepare for retirement.
	Recognize the aging process and its limitations.
	Adjust to health changes.
	Decide where to live out remaining years.
	Continue warm relationship with mate/spouse.
	Adjust living standards to retirement income.
	Maintain maximum level of health.
	Care for self physically and emotionally.
	Maintain contact with children and relatives.
	Maintain interest in people outside the family.
	Find meaning in life after retirement.
	Adjust to the death of mate/spouse or other loved ones.

never completed the developmental task of autonomy may become overly dependent on others. Failure to develop identity can result in role confusion or an unclear idea about whom one is as a person. Negotiating these developmental tasks affects how the person responds to stress and illness. Lack of success may result in feelings of inferiority, doubt, lack of confidence, and isolation—all of which can affect how a person responds to illness.

Genetics and Biologic Factors

Heredity and biologic factors are not under voluntary control. We cannot change these factors. Research has identified genetic links to several disorders. For example, some people are born with a gene associated with one type of Alzheimer's disease. Although specific genetic links have not been identified for several mental disorders (e.g., bipolar disorder, major depression, alcoholism), research has shown that these dis-

orders tend to appear more frequently in families. Genetic makeup tremendously influences a person's response to illness and perhaps even to treatment. Hence, family history and background are essential parts of the nursing assessment.

Physical Health and Health Practices

Physical health also can influence how a person responds to psychosocial stress or illness. The healthier a person is, the better he or she can cope with stress or illness. Poor nutritional status, lack of sleep, or a chronic physical illness may impair a person's ability to cope. Unlike genetic factors, how a person lives and takes care of himself or herself can alter many of these factors. For this reason, nurses must assess the client's physical health even when the client is seeking help for mental health problems.

Personal health practices, such as exercise, can influence the client's response to illness. Brugman and Ferguson

(2002) found that walking and stretching exercises diminished the negative effects of depression and anxiety. Further, when individuals participated with others in a walking group, the members of the group reported increased social support and an improved sense of well-being. This suggests that continued participation in exercise is a positive indicator of improved health, whereas cessation from participation in exercise might indicate declining mental health.

Response to Drugs

Biologic differences can affect a client's response to treatment, specifically to psychotropic drugs. Ethnic groups differ in the metabolism and efficacy of psychoactive compounds. Some ethnic groups metabolize drugs more slowly (meaning the serum level of the drug remains higher), which increases the frequency and severity of side effects. Clients who metabolize drugs more slowly generally need lower doses of a drug to produce the desired effect (Purnell & Paulanka, 2003). In general, nonwhites treated with Western dosing protocols have higher serum levels per dose and suffer more side effects. Although many non-Western countries report successful treatment with lower dosages of psychotropic drugs, Western dosage protocols continue to drive prescribing practices in the United States. When evaluating the efficacy of psychotropic medications, the nurse must be alert to side effects and serum drug levels in clients from different ethnic backgrounds.

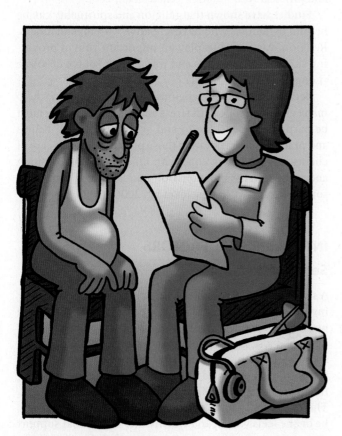

Assess client's physical health

Self-Efficacy

Self-efficacy is a belief that personal abilities and efforts affect the events in our lives. A person who believes that his or her behavior makes a difference is more likely to take action. People with high self-efficacy set personal goals, are self-motivated, cope effectively with stress, and request support from others when needed. People with low self-efficacy have low aspirations, experience much self-doubt, and may be plagued by anxiety and depression. Bandura (2004) suggested that rather than focusing on solving specific problems, treatment should focus on developing a client's skills to take control of his or her life (developing self-efficacy) so that he or she can make life changes. The four main ways to do so are as follows:

- Experience of success or mastery in overcoming obstacles
- Social modeling (observing successful people instills the idea that one also can succeed)
- Social persuasion (persuading people to believe in themselves)
- Reducing stress, building physical strength, and learning how to interpret physical sensations positively (e.g., viewing fatigue as a sign that one has accomplished something rather than as a lack of stamina)

Cutler (2005) reports a relationship between self-efficacy and the client's motivation for self-care and follow-up after discharge from treatment. Clients returning to the community with higher self-efficacy were more confident and had positive expectations about their personal success. She suggests that therapeutic interventions designed to promote the client's self-efficacy can have positive effects on interpersonal relationships and coping upon return to the community.

Hardiness

Hardiness is the ability to resist illness when under stress. First described by Kobasa (1979), hardiness has three components:

1. Commitment: active involvement in life activities
2. Control: ability to make appropriate decisions in life activities
3. Challenge: ability to perceive change as beneficial rather than just stressful

Hardiness has been found to have a moderating or buffering effect on people experiencing stress. Kobasa (1979) found that male executives who had high stress but low occurrence of illness scored higher on the hardiness scale than executives with high stress and high occurrence of illness. Study findings suggested that stressful life events caused more harm to people with low hardiness than with high hardiness.

Hardiness also has been studied in relation to chronic illness. Brooks (2003) found that higher levels of hardiness had positive outcomes in patients with chronic illness. This included better physiologic and improved psychosocial adaptation to the chronic illness.

Personal hardiness is often described as a pattern of attitudes and actions that helps the person turn stressful circumstances into opportunities for growth. Maddi (2005) found that persons with high hardiness perceived stressors more accurately and were able to problem-solve in the situation more effectively. Hardiness has been identified as an important resilience factor for families coping with the mental illness of one of their members (Greeff et al., 2006).

Some believe that the concept of hardiness is vague and indistinct and may not help everyone. Some research on hardiness suggests that its effects are not the same for men and women. In addition, hardiness may be useful only to those who value individualism, such as people from some Western cultures. For people and cultures who value relationships over individual achievement, hardiness may not be beneficial.

Resilience and Resourcefulness

Two closely related concepts, resilience and resourcefulness, help people to cope with stress and to minimize the effects of illness (Edward & Warelow, 2005). **Resilience** is defined as having healthy responses to stressful circumstances or risky situations. This concept helps to explain why one person reacts to a slightly stressful event with severe anxiety, whereas another person does not experience distress even when confronting a major disruption. Studies on resiliency first focused on factors that resulted in positive outcomes for children who were at risk because their parents had alcohol or mental health problems. Factors that enhanced outcomes were children's abilities to develop self-esteem and self-efficacy through relationships with others, have new experiences, and obtain assistance with life transitions as they matured (Krafcik, 2002).

Studies found that families who use their strengths show improved resiliency and more positive outcomes than families who view themselves as victims of multiple problems, such as poverty, unemployment, and low socioeconomic status. Family protective mechanisms that improve the resiliency of children include instilling positive family values, promoting positive communication and social interaction, maintaining flexible family roles, exercising control over children, and providing academic support to children. Family protective factors that improve the resiliency of adolescents include caring and supportive relationships with adult caregivers; high expectations for good citizenship, academic achievement, and spiritual involvement; and encouragement to participate in caring for siblings, household chores, part-time work, and carefully selected safe activities outside the home.

Resourcefulness involves using problem-solving abilities and believing that one can cope with adverse or novel situations. People develop resourcefulness through interactions with others, that is, through successfully coping with life experiences (Krafcik, 2002). Examples of resourcefulness include performing health-seeking behaviors, learning self-care, monitoring one's thoughts and feelings about stressful situations, and taking action to deal with stressful circumstances.

Spirituality

Spirituality involves the essence of a person's being and his or her beliefs about the meaning of life and the purpose for living. It may include belief in God or a higher power, the practice of religion, cultural beliefs and practices, and a relationship with the environment. Although many clients with mental disorders have disturbing religious delusions, for many in the general population, religion and spirituality are a source of comfort and help in times of stress or trauma. Studies have shown that spirituality is a genuine help to many adults with mental illness, serving as a primary coping device and a source of meaning and coherence in their lives or helping to provide a social network (Sageman, 2004).

Religious activities such as church attendance and praying and associated social support have been shown to be very important for many people and are linked with better health and a sense of well-being. These activities also have been found to help people cope with poor health. Hope and faith have been identified as critical factors in psychiatric and physical rehabilitation (Baetz et al., 2002).

Studies have shown that religion and spirituality can be helpful to families who have a relative with mental illness. Religion was found to play an important role in providing support to caregivers and was a major source of solace (Longo & Peterson, 2002).

Because spiritual or religious beliefs and practices help many clients to cope with stress and illness, the nurse must be particularly sensitive to and accepting of such beliefs and practices. Incorporating those practices into the care of clients can help them cope with illness and find meaning and purpose in the situation. Doing so can also offer a strong source of support (Huguelet et al., 2006).

INTERPERSONAL FACTORS

Sense of Belonging

A **sense of belonging** is the feeling of connectedness with or involvement in a social system or environment of which a person feels an integral part (Ross, 2002). Abraham Maslow described a sense of belonging as a basic human psychosocial need that involves both feelings of value and fit. *Value* refers to feeling needed and accepted. *Fit* refers to feeling that one meshes or fits in with the system or environment. This means that when a person belongs to a system or group, he or she feels valued and worthwhile within that support system. Examples of support systems include family, friends,

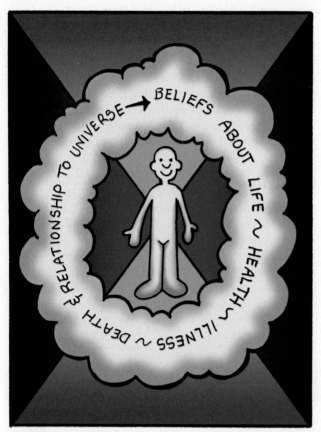

Spirituality

not supported (Vanderhorst & McLaren, 2005). Meaningful social relationships with family or friends were found to improve the health and well-being outcomes for older adults. An essential element of improved outcomes is that family or friends respond with support when it is requested. In other words, the person must be able to count on these friends or family to help or support him or her by visiting or talking on the phone. Thus, the primary components of satisfactory support are the person's ability and willingness to request support when needed and the ability and willingness of the support system to respond.

Two key components are necessary for a support system to be effective: the client's perception of the support system and the responsiveness of the support system. The client must perceive that the social support system bolsters his or her confidence and self-esteem and provides such stress-related interpersonal help as offering assistance in solving a problem. The client also must perceive that the actions of the support system are consistent with the client's desires and expectations—in other words, the support provided is what the client wants, not what the supporter believes would be good for the client. Also, the support system must be able to provide direct help or material aid (e.g., providing transportation, making a follow-up appointment). Some people have the capacity to seek help when needed, whereas a lack of well-being may cause others to withdraw from potential providers of support. The nurse can help the client to find support people who will be available and helpful and can teach the client to request support when needed.

coworkers, clubs or social groups, and even health care providers.

A person's sense of belonging is closely related to his or her social and psychological functioning. A sense of belonging was found to promote health, whereas a lack of belonging impaired health. An increased sense of belonging also was associated with decreased levels of anxiety. Persons with a sense of belonging are less alienated and isolated, have a sense of purpose, believe they are needed by others, and feel productive socially. Hence, the nurse should focus on interventions that help increase a client's sense of belonging (Granerud & Severinsson, 2006).

Social Networks and Social Support

Social networks are groups of people whom one knows and with whom one feels connected. Studies have found that having a social network can help reduce stress, diminish illness, and positively influence the ability to cope and to adapt (Chanokruthai et al., 2005). **Social support** is emotional sustenance that comes from friends, family members, and even health care providers who help a person when a problem arises. It is different from social contact, which does not always provide emotional support. An example of social contact is the friendly talk that goes on at parties.

Persons who are supported emotionally and functionally have been found to be healthier than those who are

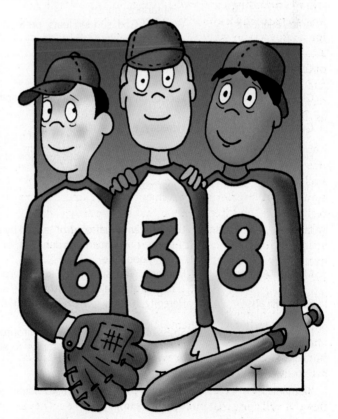

Sense of belonging

Family Support

Family as a source of social support can be a key factor in the recovery of clients with psychiatric illnesses. Although family members are not always a positive resource in mental health, they are most often an important part of recovery. Health care professionals cannot totally replace family members. The nurse must encourage family members to continue to support the client even while he or she is in the hospital and should identify family strengths, such as love and caring, as a resource for the client (Reid et al., 2005).

CULTURAL FACTORS

According to the U.S. Census Bureau, 33% of U.S. residents currently are members of nonwhite cultures. By 2050, the nonwhite population will more than triple. This changing composition of society has implications for health care professionals, who are predominantly white and unfamiliar with different cultural beliefs and practices (Purnell & Paulanka,

2003). **Culturally competent** nursing care means being sensitive to issues related to culture, race, gender, sexual orientation, social class, economic situation, and other factors.

Nurses and other health care providers must learn about other cultures and become skilled at providing care to people with cultural backgrounds that are different from their own. Finding out about another's cultural beliefs and practices and understanding their meaning is essential to providing holistic and meaningful care to the client (Table 7.3).

Beliefs About Causes of Illness

Culture has the most influence on a person's health beliefs and practices (Campinha-Bacote, 2002). Culture has been shown to influence one's concept of disease and illness. The two prevalent types of beliefs about what causes illness in non-Western cultures are personalistic and naturalistic. *Personalistic* beliefs attribute the cause of illness to the active, purposeful intervention of an outside agent, spirit, or supernatural force or deity. The *naturalistic* view

Table 7.3	CULTURAL BELIEFS ABOUT HEALTH AND ILLNESS	
Culture	**Illness Beliefs: Causes of Mental Illness**	**Concept of Health**
African American	Lack of spiritual balance	Feelings of well-being, able to fulfill role expectations, free of pain or excess stress
American Indians	Loss of harmony with natural world, breaking of taboos, ghosts	Holistic and wellness-oriented
Arab Americans	Wrath of God, sudden fears, pretending to be ill to manipulate family	Gift of God manifested by eating well, meeting social obligations, being in a good mood, having no stressors or pain
Cambodians	Khmer Rouge brutalities	Health as equilibrium, individually maintained but influenced by family and community
Chinese	Lack of harmony of emotions, evil spirits	Health maintained by balance of *yin* and *yang*, body, mind, and spirit
Cubans	Heredity, extreme stress	Fat and rosy-cheeked (traditional); fitness and staying trim (acculturated)
Filipinos	Disruption of harmonious function of individual and spirit world	Maintaining balance; good health involves good food, strength, and no pain
Haitians	Supernatural causes	Maintenance of equilibrium by eating well, paying attention to personal hygiene; prayer and good spiritual habits
Japanese Americans	Loss of mental self-control caused by evil spirits, punishment for behavior, or not living good life	Balance and harmony among oneself, society, and universe
Mexican Americans	Humoral, God, spirituality, and interpersonal relationships all can contribute	Feeling well and being able to maintain role function
Puerto Ricans	Heredity, follows *sufriamientos* (suffering)	No mental, spiritual, or physical discomforts; being clean and not being too thin
Russians	Stress and moving into new environment	Regular bowel movements and no symptoms
South Asians	Spells cast by enemy, falling prey to evil spirit	Balance of digestive fire, bodily humors, and waste products; senses functioning normally; body, mind, and spirit in harmony
Vietnamese	Disruption of harmony in individual; ancestral spirit haunting	Harmony and balance within oneself

is rooted in a belief that natural conditions or forces, such as cold, heat, wind, or dampness, are responsible for the illness (Campinha-Bacote, 2002). A sick person with these beliefs would not see the relationship between his or her behavior or health practices and the illness. Thus, he or she would try to counteract the negative forces or spirits using traditional cultural remedies rather than taking medication or changing his or her health practices.

Factors in Cultural Assessment

Giger and Davidhizar (2003) recommended a model for assessing clients using six cultural phenomena: communication, physical distance or space, social organization, time orientation, environmental control, and biologic variations (Box 7.1). Each phenomenon is discussed in more detail below and in Table 7.4.

COMMUNICATION

Verbal communication can be difficult when the client and nurse do not speak the same language. The nurse should be aware that nonverbal communication has different meanings in various cultures. For example, some cultures welcome touch and consider it supportive, whereas other cultures find touch offensive. Some Asian women avoid shaking hands with one another or men. Some Native American tribes believe that vigorous handshaking is aggressive, whereas people from Spain and France consider a firm handshake a sign of strength and good character.

Although Western cultures view direct eye contact as positive, Native American and Asian cultures may find it rude, and people from these backgrounds may avoid looking strangers in the eye when talking to them. People from Middle Eastern cultures can maintain very intense eye contact, which may appear to be glaring to those from different cultures. These differences are important to note because many people make inferences about a person's behavior based on the frequency or duration of eye contact.

Box 7.1 IMPORTANT FACTORS IN CULTURAL ASSESSMENT

Communication
Physical distance or space
Social organization
Time orientation
Environmental control
Biologic variations

Giger, J. N., & Davidhizar, R. E. (2003). Transcultural nursing: Assessment and intervention *(4th ed.). St. Louis: Mosby.*

Chapter 6 provides a detailed discussion of communication techniques.

PHYSICAL DISTANCE OR SPACE

Various cultures have different perspectives on what they consider a comfortable physical distance from another person during communication. In the United States and many other Western cultures, 2 to 3 feet is a comfortable distance. Latin Americans and people from the Middle East tend to stand closer to one another than do people in Western cultures. People from Asian and Native American cultures are usually more comfortable with distances greater than 2 or 3 feet. The nurse should be conscious of these cultural differences in space and should allow enough room for clients to be comfortable (Giger & Davidhizar, 2003).

SOCIAL ORGANIZATION

Social organization refers to family structure and organization, religious values and beliefs, ethnicity, and culture, all of which affect a person's role and, therefore, his or her health and illness behavior. In Western cultures, people may seek the advice of a friend or family member or may make most decisions independently. Many Chinese, Mexican, Vietnamese, and Puerto Rican Americans strongly value the role of family in making health care decisions. People from these backgrounds may delay making decisions until they can consult appropriate family members. Autonomy in health care decisions is an unfamiliar and undesirable concept because the cultures consider the collective to be greater than the individual.

TIME ORIENTATION

Time orientation, or whether one views time as precise or approximate, differs among cultures. Many Western countries focus on the urgency of time, valuing punctuality and precise schedules. Clients from other cultures may not perceive the importance of adhering to specific follow-up appointments or procedures or time-related treatment regimens. Health care providers can become resentful and angry when these clients miss appointments or fail to follow specific treatment regimens such as taking medications at prescribed times. Nurses should not label such clients as noncompliant when their behavior may be related to a different cultural orientation to the meaning of time. When possible, the nurse should be sensitive to the client's time orientation, as with follow-up appointments. When timing is essential, as with some medications, the nurse can explain the importance of more precise timing.

ENVIRONMENTAL CONTROL

Environmental control refers to a client's ability to control the surroundings or direct factors in the environment (Giger & Davidhizar, 2003). People who believe they have control of their health are more likely to seek care, to change their

Table 7.4	CULTURAL ASSESSMENT FACTORS OF VARIOUS CULTURES AFFECTING RESPONSE TO ILLNESS			
Culture	**Communication**	**Space**	**Social Organization**	**Time Orientation**
African American	**Nonverbal**: affectionate, hugging, touching, eye contact **Tone**: may be loud and animated	Respect privacy, respectful approach, handshake appropriate	Family: nuclear, extended, matriarchal, may include close friends	Flexible, nonlinear; life issues may take priority over keeping appointments
American Indians/ Native Americans	**Nonverbal**: respect communicated by avoiding eye contact **Tone**: quiet, reserved	Light-touch handshake	Family: vary; may be matrilineal or patrilineal clan	Flexible, nonlinear; flow with natural cycles rather than scheduled, rigid appointments
Arab American	**Nonverbal**: expressive, warm, other-oriented, shy and modest **Tone:** flowery, loud voice means message is important	Prefer closeness in space and with same sex	Family: nuclear and extended, often in same household	More past and future than present
Cambodian	**Nonverbal**: silence welcomed rather than chatter; eye contact acceptable, but "polite" women lower their eyes **Tone**: quiet	Small personal space with one another	Family-oriented, usually three generations in one house	Flexible attitude, tardiness for appointments expected, emphasis on past (remembering ancestors) but also on present because actions will determine future
Chinese	**Nonverbal**: eye contact and touching among family and friends; eye contact avoided with authority figures **Tone**: expressive and may appear loud	Keep respectful distance	Extended families common, wife expected to be part of husband's family	Being on time not valued
Cuban	**Nonverbal**: direct eye contact, outgoing, close contact and touching with family and friends **Tone**: loud in normal conversation, direct commands or requests may seem forceful	Preferences for personal space vary greatly	Family-oriented, extended families in same household	Social orientation to time varies, on time for business appointments
Filipinos	**Nonverbal**: shy and affectionate, little direct eye contact with authority figures **Tone**: soft-spoken, tone changes with emotion	Handshakes not usually practiced, personal space constricted	Family-oriented, nuclear and extended, may have several generations in one household	Both past and present orientations; tardy for social events but on time for business events like appointments

| Table 7.4 | CULTURAL ASSESSMENT FACTORS OF VARIOUS CULTURES AFFECTING RESPONSE TO ILLNESS *(Continued)* | | | |

Culture	Communication	Space	Social Organization	Time Orientation
Haitians	**Nonverbal**: polite, shy, less eye contact with authority figures, smile and nod as sign of respect **Tone**: rich and expressive, increased volume for emphasis	Very friendly and close with family, respectful handshake with others	Close, tightly knit, extended family and nuclear family, matriarchal society	Not committed to time or schedule, everyone and everything can wait
Japanese American	**Nonverbal**: quiet and polite, reserved and formal, little eye contact with authority figures **Tone**: soft, conflict avoided	Touching uncommon, small bow, handshake with younger generation	Family-oriented, self subordinate to family unit; family structure hierarchical, interdependent	Promptness important, often early for appointments
Mexican American	**Nonverbal**: avoid direct eye contact with authority figures **Tone**: respectful and polite	Touch by strangers not appreciated, handshake polite and welcomed	Mostly nuclear families with extended family and godparents; family comes first	Present-oriented, time viewed as relative to situation
Puerto Ricans	**Nonverbal**: eye contact varies greatly, desire warm and smooth interpersonal relationships **Tone**: melodic, increased volume for emphasis	Space close for family and friends, handshake with others	All activities, decisions, social and cultural standards conceived around family	May be late for appointments or want more time than allotted
Russians	**Nonverbal**: direct eye contact, nodding means approval **Tone**: sometimes loud even in pleasant conversations	Space close for family and friends and more distant for others until familiarity is established	Extended family with strong family bonds and great respect for elders	On time or early
South Asians	**Nonverbal**: direct eye contact considered rude; modesty, humility, shyness emphasized **Tone**: soft, may boss younger people	Personal space constricted; handshake acceptable for men but not common among women	Extended family common, daughter expected to move in with husband's family	Not extremely time-conscious in social situations, but on time for appointments
Vietnamese	**Nonverbal**: gentle touch may be accepted in conversation, no eye contact with authority **Tone**: soft-spoken	Personal space more distant than in European Americans	Highly family-oriented, may be nuclear or extended	Fashionably late at social functions, but understand the importance of being on time for appointments

behavior, and to follow treatment recommendations. Those who believe that illness is a result of nature or natural causes (personalistic or naturalistic view) are less likely to seek traditional health care because they do not believe it can help them.

BIOLOGIC VARIATIONS

Biologic variations exist among people from different cultural backgrounds, and research is just beginning to help us understand these variations. For example, we now know that differences related to **ethnicity**/cultural origins cause variations in response to some psychotropic drugs (discussed earlier). Biologic variations based on physical makeup are said to arise from one's **race**, whereas other cultural variations arise from ethnicity. For example, sickle cell anemia is found almost exclusively in African Americans, and Tay-Sachs disease is most prevalent in the Jewish community.

Socioeconomic Status and Social Class

Socioeconomic status refers to one's income, education, and occupation. It strongly influences a person's health, including whether or not the person has insurance and adequate access to health care or can afford prescribed treatment. People who live in poverty are also at risk for threats to health, such as inadequate housing, lead paint, gang-related violence, drug trafficking, or substandard schools.

Social class has less influence in the United States, where barriers among the social classes are loose and mobility is common: people can gain access to better schools, housing, health care, and lifestyle as they increase their income. In many other countries, however, social class is a powerful influence on social relationships and can determine how people relate to one another, even in a health care setting. For example, the caste system still exists in India, and people in the lowest caste may feel unworthy or undeserving of the same level of health care as people in higher castes. The nurse must determine whether social class is a factor in how clients relate to health care providers and the health care system.

Cultural Patterns and Differences

Knowledge of expected cultural patterns provides a starting point for the nurse to begin to relate to people with ethnic backgrounds different from his or her own (Andrews & Boyle, 2003). Being aware of the usual differences can help the nurse know what to ask or how to assess preferences and health practices. Nevertheless, variations among people from any culture are wide: Not everyone fits the general pattern. Individual assessment of each person and family is necessary to provide culturally competent care that meets the client's needs. The following information about various ethnic groups should be a starting place for the nurse in terms of learning about greetings, acceptable communication patterns and tone of voice, and beliefs regarding mental illness, healing, spirituality, and medical treatment.

AFRICAN AMERICANS

Several terms are used to refer to African Americans, such as *Afro Americans, blacks,* and *persons of color.* Therefore, it is best to ask what each client prefers.

During illness, families are often a support system for the sick person, although the client maintains his or her independence, such as making his or her own health care decisions. Families often feel comfortable demonstrating public affection such as hugging and touching one another. Conversation among family and friends may be animated and loud. Greeting a stranger usually includes a handshake, and direct eye contact indicates interest and respect. Silence may indicate a lack of trust of the caregiver or the situation (Waters & Locks, 2005).

The church is an important and valued support system for many African Americans, who may receive frequent hospital visits from ministers or congregation members. Prayer is an important part of healing. Some in the black community may view the cause of mental illness to be a spiritual imbalance or a punishment for sin. African American clients may use folk remedies in conjunction with Western medicine (Waters & Locks, 2005).

AMERICAN INDIANS OR NATIVE AMERICANS

Older adults usually prefer the term *American Indian,* whereas younger adults prefer *Native American.* Many Native Americans refer to themselves by a tribal name such as Winnebago or Navajo. A light-touch handshake is a respectful greeting with minimal direct eye contact. Communication is slow and may be punctuated by many long pauses. It is important not to rush the speaker or interrupt with questions. This culture is accustomed to communicating by telling stories, so communicating can be a long, detailed process. Family members are reluctant to provide information about the client if he or she can do so, believing it violates the client's privacy to talk about him or her. Orientation to time is flexible and does not coincide with rigidly scheduled appointments.

Mental illness is a culturally specific concept, and beliefs about causation may include ghosts, breaking taboos, or loss of harmony with the environment. Clients are often quiet and stoic, making few if any requests. Experiences that involve seeing visions or hearing voices may have spiritual meaning; thus, these clients may not view such phenomena as illness. Native Americans with traditional religious beliefs may be reluctant to discuss their beliefs and practices with strangers. If the client wears a medicine bag, the nurse should not remove it if possible. Others should not casually discuss or touch the medicine bag or other ritual healing objects. Other Native Americans belong to Christian denominations, but they may incorporate healing practices or use a spiritual healer along with Western medicine (Palacios et al., 2005).

ARAB AMERICANS

The preferred term of address may be by region, such as *Arab Americans* or *Middle Eastern Americans,* or by country of origin, such as *Egyptian* or *Palestinian*. Greetings include a smile, direct eye contact, and a social comment about family or the client. Using a loud voice indicates the importance of the topic, as does repeating the message. To appear respectful, those of Middle Eastern background commonly express agreement in front of a stranger, but it does not necessarily reflect their true feelings. Families make collective decisions with the father, eldest son, uncle, or husband as the family spokesperson. Most appointments viewed as official will be kept, although human concerns are more valued than is adhering to a schedule (Meleis, 2005).

This culture believes mental illness to result from sudden fears, attempts to manipulate family, wrath of God, or God's will, all of which focus on the individual. Loss of country, family, or friends also may cause mental illness. Such clients may seek mental health care only as a last resort after they have exhausted all family and community resources. When sick, these clients expect family or health care professionals to take care of them. The client reserves his or her energy for healing and thus is likely to practice complete rest and abdication from all responsibilities during illness. These clients view mental illness more negatively than physical illness and believe mental illness to be something the person can control. Although early immigrants were Christians, more recent immigrants are Muslims. Prayer is very important to Muslims: strict Muslims pray five times a day, wash before every prayer, and pray in silence. Western medicine is the primary treatment sought, but some may use home remedies and amulets (charms or objects used for their protective powers).

CAMBODIANS

The preferred term for people from Cambodia is *Khmer* (pronounced Kuh-meer') or *Sino-Khmer* (if Chinese Cambodian). Those who have assimilated into Western culture use a handshake for greeting, whereas others may slightly bow, bringing the palms together with the fingers pointed upward, and make no contact with the person they are greeting. Many Asians speak softly, so it is important to listen carefully rather than asking them to speak louder. Cambodian clients highly value politeness. Eye contact is acceptable, but women may lower their eyes to be polite. Silences are common and appropriate; nurses should avoid meaningless chatter. These clients may consider it impolite to disagree, so they say yes when not really agreeing or intending to comply. It is inappropriate to touch someone's head without permission because some believe the soul is in the head. Cambodian clients usually include family members in making decisions. Orientation to time can be flexible (Kulig & Prak, 2005).

Most Khmer immigrated to the United States after 1970 and believe that mental illness is the result of the Khmer Rouge war and associated brutalities. When ill, they assume a passive role, expecting others to care for them. Many may use Western medicine and traditional healing practices simultaneously. Buddhism is the primary religion, although some have converted to Christianity. An *accha* (holy person) may perform many elaborate ceremonies in the person's home but will not do so in the hospital. Healers may visit the client in the hospital but are unlikely to disclose they are healers, much less what their practices are. Some still have a naturalistic view of illness and may be reluctant to have blood drawn, believing they will lose body heat needed for harmony and balance (Kulig & Prak, 2005).

CHINESE

The Chinese are often shy in unfamiliar environments, so socializing or friendly greetings are helpful. They may avoid direct eye contact with authority figures to show respect; keeping a respectful distance is recommended. Asking questions can be a sign of disrespect; silence is a sign of respect. Chinese is an expressive language, so loudness is not necessarily a sign of agitation or anger. Traditional Chinese societies tend not to highly value time urgency. Extended families are common, with the eldest male member of the household making decisions and serving as the spokesperson for the family (Chin, 2005).

Mental illness is thought to result from a lack of harmony of emotions or from evil spirits. Health practices may vary according to how long immigrants have lived in the United States. Immigrants from 40 to 60 years ago are strong believers in Chinese folk medicine, whereas immigrants from the last 20 years combine folk and Western medicine. First- and second-generation Chinese Americans are mostly oriented to Western medicine. Many Chinese use herbalists and acupuncture, however, either before or in conjunction with Western medicine. Rarely, these clients will seek a spiritual healer for psychiatric problems to rid themselves of evil spirits. Many Chinese are Buddhists, but Catholic and Protestant religions are also common.

CUBANS

Cubans, or Cuban Americans if born in the United States, are typically outgoing and may speak loudly during normal conversation. Extended family is very important, and often more than one generation resides in a household. These clients expect direct eye contact during conversation and may view looking away as a lack of respect or honesty. Silence indicates awkwardness or uncertainty. Although orientation to social time may vary greatly, these clients view appointments as business and are punctual (Varela, 2005).

Cuban clients view stress as a cause of both physical and mental illness, and some believe mental illness is hereditary. Mental illness is a stigma for the family; thus, Cuban clients may hide or not publicly acknowledge such problems. The person in the sick role often is submissive, helpless, and dependent on others. Although Cuban clients may use herbal medicine to treat minor illness at home, they usually seek Western medicine for more serious illness. Most Cubans are Catholic or belong to other Christian denominations, so prayer and worship may be very important.

FILIPINOS

Smiles rather than handshakes are a common form of greeting. Facial expressions are animated, and clients may use them rather than words to convey emotion. Filipino clients consider direct eye contact impolite, so there is little direct eye contact with authority figures such as nurses and physicians. Typically, Filipinos are soft-spoken and avoid expressing disagreement (Rodriguez et al., 2005); however, their tone of voice may get louder to emphasize what they are saying or as a sign of anxiety or fear. They are likely to view medical appointments as business and thus be punctual.

They believe the causes of mental illness to be both religious and mystical. Filipinos are likely to view mental illness as the result of a disruption of the harmonious function of the whole person and the spiritual world. These causes can include contact with a stronger life force, ghosts, or souls of the dead; disharmony among wind, vapors, diet, and shifted body organs; or physical and emotional strain, sexual frustration, and unrequited love. Most Filipinos are Catholic; when very ill, they may want to see a priest and a physician. Prayer is important to the client and family, and they often want to receive the religious sacraments while sick. Filipinos often seek both Western medical treatment and the help of healers to remove evil spirits. The ill client assumes a passive role, and the eldest male in the household makes decisions after conferring with family members (Rodriguez et al., 2005).

HAITIANS

Haiti has two official languages, French and Creole, and a strong oral culture that uses stories as educational tools. In Haiti, 80% of the people neither read nor write, but literacy may vary among Haitians in the United States. Videos, oral teaching, and demonstrations are effective ways to communicate information. Haitians are polite but shy, especially with authority figures, and may avoid direct eye contact. Handshakes are the formal greeting of choice. Haitians may smile and nod as a sign of respect even when they do not understand what is being said. Tone of voice and hand gestures may increase to emphasize what is being said. There is little commitment to time or schedule in Haitian culture, but clients may be on time for medical appointments if the provider emphasizes the need for punctuality (Colin, 2005).

Mental illness is not well accepted in Haitian culture. These clients usually believe mental illness to have supernatural causes. The sick person assumes a passive role, and family members provide care for the individual. Home and folk remedies are often the first treatment used at home, and clients seek medical care when it is apparent the person needs medical attention. Haitians are predominantly Catholic and have a very strong belief in God's power and ability to heal (Colin, 2005).

JAPANESE AMERICANS

Japanese Americans identify themselves by the generation in which they were born. Issei, the first generation of Japanese Americans in the United States, have a strong sense of Japanese identity. Nisei, second-generation Japanese Americans born and educated in the United States, appear to be westernized but have strong roots in Japanese culture. Sansei (third generation) and Yonsei (fourth generation) are assimilated into Western culture and are less connected to Japanese culture.

Greetings tend to be formal, such as a smile or small bow for older generations and a handshake for younger generations. There is little touching and eye contact is minimal, especially with authority figures. These clients control facial expressions and avoid conflict or disagreement. Elders may nod frequently, but this does not necessarily indicate understanding or agreement. Self-disclosure is unlikely unless trust has been established, and then only if the information is directly requested. Nurses should phrase questions to elicit more than just a yes or no answer. Promptness is important, so clients are often early for appointments (Shiba et al., 2005).

Mental illness brings shame and social stigma to the family, so clients are reluctant to seek help. Evil spirits are thought to cause loss of mental self-control as a punishment for bad behavior or failure to live a good life. These clients expect themselves and others to use will power to regain their lost self-control and often perceive those with mental illness as not trying hard enough. Western psychological therapies based on self-disclosure, sharing feelings, and discussing one's family experiences are very difficult for many Japanese Americans. The nurse might incorrectly view these clients as unwilling or uncooperative (Shiba et al., 2005).

Buddhism, Shinto, and Christianity are the most common religions among Japanese Americans, and religious practices vary with the religion. Prayer and offerings are common in Buddhist and Shinto religions and are usually done in conjunction with Western medicine.

MEXICAN AMERICANS

Diversity is wide among Mexican Americans in terms of health practices and beliefs, depending on the client's education, socioeconomic status, generation, time spent in the United States, and affinity to traditional culture. It is best for the nurse to ask the client how he or she would like to be identified (e.g., Mexican American, Latino, Hispanic). Most Mexicans consider a handshake to be a polite greeting but do not appreciate other touch by strangers, although touching and embracing warmly are common among family and friends. To convey respect, Mexican clients may avoid direct eye contact with authority figures. They usually prefer polite social interaction to help establish rapport before answering health-related questions.

Generally, one or two questions will produce a wealth of information, so listening is important. Silence is often a sign of disagreement, which these clients may use in place of words. Orientation to time is flexible; the client may be 15 or 20 minutes late for an appointment but will not consider that as being late (Guarnero, 2005).

There is no clear separation of mental and physical illness. Many have a naturalistic or personalistic view of illness and believe disease is based on the imbalance of the person and the environment, including emotional, spiritual, social, and physical factors (Guarnero, 2005). Mexican Americans may seek medical care for severe symptoms while still using folk medicine to deal with spiritual or psychic influences. Between 80% and 90% of Mexican Americans are Catholic and observe the rites and sacraments of that religion.

PUERTO RICANS

Preferences for personal space vary among Puerto Ricans, so it is important to assess each individual. Typically, older and more traditional people prefer greater distance and less direct eye contact, whereas younger people prefer direct eye contact and less distance with others. Puerto Ricans desire warm and smooth interpersonal relationships and may express gratitude to health care providers with homemade traditional cooking; these clients might interpret the refusal of such an offer as an insult. There may be some difficulty being on time for appointments or limiting the length of an appointment (Juarbe, 2005).

Physical illness is seen as hereditary, punishment for sin, or lack of attention to personal health. Mental illness is believed to be hereditary or a result of *sufriamientos* (suffering). Mental illness carries great stigma, and past or present history of mental illness may not be acknowledged. Religious and spiritual practices are very important, and these clients may use spiritual healers or healing practices (Juarbe, 2005).

RUSSIANS

A formal greeting or a handshake with direct eye contact is acceptable. These clients reserve touching or embracing and kissing on the cheeks for close friends and family. Tone of voice can be loud even in pleasant conversations. Most clients are on time or early for appointments (del Puerto & Sigal, 2005).

Russians believe the cause of mental illness to be stress and moving into a new environment. Some Russian Christians believe illness is God's will or a test of faith. Sick people often put themselves on bed rest. Many Russians do not like to take any medications and will try home remedies first. Some older Russians believe that excessive drug use can be harmful and that many medicines can be more damaging than natural remedies. Primary religious affiliations are Eastern Orthodox, with a minority being Jewish or Protestant (del Puerto & Sigal, 2005).

SOUTH ASIANS

South Asians living in the United States include people from India, Pakistan, Bangladesh, Sri Lanka, Nepal, Fiji, and East Africa. Preferred terms of identification may be related to geography, such as *South Asians, East Indians, Asian Indians,* or *Indo-Americans,* or by religious affiliation, such as *Sikhs, Hindus,* or *Muslims.* Greetings are expressed orally as well as in gestures. Hindus and Sikhs press their palms together while saying *namaste* (Hindus) or *sasariyakal* (Sikhs). Muslims take the palm of the right hand to their forehead and bow slightly while saying *AsSalamOAlaikuum.* Shaking hands is common among men but not among women. Touching is not common among South Asians; rather, they express feelings through eyes and facial expressions. They may consider direct eye contact, especially with elders, rude or disrespectful. Silence usually indicates acceptance, approval, or tolerance. Most South Asians have a soft tone of voice and consider loudness to be disrespectful. Although not time conscious about social activities, most South Asians are punctual for scheduled appointments for health care (Lee et al., 2001).

South Asians believe mental illness to result from spells cast by an enemy or possession by evil spirits. Those who believe in Ayurvedic philosophy may believe a person is susceptible to mental problems related to physical imbalances in the body. Sick people usually assume a passive role and want to rest and be relieved of daily responsibilities. Hindus worship many gods and goddesses and believe in a social caste system. Hindus believe that reciting charms and performing rituals eliminate diseases, enemies, sins, and demons. Many believe that yoga eliminates certain mental illnesses. Muslims believe in one God and pray five times daily after washing their hands. They believe that reciting verses from the holy Koran eliminates diseases and eases suffering. Sikhs also believe in one God and the equality of all people. Spiritual healing practices and prayer are common, but South Asians living in the United States readily seek health care from Western physicians as well (Lee et al., 2001).

VIETNAMESE

Vietnamese greet with a smile and bow. A health care provider should not shake a woman's hand unless she offers her hand first. Touch in communication is more limited among older, more traditional people. Vietnamese may consider the head sacred and the feet profane, so the order of touching is important. As a sign of respect, many of these clients avoid direct eye contact with those in authority and elders. Personal space is more distant than it is for European Americans. Typically, the Vietnamese are soft-spoken and consider raising the voice and pointing to be disrespectful. They also may consider open expression of emotions or conflict to be in bad taste. Punctuality for appointments is usual (Nowak, 2005).

Vietnamese believe mental illness to be the result of individual disharmony or an ancestral spirit returning to haunt the person because of past bad behavior. When sick, clients assume a passive role and expect to have everything their way.

The two primary religions are Catholicism and Buddhism. Catholics recite the rosary and say prayers and may wish to see a priest daily. Buddhists pray silently to themselves.

Vietnamese people believe in both Western medicine and folk medicine. Some believe that traditional healers can exorcise evil spirits. Other health practices include coin rubbing, pinching the skin, acupuncture, and herbal medicine (Nowak, 2005).

Nurse's Role in Working With Clients of Various Cultures

To provide culturally competent care, the nurse must find out as much as possible about a client's cultural values, beliefs, and health practices. Often, the client is the best source for that information, so the nurse must ask the client what is important to him or her—for instance, "How would you like to be cared for?" or "What do you expect (or want) me to do for you?" (Andrews & Boyle, 2003).

At the initial meeting, the nurse may rely on what he or she knows about a client's particular cultural group such as preferences for greeting, eye contact, and physical distance. Based on the client's behavior, the nurse can alter that approach as needed. For example, if a client from a culture that does not usually shake hands offers the nurse his or her hand, the nurse should return the handshake. Variation among members of the same cultural group is wide, and the nurse must remain alert for these individual differences.

A client's health practices and religious beliefs are other important areas to assess. The nurse can ask, "Do you follow any dietary preferences or restrictions?" and "How can I assist you in practicing your religious or spiritual beliefs?" The nurse also can gain an understanding of the client's health and illness beliefs by asking, "How do you think this health problem came about?" and "What kinds of remedies have you tried at home?"

An open and objective approach to the client is essential. Clients will be more likely to share personal and cultural information if the nurse is genuinely interested in knowing and does not appear skeptical or judgmental.

The nurse should ask these same questions even to clients from his or her own cultural background. Again, people in a cultural group vary widely, so the nurse should not assume that he or she knows what a client believes or practices just because the nurse shares the same culture.

SELF-AWARENESS ISSUES

The nurse must be aware of the factors that influence a client's response to illness, including the individual, interpersonal, and cultural factors discussed earlier. Assessment of these factors can help guide the planning

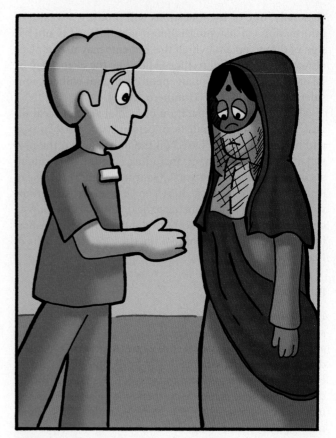

Cultural awareness

and implementation of nursing care. Biologic and hereditary factors cannot be changed. Others, such as interpersonal factors, can be changed but only with difficulty. For instance, helping a client to develop a social support system requires more than simply giving him or her a list of community contacts. The client needs to feel that these resources are valuable to him or her; must perceive them as helpful, responsive, and supportive; and must be willing to use them.

Nurses with limited experience in working with various ethnic groups may feel anxious when encountering someone from a different cultural background and worry about saying "the wrong thing" or doing something offensive or disrespectful to the client or family. Nurses may have stereotypical concepts about some ethnic groups and be unaware of them until they encounter a client from that group. It is a constant challenge to remain aware of one's feelings and to handle them effectively.

Points to Consider When Working With Individual Responses to Illness

- Approach the client with a genuine caring attitude.
- Ask the client at the beginning of the interview how he or she prefers to be addressed and ways the nurse can promote spiritual, religious, and health practices.

- Recognize any negative feelings or stereotypes and discuss them with a colleague to dispel myths and misconceptions.
- Remember that a wide variety of factors influence the client's complex response to illness.

Critical Thinking Questions

1. What is the cultural and ethnic background of your family? How does that influence your beliefs about mental illness?
2. How would you describe yourself in terms of the individual characteristics that affect one's response to illness, such as growth and development, biologic factors, self-efficacy, hardiness, resilience and resourcefulness, and spirituality?
3. Which of the categories of factors that influence the client's response to illness—individual, interpersonal, and cultural—do you think is most influential? Why?

 KEY POINTS

- Each client is unique with different biologic, psychological, and social factors that influence his or her response to illness.
- Individual factors that influence a client's response to illness include age, growth, and development; biologic and genetic factors; hardiness, resilience, and resourcefulness; and self-efficacy and spirituality.
- Biologic makeup includes the person's heredity and physical health.
- Younger clients may have difficulty expressing their thoughts and feelings so they often have poorer outcomes when experiencing stress or illness at an early age.
- People who have difficulty negotiating the tasks of psychosocial development have less effective skills to cope with illness.

- There are cultural/ethnic differences in how people respond to certain psychotropic drugs; these differences can affect dosage and side effects. Nurses must be aware of these cultural differences when treating clients. Clients from non-Western countries generally require lower doses of psychotropic drugs to produce desired effects.
- Self-efficacy is a belief that a person's abilities and efforts can influence the events in her or his life. A person's sense of self-efficacy is an important factor in coping with stress and illness.
- Hardiness is a person's ability to resist illness when under stress.
- Resilience is a person's ability to respond in a healthy manner to stressful circumstances or risky situations.
- Resourcefulness is demonstrated in one's ability to manage daily activities and is a personal characteristic acquired through interactions with others.
- Spirituality involves the inner core of a person's being and his or her beliefs about the meaning of life and the purpose for living. It may include belief in God or a higher power, the practice of religion, cultural beliefs and practices, and a relationship with the environment.
- Interpersonal factors that influence the client's response to illness include a sense of belonging, or personal involvement in a system or environment, and social networks, which provide social support or emotional sustenance.
- The increasing social and cultural diversity in the United States and Canada makes it essential for nurses to be knowledgeable about the health and cultural practices of various ethnic or racial groups. To provide competent nursing care, nurses must be sensitive to and knowledgeable about factors that influence the care of clients, including issues related to culture, race, gender, sexual orientation, and social and economic situations.
- Culture has the most influence on a person's health beliefs and behaviors.
- A model for assessing clients from various ethnic backgrounds includes six cultural phenomena: communication techniques and style, physical distance and space, social organization, time orientation, environmental control, and biologic variations.
- Socioeconomic status has a strong influence on a person's health. It may determine whether or not the person has

 INTERNET RESOURCES

RESOURCE	INTERNET ADDRESS
• Culture Med™ (Extensive bibliography of transcultural nursing articles)	http://www.sunyit.edu/library/html/culturemed/bib/transcultural
• National MultiCultural Institute	http://www.nmci.org
• Native American Cultural Society	http://www.nacs-athens.com

insurance, adequate access to health care, or the ability to afford prescribed treatment.

- Knowledge of various cultural patterns and differences helps the nurse begin to relate to persons of different ethnic backgrounds.
- Nurses who are unsure of a person's social or cultural preferences need to ask the client directly during the initial encounter about preferred terms of address and ways the nurse can help support the client's spiritual, religious, or health practices.

REFERENCES

Andrews, M. M., & Boyle, J. S. (2003). *Transcultural concepts in nursing care* (4th ed.). Philadelphia: Lippincott Williams & Wilkins.

Baetz, M., Larson, D. B., Marcoux, G., et al. (2002). Canadian psychiatric inpatient religious commitment: An association with mental health. *Canadian Journal of Psychiatry, 47*(2), 159–166.

Bandura, A. (2004). Health promotion by social cognitive means. *Health Education and Behavior, 31*(2), 143–164.

Brooks, M. V. (2003). Health-related hardiness and chronic illness: A synthesis of current research. *Nursing Forum, 38*(3), 11–20.

Brugman, T., & Ferguson, S. (2002). Physical exercise and improvements in mental health. *Journal of Psychosocial Nursing, 40*(8), 24–31.

Buchanan, B. W., & Carpenter, W. T. (2005). Concept of schizophrenia. In B. J. Sadock & V. A. Sadock (Eds.), *Comprehensive textbook of psychiatry* (Vol. 1, 8th ed., pp. 1329–1345). Philadelphia: Lippincott Williams & Wilkins.

Campinha-Bacote, J. (2002). The process of cultural competence in the delivery of health care services: A model of care. *Journal of Transcultural Nursing, 13*(3), 181–184.

Chanokruthai, C., Williams, R. A., & Hagerty, B. M. (2005). The role of sense of belonging and social support on stress and depression in individuals with depression. *Archives of Psychiatric Nursing, 19*(1), 18–29.

Chin, P. (2005). Chinese. In J. G. Lipson & S. L. Dibble (Eds.), *Culture & Clinical Care* (pp. 98–108). San Francisco: UCSF Nursing Press.

Colin, J. M. (2005). Haitians. In J. G. Lipson & S. L. Dibble (Eds.), *Culture & Clinical Care* (pp. 221–235). San Francisco: UCSF Nursing Press.

Cutler, C. G. (2005). Self-efficacy and social adjustment of patients with mood disorder. *Journal of the American Psychiatric Nurses Association, 11*(5), 283–289.

del Puerto, L. E., & Sigal, E. (2005) Russians and others from the former Soviet Union. In J. G. Lipson & S. L. Dibble (Eds.), *Culture & Clinical Care* (pp. 415–430). San Francisco: UCSF Nursing Press.

Edward, K., & Warelow, P. (2005). Resilience: When coping is emotionally intelligent. *Journal of the American Psychiatric Nurses Association, 11*(2), 101–102.

Giger, J. N., & Davidhizar, R. E. (2003). *Transcultural nursing: Assessment and intervention* (4th ed.). St. Louis: Mosby.

Granerud, A., & Severinsson, E. (2006). The struggle for social integration in the community: The experiences of people with mental health problems. *Journal of Psychiatric and Mental Health Nursing, 13*(3), 288–293.

Greeff, A. P., Vansteenween, A., & Mieke, I. (2006). Resiliency in families with a member with a psychological disorder. *American Journal of Family Therapy, 34*(4), 285–300.

Guarnero, P. A. (2005). Mexicans. In J. G. Lipson & S. L. Dibble (Eds.), *Culture & Clinical Care* (pp. 330–342). San Francisco: UCSF Nursing Press.

Huguelet, P., Mohr, S., Borras, L., Gillieron, C., & Brandt, P. (2006). Spirituality and religious practices among outpatients with schizophrenia and their clinicians. *Psychiatric Services, 57*(3), 366–372.

Juarbe, T. C. (2005). Puerto Ricans. In J. G. Lipson & S. L. Dibble (Eds.), *Culture & Clinical Care* (pp. 389–404). San Francisco: UCSF Nursing Press.

Kobasa, S. C. (1979). Stressful life events, personality, and health: An inquiry into hardiness. *Journal of Personality & Social Psychology, 37*(1), 1–11.

Krafcik, K. A. (2002). Predictors of resourcefulness in school aged children. *Issues in Mental Health Nursing, 23*(4), 385–407.

Kulig, J. C., & Prak, S. (2005). Cambodians (Khmer). In J. G. Lipson & S. L. Dibble (Eds.), *Culture & Clinical Care* (pp. 73–84). San Francisco: UCSF Nursing Press.

Lee, J., Lei, A., & Sue, S. (2001). The current state of mental health research on Asian Americans. *Journal of Human Behavior in the Social Environment, 3*(3/4), 159–178.

Longo, D. A., & Peterson, S. A. (2002). The role of spirituality in psychosocial rehabilitation. *Psychiatric Rehabilitation Journal, 25*(4), 333–340.

Maddi, S. R. (2005). On hardiness and other pathways to resilience. *American Psychologist, 60*(3), 261–262.

Meleis, A. I. (2005). Arabs. In J. G. Lipson & S. L. Dibble (Eds.), *Culture & Clinical Care* (pp. 42–57). San Francisco: UCSF Nursing Press.

Nowak, T. T. (2005) Vietnamese. In J. G. Lipson & S. L. Dibble (Eds.), *Culture & Clinical Care* (pp. 446–460). San Francisco: UCSF Nursing Press.

Palacios, J., Butterfly, R., & Strickland, C. J. (2005). American Indians/Alaskan Natives. In J. G. Lipson & S. L. Dibble (Eds.), *Culture & Clinical Care* (pp. 27–41). San Francisco: UCSF Nursing Press.

Purnell, L. D., & Paulanka, B. J. (Eds.). (2003). *Transcultural healthcare: A culturally competent approach* (2nd ed.). Philadelphia: F. A. Davis.

Reid, J., Lloyd, C., & de Groot, L. (2005). The psychoeducation needs of parents who have an adult son of daughter with a mental illness. *Australian e-Journal for the Advancement of Mental Health, 4*(2), 1–13.

Rodriguez, D. M., de Guzman, C. P., & Cantos, A. (2005). Filipinos. In J. G. Lipson & S. L. Dibble (Eds.), *Culture & Clinical Care,* (pp. 177–191). San Francisco: UCSF Nursing Press.

Ross, N. (2002). Community belonging and health. *Health Reports, 13*(3), 33–40.

Sageman, S. (2004). Breaking through the despair: Spiritually oriented group therapy as a means of healing women with severe mental illness. *Journal of the American Academy of Psychoanalysis and Dynamic Psychiatry, 32*(1), 125–141.

Shiba, G., Leong, Y. M., & Oka, R. (2005). Japanese. J. G. Lipson & S. L. Dibble (Eds.), *Culture & Clinical Care* (pp. 304–316). San Francisco: UCSF Nursing Press.

Vanderhorst, R. K., & McLaren, S. (2005). Social relationships as predictors of depression and suicidal ideation in older adults. *Aging & Mental Health, 9*(6), 517–525.

Varela, L. (2005). Cubans. In J. G. Lipson & S. L. Dibble (Eds.), *Culture & Clinical Care* (pp. 122–131). San Francisco: UCSF Nursing Press.

Waters, C. M., & Locks, S. (2005) African Americans. In J. G. Lipson & S. L. Dibble (Eds.), *Culture & Clinical Care* (pp. 14–26). San Francisco: UCSF Nursing Press.

ADDITIONAL READINGS

Chady, S. (2001). The NSF for mental health from a transcultural perspective. *British Journal of Nursing, 10*(15), 830–835.

Lowe, J. (2002). Cherokee self-reliance. *Journal of Transcultural Nursing, 13*(4), 287–295.

Shin, S., & Lukens, E. P. (2002). Effects of psychoeducation for Korean Americans with chronic mental illness. *Psychiatric Services, 53*(9), 1125–1131.

Chapter Study Guide

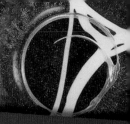

MULTIPLE-CHOICE QUESTIONS

Select the best answer for each of the following questions.

1. Which of the following is important for nurses to remember when administering psychotropic drugs to nonwhites?
   A. Lower doses may be used to produce desired effects.
   B. Fewer side effects occur with nonwhite clients.
   C. Response to the drug is similar to that in whites.
   D. No generalization can be made.

2. Which of the following states the naturalistic view of what causes illness?
   A. Illness is a natural part of life and therefore unavoidable.
   B. Illness is caused by cold, heat, wind, and dampness.
   C. Only natural agents are effective in treating illness.
   D. Outside agents, such as evil spirits, upset the body's natural balance.

3. Which of the following is most influential in determining health beliefs and practices?
   A. Cultural factors
   B. Individual factors
   C. Interpersonal factors
   D. All the above are equally influential.

4. Which of the following groups considers a firm handshake a sign of strength?
   A. White European Americans
   B. Filipinos
   C. Mexican Americans
   D. Native Americans

5. Which of the following groups considers direct eye contact a lack of respect?
   A. African Americans
   B. Arab Americans
   C. Russians
   D. Vietnamese

6. Which of the following assessments indicates positive growth and development for a 30-year-old adult?
   A. Is dissatisfied with body image
   B. Enjoys social activities with three or four close friends
   C. Frequently changes jobs to "find the right one"
   D. Plans to move from parental home in near future

7. Which of the following statements would cause concern for achievement of developmental tasks of a 55-year old woman?
   A. "I feel like I'm taking care of my parents now."
   B. "I really enjoy just sitting around visiting with friends."
   C. "My children need me now just as much as when they were small."
   D. "When I retire, I want a smaller house to take care of."

8. Which of the following client statements would indicate self-efficacy?
   A. "I like to get several opinions before deciding a course of action."
   B. "I know if I can learn to relax, I will feel better."
   C. "I'm never sure if I'm making the right decision."
   D. "No matter how hard I try to relax, something always comes up."

FILL-IN-THE-BLANK QUESTIONS

Identify the developmental task that corresponds to the following age groups, according to Erik Erikson.

_____ Infant

_____ School age

_____ Adolescence

_____ Young adult

_____ Maturity

SHORT-ANSWER QUESTIONS

1. Briefly explain culturally competent nursing care.

2. What is the result of achieving or failing to achieve a psychosocial developmental task, according to Erik Erikson?

3. What is the essential difference between hardiness and resilience?

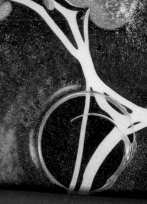

Chapter

8

Assessment

Key Terms

- abstract thinking
- affect
- automatisms
- blunted affect
- broad affect
- circumstantial thinking
- concrete thinking
- delusion
- duty to warn
- flat affect
- flight of ideas
- hallucinations
- ideas of reference
- inappropriate affect
- insight
- judgment
- labile
- loose associations
- mood
- neologisms
- psychomotor retardation
- restricted affect
- self-concept
- tangential thinking
- thought blocking
- thought broadcasting
- thought content
- thought insertion
- thought process
- thought withdrawal
- waxy flexibility
- word salad

Learning Objectives

After reading this chapter, you should be able to

1. Identify the categories used to assess the client's mental health status.

2. Formulate questions to obtain information in each category.

3. Describe the client's functioning in terms of self-concept, roles, and relationships.

4. Recognize key physiologic functions that frequently are impaired in people with mental disorders.

5. Obtain and organize psychosocial assessment data to use as a basis for planning nursing care.

6. Examine one's own feelings and any discomfort discussing suicide, homicide, or self-harm behaviors with a client.

Visit the Point http://thePoint.lww.com for NCLEX-style questions, journal articles, and more!

Assessment is the first step of the nursing process and involves the collection, organization, and analysis of information about the client's health (American Nurses Association, 2000). In psychiatric mental health nursing, this process is often referred to as a psychosocial assessment, which includes a mental status examination. The purpose of the psychosocial assessment is to construct a picture of the client's current emotional state, mental capacity, and behavioral function. This assessment serves as the basis for developing a plan of care to meet the client's needs. The assessment is also a clinical baseline used to evaluate the effectiveness of treatment and interventions or a measure of the client's progress (American Nurses Association, 2000).

FACTORS INFLUENCING ASSESSMENT

Client Participation/Feedback

A thorough and complete psychosocial assessment requires active client participation. If the client is unable or unwilling to participate, some areas of the assessment will be incomplete or vague. For example, the client who is extremely depressed may not have the energy to answer questions or complete the assessment. Clients exhibiting psychotic thought processes or impaired cognition may have an insufficient attention span or may be unable to comprehend the questions being asked. The nurse may need to have several contacts with such clients to complete the assessment or gather further information as the client's condition permits.

Client's Health Status

The client's health status also can affect the psychosocial assessment. If the client is anxious, tired, or in pain, the nurse may have difficulty eliciting the client's full participation in the assessment. The information that the nurse obtains may reflect the client's pain or anxiety rather than an accurate assessment of the client's situation. The nurse needs to recognize these situations and deal with them before continuing the full assessment. The client may need to rest, receive medications to alleviate pain, or be calmed before the assessment can continue.

Client's Previous Experiences/Misconceptions About Health Care

The client's perception of his or her circumstances can elicit emotions that interfere with obtaining an accurate psychosocial assessment. If the client is reluctant to seek treatment or has had previous unsatisfactory experiences with the health care system, he or she may have difficulty answering questions directly. The client may minimize or maximize symptoms or problems or may refuse to provide information in some areas. The nurse must address the client's feelings and perceptions to establish a trusting working relationship before proceeding with the assessment.

Client's Ability to Understand

The nurse also must determine the client's ability to hear, read, and understand the language being used in the assessment. If the client's primary language differs from that of the nurse, the client may misunderstand or misinterpret what the nurse is asking, which results in inaccurate information. A client with impaired hearing also may fail to understand what the nurse is asking. It is important that the information in the assessment reflects the client's health status; it should not be a result of poor communication.

Nurse's Attitude and Approach

The nurse's attitude and approach can influence the psychosocial assessment. If the client perceives the nurse's questions to be short and curt or feels rushed or pressured to complete the assessment, he or she may provide only superficial information or omit discussing problems in some areas altogether. The client also may refrain from providing sensitive information if he or she perceives the nurse as nonaccepting, defensive, or judgmental. For example, a client may be reluctant to relate instances of child abuse or domestic violence if the nurse seems uncomfortable or nonaccepting. The nurse must be aware of his or her own feelings and responses and approach the assessment matter-of-factly.

HOW TO CONDUCT THE INTERVIEW

Environment

The nurse should conduct the psychosocial assessment in an environment that is comfortable, private, and safe for both the client and the nurse. An environment that is fairly quiet with few distractions allows the client to give his or her full attention to the interview. Conducting the interview in a place such as a conference room ensures the client that no one will overhear what is being discussed. The nurse should not choose an isolated location for the interview, however, particularly if the client is unknown to the nurse or has a history of any threatening behavior. The nurse must ensure the safety of self and client even if that means another person is present during the assessment.

Input From Family and Friends

If family members, friends, or caregivers have accompanied the client, the nurse should obtain their perceptions of the client's behavior and emotional state. How this is accomplished depends on the situation. Sometimes the client does not give permission for the nurse to conduct separate interviews with family members. The nurse should then be aware that friends or family may not feel comfortable talking about the client in his or her presence and may provide limited information. Or the client may not feel comfortable participating in the assessment without family or friends. This, too, may limit the amount or type of information the nurse obtains. It is desirable to conduct at least part of the assessment without others, especially in cases of suspected abuse or intimidation. The nurse should make every effort to assess the client in privacy in cases of suspected abuse.

How to Phrase Questions

The nurse may use open-ended questions to start the assessment (see Chapter 6). Doing so allows the client to begin as he or she feels comfortable and also gives the nurse an idea about the client's perception of his or her situation. Examples of open-ended questions are as follows:

- What brings you here today?
- Tell me what has been happening to you.
- How can we help you?

If the client cannot organize his or her thoughts, or has difficulty answering open-ended questions, the nurse may need to use more direct questions to obtain information. Questions need to be clear, simple, and focused on one specific behavior or symptom; they should not cause the client to remember several things at once. Questions regarding several different behaviors or symptoms—"How are your eating and sleeping habits and have you been taking any over-the-counter medications that affect your eating and sleeping?"—can be confusing to the client. The following are examples of focused or closed-ended questions:

- How many hours did you sleep last night?
- Have you been thinking about suicide?
- How much alcohol have you been drinking?
- How well have you been sleeping?
- How many meals a day do you eat?
- What over-the-counter medications are you taking?

The nurse should use a nonjudgmental tone and language, particularly when asking about sensitive information such as drug or alcohol use, sexual behavior, abuse or violence, and childrearing practices. Using nonjudgmental language and a matter-of-fact tone avoids giving the client verbal cues to become defensive or to not tell the truth. For example, when asking a client about his or her parenting role, the nurse should ask, "What types of discipline do you use?" rather than, "How often do you physically punish your child?" The first question is more likely to elicit honest and accurate information; the second question gives the impression that physical discipline is wrong, and it may cause the client to respond dishonestly.

CONTENT OF THE ASSESSMENT

The information gathered in a psychosocial assessment can be organized in many different ways. Most assessment tools or conceptual frameworks contain similar categories with some variety in arrangement or order. The nurse should use some kind of organizing framework so that he or she can assess the client in a thorough and systematic way that lends itself to analysis and serves as a basis for the client's care. The framework for psychosocial assessment discussed here and used throughout this textbook contains the following components:

- History
- General appearance and motor behavior
- Mood and affect
- Thought process and content
- Sensorium and intellectual processes
- Judgment and insight
- Self-concept
- Roles and relationships
- Physiologic and self-care concerns

Box 8.1 lists the factors the nurse should include in each of these areas of the psychosocial assessment.

History

Background assessments include the client's history, age and developmental stage, cultural and spiritual beliefs, and beliefs about health and illness. The history of the client, as well as his or her family, may provide some insight into the client's current situation. For example, has the client experienced similar difficulties in the past? Has the client been admitted to the hospital, and, if so, what was that experience like? A family history that is positive for alcoholism, bipolar disorder, or suicide is significant because it increases the client's risk for these problems.

The client's chronologic age and developmental stage are important factors in the psychosocial assessment. The nurse evaluates the client's age and developmental level for congruence with expected norms. For example, a client may be struggling with personal identity and attempting to achieve independence from his or her parents. If the client is 17 years old, these struggles are normal and anticipated because these are two of the primary developmental tasks for the adolescent. If the client is 35 years old and still struggling with these issues of self-identity and independence, the nurse will need to explore the situation. The client's age and developmental level also may be incongruent with expected norms if the client has a developmental delay or mental retardation.

The nurse must be sensitive to the client's cultural and spiritual beliefs to avoid making inaccurate assumptions about his or her psychosocial functioning (Schultz & Videbeck, 2005). Many cultures have beliefs and values about a person's role in society or acceptable social or personal behavior that may differ from those of the nurse. Western cultures generally expect that as a person reaches adulthood, he or she becomes financially independent, leaves home, and makes his or her own life decisions. In contrast, in some Eastern cultures, three generations may live in one household, and elders of the family make major life decisions for all. Another example is the assessment of

Box 8.1   PSYCHOSOCIAL ASSESSMENT COMPONENTS

History
  Age
  Developmental stage
  Cultural considerations
  Spiritual beliefs
  Previous history
General assessment and motor behavior
  Hygiene and grooming
  Appropriate dress
  Posture
  Eye contact
  Unusual movements or mannerisms
  Speech
Mood and affect
  Expressed emotions
  Facial expressions
Thought process and content
  Content (what client is thinking)
  Process (how client is thinking)
  Clarity of ideas
  Self-harm or suicide urges
Sensorium and intellectual processes
  Orientation
  Confusion

Memory
  Abnormal sensory experiences or misperceptions
  Concentration
  Abstract thinking abilities
Judgment and insight
  Judgment (interpretation of environment)
  Decision-making ability
  Insight (understanding one's own part in current situation)
Self-concept
  Personal view of self
  Description of physical self
  Personal qualities or attributes
Roles and relationships
  Current roles
  Satisfaction with roles
  Success at roles
  Significant relationships
  Support systems
Physiologic and self-care considerations
  Eating habits
  Sleep patterns
  Health problems
  Compliance with prescribed medications
  Ability to perform activities of daily living

eye contact. Western cultures consider good eye contact to be a positive characteristic indicating self-esteem and paying attention. People from other cultures, such as Japan, consider such eye contact to be a sign of disrespect.

The nurse must not stereotype clients. Just because a person's physical characteristics are consistent with a particular race, he or she may not have the attitudes, beliefs, and behaviors traditionally attributed to that group. For example, many people of Asian ancestry have beliefs and values that are more consistent with Western beliefs and values than with those typically associated with Asian countries. To avoid making inaccurate assumptions, the nurse must ask clients about the beliefs or health practices that are important to them or how they view themselves in the context of society or relationships (see Cultural Patterns and Differences in Chapter 7).

The nurse also must consider the client's beliefs about health and illness when assessing the client's psychosocial functioning. Some people view emotional or mental problems as family concerns to be handled only among family members. They may view seeking outside or professional help as a sign of individual weakness. Others may believe that their problems can be solved only with the right medication, and they will not accept other forms of therapy.

Another common problem is the misconception that one should take medication only when feeling sick. Many mental disorders, like some medical conditions, may require clients to take medications on a long-term basis, perhaps even for a lifetime. Just like people with diabetes must take insulin and people with hypertension need antihypertensive medications, people with recurrent depression may need to take antidepressants on a long-term basis.

General Appearance and Motor Behavior

The nurse assesses the client's overall appearance, including dress, hygiene, and grooming. Is the client appropriately dressed for his or her age and the weather? Is the client unkempt or disheveled? Does the client appear to be his or her stated age? The nurse also observes the client's posture, eye contact, facial expression, and any unusual tics or tremors. He or she documents observations and examples of behaviors to avoid personal judgment or misinterpretation. Specific terms used in making assessments of general appearance and motor behavior include the following:

- **Automatisms:** repeated purposeless behaviors often indicative of anxiety, such as drumming fingers, twisting locks of hair, or tapping the foot

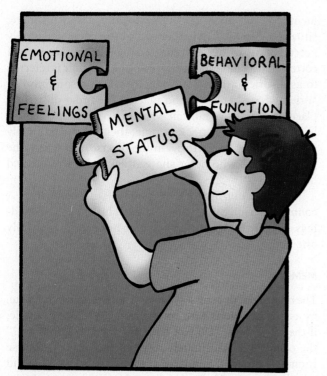

Building a picture of your client through psychosocial assessment

- **Psychomotor retardation:** overall slowed movements
- **Waxy flexibility:** maintenance of posture or position over time even when it is awkward or uncomfortable

The nurse assesses the client's speech for quantity, quality, and any abnormalities. Does the client talk nonstop? Does the client perseverate (seem to be stuck on one topic and unable to move to another idea)? Are responses a minimal "yes" or "no" without elaboration? Is the content of the client's speech relevant to the question being asked? Is the rate of speech fast or slow? Is the tone audible or loud? Does the client speak in a rhyming manner? Does the client use **neologisms** (invented words that have meaning only for the client)? The nurse notes any speech difficulties such as stuttering or lisping.

Mood and Affect

Mood refers to the client's pervasive and enduring emotional state. **Affect** is the outward expression of the client's emotional state. The client may make statements about feelings, such as "I'm depressed" or "I'm elated," or the nurse may infer the client's mood from data such as posture, gestures, tone of voice, and facial expression. The nurse also assesses for consistency among the client's mood, affect, and situation. For instance, the client may have an angry facial expression but deny feeling angry or upset in any way. Or the client may be talking about the recent loss of a family member while laughing and smiling. The nurse must note such inconsistencies.

Common terms used in assessing affect include the following:

- **Blunted affect:** showing little or a slow-to-respond facial expression
- **Broad affect:** displaying a full range of emotional expressions
- **Flat affect:** showing no facial expression
- **Inappropriate affect:** displaying a facial expression that is incongruent with mood or situation; often silly or giddy regardless of circumstances
- **Restricted affect:** displaying one type of expression, usually serious or somber

The client's mood may be described as happy, sad, depressed, euphoric, anxious, or angry. When the client exhibits unpredictable and rapid mood swings from depressed and crying to euphoria with no apparent stimuli, the mood is called **labile** (rapidly changing).

The nurse may find it helpful to ask the client to estimate the intensity of his or her mood. The nurse can do so by asking the client to rate his or her mood on a scale of 1 to 10. For example, if the client reports being depressed, the nurse might ask, "On a scale of 1 to 10, with 1 being least depressed and 10 being most depressed, where would you place yourself right now?"

Thought Process and Content

Thought process refers to how the client thinks. The nurse can infer a client's thought process from speech and speech patterns. **Thought content** is what the client actually says. The nurse assesses whether or not the client's verbalizations make sense, that is, if ideas are related and flow logically from one to the next. The nurse also must determine whether the client seems preoccupied, as if talking or paying attention to someone or something else. When the nurse encounters clients with marked difficulties in thought process and content, he or she may find it helpful to ask focused questions requiring short answers. Common terms related to the assessment of thought process and content include the following (American Psychiatric Association, 2000):

- **Circumstantial thinking:** a client eventually answers a question but only after giving excessive unnecessary detail
- **Delusion:** a fixed false belief not based in reality
- **Flight of ideas:** excessive amount and rate of speech composed of fragmented or unrelated ideas
- **Ideas of reference:** client's inaccurate interpretation that general events are personally directed to him or her, such as hearing a speech on the news and believing the message had personal meaning
- **Loose associations:** disorganized thinking that jumps from one idea to another with little or no evident relation between the thoughts
- **Tangential thinking:** wandering off the topic and never providing the information requested
- **Thought blocking:** stopping abruptly in the middle of a sentence or train of thought; sometimes unable to continue the idea
- **Thought broadcasting:** a delusional belief that others can hear or know what the client is thinking

- **Thought insertion:** a delusional belief that others are putting ideas or thoughts into the client's head—that is, the ideas are not those of the client
- **Thought withdrawal:** a delusional belief that others are taking the client's thoughts away and the client is powerless to stop it
- **Word salad:** flow of unconnected words that convey no meaning to the listener

ASSESSMENT OF SUICIDE OR HARM TOWARD OTHERS

The nurse must determine whether the depressed or hopeless client has suicidal ideation or a lethal plan. The nurse does so by asking the client directly "Do you have thoughts of suicide?" or "What thoughts of suicide have you had?" Box 8.2 lists assessment questions the nurse should ask any client who has suicidal ideas.

Likewise, if the client is angry, hostile, or making threatening remarks about a family member, spouse, or anyone else, the nurse must ask if the client has thoughts or plans about hurting that person. The nurse does so by questioning the client directly:

- What thoughts have you had about hurting [person's name]?
- What is your plan?
- What do you want to do to [person's name]?

When a client makes specific threats or has a plan to harm another person, health care providers are legally obligated to warn the person who is the target of the threats or plan. The legal term for this is **duty to warn.** This is one situation in which the nurse must breach the client's confidentiality to protect the threatened person.

Sensorium and Intellectual Processes

ORIENTATION

Orientation refers to the client's recognition of person, place, and time—that is, knowing who and where he or she is and the correct day, date, and year. This is often docu-

mented as "oriented × 3." Occasionally, a fourth sphere, situation, is added (whether or not the client accurately perceives his or her current circumstances). Absence of correct information about person, place, and time is referred to as disorientation, or "oriented × 1" (person only) or "oriented × 2" (person and place). The order of person, place, and time is significant. When a person is disoriented, he or she first loses track of time, then place, and finally person. Orientation returns in the reverse order: first, the person knows who he or she is, then realizes place, and finally time.

Disorientation is not synonymous with confusion. A confused person cannot make sense of his or her surroundings or figure things out even though he or she may be fully oriented.

MEMORY

The nurse directly assesses memory, both recent and remote, by asking questions with verifiable answers. For example, if the nurse asks, "Do you have any memory problems?" the client may inaccurately respond "no," and the nurse cannot verify that. Similarly, if the nurse asks "What did you do yesterday?" the nurse may be unable to verify the accuracy of the client's responses. Hence, questions to assess memory generally include the following:

- What is the name of the current president?
- Who was the president before that?
- In what county do you live?
- What is the capital of this state?
- What is your social security number?

ABILITY TO CONCENTRATE

The nurse assesses the client's ability to concentrate by asking the client to perform certain tasks:

- Spell the word *world* backward.
- Begin with the number 100, subtract 7, subtract 7 again, and so on. This is called "serial sevens."
- Repeat the days of the week backward.
- Perform a three-part task, such as "Take a piece of paper in your right hand, fold it in half, and put it on the floor." (The nurse should give the instructions at one time.)

ABSTRACT THINKING AND INTELLECTUAL ABILITIES

When assessing intellectual functioning, the nurse must consider the client's level of formal education. Lack of formal education could hinder performance in many tasks in this section.

The nurse assesses the client's ability to use **abstract thinking,** which is to make associations or interpretations about a situation or comment. The nurse usually can do so by asking the client to interpret a common proverb such as "a stitch in time saves nine." If the client can explain the proverb correctly, his or her abstract thinking abilities are intact. If the client provides a literal explanation of the proverb and cannot interpret its meaning, abstract thinking

---

Box 8.2   SUICIDE ASSESSMENT QUESTIONS

Ideation: "Are you thinking about killing yourself?"

Plan: "Do you have a plan to kill yourself?"

Method: "How do you plan to kill yourself?"

Access: "How would you carry out this plan? Do you have access to the means to carry out the plan?"

Where: "Where would you kill yourself?"

When: "When do you plan to kill yourself?"

Timing: "What day or time of day do you plan to kill yourself?"

abilities are lacking. When the client continually gives literal translations, this is evidence of **concrete thinking**. For instance,

- *Proverb:* A stitch in time saves nine.
    Abstract meaning: If you take the time to fix something now, you'll avoid bigger problems in the future.
    Literal translation: Don't forget to sew up holes in your clothes (concrete thinking).
- *Proverb:* People who live in glass houses shouldn't throw stones.
    Abstract meaning: Don't criticize others for things you also may be guilty of doing.
    Literal translation: If you throw a stone at a glass house, the glass will break (concrete thinking).

The nurse also may assess the client's intellectual functioning by asking him or her to identify the similarities between pairs of objects, for example, "What is similar about an apple and an orange?" or "What do the newspaper and the television have in common?"

Sensory-Perceptual Alterations

Some clients experience **hallucinations** (false sensory perceptions or perceptual experiences that do not really exist). Hallucinations can involve the five senses and bodily sensations. Auditory hallucinations (hearing voices) are the most common; visual hallucinations (seeing things that don't really exist) are the second most common. Initially, clients perceive hallucinations as real experiences, but later in the illness, they may recognize them as hallucinations.

Judgment and Insight

Judgment refers to the ability to interpret one's environment and situation correctly and to adapt one's behavior and decisions accordingly. Problems with judgment may be evidenced as the client describes recent behavior and activities that reflect a lack of reasonable care for self or others. For example, the client may spend large sums of money on frivolous items when he or she cannot afford basic necessities such as food or clothing. Risky behaviors such as picking up strangers in bars or engaging in unprotected sexual activity also may indicate poor judgment. The nurse also may assess a client's judgment by asking the client hypothetical questions, such as "If you found a stamped addressed envelope on the ground, what would you do?"

Insight is the ability to understand the true nature of one's situation and accept some personal responsibility for that situation. The nurse frequently can infer insight from the client's ability to describe realistically the strengths and weaknesses of his or her behavior. An example of poor insight would be a client who places all blame on others for his own behavior, saying "It's my wife's fault that I drink and get into fights, because she nags me all the time." This client is not accepting responsibility for his drinking and fighting. Another example of poor insight would be the client who expects all problems to be solved with little or no personal effort: "The problem is my medication. As soon as the doctor gets the medication right, I'll be just fine."

Self-Concept

Self-concept is the way one views oneself in terms of personal worth and dignity. To assess a client's self-concept, the nurse can ask the client to describe himself or herself and what characteristics he or she likes and what he or she would change. The client's description of self in terms of physical characteristics gives the nurse information about the client's body image, which is also part of self-concept.

Also included in an assessment of self-concept are the emotions that the client frequently experiences, such as sadness or anger, and whether or not the client is comfortable with those emotions. The nurse also must assess the client's coping strategies. He or she can do so by asking, "What do you do when you have a problem? How do you solve it? What usually works to deal with anger or disappointment?"

Roles and Relationships

People function in their community through various roles such as mother, wife, son, daughter, teacher, secretary, or volunteer. The nurse assesses the roles the client occupies,

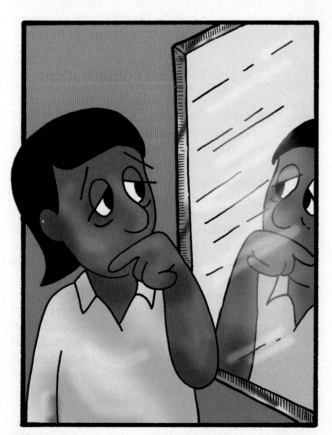

Self-concept

client satisfaction with those roles, and whether the client believes he or she is fulfilling the roles adequately (Hanna & Roy, 2001). The number and type of roles may vary, but they usually include family, occupation, and hobbies or activities. Family roles include son or daughter, sibling, parent, child, and spouse or partner. Occupation roles can be related to a career, school, or both. The ability to fulfill a role or the lack of a desired role is often central to the client's psychosocial functioning. Changes in roles also may be part of the client's difficulty.

Relationships with other people are important to one's social and emotional health. Relationships vary in terms of significance, level of intimacy or closeness, and intensity. The inability to sustain satisfying relationships can result from mental health problems or can contribute to the worsening of some problems. The nurse must assess the relationships in the client's life, the client's satisfaction with those relationships, or any loss of relationships. Common questions include the following:

- Do you feel close to your family?
- Do you have or want a relationship with a significant other?
- Are your relationships meeting your needs for companionship or intimacy?
- Can you meet your sexual needs satisfactorily?
- Have you been involved in any abusive relationships?

If the client's family relationships seem to be a significant source of stress or if the client is closely involved with his or her family, a more in-depth assessment of this area may be useful. Box 8.3 is the McMaster Family Assessment Device, an example of such an in-depth family assessment.

Physiologic and Self-Care Considerations

When doing a psychosocial assessment, the nurse must include physiologic functioning. Although a full physical health assessment may not be indicated, emotional problems often affect some areas of physiologic function. Emotional problems can greatly affect eating and sleeping patterns: Under stress, people may eat excessively or not at all and may sleep up to 20 hours a day or may be unable to sleep more than 2 or 3 hours a night. Clients with bipolar disorder may not eat or sleep for days. Clients with major depression may not be able to get out of bed. Therefore, the nurse must assess the client's usual patterns of eating and sleeping and then determine how those patterns have changed.

The nurse also asks the client if he or she has any major or chronic health problems and if he or she takes prescribed medications as ordered and follows dietary recommendations. The nurse also explores the client's use of alcohol and over-the-counter or illicit drugs. Such questions require nonjudgmental phrasing; the nurse must reassure the client that truthful information is crucial in determining the client's plan of care.

Noncompliance with prescribed medications is an important area. If the client has stopped taking medication or is taking medication other than as prescribed, the nurse must help the client feel comfortable enough to reveal this information. The nurse also explores the barriers to compliance. Is the client choosing noncompliance because of undesirable side effects? Has the medication failed to produce the desired results? Does the client have difficulty obtaining the medication? Is the medication too expensive for the client?

DATA ANALYSIS

After completing the psychosocial assessment, the nurse analyzes all the data that he or she has collected. Data analysis involves thinking about the overall assessment rather than focusing on isolated bits of information. The nurse looks for patterns or themes in the data that lead to conclusions about the client's strengths and needs and to a particular nursing diagnosis. No one statement or behavior is adequate to reach such a conclusion. The nurse also must consider the congruence of all information provided by the client, family, or caregivers, as well as his or her own observations. It is not uncommon for the client's perception of his or her behavior and situation to differ from that of others. Assessments in a variety of areas are necessary to support nursing diagnoses such as Chronic Low Self-Esteem or Ineffective Coping.

Traditionally, data analysis leads to the formulation of nursing diagnoses as a basis for the client's plan of care. Nursing diagnoses have been an integral part of the nursing process for many years. With the sweeping changes occurring in health care, however, the nurse also must articulate the client's needs in ways that are clear to health team members in other disciplines as well as to families and caregivers. For example, a multidisciplinary treatment plan or critical pathway may be the vehicle for planning care in some agencies. A plan of care that is useful to the client's family for home care may be necessary. The nurse must describe and document goals and interventions that many others, not just professional nurses, can understand. The descriptions must contain no jargon or terms that are unclear to the client, family, or other providers of care.

Psychological Tests

Psychological tests are another source of data for the nurse to use in planning care for the client. Two basic types of tests are intelligence tests and personality tests. *Intelligence tests* are designed to evaluate the client's cognitive abilities and intellectual functioning. *Personality tests* reflect the client's personality in areas such as self-concept, impulse control, reality testing, and major defenses (Adams & Culbertson, 2005). Personality tests may be objective (constructed of true and false or multiple-choice questions). Table 8.1 describes selected objective personality tests. The nurse compares the client's answers with standard answers or criteria and obtains a score or scores.

Box 8.3   McMASTER FAMILY ASSESSMENT DEVICE

Instructions: Following are a number of statements about families. Please read each statement carefully, and decide how well it describes your own family. You should answer according to how you see your family. For each statement, there are four (4) possible responses:

Strongly Agree (SA)   Check SA if you believe the statement describes your family very accurately.
Agree (A)   Check A if you believe the statement describes your family for the most part.
Disagree (D)   Check D if you believe the statement does not describe your family for the most part.
Strongly Disagree (SD)   Check SD if you believe the statement does not describe your family at all.

Try not to spend too much time thinking about each statement, but respond as quickly and honestly as you can. If you have trouble with one, answer with your first reaction. Please be sure to answer every statement, and mark all your answers in the space provided next to each statement.

Statements	SA	A	D	SD
1. Planning family activities is difficult because we misunderstand each other.	___	___	___	___
2. We resolve most everyday problems around the house.	___	___	___	___
3. When someone is upset the others know why.	___	___	___	___
4. When you ask someone to do something, you have to check that they did it.	___	___	___	___
5. If someone is in trouble, the others become too involved.	___	___	___	___
6. In times of crisis we can turn to each other for support.	___	___	___	___
7. We don't know what to do when an emergency comes up.	___	___	___	___
8. We sometimes run out of things that we need.	___	___	___	___
9. We are reluctant to show our affection to each other.	___	___	___	___
10. We make sure members meet their family responsibilities.	___	___	___	___
11. We cannot talk to each other about the sadness we feel.	___	___	___	___
12. We usually act on our decisions regarding problems.	___	___	___	___
13. You only get the interest of others when something is important to them.	___	___	___	___
14. You can't tell how a person is feeling from what they are saying.	___	___	___	___
15. Family tasks don't get spread around enough.	___	___	___	___
16. Individuals are accepted for what they are.	___	___	___	___
17. You can easily get away with breaking the rules.	___	___	___	___
18. People come right out and say things instead of hinting at them.	___	___	___	___
19. Some of us just don't respond emotionally.	___	___	___	___
20. We know what to do in an emergency.	___	___	___	___
21. We avoid discussing our fears and concerns.	___	___	___	___
22. It is difficult to talk to each other about tender feelings.	___	___	___	___
23. We have trouble meeting our bills.	___	___	___	___
24. After our family tries to solve a problem, we usually discuss whether it worked or not.	___	___	___	___
25. We are too self-centered.	___	___	___	___
26. We can express our feelings to each other.	___	___	___	___
27. We have no clear expectations about toilet habits.	___	___	___	___
28. We do not show our love for each other.	___	___	___	___
29. We talk to people directly rather than through go-betweens.	___	___	___	___
30. Each of us has particular duties and responsibilities.	___	___	___	___
31. There are lots of bad feelings in the family.	___	___	___	___
32. We have rules about hitting people.	___	___	___	___
33. We get involved with each other only when something interests us.	___	___	___	___
34. There's little time to explore personal interests.	___	___	___	___
35. We often don't say what we mean.	___	___	___	___

continued ···▷

Box 8.3: McMaster Family Assessment Device, cont.

Statements	SA	A	D	SD
36. We feel accepted for what we are.	___	___	___	___
37. We show interest in each other when we can get something out of it personally.	___	___	___	___
38. We resolve most emotional upsets that come up.	___	___	___	___
39. Tenderness takes second place to other things in our family.	___	___	___	___
40. We discuss who is to do household jobs.	___	___	___	___
41. Making decisions is a problem for our family.	___	___	___	___
42. Our family shows interest in each other only when they can get something out of it.	___	___	___	___
43. We are frank with each other.	___	___	___	___
44. We don't hold to any rules or standards.	___	___	___	___
45. If people are asked to do something, they need reminding.	___	___	___	___
46. We are able to make decisions about how to solve problems.	___	___	___	___
47. If the rules are broken, we don't know what to expect.	___	___	___	___
48. Anything goes in our family.	___	___	___	___
49. We express tenderness.	___	___	___	___
50. We control problems involving feelings.	___	___	___	___
51. We don't get along well together.	___	___	___	___
52. We don't talk to each other when we are angry.	___	___	___	___
53. We are generally dissatisfied with the family duties assigned to us.	___	___	___	___
54. Even though we mean well, we intrude too much into each other's lives.	___	___	___	___
55. There are rules about dangerous situations.	___	___	___	___
56. We confide in each other.	___	___	___	___
57. We cry openly.	___	___	___	___
58. We don't have reasonable transport.	___	___	___	___
59. When we don't like what someone has done, we tell them.	___	___	___	___
60. We try to think of different ways to solve problems.	___	___	___	___

From Schutle, N. S., & Malouff, J. M. (1995). Sourcebook of adult assessment strategies. *New York: Plenum Press, Brown University/ Butler Hospital Family Research Program,* © 1982.

Other personality tests, called projective tests, are unstructured and are usually conducted by the interview method. The stimuli for these tests, such as pictures or Rorschach's ink blots, are standard, but clients may respond with answers that are very different. The evaluator analyzes the client's responses and gives a narrative result of the testing. Table 8.2 lists commonly used projective personality tests.

Both intelligence tests and personality tests are frequently criticized as being culturally biased. It is important to consider the client's culture and environment when evaluating the importance of scores or projections from any of these tests; they can provide useful information about the client in some circumstances but may not be suitable for all clients.

Psychiatric Diagnoses

Medical diagnoses of psychiatric illness are found in the *Diagnostic and Statistical Manual of Mental Disorders, 4th edi-*tion, *Text Revision (DSM-IV-TR).* This taxonomy is universally used by psychiatrists and by some therapists in the diagnosis of psychiatric illnesses. The *DSM-IV-TR* classifies mental disorders into categories. It describes each disorder and provides diagnostic criteria to distinguish one from another. Although the *DSM-IV-TR* is not a substitute for a thorough psychosocial nursing assessment, the descriptions of disorders and related behaviors can be a valuable resource for the nurse to use as a guide. The *DSM-IV-TR* uses a multiaxial system to provide the format for a complete psychiatric diagnosis:

- Axis I: clinical disorders, other conditions that may be a focus of clinical attention
- Axis II: personality disorders, mental retardation
- Axis III: general medical conditions
- Axis IV: psychosocial and environmental problems
- Axis V: global assessment of functioning (GAF)

The psychosocial and environmental problems categorized on axis IV include educational, occupational, housing, finan-

Table 8.1 OBJECTIVE MEASURES OF PERSONALITY

Test	Description
Minnesota Multiphasic Personality Inventory (MMPI)	566 multiple-choice items; provides scores on 10 clinical scales such as hypochondriasis, depression, hysteria, paranoia; 4 special scales such as anxiety and alcoholism; 3 validity scales to evaluate the truth and accuracy of responses
MMPI-2	Revised version of MMPI with 567 multiple-choice items; provides scores on same areas as MMPI
Milton Clinical Multiaxial Inventory (MCMI) and MCMI-II (revised version)	175 true-false items; provides scores on various personality traits and personality disorders
Psychological Screening Inventory (PSI)	103 true-false items; used to screen for the need for psychological help
Beck Depression Inventory (BDI)	21 items rated on scale of 0–3 to indicate level of depression
Tennessee Self-Concept Scale (TSCS)	100 true-false items; provides information on 14 scales related to self-concept

Adams, R. L., & Culbertson, J. L. (2005). Personality assessment: Adults and children. In B. J. Sadock & V. A. Sadock (Eds.), *Comprehensive textbook of psychiatry* (*Vol. 1,* 8th ed., pp. 874–895). Philadelphia: Lippincott Williams & Wilkins.

Table 8.2 PROJECTIVE MEASURES OF PERSONALITY

Test	Description
Rorschach test	10 stimulus cards of ink blots; client describes perceptions of ink blots; narrative interpretation discusses areas such as coping styles, interpersonal attitudes, characteristics of ideation
Thematic Apperception Test (TAT)	20 stimulus cards with pictures; client tells a story about the picture; narrative interpretation discusses themes about mood state, conflict, quality of interpersonal relationships
Sentence completion test	Client completes a sentence from beginnings such as "I often wish," "Most people," and "When I was young."

Adams, R. L., & Culbertson, J. L. (2005). Personality assessment: Adults and children. In B. J. Sadock & V. A. Sadock (Eds.), *Comprehensive textbook of psychiatry* (*Vol. 1,* 8th ed., pp. 874–895). Philadelphia: Lippincott Williams & Wilkins.

cial, and legal problems as well as difficulties with the social environment, relationships, and access to health care.

The GAF is used to make a judgment about the client's overall level of functioning (Box 8.4). The GAF score given to the client may describe his or her current level of functioning as well as the highest level of functioning in the past year or 6 months. This information is useful in setting appropriate goals for the client's care.

Mental Status Exam

Often, psychiatrists, therapists, or other clinicians perform a cursory abbreviated exam that focuses on the client's cognitive abilities. These exams usually include items such as orientation to person, time, place, date, season, and day of the week; ability to interpret proverbs; ability to perform math calculations; memorization and short-term recall; naming common objects in the environment; ability to follow multistep commands; and ability to write or copy a simple drawing. The fewer tasks the client completes accurately, the greater the cognitive deficit. Because this exam assesses

cognitive ability, it is often used to screen for dementia. However, cognition may also be impaired (usually temporarily) when clients are depressed or psychotic.

SELF-AWARENESS ISSUES

Self-awareness is crucial when a nurse is trying to obtain accurate and complete information from the client during the assessment process. The nurse must be aware of any feelings, biases, and values that could interfere with the psychosocial assessment of a client with different beliefs, values, and behaviors. The nurse cannot let personal feelings and beliefs influence the client's treatment. Self-awareness does not mean the nurse's beliefs are wrong or must change, but it does help the nurse to be open and accepting of others' beliefs and behaviors even when the nurse does not agree with them.

Two areas that may be uncomfortable or difficult for the nurse to assess are sexuality and self-harm behaviors. The beginning nurse may feel uncomfortable, as if prying into personal matters, when asking questions about a client's intimate relationships and behavior and any self-harm behaviors or thoughts of suicide. Asking such questions, however, is essential to obtaining a thorough and complete assessment. The nurse needs to remember that it may be uncomfortable for the client to discuss these topics as well.

The nurse may hold beliefs that differ from the client's, but he or she must not make judgments about the client's

Box 8.4   GLOBAL ASSESSMENT OF FUNCTIONING (GAF) SCALE

Consider psychological, social, and occupational functioning on a hypothetical continuum of mental health to illness. Do not include impairment in functioning due to physical (or environmental) limitations. (Note: Use intermediate codes when appropriate, e.g., 45, 68, 72.)

CODE

100 | 91	Superior functioning in a wide range of activities; life's problems never seem to get out of hand; is sought out by others because of his or her many positive qualities. No symptoms.
90 | 81	Absent or minimal symptoms (e.g., mild anxiety before an exam), good functioning in all areas, interested and involved in a wide range of activities, socially effective, generally satisfied with life; no more than everyday problems or concerns (e.g., an occasional argument with family members).
80 | 71	If symptoms are present, they are transient and expectable reactions to psychosocial stressors (e.g., difficulty concentrating after family argument); no more than slight impairment in social, occupational, or school functioning (e.g., temporarily falling behind in schoolwork).
70 | 61	Some mild symptoms (e.g., depressed mood and mild insomnia) OR some difficulty in social, occupational, or school functioning (e.g., occasional truancy, or theft within the household), but generally functioning pretty well; has some meaningful interpersonal relationships.
60 | 51	Moderate symptoms (e.g., flat affect and circumstantial speech, occasional panic attacks) OR moderate difficulty in social, occupational, or school functioning (e.g., few friends, conflicts with peers or coworkers).
50 | 41	Serious symptoms (e.g., suicidal ideation, severe obsessional rituals, frequent shoplifting) OR any serious impairment in social, occupational, or school functioning (e.g., no friends, unable to keep a job).
40 | 31	Some impairment in reality testing or communication (e.g., speech is at times illogical, obscure, or irrelevant) OR major impairment in several areas such as work or school, family relations, judgment, thinking, or mood (e.g., depressed man avoids friends, neglects family, and is unable to work; child frequently beats up younger children, is defiant at home, and is failing at school).
30 | 21	Behavior is considerably influenced by delusions or hallucinations OR serious impairment in communication or judgment (e.g., sometimes incoherent, acts grossly inappropriately, suicidal preoccupation) OR inability to function in almost all areas (e.g., stays in bed all day; no job, home, or friends).
20 | 11	Some danger of hurting self or others (e.g., suicide attempts without clear expectation of death; frequently violent; manic excitement) OR occasionally fails to maintain minimal personal hygiene (e.g., smears feces) OR gross impairment in communication (e.g., largely incoherent or mute).
10 | 1	Persistent danger of severely hurting self or others (e.g., recurrent violence) OR persistent inability to maintain minimal personal hygiene OR serious suicidal act with clear expectation of death.
0	Inadequate information.

The rating of overall psychological functioning on a scale of 0–100 was operationalized by Luborsky in the Health-Sickness Rating Scale (Luborsky L.: "Clinicians' Judgments of Mental Health." Archives of General Psychiatry 7:407–417, 1962). Spitzer and colleagues developed a revision of the Health-Sickness Rating Scale called the Global Assessment Scale (GAS) (Endicott J., Spitzer R. L., Fleiss J. L., Cohen J.: "The Global Assessment Scale: A Procedure for Measuring Overall Severity of Psychiatric Disturbance." Archives of General Psychiatry 33:766–771, 1976). A modified version of the GAS was included in DSM-III-R as the Global Assessment of Functioning (GAF) Scale.

practices. For example, the nurse may believe abortion is a sin, but the client might have had several elective abortions. Or the nurse may believe that adultery is wrong, but, during the course of an assessment, he or she may discover that a client has had several extramarital affairs.

Being able to listen to the client without judgment and to support the discussion of personal topics takes practice and usually gets easier with experience. Talking to more experienced colleagues about such discomfort and methods to alleviate it often helps. It may also help for the nurse to preface uncomfortable questions by saying to the client, "I need to ask you some personal questions. Remember, this is information that will help the staff provide better care for you."

The nurse must assess the client for suicidal thoughts. Some beginning nurses feel uncomfortable discussing suicide or believe that asking about suicide might suggest it to a client who had not previously thought about it. This is not the case. It has been shown that the safest way to assess a client with suspected mental disorders is to ask him or her clearly and directly about suicidal ideas. It is the nurse's professional responsibility to keep the client's safety needs first and foremost, and this includes overcoming any personal discomfort in talking about suicide (Schultz & Videbeck, 2005).

Points to Consider When Doing a Psychosocial Assessment

- The nurse is trying to gain all the information needed to help the client. Judgments are not part of the assessment process.
- Being open, clear, and direct when asking about personal or uncomfortable topics helps to alleviate the client's anxiety or hesitancy about discussing the topic.
- Examining one's own beliefs and gaining self-awareness is a growth-producing experience for the nurse.
- If the nurse's beliefs differ strongly from those of the client, the nurse should express his or her feelings to colleagues or discuss the differences with them. The nurse must not allow personal beliefs to interfere with the nurse–client relationship and the assessment process.

Critical Thinking Questions

1. The nurse is preparing to do a psychosocial assessment for a client who is seeking help because she has been physically abusive to her children. What feelings might the nurse experience? How does the nurse view this client?
2. The nurse has discovered through the assessment process that the client drinks a quart of vodka every 2 days. The client states this is not a problem. How does the nurse proceed? What could the nurse say to this client?
3. The nurse is assessing a client who is illiterate. How will the nurse assess the intellectual functioning of this client? What other areas of a psychosocial assessment might be impaired by the client's inability to read or write?

KEY POINTS

- The purpose of the psychosocial assessment is to construct a picture of the client's current emotional state, mental capacity, and behavioral function. This baseline clinical picture serves as the basis for developing a plan of care to meet the client's needs.
- The components of a thorough psychosocial assessment include the client's history, general appearance and motor behavior, mood and affect, thought process and content, sensorium and intellectual process, judgment and insight, self-concept, roles and relationships, and physiologic and self-care considerations.
- Several important factors in the client can influence the psychosocial assessment: ability to participate and give feedback, physical health status, emotional well-being and perception of the situation, and ability to communicate.
- The nurse's attitude and approach can greatly influence the psychosocial assessment. The nurse must conduct the assessment professionally, nonjudgmentally, and matter-of-factly while not allowing personal feelings to influence the interview.
- To avoid making inaccurate assumptions about the client's psychosocial functioning, the nurse must be sensitive to the client's cultural and spiritual beliefs. Many cultures have values and beliefs about a person's role in society or acceptable social or personal behavior that may differ from the beliefs and values of the nurse.
- Accurate analysis of assessment data involves considering the entire assessment and identifying patterns of behavior as well as congruence among components and sources of information.
- Self-awareness on the nurse's part is crucial to obtain an accurate, objective, and thorough psychosocial assessment.
- Areas that are often difficult for nurses to assess include sexuality and self-harm behaviors and suicidality. Discussion with colleagues and experience with clients can help the nurse to deal with uncomfortable feelings.
- The client's safety is a priority; therefore, asking clients clearly and directly about suicidal ideation is essential.

REFERENCES

Adams, R. L., & Culbertson, J. L. (2005). Personality assessment: Adults and children. In B. J. Sadock & V. A. Sadock (Eds.), *Comprehensive textbook of psychiatry* (Vol. 1, 8th ed., pp. 874–895). Philadelphia: Lippincott Williams & Wilkins.

American Nurses Association. (2000). *Statement on psychiatric-mental health nursing practice and standards of psychiatric and mental health nursing practice.* Washington, DC: American Nurses Publishing.

American Psychiatric Association. (2000). *Diagnostic and statistical manual of mental disorders* (4th ed., text revision). Washington, DC: American Psychiatric Association.

Hanna, D. R., & Roy, C. Sr. (2001). Roy adaptation model and perspectives on family. *Nursing Science Quarterly, 14*(1), 9–13.

Schultz, J. M., & Videbeck, S. (2005). *Lippincott's manual of psychiatric nursing care plans* (7th ed.). Philadelphia: Lippincott Williams & Wilkins.

Chapter Study Guide

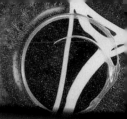

MULTIPLE-CHOICE QUESTIONS

Select the best answer for each of the following questions.

1. Which of the following is an example of an open-ended question?
   A. Who is the current president of the United States?
   B. What concerns you most about your health?
   C. What is your address?
   D. Have you lost any weight recently?

2. Which of the following is an example of a closed-ended question?
   A. How have you been feeling lately?
   B. How is your relationship with your wife?
   C. Have you had any health problems recently?
   D. Where are you employed?

3. Which of the following is not included in the assessment of sensorium and intellectual processes?
   A. Concentration
   B. Memory
   C. Judgment
   D. Orientation

4. Assessment data about the client's speech patterns are categorized in which of the following areas?
   A. History
   B. General appearance and motor behavior
   C. Sensorium and intellectual processes
   D. Self-concept

5. When the nurse is assessing whether or not the client's ideas are logical and make sense, the nurse is examining which of the following?
   A. Thought content
   B. Thought process
   C. Memory
   D. Sensorium

6. The client's belief that a news broadcast has special meaning for him or her is an example of
   A. Abstract thinking
   B. Flight of ideas
   C. Ideas of reference
   D. Thought broadcasting

7. The client who believes everyone is out to get him or her is experiencing a(n)
   A. Delusion
   B. Hallucination
   C. Idea of reference
   D. Loose association

8. To assess the client's ability to concentrate, the nurse would instruct the client to do which of the following?
   A. Explain what "a rolling stone gathers no moss" means.
   B. Name the last three presidents.
   C. Repeat the days of the week backward.
   D. Tell what a typical day is like.

FILL-IN-THE-BLANK QUESTIONS

Identify each of the following terms being described.

_____ 1. Repeated purposeless behaviors often indicating anxiety

_____ 2. The belief that others can read one's thoughts

_____ 3. Generally slowed body movements

_____ 4. Flow of unconnected words that have no meaning

SHORT-ANSWER QUESTIONS

Identify a question that the nurse might ask to assess each of the following.

1. Abstract thinking ability

2. Insight

3. Self-concept

4. Judgment

5. Mood

6. Orientation

CLINICAL EXAMPLE

The nurse at a mental health clinic is meeting a new client for the first time and plans to do a psychosocial assessment. When the client arrives, the nurse finds a young woman who looks somewhat apprehensive and is crying and twisting facial tissues in her hands. The client can tell the nurse her name and age but begins crying before she can provide any other information. The nurse knows it is essential to obtain information from this young woman, but it is clear she will have trouble answering all interview questions at this time.

1. How should the nurse approach the crying client? What should the nurse say and do?

2. Identify five questions that the nurse would choose to ask this client initially. Give a rationale for the chosen questions.

3. What, if any, assumptions might the nurse make about this client and her situation?

4. If the client decided to leave the clinic before the assessment formally began, what would the nurse need to do?

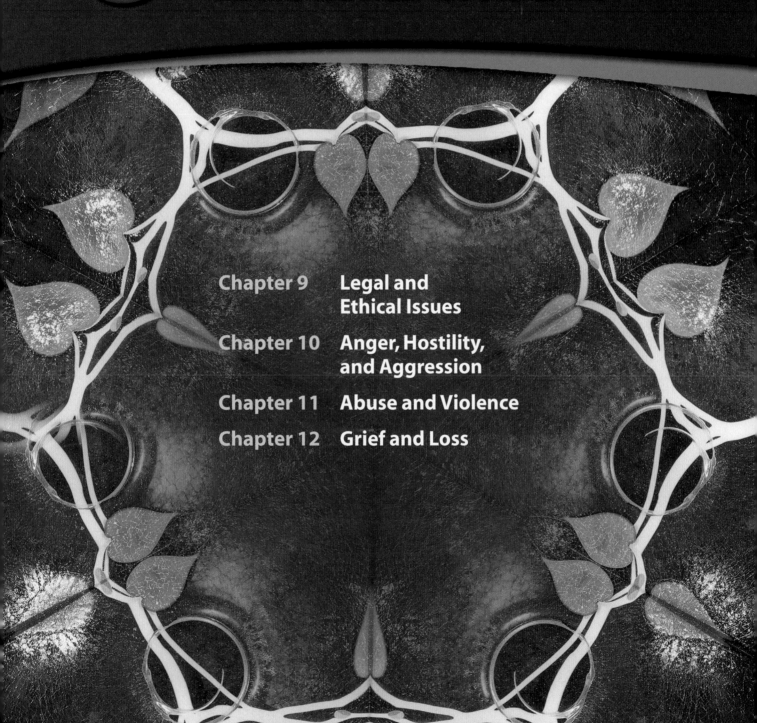

3 Current Social and Emotional Concerns

Legal and Ethical Issues

Key Terms

- assault
- autonomy
- battery
- beneficence
- breach of duty
- causation
- deontology
- duty
- duty to warn
- ethical dilemma
- ethics
- false imprisonment
- fidelity
- injury or damage
- justice
- least restrictive environment
- malpractice
- mandatory outpatient treatment
- negligence
- nonmaleficence
- restraint
- seclusion
- standards of care
- tort
- utilitarianism
- veracity

Learning Objectives

After reading this chapter, you should be able to

1. Describe the rights of the client in a psychiatric setting.

2. Discuss the legal and ethical issues related to seclusion and restraint.

3. Describe the components of malpractice.

4. Identify pertinent ethical issues in the practice of psychiatric nursing.

5. Discuss the meaning of *standard of care*.

6. Describe the most common types of torts in the mental health setting.

Historically, clients with mental illness had few rights and were subjected to institutionalization, warehousing, and inhumane treatment (see Chapter 1). In the 1970s, recognition of patient's rights and changes in laws governing commitment improved the rights of clients. This chapter discusses the legal considerations related to mental health treatment and ethical issues that commonly arise in mental health settings.

LEGAL CONSIDERATIONS

Rights of Clients and Related Issues

Clients receiving mental health care retain all civil rights afforded to all people except the right to leave the hospital in the case of involuntary commitment (discussed later). They have the right to refuse treatment, to send and to receive sealed mail, and to have or to refuse visitors. Any restrictions (e.g., mail, visitors, clothing) must be made by a court or a physician's order for a verifiable, documented reason. Examples include the following:

- A suicidal client may not be permitted to keep a belt, shoelaces, or scissors because he or she may use these items for self-harm.
- A client who becomes aggressive after having a particular visitor may have that person restricted from visiting for a period of time.
- A client making threatening phone calls to others outside the hospital may be permitted only supervised phone calls until his or her condition improves.

The American Psychiatric Association (APA) developed Principles for the Provision of Mental Health and Substance Abuse Treatment Services. This mental health patient's bill of rights is summarized in Box 9.1. The entire document can be accessed at http://www.apa.org/pubinfo/rights/rights.html.

INVOLUNTARY HOSPITALIZATION

Most clients are admitted to inpatient settings on a *voluntary* basis, which means they are willing to seek treatment and agree to be hospitalized. Some clients, however, do not wish to be hospitalized and treated. Health care professionals respect these wishes unless clients are a danger to themselves or others (i.e., they are threatening or have attempted suicide or represent a danger to others). Clients hospitalized against their will under these conditions are committed to a facility for psychiatric care until they no longer pose a danger to themselves or to anyone else. Each state has laws that govern the civil commitment process, but such laws are similar across all 50 states. Civil commitment or involuntary hospitalization curtails the client's right to freedom (the ability to leave the hospital when he or she wishes). All other client rights, however, remain intact.

A person can be detained in a psychiatric facility for 48 to 72 hours on an emergency basis until a hearing can be conducted to determine whether or not he or she should be committed to a facility for treatment for a specified period.

Box 9.1 | HIGHLIGHTS OF PATIENT'S BILL OF RIGHTS

- To be informed about benefits, qualifications of all providers, available treatment options, and appeals and grievance procedures
- Confidentiality
- Choice of providers
- Treatment determined by professionals, not third-party payers
- Parity
- Nondiscrimination
- All benefits within scope of benefit plan
- Treatment that affords greatest protection and benefit
- Fair and valid treatment review processes
- Treating-professionals and payers held accountable for any injury caused by gross incompetence, negligence, or clinically unjustified decisions

Many states have similar laws governing the commitment of clients with substance abuse problems who represent a danger to themselves or others when under the influence.

RELEASE FROM THE HOSPITAL

Clients admitted to the hospital voluntarily have the right to leave, provided they do not represent a danger to themselves or others. They can sign a written request for discharge and can be released from the hospital against medical advice. If a voluntary client who is dangerous to himself or herself or others signs a request for discharge, the psychiatrist may file for a civil commitment to detain the client against his or her will until a hearing can take place to decide the matter.

While in the hospital, the committed client may take medications and improve fairly rapidly, making him or her eligible for discharge when he or she no longer represents a danger. Some clients stop taking their medications after discharge and once again become threatening, aggressive, or dangerous. Mental health clinicians increasingly have been held legally liable for the criminal actions of such clients; this situation contributes to the debate about extended civil commitment for dangerous clients.

MANDATORY OUTPATIENT TREATMENT

Legally **mandated outpatient treatment** (MOT) is the requirement that clients continue to participate in treatment on an involuntary basis after their release from the hospital into the community. This may involve taking prescribed medication, keeping appointments with health care providers for follow-up, and attending specific treatment programs or groups (Wysocker et al., 2004). In the United States, all but eight states have laws for some type of mandatory outpatient treatment. A complete list can be obtained on the Web site for the Treatment Advocacy Center (2006). Benefits of MOT include shorter inpatient hospital stays, although these individuals may be hospitalized more frequently (Segal & Burgess, 2006a); reduced mortality risk for clients considered dangerous to self or others (Segal & Burgess, 2006b); and protection of clients from criminal victimization by others (Hiday et al., 2002).

MOT is sometimes also called conditional release or outpatient commitment. Court-ordered outpatient treatment is most common among persons with severe and persistent metal illness who have had frequent and multiple contacts with mental health, social welfare, and criminal justice agencies (Swartz et al., 2006). This supports the notion that clients are given several opportunities to voluntarily comply with outpatient treatment recommendations, and that court-ordered treatment is considered when those attempts have been repeatedly unsuccessful. The court's concern is that clients with psychiatric disorders have civil rights and should not be unreasonably required to participate in any activities against their will. Communities counter that they deserve protection against dangerous people with histories of not taking their medications and who may become threats.

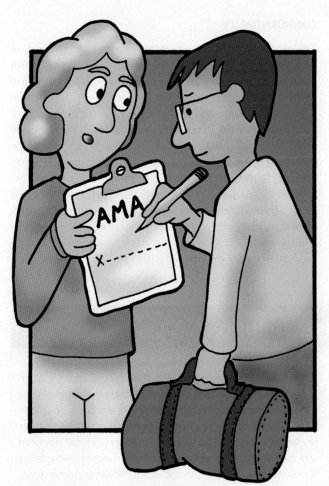

Voluntary clients may sign a written request for discharge against medical advice.

CONSERVATORSHIP

The appointment of a *conservator* or legal guardian is a separate process from civil commitment. People who are gravely disabled; are found to be incompetent; cannot provide food, clothing, and shelter for themselves even when resources exist; and cannot act in their own best interests may require appointment of a conservator. In these cases, the court appoints a person to act as a legal guardian who assumes many responsibilities for the person, such as giving informed consent, writing checks, and entering contracts. The client with a guardian loses the right to enter into legal contracts or agreements that require a signature (e.g., marriage, mortgage). This affects many daily activities usually taken for granted. Because conservators or guardians speak for clients, the nurse must obtain consent or permission from the conservator.

LEAST RESTRICTIVE ENVIRONMENT

Clients have the right to treatment in the **least restrictive environment** appropriate to meet their needs. This concept was central to the deinstitutionalization movement discussed in Chapters 1 and 4. It means that a client does not have to be hospitalized if he or she can be treated in an outpatient setting or in a group home. It also means that the client must be free of restraint or seclusion unless it is necessary.

Restraint is the direct application of physical force to a person, without his or her permission, to restrict his or her freedom of movement. The physical force may be human, mechanical, or both. *Human restraint* is when staff members physically control the client and move him or her to a seclusion room. *Mechanical restraints* are devices, usually ankle and wrist restraints, fastened to the bed frame to curtail the client's physical aggression, such as hitting, kicking, and hair pulling.

Seclusion is the involuntary confinement of a person in a specially constructed, locked room equipped with a security window or camera for direct visual monitoring. For safety, the room often has a bed bolted to the floor and a mattress. Any sharp or potentially dangerous objects, such as pens, glasses, belts, and matches, are removed from the client as a safety precaution. Seclusion decreases stimulation, protects others from the client, prevents property destruction, and provides privacy for the client. The goal is to give the client the opportunity to regain physical and emotional self-control.

Short-term use of restraint or seclusion is permitted only when the client is imminently aggressive and dangerous to himself or herself or to others. Use of restraint and seclusion requires a face-to-face evaluation by a licensed independent practitioner within 1 hour of restraint or seclusion, a physician's order every 4 hours, documented assessment by the nurse every 1 to 2 hours, and close supervision of the client. The nurse assesses the client for any injury and provides treatment as needed. Staff must monitor a client in restraints continuously on a 1:1 basis for the duration of the restraint

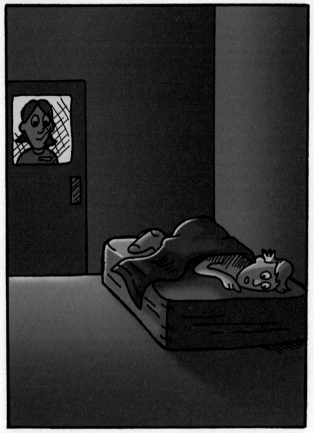

Seclusion

As soon as possible, staff members must inform the client of the behavioral criteria that will be used to determine whether to decrease or to end the use of restraint or seclusion. Criteria may include the client's ability to verbalize feelings and concerns rationally, to make no verbal threats, to have decreased muscle tension, and to demonstrate self-control. If a client remains in restraints for 1 to 2 hours, two staff members can free one limb at a time for movement and exercise. Frequent contact by the nurse promotes ongoing assessment of the client's well-being and self-control. It also provides an opportunity for the nurse to reassure the client that restraint is a restorative, not a punitive, procedure.

The nurse also should offer support to the client's family, who may be angry or embarrassed when the client is restrained or secluded. A careful and thorough explanation about the client's behavior and subsequent use of restraint or seclusion is important. If the client is an adult, however, such discussion requires a signed release of information. In the case of minor children, signed consent is not required to inform parents or guardians about the use of restraint or seclusion. Providing the family with information may help prevent legal or ethical difficulties. It also keeps the family involved in the client's treatment.

CONFIDENTIALITY

The protection and privacy of personal health information is regulated by the federal government through the Health Insurance Portability and Accountability Act (HIPAA) of 1996. The law guarantees the privacy and protection of health information and outlines penalties for violations.

Mandatory compliance with the Final HIPAA Privacy rule took effect on April 14, 2003, for all health care providers, including individuals and organizations that provide or pay for care. Both civil (fines) and criminal (prison sentences) penalties exist for violation of patient privacy. Protected Health Information is any individually identifiable health information in oral, written, or electronic form. Mental health and substance abuse records have additional special protection under the privacy rules.

period. A client in seclusion is monitored 1:1 for the first hour and then may be monitored by audio and video equipment. The nurse monitors and documents the client's skin condition, blood circulation in hands and feet (for the client in restraints), and emotional well-being. He or she observes the client closely for side effects of medications, which may be given in large doses in emergencies. The nurse also implements and documents offers of food, fluids, and opportunities to use the bathroom per facility policies and procedures (Joint Commission on Accreditation of Healthcare Organizations, 2005).

CLINICAL VIGNETTE: SECLUSION

The goal of seclusion is to give the client the opportunity to regain self-control, both emotionally and physically. Most clients who have been secluded, however, have very different feelings and thoughts about seclusion. Clients report feeling angry, agitated, bored, frustrated, helpless, and afraid while in seclusion. They perceive seclusion as a punishment and receive the message that they were "bad." Many clients are not clear about the reasons for seclusion or the criteria for exiting seclusion, and they believe that seclusion lasted too long. In general, clients think that other interventions such as interaction with staff, a place to calm down or scream when needed, or the presence of a family member could reduce or eliminate the need for seclusion. Clients who had not been secluded describe the seclusion of others in more positive terms such as *helpful, caring, fair,* and *good.* However, these clients also express the wish that "that never happens to me."

Some believe that these strict confidentiality policies may pose a barrier to collaboration among providers and families (Marshall & Solomon, 2003). In community mental health settings, compliance with the privacy rule has decreased communication and collaboration among providers, which may have a negative impact on patient care (Touchet et al., 2004). Marshall and Solomon, as well as Touchet and colleagues, recommended a vigorous education program for clients and families about the privacy regulation as well as establishing open lines of communication between clients and families before a crisis occurs.

DUTY TO WARN THIRD PARTIES

One exception to the client's right to confidentiality is the **duty to warn,** based on the California Supreme Court decision in *Tarasoff vs. Regents of the University of California* (Box 9.2). As a result of this decision, mental health clinicians have a duty to warn identifiable third parties of threats made by clients, even if these threats were discussed during therapy sessions otherwise protected by privilege. Based on the Tarasoff decision, many states have enacted laws regarding warning a third party of threats or danger. The clinician must base his or her decision to warn others on the following:

- Is the client dangerous to others?
- Is the danger the result of serious mental illness?
- Is the danger serious?
- Are the means to carry out the threat available?
- Is the danger targeted at identifiable victims?
- Is the victim accessible?

> ### Box 9.2 TARASOFF VS. REGENTS OF THE UNIVERSITY OF CALIFORNIA (1976)
>
> In 1969, a graduate student at the University of California, Prosenjit Poddar, dated a young woman named Tatiana Tarasoff for a short time. After the brief relationship ended, Poddar sought counseling with a psychologist at the university. He confided to the therapist that he intended to kill his former girlfriend when she returned from Brazil at the end of the summer. The psychologist contacted the university campus police, who detained and questioned Poddar. He was released because he appeared rational, promised to stay away from Tarasoff, and claimed he would not harm her. Two months later, shortly after her return from Brazil, Tatiana Tarasoff was murdered by Poddar on Oct. 27, 1969. Her parents sued the University of California, claiming that the therapist had a duty to warn their daughter of Poddar's threats. The California Supreme Court concluded that the protective privilege ends where the public peril begins.

For example, if a man were admitted to a psychiatric facility stating he was going to kill his wife, the duty to warn his wife is clear. If, however, a client with paranoia were admitted saying, "I'm going to get them before they get me," but providing no other information, there is no specific third party to warn. Decisions about the duty to warn third parties usually are made by psychiatrists or by qualified mental health therapists in outpatient settings.

Insanity Defense

One legal issue that sparks controversy is the insanity defense, with *insanity* having a legal meaning but no medical definition. The argument that a person accused of a crime is not guilty because that person cannot control his or her actions or cannot understand the wrongfulness of the act is known as the M'Naghten rule. When the person meets the criteria, he or she may be found not guilty by reason of insanity. The public perception of the insanity defense is that it is used in 33% to 45% of major criminal cases and that it is usually successful; that is, the person accused of the crime "gets off" and is free immediately (Melton et al., 1997). In actuality, this defense is used in only 0.9% (9 in 1000) of all criminal cases and is successful in less than 20% of those cases.

Four states—Idaho, Kansas, Montana, and Utah—have abolished the insanity defense. Thirteen states, including Montana and Utah, have a law allowing a verdict of guilty but insane. Ideally, this means that the person is held responsible for the criminal behavior but can receive treatment for mental illness. Critics of this verdict, including the APA, argue that people do not always receive needed psychiatric treatment and that this verdict absolves the legal system of its responsibility.

Nursing Liability

Nurses are responsible for providing safe, competent, legal, and ethical care to clients and families. Professional guidelines such as the American Nurses Association's (ANA's) *Code of Ethics for Nurses with Interpretive Statements* (2001) and the ANA's *Scope and Standards of Psychiatric-Mental Health Nursing Practice* (2000) outline the nurse's responsibilities and provide guidance (see Chapter 1). Nurses are expected to meet **standards of care,** meaning the care they provide to clients meets set expectations and is what any nurse in a similar situation would do. Standards of care are developed from professional standards (cited earlier in this paragraph), state nurse practice acts, federal agency regulations, agency policies and procedures, job descriptions, and civil and criminal laws.

TORTS

A **tort** is a wrongful act that results in injury, loss, or damage. Torts may be either unintentional or intentional.

Unintentional Torts: Negligence and Malpractice. **Negligence** is an unintentional tort that involves causing harm by failing to do what a reasonable and prudent person would do in similar circumstances. **Malpractice** is a type of negligence that refers specifically to professionals such as nurses and physicians (*Nurses' Legal Handbook,* 2004). Clients or families can file malpractice lawsuits in any case of injury, loss, or death. For a malpractice suit to be successful, that is, for the nurse, physician, or hospital or agency to be liable, the client or family needs to prove the following four elements:

1. **Duty:** A legally recognized relationship (i.e., physician to client, nurse to client) existed. The nurse had a duty to the client, meaning that the nurse was acting in the capacity of a nurse.
2. **Breach of duty:** The nurse (or physician) failed to conform to standards of care, thereby breaching or failing the existing duty. The nurse did not act as a reasonable, prudent nurse would have acted in similar circumstances.
3. **Injury or damage:** The client suffered some type of loss, damage, or injury.
4. **Causation:** The breach of duty was the direct cause of the loss, damage, or injury. In other words, the loss, damage, or injury would not have occurred if the nurse had acted in a reasonable, prudent manner.

Not all injury or harm to a client can be prevented, nor do all client injuries result from malpractice. The issues are whether or not the client's actions were predictable or foreseeable (and, therefore, preventable) and whether or not the nurse carried out appropriate assessment, interventions, and evaluation that met the standards of care. In the mental health setting, lawsuits most often are related to suicide and suicide attempts. Other areas of concern include clients harming others (staff, family, other clients), sexual assault, and medication errors.

Intentional Torts. Psychiatric nurses also may be liable for intentional torts or voluntary acts that result in harm to the client. Examples include assault, battery, and false imprisonment.

Assault involves any action that causes a person to fear being touched in a way that is offensive, insulting, or physically injurious without consent or authority. Examples include making threats to restrain the client to give him or her an injection for failure to cooperate. **Battery** involves harmful or unwarranted contact with a client; actual harm or injury may or may not have occurred. Examples include touching a client without consent or unnecessarily restraining a client. **False imprisonment** is defined as the unjustifiable detention of a client such as the inappropriate use of restraint or seclusion.

Proving liability for an intentional tort involves three elements (*Nurses' Legal Handbook,* 2004):

1. The act was willful and voluntary on the part of the defendant (nurse).

2. The nurse intended to bring about consequences or injury to the person (client).
3. The act was a substantial factor in causing injury or consequences.

PREVENTION OF LIABILITY

Nurses can minimize the risk for lawsuits through safe, competent nursing care and descriptive, accurate documentation. Box 9.3 highlights ways to minimize the risk for liability.

ETHICAL ISSUES

Ethics is a branch of philosophy that deals with values of human conduct related to the rightness or wrongness of actions and to the goodness and badness of the motives and ends of such actions (King, 1984). Ethical theories are sets of principles used to decide what is morally right or wrong.

Utilitarianism is a theory that bases decisions on "the greatest good for the greatest number." Decisions based on utilitarianism consider which action would produce the greatest benefit for the most people. **Deontology** is a theory that says decisions should be based on whether or not an action is morally right with no regard for the result or consequences. Principles used as guides for decision-making in deontology include autonomy, beneficence, nonmaleficence, justice, veracity, and fidelity.

Autonomy refers to the person's right to self-determination and independence. **Beneficence** refers to one's duty to benefit or to promote good for others. **Nonmaleficence** is the requirement to do no harm to others either intentionally or unintentionally. **Justice** refers to fairness; that is, treating all people fairly and equally without regard for social or economic status, race, sex, marital status, religion, ethnicity, or cultural beliefs. **Veracity** is the duty to be hon-

---

Box 9.3   STEPS TO AVOID LIABILITY

Practice within the scope of state laws and nurse practice act.

Collaborate with colleagues to determine the best course of action.

Use established practice standards to guide decisions and actions.

Always put the client's rights and welfare first.

Develop effective interpersonal relationships with clients and families.

Accurately and thoroughly document all assessment data, treatments, interventions, and evaluations of the client's response to care.

est or truthful. **Fidelity** refers to the obligation to honor commitments and contracts.

All these principles have meaning in health care. The nurse respects the client's autonomy through patient's rights, informed consent, and encouraging the client to make choices about his or her health care. The nurse has a duty to take actions that promote the client's health (beneficence) and that do not harm the client (nonmaleficence). The nurse must treat all clients fairly (justice), be truthful and honest (veracity), and honor all duties and commitments to clients and families (fidelity).

Ethical Dilemmas in Mental Health

An **ethical dilemma** is a situation in which ethical principles conflict or when there is no one clear course of action in a given situation. For example, the client who refuses medication or treatment is allowed to do so based on the principle of autonomy. If the client presents an imminent threat of danger to self or others, however, the principle of nonmaleficence (do no harm) is at risk. To protect the client or others from harm, the client may be involuntarily committed to a hospital, even though some may argue that this action violates his or her right to autonomy. In this example, the utilitarian theory of doing the greatest good for the greatest number (involuntary commitment) overrides the individual client's autonomy (right to refuse treatment). Ethical dilemmas are often complicated and charged with emotion, making it difficult to arrive at fair or "right" decisions.

Many dilemmas in mental health involve the client's right to self-determination and independence (autonomy) and concern for the "public good" (utilitarianism). Examples include the following:

- Once a client is stabilized on psychotropic medication, should the client be forced to remain on medication through the use of enforced depot injections or through outpatient commitment?
- Are clients who are psychotic necessarily incompetent, or do they still have the right to refuse hospitalization and medication?
- Can consumers of mental health care truly be empowered if health care professionals "step in" to make decisions for them "for their own good"?
- Should physicians break confidentiality to report clients who drive cars at high speeds and recklessly?
- Should a client who is loud and intrusive to other clients on a hospital unit be secluded from the others?
- A health care worker has an established relationship with a person who later becomes a client in the agency where the health care worker practices. Can the health care worker continue the relationship with the person who is now a client?
- To protect the public, can clients with a history of violence toward others be detained after their symptoms are stable?

- When a therapeutic relationship has ended, can a health care professional ever have a social or intimate relationship with someone he or she met as a client?
- Is it possible to maintain strict professional boundaries (i.e., no previous, current, or future personal relationships with clients) in small communities and rural areas where all people in the community know one another?

The nurse will confront some of these dilemmas directly, and he or she will have to make decisions about a course of action. For example, the nurse may observe behavior between another health care worker and a client that seems flirtatious or inappropriate. Another dilemma might represent the policies or common practice of the agency where the nurse is employed; the nurse may have to decide whether he or she can support those practices or seek a position elsewhere. An example would be an agency that takes clients with a history of medication noncompliance only if they are scheduled for depot injections or remain on an outpatient commitment status. Yet other dilemmas are in the larger social arena; the nurse's decision is whether to support current practice or to advocate for change on behalf of clients, such as laws permitting people to be detained after treatment is completed when there is a potential of future risk for violence.

Ethical Decision-Making

The ANA published a *Code of Ethics for Nurses* (2001) to guide choices about ethical actions (Box 9.4). Models for ethical decision-making include gathering information, clarifying values, identifying options, identifying legal considerations and practical restraints, building consensus for the decision reached, and reviewing and analyzing the decision to determine what was learned (Abma & Widdershoven, 2006).

SELF-AWARENESS ISSUES

All nurses have beliefs about what is right or wrong and good or bad. That is, they have values just like all other people. Being a member of the nursing profession, however, presumes a duty to clients and families under the nurse's care: a duty to protect rights, to be an advocate, and to act in the clients' best interests even if that duty is in conflict with the nurse's personal values and beliefs. The nurse is obligated to engage in self-awareness by identifying clearly and examining his or her own values and beliefs so they do not become confused with or overshadow a client's. For example, if a client is grieving over her decision to have an abortion, the nurse must be able to provide support to her even though the nurse may be opposed to abortion. If the nurse cannot do that, then he or she should talk to colleagues to find someone who can meet that client's needs.

Box 9.4   AMERICAN NURSES ASSOCIATION CODE OF ETHICS FOR NURSES

1. The nurse, in all professional relationships, practices with compassion and respect for the inherent dignity, worth, and uniqueness of every individual, unrestricted by considerations of social or economic status, personal attributes, or the nature of health problems.
2. The nurse's primary commitment is to the patient, whether an individual, family, group, or community.
3. The nurse promotes, advocates for, and strives to protect the health, safety, and rights of the patient.
4. The nurse is responsible and accountable for individual nursing practice and determines the appropriate delegation of tasks consistent with the nurse's obligation to provide optimum patient care.
5. The nurse owes the same duties to self as to others, including the responsibility to preserve integrity and safety, to maintain competence, and to continue personal and professional growth.
6. The nurse participates in establishing, maintaining, and improving health care environments and conditions of employment conducive to the provision of quality health care and consistent with the values of the profession through individual and collective action.
7. The nurse participates in the advancement of the profession through contributions to practice, education, administration, and knowledge development.
8. The nurse collaborates with other health professionals and the public in promoting community, national, and international efforts to meet health needs.
9. The profession of nursing, as represented by associations and their members, is responsible for articulating nursing values, for maintaining the integrity of the profession and its practice, and for shaping social policy.

American Nurses Association. (2001). Code of ethics for nurses. *Washington, DC: American Nurses Publishing.*

Points to Consider When Confronting Ethical Dilemmas

- Talk to colleagues or seek professional supervision. Usually, the nurse does not need to resolve an ethical dilemma alone.
- Spend time thinking about ethical issues and determine what your values and beliefs are regarding situations before they occur.
- Be willing to discuss ethical concerns with colleagues or managers. Being silent is condoning the behavior.

Critical Thinking Questions

1. Some clients with psychiatric disorders make headlines when they commit crimes against others that involve serious injury or death. With treatment and medication, these clients are rational and represent no threat to others, but they have a history of stopping their medications when released from treatment facilities. Where and how should these clients be treated? What measures can protect their individual rights as well as the public right to safety?
2. Some critics of deinstitutionalization argue that taking people who are severely and persistently mentally

ill out of institutions and closing some or all those institutions have worsened the mental health crisis. These closings have made it difficult for this minority of mentally ill clients to receive necessary inpatient treatment. Opponents counter that institutions are harmful because they segregate the mentally ill from the community, limit autonomy, and contribute to the loss of social skills. With which viewpoint do you agree? Why?

KEY POINTS

- Clients can be involuntarily hospitalized if they present an imminent danger of harm to themselves or others.
- Patients' rights include the right to receive and refuse treatment, to be involved in the plan of care, to be treated in the least restrictive environment, to refuse to participate in research, and to have unrestricted visitors, mail, and phone calls.
- The use of seclusion (confinement in a locked room) and restraint (direct application of physical force) falls under the domain of the patient's right to the least restrictive

INTERNET RESOURCES

RESOURCE	INTERNET ADDRESS
• American Academy of Psychiatry and the Law	http://www.aapl.org
• ADA (Americans With Disabilities Act) Information Center	http://www.adainfo.org
• Institute of Law, Psychiatry, and Public Policy	http://www.ilppp.virginia.edu
• Mental Health Matters Mental Health Advocacy and Legal Center	http://www.mental-health-matters.com/ advocacy/index.php
• Mental Health Patient's Bill of Rights	http://www.apa.org/pubinfo/rights

environment. Short-term use is permitted only if the client is imminently aggressive and dangerous to himself or herself or to others.

- Mental health clinicians have a legal obligation to breach client confidentiality to warn a third party of direct threats made by the client.
- Nurses have the responsibility to provide safe, competent, legal, and ethical care as outlined in nurse practice acts, the *Scope and Standards of Psychiatric-Mental Health Nursing Practice,* and the *Code of Ethics for Nurses.*
- A tort is a wrongful act that results in injury, loss, or damage. Negligence is an unintentional tort causing harm through failure to act.
- Malpractice is negligence by health professionals in cases in which they have a duty to the client that is breached, thereby causing injury or damage to the client.
- Intentional torts include assault, battery, and false imprisonment.
- Ethical theories are sets of principles used to decide what is morally right or wrong, such as utilitarianism (the greatest good for the greatest number) and deontology (using principles such as autonomy, beneficence, nonmaleficence, justice, veracity, and fidelity), to make ethical decisions.
- Ethical dilemmas are situations that arise when principles conflict or when there is no single clear course of action in a given situation.
- Many ethical dilemmas in mental health involve a conflict between the client's autonomy and concerns for the public good (utilitarianism).

REFERENCES

Abma, T. A., & Widdershoven, G. A. (2006). Moral deliberation in psychiatric nursing practice. *Nursing Ethics, 13*(5), 546–557.

American Nurses Association. (2000). *Scope and standards of psychiatric-mental health nursing practice.* Washington, DC: American Nurses Publishing, American Nurses Foundation/American Nurses Association.

American Nurses Association. (2001). *Code of ethics for nurses with interpretive statements.* Washington, DC: American Nurses Publishing.

Hiday, V. A., Swartz, M. S., Swanson, J. W., Borum, R., & Wagner, H. R. (2002). Impact of outpatient commitment on victimization of people with severe mental illness. *American Journal of Psychiatry, 159*(8), 1403–1411.

Joint Commission on Accreditation of Healthcare Organizations. (2005). *Restraint and seclusion standards for behavioral health.* Oakbrook, IL: Joint Commission Resources.

King, E. C. (1984). *Affective education in nursing: A guide to teaching and assessment.* Rockville, MD: Aspen Systems.

Marshall, T., & Solomon, P. (2003). Professionals' responsibilities in releasing information to families of adults with mental illness. *Psychiatric Services, 54*(12), 1622–1628.

Melton, G., Petrila, J., Poythree, N, & Slobogin, C. (1997). *Psychological evaluations for the courts: A handbook for mental health professionals and lawyers* (2nd ed.). New York: Guilford Press.

Segal, S. P., & Burgess, P. M. (2006a). Conditional release: A less restrictive alternative to hospitalization? *Psychiatric Services, 57*(11), 1600–1606.

Segal, S. P., & Burgess, P. M. (2006b). Effect of conditional release from hospitalization on mortality risk. *Psychiatric Services, 57*(11), 1607–1613.

Springhouse. (2004). *Nurses' legal handbook* (5th ed.) Philadelphia: Lippincott Williams & Wilkins.

Swartz, M. S., Swanson, J. W., Kim, M., & Petrila, J. (2006). Use of outpatient commitment or related civil court treatment orders in 5 U.S. communities. *Psychiatric Services, 57*(3), 343–349.

Touchet, B. K., Drummond, S. R., & Yates, W. R. (2004). The impact of fear of HIPAA violation on patient care. *Psychiatric Services, 55*(5), 575–576.

Treatment Advocacy Center. (2006). Standards for assisted treatment: State-by-state summary. Retrieved December 31, 2006: http://www.psychlaws.org/LegalResources/statechart.htm.

Wysocker, A., Agrati, G., Collins, J., Marcus, P., & Thelander, T. (2004). Mandatory outpatient treatment. *Journal of the American Psychiatric Nurses Association, 10*(5), 247–250.

ADDITIONAL READINGS

Appelbaum, P. S. (2005). Assessing Kendra's law: Five years of outpatient commitment in New York. *Psychiatric Services, 56*(7), 791–792.

Appelbaum, P. S. (2006). Insanity, guilty minds, and psychiatric testimony. *Psychiatric Services, 57*(10), 1370–1372.

Campbell, R. J., Yonge, O., & Austin, W. (2005). Intimacy boundaries between mental health nurses & psychiatric patients. *Journal of Psychosocial Nursing, 43*(5), 32–39.

Seeman, M. V. (2004). Relational ethics: When mothers suffer from psychosis. *Archives of Women's Mental Health, 7*(3), 201–210.

Vukovich, P. K. (2000). The ethics of involuntary procedures. *Perspectives in Psychiatric Care, 36*(4), 111–112.

Williamson, T. (2002). Ethics of assertive outreach (assertive community treatment teams). *Current Opinion in Psychiatry, 15*(5), 543–547.

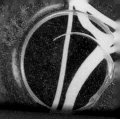

Chapter Study Guide

MULTIPLE-CHOICE QUESTIONS

Select the best answer for each of the following questions.

1. The client who is involuntarily committed to an inpatient psychiatric unit loses which of the following rights?
   A. Right to freedom
   B. Right to refuse treatment
   C. Right to sign legal documents
   D. The client loses no rights.

2. A client has a prescription for Haloperidol, 5 mg orally two times a day, as ordered by the physician. The client is suspicious and refuses to take the medication. The nurse says, "If you don't take this pill, I'll get an order to give you an injection." The nurse's statement is an example of
   A. Assault
   B. Battery
   C. Malpractice
   D. Unintentional tort

3. A hospitalized client is delusional, yelling "The world is coming to an end. We must all run to safety!" When other clients complain that this client is loud and annoying, the nurse decides to put the client in seclusion. The client has made no threatening gestures or statements to anyone. The nurse's action is an example of
   A. Assault
   B. False imprisonment
   C. Malpractice
   D. Negligence

4. Which of the following would indicate a duty to warn a third party?
   A. A client with delusions states, "I'm going to get them before they get me."
   B. A hostile client says, "I hate all police."
   C. A client says he plans to blow up the federal government.
   D. A client states, "If I can't have my girlfriend back, then no one can have her."

5. The nurse gives the client quetiapine (Seroquel) in error when olanzapine (Zyprexa) was ordered. The client has no ill effects from the quetiapine. In addition to making a medication error, the nurse has committed which of the following?
   A. Malpractice
   B. Negligence
   C. Tort (unintentional)
   D. None of the above

FILL-IN-THE-BLANK QUESTIONS

Identify the deontological principle being described.

_____	Telling the truth
_____	Doing no harm
_____	Keeping commitments
_____	Promoting good
_____	Being fair
_____	Exhibiting self-determination

SHORT-ANSWER QUESTIONS

1. Describe the concept of the least restrictive environment.

2. Discuss the elements involved in the clinician's duty to warn.

3. Identify the steps involved in the ethical decision-making process.

4. Discuss the standard of care for nursing.

5. Discuss the elements necessary to prove liability in malpractice lawsuits.

Anger, Hostility, and Aggression

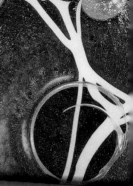

Key Terms

- acting out
- anger
- catharsis
- hostility
- impulse control
- physical aggression

Learning Objectives

After reading this chapter, you should be able to

1. Discuss anger, hostility, and aggression.

2. Describe psychiatric disorders that may be associated with an increased risk for hostility and physical aggression in clients.

3. Describe the signs, symptoms, and behaviors associated with the five phases of aggression.

4. Discuss appropriate nursing interventions for the client during the five phases of aggression.

5. Describe important issues for nurses to be aware of when working with angry, hostile, or aggressive clients.

Anger, a normal human emotion, is a strong, uncomfortable, emotional response to a real or perceived provocation. Anger results when a person is frustrated, hurt, or afraid. Handled appropriately and expressed assertively, anger can be a positive force that helps a person to resolve conflicts, solve problems, and make decisions (Dunbar, 2004). Anger energizes the body physically for self-defense, when needed, by activating the "fight-or-flight" response mechanisms of the sympathetic nervous system. When expressed inappropriately or suppressed, however, anger can cause physical or emotional problems or interfere with relationships.

Hostility, also called *verbal aggression*, is an emotion expressed through verbal abuse, lack of cooperation, violation of rules or norms, or threatening behavior (Schultz & Videbeck, 2005). A person may express hostility when he or she feels threatened or powerless. Hostile behavior is intended to intimidate or cause emotional harm to another, and it can lead to physical aggression. Physical aggression is behavior in which a person attacks or injures another person or that involves destruction of property. Both verbal and physical aggression are meant to harm or punish another person or to force someone into compliance. Some clients with psychiatric disorders display hostile or physically aggressive behavior that represents a challenge to nurses and other staff members.

Violence and abuse are discussed in Chapter 11, and self-directed aggression such as suicidal behavior is presented in Chapter 15. The focus of this chapter is the nurse's role in recognizing and managing hostile and aggressive behavior that clients direct toward others within psychiatric settings.

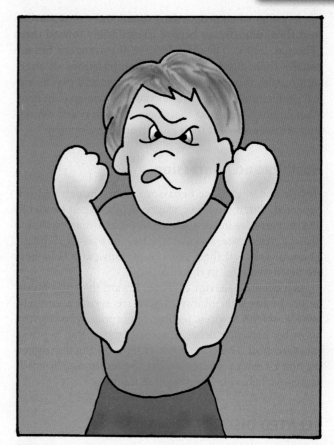

Hostility

ONSET AND CLINICAL COURSE

Anger

Although anger is normal, it often is perceived as a negative feeling. Many people are not comfortable expressing anger directly. Nevertheless, anger can be a normal and healthy reaction when situations or circumstances are unfair or unjust, personal rights are not respected, or realistic expectations are not met. If the person can express his or her anger assertively, problem-solving or conflict resolution is possible.

Anger becomes negative when the person denies it, suppresses it, or expresses it inappropriately. A person may deny or suppress (i.e., hold in) angry feelings if he or she is uncomfortable expressing anger. Possible consequences are physical problems such as migraine headaches, ulcers, or coronary artery disease and emotional problems such as depression and low self-esteem.

Anger that is expressed inappropriately can lead to hostility and aggression. The nurse can help clients express anger appropriately by serving as a model and by role-playing assertive communication techniques. Assertive communication uses "I" statements that express feelings and are specific to the situation, for example, "I feel angry when you interrupt me," or "I am angry that you changed the

work schedule without talking to me." Statements such as these allow appropriate expression of anger and can lead to productive problem-solving discussions and reduced anger.

Some people try to express their angry feelings by engaging in aggressive but safe activities such as hitting a punching bag or yelling. Such activities, called catharsis, are supposed to provide a release for anger. However, catharsis can increase rather than alleviate angry feelings. Therefore, cathartic activities may be contraindicated for angry clients. Activities that are not aggressive, such as walking or talking with another person, are more likely to be effective in decreasing anger (Jacob & Pelham, 2005).

Shapiro (2005) reported that high hostility is associated with increased risk for coronary artery disease and hypertension. Hostility can lead to angry outbursts that are not effective for anger expression. Effective methods of anger expression, such as using assertive communication, to express anger should replace angry aggressive outbursts of temper such as yelling or throwing things. Controlling one's temper or managing anger effectively should not be confused with suppressing angry feelings, which can lead to the problems described earlier.

Anger suppression is especially common in women, who have been socialized to maintain and enhance relationships with others and to avoid the expression of so-called negative or unfeminine emotions such as anger. Women's anger often results when people deny them power or resources, treat them unjustly, or behave irresponsibly toward them (Thomas, 2005). The offenders are not strangers, but are usually their closest intimates. Manifestations of anger suppression through somatic complaints and psychological problems are more common among women than men. Women must recognize that anger awareness and expression are necessary for their growth and development.

Hostility and Aggression

Hostile and aggressive behavior can be sudden and unexpected. Often, however, stages or phases can be identified in aggressive incidents: a triggering phase, an escalation phase, a crisis phase, a recovery phase, and a postcrisis phase. These phases and their signs, symptoms, and behaviors are discussed later in the chapter.

As a client's behavior escalates toward the crisis phase, he or she loses the ability to perceive events accurately, solve problems, express feelings appropriately, or control his or her behavior; behavior escalation may lead to physical aggression. Therefore, interventions during the triggering and escalation phases are key to preventing physically aggressive behavior (discussion to follow).

RELATED DISORDERS

The media gives a great deal of attention to people with mental illness who commit aggressive acts. This gives the general public the mistaken idea that most people with mental illness are aggressive and should be feared. In reality, clients with psychiatric disorders are much more likely to hurt themselves than other people.

Although most clients with psychiatric disorders are not aggressive, clients with a variety of psychiatric diagnoses can exhibit angry, hostile, and aggressive behavior. Clients with paranoid delusions may believe others are out to get them; believing they are protecting themselves, they retaliate with hostility or aggression. Some clients have auditory hallucinations that command them to hurt others. Aggressive behavior also is seen in clients with dementia, delirium, head injuries, intoxication with alcohol or other drugs, and antisocial and borderline personality disorders. Overall, Buckley and colleagues (2004) found that violent patients were more symptomatic, had poorer functioning, and had a marked lack of insight compared with nonviolent patients.

Some clients with depression have anger attacks. These sudden intense spells of anger typically occur in situations in which the depressed person feels emotionally trapped. Anger attacks involve verbal expressions of anger or rage but no physical aggression. Clients described these anger attacks as uncharacteristic behavior that was inappropriate for the situation and was followed by remorse. The anger attacks seen in some depressed clients may be related to irritable mood, overreaction to minor annoyances, and decreased coping abilities (Akiskal, 2005).

Intermittent explosive disorder is a rare psychiatric diagnosis characterized by discrete episodes of aggressive impulses that result in serious assaults or destruction of property. The aggressive behavior the person displays is grossly disproportionate to any provocation or precipitating factor. This diagnosis is made only if the client has no other comorbid psychiatric disorders, as previously discussed. The person describes a period of tension or arousal that the aggressive outburst seems to relieve. Afterward, however, the person is remorseful and embarrassed, and there are no signs of aggressiveness between episodes (Greenberg, 2005). Intermittent explosive disorder develops between late adolescence and the third decade of life (American Psychiatric Association, 2000). Clients with intermittent explosive disorder typically are large men with dependent personality features who respond to feelings of uselessness or ineffectiveness with violent outbursts.

Acting out is an immature defense mechanism by which the person deals with emotional conflicts or stressors through actions rather than through reflection or feelings. The person engages in acting-out behavior, such as verbal or physical aggression, to feel temporarily less helpless or powerless. Children and adolescents often "act out" when they cannot handle intense feelings or deal with emotional conflict verbally. To understand acting-out behaviors, it is important to consider the situation and the person's ability to deal with feelings and emotions.

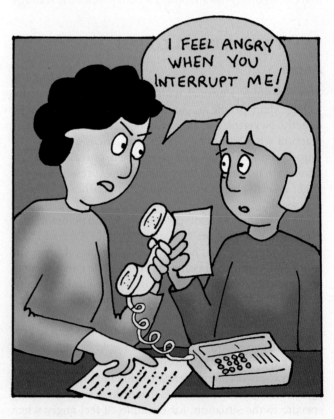

Assertive communication

ETIOLOGY

Neurobiologic Theories

Researchers have examined the role of neurotransmitters in aggression in animals and humans, but they have been unable to identify a single cause. Findings reveal that serotonin plays a major inhibitory role in aggressive behavior; therefore, low serotonin levels may lead to increased aggressive behavior (Johnson, 2004). This finding may be related to the anger attacks seen in some clients with depression. In addition, increased activity of dopamine and norepinephrine in the brain is associated with increased impulsively violent behavior. Further, structural damage to the limbic system and the frontal and temporal lobes of the brain may alter the person's ability to modulate aggression; this can lead to aggressive behavior.

Psychosocial Theories

Infants and toddlers express themselves loudly and intensely, which is normal for these stages of growth and development. Temper tantrums are a common response from toddlers whose wishes are not granted. As a child matures, he or she is expected to develop **impulse control** (the ability to delay gratification) and socially appropriate behavior. Positive relationships with parents, teachers, and peers; success in school; and the ability to be responsible for oneself foster development of these qualities. Children in dysfunctional families with poor parenting, children who receive inconsistent responses to their behavior, and children whose families are of lower socioeconomic status are at increased risk for failing to develop socially appropriate behavior; this lack of development can result in a person who is impulsive, easily frustrated, and prone to aggressive behavior.

Leary and colleagues (2006) found a relationship between interpersonal rejection and aggression. Rejection can lead to anger and aggression when that rejection causes the individual emotional pain or frustration, or is a threat to self-esteem. Aggressive behavior was often seen as a means of re-establishing control, improving mood, or achieving retribution.

CULTURAL CONSIDERATIONS

What a culture considers acceptable strongly influences the expression of anger. The nurse must be aware of cultural norms to provide culturally competent care. In the United States, women traditionally were not permitted to express anger openly and directly because doing so would not be "feminine" and would challenge male authority. That cultural norm has changed slowly during the past 25 years. Some cultures, such as Asian and Native American, see expressing anger as rude or disrespectful and avoid it at all costs. In these cultures, trying to help a client express anger verbally to an authority figure would be unacceptable.

Spector (2001) conducted a literature review to study whether or not racial bias influences clinicians' perceptions of patient dangerousness in Britain and the United States. She found that clinicians generally perceived patients with black skin (regardless of ethnicity or place of birth) as being more dangerous; this bias influenced treatment decisions (e.g., more compulsory hospitalizations, increased use of restraint and seclusion).

Two culture-bound syndromes involve aggressive behavior. *Bouffée delirante,* a condition observed in West Africa and Haiti, is characterized by a sudden outburst of agitated and aggressive behavior, marked confusion, and psychomotor excitement. These episodes may include visual and auditory hallucinations and paranoid ideation that resemble brief psychotic episodes. Amok is a dissociative episode characterized by a period of brooding followed by an outburst of violent, aggressive, or homicidal behavior directed at other people and objects. This behavior is precipitated by a perceived slight or insult and is seen only in men. Originally reported from Malaysia, similar behavior patterns are seen in Laos, the Philippines, Papua New Guinea, Polynesia (*cafard*), Puerto Rico (*mal de pelea*), and among the Navajo (*iich'aa*) (Moitabai, 2005).

TREATMENT

The treatment of aggressive clients often focuses on treating the underlying or comorbid psychiatric diagnosis such as schizophrenia or bipolar disorder. Successful treatment of comorbid disorders results in successful treatment of aggressive behavior. Lithium has been effective in treating aggressive clients with bipolar disorder, conduct disorders (in children), and mental retardation. Carbamazepine (Tegretol) and valproate (Depakote) are used to treat aggression associated with dementia, psychosis, and personality disorders. Atypical antipsychotic agents such as clozapine (Clozaril), risperidone (Risperdal), and olanzapine (Zyprexa) have been effective in treating aggressive clients with dementia, brain injury, mental retardation, and personality disorders. Benzodiazepines can reduce irritability and agitation in older adults with dementia, but they can result in the loss of social inhibition for other aggressive clients, thereby increasing rather than reducing their aggression.

For aggressive clients with psychoses, rapid tranquilization can be used to decrease agitation and aggression and provide sedation. Haloperidol (Haldol) and lorazepam (Ativan) are commonly used in combination to decrease agitation or aggression and psychotic symptoms. Midazolam (Versed) can be effective to decrease agitation (TREC Collaborative Group, 2003). Goedhard and associates (2006) found that atypical antipsychotics were more effective than conventional antipsychotics for aggressive, psychotic clients. Use of antipsychotic medications requires careful assessment for the development of extrapyramidal side effects, which can be quickly treated with benztropine (Cogentin). Chapter 2 provides a full discussion of these medications and their side effects.

Although not a treatment per se, the short-term use of seclusion or restraint may be required during the crisis phase of the aggression cycle to protect the client and others from injury. Many legal and ethical safeguards govern the use of seclusion and restraint (see Chapter 9).

APPLICATION OF THE NURSING PROCESS

Assessment and effective intervention with angry or hostile clients can often prevent aggressive episodes. Early assessment, judicious use of medications, and verbal interaction with an angry client can often prevent anger from escalating into physical aggression.

Assessment

The nurse should be aware of factors that influence aggression in the psychiatric environment, or unit milieu. Huckshorn (2004) found that aggressive behavior was less common on psychiatric units with strong psychiatric leadership, clear staff roles, and planned and adequate events such as staff–client interaction, group interaction, and activities. Conversely, when predictability of meetings or groups and staff–client interactions were lacking, clients often felt frustrated and bored, and aggression was more common and intense. A lack of psychological space—

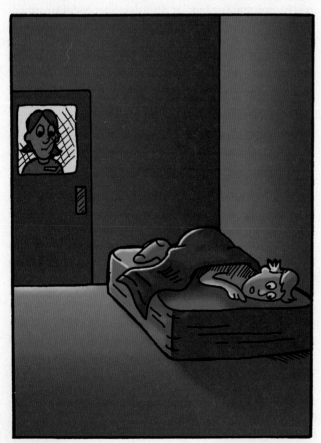

Seclusion

having no privacy, being unable to get sufficient rest—may be more important in triggering aggression than a lack of physical space.

In addition to assessing the unit milieu, the nurse needs to assess individual clients carefully. A history of violent or aggressive behavior is one of the best predictors of future aggression. Determining how the client with a history of aggression handles anger and what the client believes is helpful is important in assisting him or her to control or nonaggressively manage angry feelings. Clients who are angry and frustrated and believe that no one is listening to them are more prone to behave in a hostile or aggressive manner. In addition to a past history of violence, a history of being personally victimized and one of substance abuse increase a client's likelihood of aggressive behavior. Individual cues can help the nurse recognize when aggressive behavior is imminent (Pryor, 2005). These cues include what the client is saying; changes in the client's voice—volume, pitch, speed; changes in the client's facial expression; and changes in the client's behavior.

The nurse should assess the client's behavior to determine which phase of the aggression cycle he or she is in so that appropriate interventions can be implemented. The five phases of aggression and their signs, symptoms, and behaviors are presented in Table 10.1. Assessment of clients must take place at a safe distance. The nurse can approach the client while maintaining an adequate distance so that the client does not feel trapped or threatened. To ensure staff safety and exhibit teamwork, it may be prudent for two staff members to approach the client.

Data Analysis

Nursing diagnoses commonly used when working with aggressive clients include the following:
- Risk for Other-Directed Violence
- Ineffective Coping

If the client is intoxicated, depressed, or psychotic, additional nursing diagnoses may be indicated.

Outcome Identification

Expected outcomes for aggressive clients may include the following:

1. The client will not harm or threaten others.
2. The client will refrain from behaviors that are intimidating or frightening to others.
3. The client will describe his or her feelings and concerns without aggression.
4. The client will comply with treatment.

Intervention

Hostility or verbally aggressive behavior can be intimidating or frightening even for experienced nurses. Clients exhibiting these behaviors are also threatening to other clients, staff,

Table 10.1 FIVE-PHASE AGGRESSION CYCLE

Phase	Definition	Signs, Symptoms, and Behaviors
Triggering	An event or circumstances in the environment initiates the client's response, which is often anger or hostility.	Restlessness, anxiety, irritability, pacing, muscle tension, rapid breathing, perspiration, loud voice, anger
Escalation	Client's responses represent escalating behaviors that indicate movement toward a loss of control.	Pale or flushed face, yelling, swearing, agitated, threatening, demanding, clenched fists, threatening gestures, hostility, loss of ability to solve the problem or think clearly
Crisis	During a period of emotional and physical crisis, the client loses control.	Loss of emotional and physical control, throwing objects, kicking, hitting, spitting, biting, scratching, shrieking, screaming, inability to communicate clearly
Recovery	Client regains physical and emotional control.	Lowering of voice; decreased muscle tension; clearer, more rational communication; physical relaxation
Postcrisis	Client attempts reconciliation with others and returns to the level of functioning before the aggressive incident and its antecedents.	Remorse; apologies; crying; quiet, withdrawn behavior

Adapted from Keltner, N. L., Schwecke, L. H., & Bostrom, C. E. (2007). *Psychiatric nursing* (5th ed.). St. Louis: Mosby, Inc.

and visitors. In social settings, the most frequent response to hostile people is to get as far away from them as possible. In the psychiatric setting, however, engaging the hostile person in dialogue is most effective to prevent the behavior from escalating to physical aggression.

Interventions are most effective and least restrictive when implemented early in the cycle of aggression. This section presents interventions for the management of the milieu (which benefit all clients regardless of setting) and specific interventions for each phase of the aggression cycle.

MANAGING THE ENVIRONMENT

It is important to consider the environment for all clients when trying to reduce or eliminate aggressive behavior. Group and planned activities such as playing card games, watching and discussing movies, or participating in informal discussions give clients the opportunity to talk about events or issues when they are calm. Activities also engage clients in the therapeutic process and minimize boredom. Scheduling one-to-one interactions with clients indicates the nurse's genuine interest in the client and a willingness to listen to the client's concerns, thoughts, and feelings. Knowing what to expect enhances the client's feelings of security.

If clients have a conflict or dispute with one another, the nurse can offer the opportunity for problem-solving or conflict resolution. Expressing angry feelings appropriately, using assertive communication statements, and negotiating a solution are important skills clients can practice. These skills will be useful for the client when he or she returns to the community.

If a client is psychotic, hyperactive, or intoxicated, the nurse must consider the safety and security of other clients, who may need protection from the intrusive or threatening

demeanor of that client. Talking with other clients about their feelings is helpful, and close supervision of the client who is potentially aggressive is essential.

MANAGING AGGRESSIVE BEHAVIOR

In the *triggering phase*, the nurse should approach the client in a nonthreatening, calm manner in order to de-escalate the client's emotion and behavior. Conveying empathy for the client's anger or frustration is important. The nurse can encourage the client to express his or her angry feelings verbally, suggesting that the client is still in control and can maintain that control. Use of clear, simple, short statements is helpful. The nurse should allow the client time to express himself or herself. The nurse can suggest that the client go to a quiet area or may get assistance to move other clients to decrease stimulation. Medications (PRN, or as needed) should be offered, if ordered. As the client's anger subsides, the nurse can help the client to use relaxation techniques and look at ways to solve any problem or conflict that may exist (Marder, 2006). Physical activity, such as walking, also may help the client relax and become calmer.

If these techniques are unsuccessful and the client progresses to the *escalation phase*, the nurse must take control of the situation. The nurse should provide directions to the client in a calm, firm voice. The client should be directed to take a time-out for cooling off in a quiet area or his or her room. The nurse should tell the client that aggressive behavior is not acceptable and that the nurse is there to help the client regain control. If the client refused medications during the triggering phase, the nurse should offer them again.

If the client's behavior continues to escalate and he or she is unwilling to accept direction to a quiet area, the nurse should obtain assistance from other staff members. Initially, four to six staff members should remain ready within sight of the client but not as close as the primary nurse talking with the client. This technique, sometimes called a "show of force," indicates to the client that the staff will control the situation if the client cannot do so. Sometimes the presence of additional staff convinces the client to accept medication and take the time-out necessary to regain control.

When the client becomes physically aggressive (*crisis phase*), the staff must take charge of the situation for the safety of the client, staff, and other clients. Psychiatric facilities offer training and practice in safe techniques for managing behavioral emergencies, and only staff with such training should participate in the restraint of a physically aggressive client. The nurse's decision to use seclusion or restraint should be based on the facility's protocols and standards for restraint and seclusion. The nurse should obtain a physician's order as soon as possible after deciding to use restraint or seclusion.

Four to six trained staff members are needed to restrain an aggressive client safely. Children, adolescents, and female clients can be just as aggressive as adult male clients. The client is informed that his or her behavior is out of control and that the staff is taking control to provide safety and prevent injury. Four staff members each take a limb, one staff member protects the client's head, and one staff member helps control the client's torso, if needed. The client is transported by gurney or carried to a seclusion room, and restraints are applied to each limb and fastened to the bed frame. If PRN medication has not been taken earlier, the nurse may obtain an order for intramuscular (IM) medication in this type of emergency situation. As noted previously, the nurse performs close assessment of the client in seclusion or restraint and documents the actions.

As the client regains control (*recovery phase*), he or she is encouraged to talk about the situation or triggers that led to the aggressive behavior. The nurse should help the client relax, perhaps sleep, and return to a calmer state. It is important to help the client explore alternatives to aggressive behavior by asking what the client or staff can do next time to avoid an aggressive episode. The nurse also should assess staff members for any injuries and complete the required documentation such as incident reports and flow sheets. The staff usually has a debriefing session to discuss the aggressive episode, how it was handled, what worked well or needed improvement, and how the situation could have been defused more effectively. It also is important to encourage other clients to talk about their feelings regarding the incident. However, the aggressive client should not be discussed in detail with other clients.

In the *postcrisis phase*, the client is removed from restraint or seclusion as soon as he or she meets the behavioral criteria. The nurse should not lecture or chastise the client for the aggressive behavior but should discuss the behavior in a calm, rational manner. The client can be given feedback for regaining control, with the expectation that he or she will be able to handle feelings or events in a nonaggressive manner in the future. The client should be reintegrated into the milieu and its activities as soon as he or she can participate.

Evaluation

Care is most effective when the client's anger can be defused in an earlier stage, but restraint or seclusion is sometimes necessary to handle physically aggressive behavior. The goal is to teach angry, hostile, and potentially aggressive clients to express their feelings verbally and safely without threats or harm to others or destruction of property.

COMMUNITY-BASED CARE

For many clients with aggressive behavior, effective management of the comorbid psychiatric disorder is the key to controlling aggression. Regular follow-up appointments, compliance with prescribed medication, and participation in community support programs help the client to achieve stability. Anger management groups are available to help clients express their feelings and to learn problem-solving and conflict-resolution techniques.

Studies of client assaults on staff in the community become increasingly important as more clients experience

---

CLINICAL VIGNETTE: ESCALATION PHASE

John, 35 years of age, was admitted to the hospital for schizophrenia. John has a history of aggressive behavior, usually precipitated by voices telling him he will be harmed by staff and must kill them to protect himself. John had not been taking his prescribed medication for 2 weeks before hospitalization. The nurse observes John pacing in the hall, muttering to himself, and avoiding close contact with anyone else.

Suddenly, John begins to yell, "I can't take it. I can't stay here!" His fists are clenched, and he is very agitated. The nurse approaches John, remaining 6 feet away from him, and says, "John, tell me what is happening." John runs to the end of the hall and will not talk to the nurse. The nurse asks John to take a PRN medication and go to his room. He refuses both. As he begins to pick up objects from a nearby table, the nurse summons other staff to assist.

rapid discharge from inpatient or acute care settings. Assaults by clients in the community were caused partly by stressful living situations, increased access to alcohol and drugs, availability of lethal weapons, and noncompliance with medications. Episodes of assault were often precipitated by denial of services, acute psychosis, and excessive stimulation (Flannery et al., 2006b).

Flannery and colleagues (2006a) studied assaults by clients in community residences, including physical or sexual assaults, nonverbal intimidation, and verbal threats. Clients who were assaultive were most likely to be older male clients with schizophrenia and younger clients with personality disorders. These authors described the assaulted staff action program (ASAP) established in Massachusetts to help staff victims cope with the psychological sequelae of assaults by clients in community-based residential programs. In addition, ASAP works with staff to determine better methods of handling situations with aggressive clients and ways to improve safety in community settings. It is their belief that similar programs would be beneficial to staff in residential settings in other states.

SELF-AWARENESS ISSUES

The nurse must be aware of how he or she deals with anger before helping clients do so. The nurse who is afraid of angry feelings may avoid a client's anger, which allows the client's behavior to escalate. If the nurse's response is angry, the situation can escalate into a power struggle, and the nurse loses the opportunity to "talk down" the client's anger.

It is important to practice and gain experience in using techniques for restraint and seclusion before attempting them with clients in crisis. There is a risk for staff injury whenever a client is aggressive. Ongoing education and practice of safe techniques are essential to minimize or avoid injury to both staff and clients. The nurse must be calm, nonjudgmental, and nonpunitive when using techniques to control a client's aggressive behavior. Inexperienced nurses can learn from watching experienced nurses deal with clients who are hostile or aggressive.

When verbal techniques fail to defuse a client's anger and the client becomes aggressive, the nurse may feel frustrated or angry, as if he or she failed. The client's aggressive behavior, however, does not necessarily reflect the nurse's skills and abilities. Some clients have a limited capacity to control their aggressive behaviors, and the nurse can help them to learn alternative ways to handle angry or aggressive impulses.

Points to Consider When Working With Clients Who Are Angry, Hostile, or Aggressive

- Identify how you handle angry feelings; assess your use of assertive communication and conflict resolution.

Increasing your skills in dealing with your angry feelings will help you to work more effectively with clients.
- Discuss situations or the care of potentially aggressive clients with experienced nurses.
- Do not take the client's anger or aggressive behavior personally or as a measure of your effectiveness as a nurse.

Critical Thinking Questions

1. Many community-based residential programs will not admit a client with a recent history of aggression. Is this fair to the client? What factors should influence such decisions?
2. If an aggressive client injures another client or a staff person, should criminal charges be filed against the client? Why or why not?

KEY POINTS

- Anger, expressed appropriately, can be a positive force that helps the person solve problems and make decisions.
- Hostility, also called verbal aggression, is behavior meant to intimidate or cause emotional harm to another and can lead to physical aggression.
- Physical aggression is behavior meant to harm, punish, or force into compliance another person.
- Most clients with psychiatric disorders are not aggressive. Clients with schizophrenia, bipolar disorder, dementia, head injury, antisocial or borderline personality disorders, or conduct disorder, and those intoxicated with alcohol or other drugs, may be aggressive. Rarely, clients may be diagnosed with intermittent explosive disorder.
- Treatment of aggressive clients often involves treating the comorbid psychiatric disorder with mood stabilizers or antipsychotic medications.
- Assessment and effective intervention with angry or hostile clients can often prevent aggressive episodes.
- Aggressive behavior is less common and less intense on units with strong psychiatric leadership, clear staff roles, and planned and adequate events such as staff–client interaction, group interaction, and activities.
- The nurse must be familiar with the signs, symptoms, and behaviors associated with the triggering, escalation, crisis, recovery, and postcrisis phases of the aggression cycle.
- In the triggering phase, nursing interventions include speaking calmly and nonthreateningly, conveying empathy, listening, offering PRN medication, and suggesting retreat to a quiet area.
- In the escalation phase, interventions include using a directive approach, taking control of the situation, using

(text continues on p. 186)

Nursing Care Plan *Aggressive Behavior*

Nursing Diagnosis

Risk for Other-Directed Violence: *At risk for behaviors in which an individual demonstrates that he/she can be physically, emotionally, and/or sexually harmful to others.*

RISK FACTORS

- Actual or potential physical acting out of violence
- Destruction of property
- Homicidal or suicidal ideation
- Physical danger to self or others
- History of assaultive behavior or arrests
- Neurologic illness
- Disordered thoughts
- Agitation or restlessness
- Lack of impulse control
- Delusions, hallucinations, or other psychotic symptoms
- Personality disorder or other psychiatric symptoms
- Manic behavior
- Conduct disorder
- Posttraumatic stress disorder
- Substance use

EXPECTED OUTCOMES

Immediate
The client will
- Not harm others or destroy property
- Be free of self-inflicted harm
- Decrease acting out behavior
- Experience decreased restlessness or agitation
- Experience decreased fear, anxiety, or hostility

Stabilization
The client will
- Demonstrate the ability to exercise internal control over his or her behavior
- Be free of psychotic behavior
- Identify ways to deal with tension and aggressive feelings in a nondestructive manner
- Express feelings of anxiety, fear, anger, or hostility verbally or in a nondestructive manner
- Verbalize an understanding of aggressive behavior, associated disorder(s), and medications, if any

Community
The client will
- Participate in therapy for underlying or associated psychiatric problems
- Demonstrate internal control of behavior when confronted with stress

IMPLEMENTATION

Nursing Interventions *denotes collaborative interventions

Build a trust relationship with this client as soon as possible, ideally well in advance of aggressive episodes.

Be aware of factors that increase the likelihood of violent behavior or that signify a build-up of agitation. Use verbal communication or PRN medication to intervene before the client's behavior reaches a destructive or violent point and physical restraint becomes necessary.

Rationale

Familiarity with and trust in the staff members can decrease the client's fears and facilitate communication.

A period of building tension often precedes acting out or violent behavior; however, a client who is intoxicated or psychotic may become violent without warning. Signs of increasing agitation include increased restlessness, verbal cues, motor activity (e.g., pacing), voice volume, verbal cues ("I'm afraid of losing control."), threats, decreased frustration tolerance, and frowning or clenching fists.

continued ⋯⋯▷

Nursing Care Plan: Aggressive Behavior, cont.

IMPLEMENTATION

Nursing Interventions *denotes collaborative interventions	**Rationale**
Decrease environmental stimulation by turning stereo or television off or lowering the volume; lowering the lights; asking other clients, visitors, or others to leave the area (or you can go with the client to another room).	If the client is feeling threatened, he or she can perceive any stimulus as a threat. The client is unable to deal with excess stimuli when agitated.
If the client tells you (verbally or nonverbally) that he or she feels hostile or destructive, try to help the client express these feelings in nondestructive ways (e.g., use communication techniques, or take the client to the gym for physical exercise).	The client may need to learn nondestructive ways to express feelings. The client can try out new behaviors with you in a nonthreatening environment and learn to focus on expressing emotions rather than acting out.
Calmly and respectfully assure the client that you (the staff) will provide control if he or she cannot control himself or herself, but do not threaten the client.	The client may fear loss of control and may be afraid of what he or she may do if he or she begins to express anger. Showing that you are in control without competing with the client can reassure the client without lowering his or her self-esteem.
Be aware of PRN medication and procedures for obtaining seclusion or restraint orders.	In an aggressive situation you will need to make decisions and act quickly. If the client is severely agitated, medication may be necessary to decrease the agitation.
Be familiar with restraint, seclusion, and staff assistance procedures and legal requirements.	You must be prepared to act and direct other staff in the safe management of the client. You are legally accountable for your decisions and actions.
Always maintain control of yourself and the situation; remain calm. If you do not feel competent in dealing with a situation, obtain assistance as soon as possible.	Your behavior provides a role model for the client and communicates that you can and will provide control.
If you are not properly trained or skilled in dealing safely with a client who has a weapon, do not attempt to remove the weapon. Keep something (like a pillow, mattress, or a blanket wrapped around your arm) between you and the weapon.	Avoiding personal injury, summoning help, leaving the area, or protecting other clients may be the only things you can realistically do. You may risk further danger by attempting to remove a weapon or subdue an armed client.
If it is necessary to remove the weapon, try to kick it out of the client's hand. (Never reach for a knife or other weapon with your hand.)	Reaching for a weapon increases your physical vulnerability.
Distract the client momentarily to remove the weapon (throw water in the client's face, or yell suddenly).	Distracting the client's attention may give you an opportunity to remove the weapon or subdue the client.
*You may need to summon outside assistance (especially if the client has a gun). When this is done, total responsibility is delegated to the outside authorities.	Exceeding your abilities may place you in grave danger. It is not necessary to try to deal with a situation beyond your control or to assume personal risk.
*Notify the charge nurse and supervisor as soon as possible in a (potentially) aggressive situation; tell them your assessment of the situation and the need for help, the client's name, care plan, and orders for medication, seclusion, or restraint.	You may need assistance from staff members who are unfamiliar with this client. They will be able to help more effectively and safely if they are aware of this information.

continued ⋯⇢

Nursing Care Plan: Aggressive Behavior, cont.

IMPLEMENTATION

Nursing Interventions *denotes collaborative
  interventions

Rationale	

*Follow the hospital staff assistance plan (e.g., use intercom system to page "Code _____, [area]"); then, if possible, have one staff member meet the additional staff at the unit door to give them the client's name, situation, goal, plan, and so forth).

The need for help may be immediate in an emergency situation. Any information that can be given to arriving staff will be helpful in ensuring safety and effectiveness in dealing with this client.

Do not use physical restraints or techniques without sufficient reason.

The client has a right to the fewest restrictions possible within the limits of safety and prevention of destructive behavior.

Remain aware of the client's body space or territory; do not trap the client.

Potentially violent people have a body space zone up to four times larger than that of other people. That is, you need to stay farther away from them for them to not feel trapped or threatened.

Allow the client freedom to move around (within safe limits) unless you are trying to restrain him or her.

Interfering with the client's mobility without the intent of restraint may increase the client's frustration, fears, or perception of threat.

Talk with the client in a low, calm voice. Call the client by name, tell the client your name, where you are, and so forth.

Using a low voice may help prevent increasing agitation. The client may be disoriented or unaware of what is happening.

Tell the client what you are going to do and what you are doing. Use simple, clear, direct speech; repeat if necessary. Do not threaten the client, but state limits and expectations.

The client's ability to understand the situation and to process information is impaired. Clear limits let the client know what is expected of him or her.

*When a decision has been made to subdue or restrain the client, act quickly and cooperatively with other staff members. Tell the client in a matter-of-fact manner that he or she will be restrained, subdued, or secluded; allow no bargaining after the decision has been made. Reassure the client that he or she will not be hurt and that restraint or seclusion is to ensure safety.

Firm limits must be set and maintained. Bargaining interjects doubt and will undermine the limit.

*While subduing or restraining the client, talk with other staff members to ensure coordination of effort (e.g., do not attempt to carry the client until you are sure that everyone is ready).

Direct verbal communication will promote cooperation and safety.

Do not strike the client.

Physical safety of the client is a priority.

Do not help to restrain or subdue the client if you are angry (if enough other staff members are present). Do not restrain or subdue the client as a punishment.

Staff members must maintain self-control at all times and act in the client's best interest. There is no justification for being punitive to a client.

Do not recruit or allow other clients to help in restraining or subduing a client.

Physical safety of all clients is a priority. Other clients are not responsible for controlling the behavior of a client and should not assume a staff role.

If possible, do not allow other clients to watch staff subduing the client. Take them to a different area, and involve them in activities or discussion.

Other clients may be frightened, agitated, or endangered by an aggressive client. They need safety and reassurance at this time.

continued --->

Nursing Care Plan: Aggressive Behavior, cont.

IMPLEMENTATION

Nursing Interventions *denotes collaborative interventions

*Develop and practice consistent techniques of restraint as part of nursing orientation and continuing education.

*Develop instructions in safe techniques for carrying clients. Obtain additional staff assistance when needed. Have someone clear furniture and so forth from the area through which you will be carrying the client.

When placing the client in restraints or seclusion, tell the client what you are doing and the reason (e.g., to regain control or protect the client from injuring himself, herself, or others). Use simple, concise language in a nonjudgmental, matter-of-fact manner.

Tell the client where he or she is, that he or she will be safe, and that staff members will check on him or her. Tell the client how to summon the staff. Reorient the client or remind him or her of the reason for restraint as necessary.

Reassess the client's need for continued seclusion or restraint and release the client or decrease restraint as soon as it is safe and therapeutic. Base your decisions on the client's, not the staff's, needs.

Remain aware of the client's feelings (including fear), dignity, and rights.

Carefully observe the client, and promptly complete documentation in keeping with hospital policy. Bear in mind possible legal implications.

Administer medications safely; take care to prepare correct dosage, identify correct sites for administration, withdraw plunger to aspirate for blood, and so forth.

Take care to avoid needlestick injury and other injuries that may involve exposure to the client's blood or body fluids.

Monitor the client for effects of medications, and intervene as appropriate.

Talk with other clients after the situation is resolved; allow them to express feelings about the situation.

Rationale

Consistent techniques let each staff person know what is expected and will increase safety and effectiveness.

Consistent techniques increase safety and effectiveness. Transporting a client who is agitated can be dangerous if attempted without sufficient help and sufficient space.

The client's ability to understand what is happening to him or her may be impaired.

Being placed in seclusion or restraints can be terrifying to a client. Your assurances may help alleviate the client's fears.

The client has a right to the least restrictions possible within the limits of safety and prevention of destructive behavior.

The client is a worthwhile person regardless of his or her unacceptable behavior.

Accurate, complete documentation is essential, as restraint, seclusion, assault, and so forth are situations that may result in legal action.

When you are in a stressful situation and under pressure to move quickly, the possibility of errors in dosage or administration of medication is increased.

Hepatitis C, HIV, and other diseases are transmitted by exposure to blood or body fluids.

Psychoactive drugs can have adverse effects such as allergic reactions, hypotension, and pseudoparkinsonian symptoms.

The other clients have their own needs and problems. Be careful not to give attention only to the client who is acting out.

Adapted from Schultz, J. M., & Videbeck, S. L. (2005). Lippincott's manual of psychiatric nursing care plans (7th ed). Philadelphia: Lippincott Williams & Wilkins.

a calm, firm voice for giving directions, directing the client to take a time-out in a quiet place, offering PRN medication, and making a "show of force."

• In the crisis phase, experienced, trained staff can use the techniques of seclusion or restraint to deal quickly with the client's aggression.

• During the recovery phase, interventions include helping clients to relax, assisting them to regain self-control, and discussing the aggressive event rationally.

• In the postcrisis phase, the client is reintegrated into the milieu.

• Important self-awareness issues include examining how one handles angry feelings and deals with one's own reactions to angry clients.

REFERENCES

Akiskal, H. S. (2005). Mood disorders: Historical introduction and conceptual overview. In B. J. Sadock & V. A. Sadock (Eds.), *Comprehensive textbook of psychiatry* (Vol. 1, 8th ed., pp. 1559–1575). Philadelphia: Lippincott Williams & Wilkins.

American Psychiatric Association. (2000). *Diagnostic and statistical manual of mental disorders* (4th ed., text revision). Washington, DC: American Psychiatric Association.

Buckley, P. F., Hrouda, D. R., Friedman, L., et al. (2004). Insight and its relationship to violent behavior in patients with schizophrenia. *American Journal of Psychiatry, 161*(9), 1712–1714.

Dunbar, B. (2004). Anger management: A holistic approach. *Journal of the American Psychiatric Nurses Association, 10*(1), 16–23.

Flannery, R. J., Jr., Juliano, J., Cronin, S., & Walker, A. P. (2006a). Characteristics of assaultive patients: Fifteen-year analysis of the Assaulted Staff Action Program (ASAP). *Psychiatric Quarterly, 77*(3), 239–249.

Flannery, R. J., Jr., Laudani, L., Levitre, V., & Walker, A. P. (2006b). Precipitants of psychiatric patient assaults on staff: Three-year empirical inquiry of the Assaulted Staff Action Program (ASAP). *International Journal of Emergency Mental Health, 8*(1), 15–22.

Goedhard, L. E., Stolker, J. J., Heerdink, E. R., et al. (2006). Pharmacotherapy for the treatment of aggressive behavior in general adult psychiatry: A systematic review. *Journal of Clinical Psychiatry, 67*(7), 1013–1024.

Greenberg, H. A. (2005). Impulse-control disorders not elsewhere specified. In B. J. Sadock & V. A. Sadock (Eds.), *Comprehensive textbook of psychiatry* (Vol. 1, 8th ed., pp. 2035–2054). Philadelphia: Lippincott Williams & Wilkins.

Huckshorn, K. A. (2004). Reducing seclusion and restraint use in mental health settings: Core strategies for prevention. *Journal of Psychosocial Nursing, 42*(9), 22–33.

Jacob, R. G., & Pelham, W. E. (2005). Behavior therapy. In B. J. Sadock & V. A. Sadock (Eds.), *Comprehensive textbook of psychiatry* (Vol. 2, 8th ed., pp. 2498–2548). Philadelphia: Lippincott Williams & Wilkins.

Johnson, M. E. (2004). Violence on inpatient psychiatric units: State of the science. *Journal of the American Psychiatric Nurses Association, 10*(3), 113–121.

Keltner, N. L., Schwecke, L. H., & Bostrom, C. E. (2007). *Psychiatric nursing* (5th ed.). St. Louis: Mosby.

Leary, M. R., Twenge, J. M., & Quinlivan, E. (2006). Interpersonal rejection as a determinant of anger and aggression. *Personality and Social Psychology Review, 10*(2), 1111–1132.

Marder, S. R. (2006). A review of agitation in mental illness: Treatment guidelines and current therapies. *Journal of Clinical Psychiatry, 67*(Suppl 10), 13–21.

Moitabai, R. (2005). Culture-bound syndromes with psychotic features. In B. J. Sadock & V. A. Sadock (Eds.), *Comprehensive textbook of psychiatry* (Vol. 1, 8th ed., pp. 1538–1542). Philadelphia: Lippincott Williams & Wilkins.

Pryor, J. (2005). What cues do nurses use to predict aggression in people with acquired brain injury? *Journal of Neuroscience Nursing, 37*(2), 117–121.

Schultz, J. M., & Videbeck, S. L. (2005). *Lippincott's manual of psychiatric nursing care plans* (7th ed.). Philadelphia: Lippincott Williams & Wilkins.

Shapiro, P. A. (2005). Cardiovascular disorders. In B. J. Sadock & V. A. Sadock (Eds.), *Comprehensive textbook of psychiatry* (Vol. 2, 8th ed., pp. 2136–2148). Philadelphia: Lippincott Williams & Wilkins.

Spector, R. (2001). Is there racial bias in clinicians' perceptions of the dangerousness of psychiatric patients? A review of the literature. *Journal of Mental Health, 10*(1), 5–15.

Thomas, S. P. (2005). Women's anger, aggression, and violence. *Health Care for Women International, 26*(6), 504–522.

TREC Collaborative Group. (2003). Rapid tranquillisation for agitated patients in emergency psychiatric rooms: A randomized trial of midazolam versus Haloperidol plus promethazine. *British Medical Journal, 327*(7414), 708–713.

ADDITIONAL READINGS

Champagne, T., & Stromberg, N. (2004). Sensory approaches in inpatient psychiatric settings: Innovative alternatives to seclusion & restraint. *Journal of Psychosocial Nursing, 42*(9), 35–44.

Chang, J., & Lee, C. (2004). Risk factors for aggressive behavior among psychiatric inpatients. *Psychiatric Services, 55*(11), 1305–1307.

Ilkiw-Lavalle, O., & Grenyer, B. F. S. (2003). Differences between patient and staff perceptions of aggression in mental health units. *Psychiatric Services, 54*(3), 389–393.

Needham, I., Abderhalden, C., Halfens, R. J., et al. (2005) Non-somatic effects of patient aggression on nurses: A systematic review. *Journal of Advanced Nursing, 49*(3), 283–296.

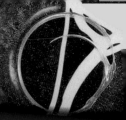

Chapter Study Guide

MULTIPLE-CHOICE QUESTIONS

Select the best answer for each of the following questions.

1. Which of the following is an example of assertive communication?
   A. "I wish you would stop making me angry."
   B. "I feel angry when you walk away when I'm talking."
   C. "You never listen to me when I'm talking."
   D. "You make me angry when you interrupt me."

2. Which of the following statements about anger is true?
   A. Expressing anger openly and directly usually leads to arguments.
   B. Anger results from being frustrated, hurt, or afraid.
   C. Suppressing anger is a sign of maturity.
   D. Angry feelings are a negative response to a situation.

3. Which of the following types of drugs requires cautious use with potentially aggressive clients?
   A. Antipsychotic medications
   B. Benzodiazepines
   C. Mood stabilizers
   D. Lithium

4. A client is pacing in the hallway with clenched fists and a flushed face. He is yelling and swearing. Which phase of the aggression cycle is he in?
   A. Anger
   B. Triggering
   C. Escalation
   D. Crisis

5. The nurse observes a client muttering to himself and pounding his fist in his other hand while pacing in the hallway. Which of the following principles should guide the nurse's action?
   A. Only one nurse should approach an upset client to avoid threatening the client.
   B. Clients who can verbalize angry feelings are less likely to become physically aggressive.
   C. Talking to a client with delusions is not helpful, because the client has no ability to reason.
   D. Verbally aggressive clients often calm down on their own if staff members don't bother them.

SHORT-ANSWER QUESTIONS

1. Describe the medication administration techniques of cocktail and chaser.

2. Discuss interventions the nurse might use for a client who becomes aggressive without warning.

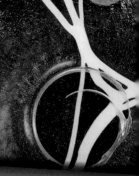

Chapter 11

Abuse and Violence

Key Terms

- abuse
- acute stress disorder
- child abuse
- cycle of violence
- date rape (acquaintance rape)
- dissociation
- dissociative disorders
- elder abuse
- family violence
- grounding techniques
- intergenerational transmission process
- neglect
- physical abuse
- posttraumatic stress disorder
- psychological abuse (emotional abuse)
- rape
- repressed memories
- restraining order
- sexual abuse
- sodomy
- spouse or partner abuse
- stalking
- survivor

Learning Objectives

After reading this chapter, you should be able to

1. Discuss the characteristics, risk factors, and family dynamics of abusive and violent behavior.

2. Examine the incidences of and trends in domestic violence, child and elder abuse, and rape.

3. Describe responses to abuse, specifically posttraumatic stress disorder and dissociative identity disorder.

4. Apply the nursing process to the care of clients who have survived abuse and violence.

5. Provide education to clients, families, and communities to promote prevention and early intervention of abuse and violence.

6. Evaluate your own experiences, feelings, attitudes, and beliefs about abusive and violent behavior.

Visit the Point. http://thePoint.lww.com for NCLEX-style questions, journal articles, and more!

Violent behavior has been identified as a national health concern and a priority for intervention in the United States, where occurrences exceed 2 million per year. The most alarming statistics relate to violence in the home and **abuse**, or the wrongful use and maltreatment of another person. Statistics show that most abuse is perpetrated by someone the victim knows. Victims of abuse are found across the life span, and they can be spouses or partners, children, or elderly parents.

This chapter discusses domestic abuse (spouse abuse, child abuse/neglect, elder abuse) and rape. Because many survivors of abuse suffer long-term emotional trauma, it also discusses disorders associated with abuse and violence: posttraumatic stress disorder (PTSD) and dissociative disorders. Other long-term problems associated with abuse and trauma include substance abuse (see Chapter 17) and depression (see Chapter 15).

CLINICAL PICTURE OF ABUSE AND VIOLENCE

Victims of abuse or violence certainly can have physical injuries needing medical attention, but they also experience psychological injuries with a broad range of responses. Some clients are agitated and visibly upset; others are withdrawn and aloof, appearing numb or oblivious to their surroundings. Often, domestic violence remains undisclosed for months or even years because victims fear their abusers. Victims frequently suppress their anger and resentment and do not tell anyone. This is particularly true in cases of childhood sexual abuse.

Survivors of abuse often suffer in silence and continue to feel guilt and shame. Children particularly come to believe that somehow they are at fault and did something to deserve or provoke the abuse. They are more likely to miss school, are less likely to attend college, and continue to have problems through adolescence into adulthood. As adults, they usually feel guilt or shame for not trying to stop the abuse. Survivors feel degraded, humiliated, and dehumanized. Their self-esteem is extremely low, and they view themselves as unlovable. They believe they are unacceptable to others, contaminated, or ruined. Depression, suicidal behavior, and marital and sexual difficulties are common (National Institutes of Health, 2006).

Victims and survivors of abuse may have problems relating to others. They find trusting others, especially authority figures, to be difficult. In relationships, their emotional reactions are likely to be erratic, intense, and perceived as unpredictable. Intimate relationships may trigger extreme emotional responses such as panic, anxiety, fear, and terror. Even when survivors of abuse desire closeness with another person, they may perceive actual closeness as intrusive and threatening.

Nurses should be particularly sensitive to the abused client's need to feel safe, secure, and in control of his or her body. They should take care to maintain the client's personal space, assess the client's anxiety level, and ask

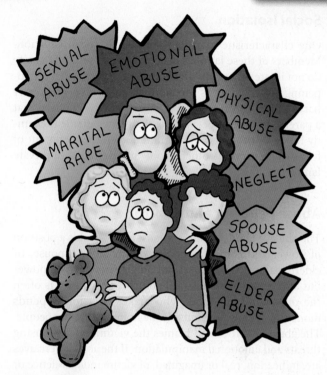

Family violence

permission before touching him or her for any reason. Because the nurse may not always be aware of a history of abuse when initially working with a client, he or she should apply these cautions to all clients in the mental health setting.

CHARACTERISTICS OF VIOLENT FAMILIES

Family violence encompasses spouse battering; neglect and physical, emotional, or sexual abuse of children; elder abuse; and marital rape. In many cases, family members tolerate abusive and violent behavior from relatives they would never accept from strangers. In violent families, the home, which is normally a safe haven of love and protection, may be the most dangerous place for victims.

Research studies have identified some common characteristics of violent families regardless of the type of abuse that exists. They are discussed next and in Box 11.1.

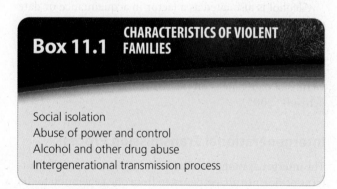

Box 11.1 CHARACTERISTICS OF VIOLENT FAMILIES

Social isolation
Abuse of power and control
Alcohol and other drug abuse
Intergenerational transmission process

Social Isolation

One characteristic of violent families is social isolation. Members of these families keep to themselves and usually do not invite others into the home or tell them what is happening. Often, abusers threaten victims with even greater harm if they reveal the secret. They may tell children that a parent, sibling, or pet will die if anyone outside the family learns of the abuse. So, children keep the secret out of fear, which prevents others from "interfering with private family business."

Abuse of Power and Control

The abusive family member almost always holds a position of power and control over the victim (child, spouse, or elderly parent). The abuser not only exerts physical power but also economic and social control. The abuser is often the only family member who makes decisions, spends money, or spends time outside the home with other people. The abuser belittles and blames the victim, often by using threats and emotional manipulation. If the abuser perceives any indication, real or imagined, of victim independence or disobedience, violence usually escalates. Twenty-two percent of nonfatal violence against women is perpetrated by an intimate partner, compared with only 3% of men injured by an intimate partner. Intimate partners are responsible for 30% of female homicides, whereas only 3% of male homicides are committed by a female intimate partner (Bureau of Justice, 2006).

Alcohol and Other Drug Abuse

Substance abuse, especially alcoholism, has been associated with family violence. This finding does not imply a cause-and-effect relationship. Alcohol does not cause the person to be abusive; rather, an abusive person also is likely to use alcohol or other drugs. Two-thirds of victims of intimate violence report that alcohol was involved in the violent incident. Women whose partners abused alcohol were 3.6 times more likely than other women to be assaulted by their partners (Marin Institute, 2006). Although alcohol may not cause the abuse, many researchers believe that alcohol may diminish inhibitions and make violent behavior more intense or frequent.

Alcohol is also cited as a factor in acquaintance or date rape. According to the Marin Institute (2006), 40% of convicted rape and sexual assault offenders reported drinking alcohol at the time of their crime. In addition, use of the illegal drug flunitrazepam (Rohypnol) to subdue potential victims of date rape is on the rise in the United States (van der Kolk, 2005).

Intergenerational Transmission Process

The **intergenerational transmission process** shows that patterns of violence are perpetuated from one generation to the next through role-modeling and social learning (van der Kolk, 2005). Intergenerational transmission suggests that family violence is a learned pattern of behavior. For example, children who witness violence between their parents learn that violence is a way to resolve conflict and is an integral part of a close relationship. Statistics show that one third of abusive men are likely to have come from violent homes where they witnessed wife-beating or were abused themselves. Women who grew up in violent homes are 50% more likely to expect or accept violence in their own relationships. Not all persons exposed to family violence, however, become abusive or violent as adults. Therefore, this single factor does not explain the perpetuation of violent behavior.

CULTURAL CONSIDERATIONS

Although domestic violence affects families of all ethnicities, races, ages, national origins, sexual orientations, religions, and socioeconomic backgrounds, a specific population is particularly at risk: immigrant women. Battered immigrant women face legal, social, and economic problems different from U.S. citizens who are battered and from people of other cultural, racial, and ethnic origins who are not battered:

- The battered woman may come from a culture that accepts domestic violence.
- She may believe she has less access to legal and social services than do U.S. citizens.
- If she is not a citizen, she may be forced to leave the United States if she seeks legal sanctions against her husband or attempts to leave him.
- She is isolated by cultural dynamics that do not permit her to leave her husband; economically, she may be unable to gather the resources to leave, work, or go to school.
- Language barriers may interfere with her ability to call 911, learn about her rights or legal options, and obtain shelter, financial assistance, or food.

It may be necessary for the nurse to obtain the assistance of an interpreter whom the woman trusts, make referrals to legal services, and assist the woman to contact the Department of Immigration to deal with these additional concerns.

SPOUSE OR PARTNER ABUSE

Spouse or partner abuse is the mistreatment or misuse of one person by another in the context of an intimate relationship. The abuse can be emotional or psychological, physical, sexual, or a combination (which is common). **Psychological abuse (emotional abuse)** includes name-calling, belittling, screaming, yelling, destroying property, and making threats as well as subtler forms such as refusing to speak to or ignoring the victim. **Physical abuse** ranges from shoving and pushing to severe battering and choking and may involve broken limbs and ribs, internal bleeding, brain damage, and even homicide. Sexual abuse includes assaults during sexual relations such as biting nipples, pulling hair, slapping and hitting, and rape (discussed later).

Ninety percent to 95% of domestic violence victims are women, and estimates are that one in three women in the United States has been beaten by a spouse at least once. Each year, as many as 5.3 million women in the United States experience a serious assault by a partner. Eight percent of U.S. homicides involve one spouse killing another, and 3 of every 10 female homicide victims are murdered by their spouse, ex-spouse, boyfriend, or ex-boyfriend (CDC, 2004).

An estimated 324,000 women experience violence while pregnant. Battering during pregnancy leads to adverse outcomes, such as miscarriage and stillbirth, as well as to further physical and psychological problems for the woman. The increase in violence is often due to the partner's jealousy, possessiveness, insecurity, and lessened physical and emotional availability of the pregnant woman (Bacchus et al., 2006).

Domestic violence occurs in same-sex relationships with the same statistical frequency as in heterosexual relationships and affects 50,000 lesbian women and 500,000 gay men each year. Although same-sex battering mirrors heterosexual battering in prevalence, its victims receive fewer protections. Seven states define domestic violence in a way that excludes same-sex victims. Twenty-one other states have sodomy laws that designate **sodomy** (anal intercourse) as a crime; thus, same-sex victims must first confess to the crime of sodomy to prove a domestic relationship between partners. The same-sex batterer has an additional weapon to use against the victim: the threat of revealing the partner's homosexuality to friends, family, employers, or the community.

Clinical Picture

Because abuse often is perpetrated by a husband against a wife, that example is used in this section. These same patterns are consistent, however, between partners who are not married, between same-sex partners, and with wives who abuse their husbands.

An abusive husband often believes his wife belongs to him (like property) and becomes increasingly violent and abusive if she shows any sign of independence, such as getting a job or threatening to leave. Typically, the abuser has strong feelings of inadequacy and low self-esteem as well as poor problem-solving and social skills. He is emotionally immature, needy, irrationally jealous, and possessive. He may even be jealous of his wife's attention to their own children or may beat both his children and wife. By bullying and physically punishing the family, the abuser often experiences a sense of power and control, a feeling that eludes him outside the home. Therefore, the violent behavior often is rewarding and boosts his self-esteem.

Dependency is the trait most commonly found in abused wives who stay with their husbands. Women often cite personal and financial dependency as reasons why they find leaving an abusive relationship extremely difficult. Regardless of the victim's talents or abilities, she perceives herself as unable to function without her husband. She too often suffers from low self-esteem and defines her success as a person by her ability to remain loyal to her marriage and "make it work." Some women internalize the criticism they receive and mistakenly believe they are to blame. Women also fear their abuser will kill them if they try to leave. This fear is realistic, given that national statistics show 65% of women murdered by spouses or boyfriends were attempting to leave or had left the relationships (Bureau of Justice, 2006).

Cycle of Abuse and Violence

The **cycle of violence** or abuse is another reason often cited for why women have difficulty leaving abusive relationships. A typical pattern exists: Usually, the initial episode of battering or violence is followed by a period of the abuser expressing regret, apologizing, and promising it will never happen again. He professes his love for his wife and may even engage in romantic behavior (e.g., buying gifts and flowers). This period of contrition or remorse sometimes is called the *honeymoon period*. The woman naturally wants to believe her husband and hopes the violence was an isolated incident. After this honeymoon period, the tension-building phase begins; there may be arguments, stony silence, or complaints from the husband. The tension ends in another violent episode after which the abuser once again feels regret and remorse and promises to change. This cycle continually repeats itself. Each time, the victim keeps hoping the violence will stop.

Initially, the honeymoon period may last weeks or even months, causing the woman to believe that the relationship has improved and her husband's behavior has changed. Over time, however, the violent episodes are more frequent, the period of remorse disappears altogether, and the level of violence and severity of injuries worsen. Eventually, the violence is routine—several times a week or even daily.

Assessment

Because most abused women do not seek direct help for the problem, nurses must help identify abused women in various settings. Nurses may encounter abused women in emergency rooms, clinics, or pediatricians' offices. Some victims may be seeking treatment for other medical conditions not directly related to the abuse or for pregnancy. Identifying abused women who need assistance is a top priority of the Department of Health and Human Services. The generalist nurse is not expected to deal with this complicated problem alone. He or she can, however, make referrals and contact appropriate health care professionals experienced in working with abused women. Above all, the nurse can offer caring and support throughout. Table 11.1

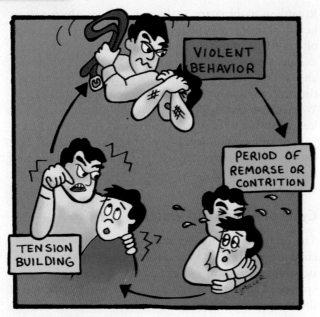

Cycle of violence

Box 11.2   SAFE QUESTIONS

- **S**tress/**S**afety: What stress do you experience in your relationships? Do you feel safe in your relationships? Should I be concerned for your safety?
- **A**fraid/**A**bused: Have there been situations in your relationships where you have felt afraid? Has your partner ever threatened or abused you or your children? Have you ever been physically hurt or threatened by your partner? Are you in a relationship like that now? Has your partner ever forced you to engage in sexual intercourse that you did not want? People in relationships/marriages often fight; what happens when you and your partner disagree?
- **F**riends/**F**amily: Are your friends aware that you have been hurt? Do your parents or siblings know about this abuse? Do you think you could tell them, and would they be able to give you support?
- **E**mergency plan: Do you have a safe place to go and the resources you (and your children) need in an emergency? If you are in danger now, would you like help in locating a shelter? Would you like to talk to a social worker/a counselor/me to develop an emergency plan?

Ashur, M. L. C. (1993). Asking about domestic violence: SAFE questions. JAMA, 269(18), 2367. © American Medical Association.

summarizes techniques for working with victims of partner violence.

Many hospitals, clinics, and doctors' offices ask women about safety issues as part of all health histories or intake interviews. Because this issue is delicate and sensitive and many abused women are afraid or embarrassed to admit the problem, nurses must be skilled in asking appropriate questions about abuse. Box 11.2 gives an example of questions to ask using the acronym SAFE (Stress/Safety, Afraid/Abused, Friends/Family, and Emergency plan). The first two categories are designed to detect abuse. The nurse should ask questions in the other two categories if abuse is present. He or she should ask these questions when the woman is alone; the nurse can paraphrase or edit the questions as needed for any given situation.

Treatment and Intervention

Every state in the United States allows police to make arrests in cases of domestic violence; more than half the states have laws requiring police to make arrests for at least some domestic violence crimes. Sometimes after police have been

Table 11.1   DO'S AND DON'TS OF WORKING WITH VICTIMS OF PARTNER ABUSE

Don'ts	Do's
Don't disclose client communications without the client's consent.	Do ensure and maintain the client's confidentiality.
Don't preach, moralize, or imply that you doubt the client.	Do listen, affirm, and say, "I am sorry you have been hurt."
Don't minimize the impact of violence.	Do express, "I'm concerned for your safety."
Don't express outrage with the perpetrator.	Do tell the victim, "You have a right to be safe and respected."
Don't imply that the client is responsible for the abuse.	Do say, "The abuse is not your fault."
Don't recommend couples' counseling.	Do recommend a support group or individual counseling.
Don't direct the client to leave the relationship.	Do identify community resources and encourage the client to develop a safety plan.
Don't take charge and do everything for the client.	Do offer to help the client contact a shelter, the police, or other resources.

Commission on Domestic Violence (2004). Domestic Violence Resources. http://www.abanet.org.domviol/home.html.

CLINICAL VIGNETTE: SPOUSE ABUSE

Darlene sat in the bathroom trying to regain her balance and holding a cold washcloth to her face. She looked in the mirror and saw a large, red, swollen area around her eye and cheek where her husband, Frank, had hit her. They had been married for only 6 months, and this was the second time that he had gotten angry and struck her in the face before storming out of the house. Last time, he was so sorry the day after it happened that he brought her flowers and took her out to dinner to apologize. He said he loved her more than ever and felt terrible about what had happened. He said it was because he had had an argument with his boss over getting a raise and went out drinking after work before coming home. He had promised not to go out drinking anymore and that it would never happen again. For several weeks after he quit drinking, he was wonderful, and it felt like it was before they got married. She remembered thinking that she must try harder to keep him happy because she knew he really did love her.

But during the past 2 weeks, he had been increasingly silent and sullen, complaining about everything. He didn't like the dinners she cooked and said he wanted to go out to eat even though money was tight and their credit cards were loaded with charges they couldn't pay off. He began drinking again. After a few hours of drinking tonight, he yelled at her and said she was the cause of all his money problems. She tried to reason with him, but he hit her and this time he knocked her to the floor and her head hit the table. She was really frightened now, but what should she do? She couldn't move out; she had no money of her own and her job just didn't pay enough to support her. Should she go to her parents? She couldn't tell them about what happened because they never wanted her to marry Frank in the first place. They would probably say, "We told you so and you didn't listen. Now you married him and you'll have to deal with his problems." She was too embarrassed to tell her friends, most of whom were "their" friends and had never seen this violent side of Frank. They probably wouldn't believe her. What should she do? Her face and head were really beginning to hurt now. "I'll talk to him tomorrow when he is sober and tell him he must get some help for the drinking problem. When he's sober, he is reasonable and he'll see that this drinking is causing a big problem for our marriage," she thought.

called to the scene, the abuser is allowed to remain at home after talking with police and calming down. If an arrest is made, sometimes the abuser is held only for a few hours or overnight. Often the abuser retaliates upon release; hence, women have a legitimate fear of calling the police. Studies have shown that arresting the batterer may reduce short-term violence but may increase long-term violence.

A woman can obtain a **restraining order** (protection order) from her county of residence that legally prohibits the abuser from approaching or contacting her. Nevertheless, a restraining order provides only limited protection. The abuser may decide to violate the order and severely injure or kill the woman before police can intervene. Civil orders of protection are more effective in preventing future violence when linked with other interventions such as advocacy counseling, shelter, talking with their health care provider (McCloskey et al., 2006). Women who left their abusive relationships were more likely to be successful if they were younger aged, had an abuse-related physician visit, had attempted to leave previously, and had a civil order of protection (Koepsell et al., 2006).

Even after a victim of battering has "ended" the relationship, problems may continue. **Stalking**, or repeated and persistent attempts to impose unwanted communication or contact on another person, is a problem. Stalkers usually are "would-be lovers," pursuing relationships that have ended or never even existed. Twenty-five percent of women and 10% of men can expect to be victims of ongoing unwanted pursuit. Nearly 1 in 22 adults, almost 10 million people, have been stalked in the United States, with 80% of the victims being female (Basile et al., 2006).

Battered women's shelters can provide temporary housing and food for abused women and their children when they decide to leave the abusive relationship. In many cities, however, shelters are crowded, some have waiting lists, and the relief they provide is temporary. The woman leaving an abusive relationship may have no financial support and limited job skills or experience. Often she has dependent children. These barriers are difficult to overcome, and public or private assistance is limited.

In addition to the many physical injuries that abused women may experience, there are emotional and psychological consequences. Individual psychotherapy or counseling, group therapy, or support and self-help groups can help abused women deal with their trauma and begin to build new, healthier relationships. Battering also may result in posttraumatic stress disorder (PTSD), which is discussed later in this chapter.

CHILD ABUSE

Child abuse or maltreatment generally is defined as the intentional injury of a child. It can include physical abuse or injuries, neglect or failure to prevent harm, failure to provide adequate physical or emotional care or supervision, abandonment, sexual assault or intrusion, and overt torture or maiming (Bernet, 2005). In the United States, each state defines child maltreatment, identifies specific reporting procedures, and establishes service delivery systems. Although similarities exist among the laws of the 50 states, there is also a great deal of variation. For this reason, accurate data on the type, frequency, and severity of child maltreatment across the country are difficult to obtain.

During 2001 in the United States, 903,000 children experienced or were at risk for child abuse or neglect. Fifty-nine percent of child maltreatment victims suffered neglect, 19% were physically abused, 10% were sexually abused, and 7% were psychologically or emotionally abused. Thirteen hundred children died from maltreatment: 35% of the deaths were from neglect and 25% were from physical abuse (CDC, 2004).

Fathers, stepfathers, uncles, older siblings, and live-in partners of the child's mother often perpetrate abuse on girls. About 75% of reported cases involve father–daughter incest; mother–son incest is much less frequent. Estimates are that 15 million women in the United States were sexually abused as children, and one third of all sexually abused victims were molested when they were younger than 9 years of age. Accurate statistics on sexual abuse are difficult to obtain because many incidences are unreported as a result of shame and embarrassment. In other cases, women do not acknowledge sexual abuse until they are adults. Risk for depression, suicide attempts, marital problems, and marriage to an alcoholic are increased among adults with a history of childhood sexual abuse (Dube et al., 2005).

Types of Child Abuse

Physical abuse of children often results from unreasonably severe corporal punishment or unjustifiable punishment such as hitting an infant for crying or soiling his or her diapers. Intentional, deliberate assaults on children include burning, biting, cutting, poking, twisting limbs, or scalding with hot water. The victim often has evidence of old injuries (e.g., scars, untreated fractures, multiple bruises of various ages) that the history given by parents or caregivers does not explain adequately.

Sexual abuse involves sexual acts performed by an adult on a child younger than 18 years. Examples include incest, rape, and sodomy performed directly by the person or with an object, oral–genital contact, and acts of molestation such as rubbing, fondling, or exposing the adult's genitals. Sexual abuse may consist of a single incident or multiple episodes over a protracted period. A second type of sexual abuse involves exploitation, such as making, promoting, or selling pornography involving minors, and coercion of minors to participate in obscene acts.

Neglect is malicious or ignorant withholding of physical, emotional, or educational necessities for the child's well-being. Child abuse by neglect is the most prevalent type of maltreatment and includes refusal to seek health care or delay doing so; abandonment; inadequate supervision; reckless disregard for the child's safety; punitive, exploitive, or abusive emotional treatment; spousal abuse in the child's presence; giving the child permission to be truant; or failing to enroll the child in school.

Psychological abuse (emotional abuse) includes verbal assaults, such as blaming, screaming, name-calling, and using sarcasm; constant family discord characterized by fighting, yelling, and chaos; and emotional deprivation or withholding of affection, nurturing, and normal experiences that engender acceptance, love, security, and self-worth. Emotional abuse often accompanies other types of abuse (e.g., physical or sexual abuse). Exposure to parental alcoholism, drug use, or prostitution—and the neglect that results—also fall within this category.

Clinical Picture

Parents who abuse their children often have minimal parenting knowledge and skills. They may not understand or know what their children need, or they may be angry or frustrated because they are emotionally or financially unequipped to meet those needs. Although lack of education and poverty contribute to child abuse and neglect, they by no means explain the entire phenomenon. Many incidences of abuse and violence occur in families who seem to have everything—the parents are well-educated with successful careers, and the family is financially stable.

Parents who abuse their children often are emotionally immature, needy, and incapable of meeting their own needs much less those of a child. As in spousal abuse, the abuser frequently views his or her children as property belonging to the abusing parent. The abuser does not value the children as people with rights and feelings. In some instances, the parent feels the need to have children to replace his or her own faulty and disappointing childhood; the parent wants to feel the love between child and parent that he or she missed as a child. The reality of the tremendous emotional, physical, and financial demands that comes with raising children usually shatters these unrealistic expectations. When the parent's unrealistic expectations are not met, he or she often reverts to using the same methods his or her parents used.

This tendency for adults to raise their children in the same way they were raised perpetuates the cycle of family violence. Adults who were victims of abuse as children frequently abuse their own children (Bernet, 2005).

Assessment

As with all types of family violence, detection and accurate identification are the first steps. Box 11.3 lists signs that might lead the nurse to suspect neglect or abuse. Burns or scalds may have an identifiable shape, such as cigarette marks, or may have a "stocking and glove" distribution, indicating scalding. The parent of an infant with a severe skull fracture may report that he or she "rolled off the couch," even though the child is too young to do so or the injury is much too severe for a fall of 20 inches. Bruises may

CLINICAL VIGNETTE: CHILD ABUSE

Johnny, 7 years old, has been sent to the school nurse because of a large bruise on his face. The teacher says Johnny is quiet, shy, and reluctant to join games or activities with others at recess. He stumbled around with no good explanation of what happened to his face when the teacher asked him about it this morning.

The nurse has seen Johnny before for a variety of bruises, injuries, and even a burn on his hands. In the past, Johnny's mother has described him as clumsy, always tripping and falling down. She says he's a "daredevil," always trying stunts with his bike or Rollerblades or climbing trees and falling or jumping to the ground. She says she has tried everything but can't slow him down.

When the nurse talks to Johnny, he is reluctant to discuss the bruise on his face. He does not make eye contact with the nurse and gives a vague explanation for his bruise: "I guess I ran into something." The nurse suspects that someone in the home is abusing Johnny.

have familiar, recognizable shapes such as belt buckles or teeth marks (Ryan, 2003).

Children who have been sexually abused may have urinary tract infections; bruised, red, or swollen genitalia; tears of the rectum or vagina; and bruising. The emotional response of these children varies widely. Often, these children talk or behave in ways that indicate more advanced knowledge of sexual issues than would be expected for their ages. Other times, they are frightened and anxious and may either cling to an adult or reject adult attention entirely. The key is to recognize when the child's behavior is outside what is normally expected for his or her age and developmental stage. Seemingly unexplained behavior, from refusal to eat to aggressive behavior with peers, may indicate abuse.

Box 11.3 WARNING SIGNS OF ABUSED/NEGLECTED CHILDREN

- Serious injuries such as fractures, burns, or lacerations with no reported history of trauma
- Delay in seeking treatment for a significant injury
- Child or parent gives a history inconsistent with severity of injury, such as a baby with *contrecoup* injuries to the brain (shaken baby syndrome) that the parents claim happened when the infant rolled off the sofa
- Inconsistencies or changes in the child's history during the evaluation by either the child or the adult
- Unusual injuries for the child's age and level of development, such as a fractured femur on a 2-month-old or a dislocated shoulder in a 2-year-old
- High incidence of urinary tract infections; bruised, red, or swollen genitalia; tears or bruising of rectum or vagina
- Evidence of old injuries not reported, such as scars, fractures not treated, multiple bruises that parent/caregiver cannot explain adequately

The nurse does not have to decide with certainty that abuse has occurred. Nurses are responsible for reporting suspected child abuse with accurate and thorough documentation of assessment data. All 50 states have laws, often called mandatory reporting laws, that require nurses to report suspected abuse. The nurse alone or in consultation with other health team members (e.g., physicians or social workers) may report suspected abuse to appropriate local governmental authorities. In some states, that authority is Child Protective Services, Children and Family Services, or the Department of Health. The number to call can be located in the local telephone book. The reporting person may remain anonymous if desired. People who work in such agencies have special education in the investigation of abuse. Questions must be asked in ways that do not further traumatize the child or impede any possible legal actions. The generalist nurse should not pursue investigation with the child: it may do more harm than good.

Treatment and Intervention

The first part of treatment for child abuse or neglect is to ensure the child's safety and well-being (Bernet, 2005). This may involve removing the child from the home, which also can be traumatic. Given the high risk for psychological problems, a thorough psychiatric evaluation also is indicated. A relationship of trust between the therapist and child is crucial to help the child deal with the trauma of abuse. Depending on the severity and duration of abuse and the child's response, therapy may be indicated over a significant period.

Long-term treatment for the child usually involves professionals from several disciplines, such as psychiatry, social work, and psychology. The very young child may communicate best through play therapy, where he or she draws or acts out situations with puppets or dolls rather than talks about what has happened or his or her feelings. Social service agencies are involved in determining whether returning the child to the parental home is possible based on whether parents can show benefit from treatment. Family therapy may be indicated if reuniting the family is feasible. Parents may require psychiatric or substance abuse treatment. If the child is unlikely to return home, short-term or long-term foster care services may be indicated.

ELDER ABUSE

Elder abuse is the maltreatment of older adults by family members or caregivers. It may include physical and sexual abuse, psychological abuse, neglect, self-neglect, financial exploitation, and denial of adequate medical treatment. Estimates are that people over age 65 are injured, exploited, abused, or neglected by their caregivers and that only 1 in 14 elder maltreatment cases are reported (Muehlbauer & Crane, 2006). Nearly 60% of the perpetrators are spouses, 20% are adult children, and 20% are others such as siblings, grandchildren, and boarders.

Most victims of elder abuse are 75 years or older; 60% to 65% are women. Abuse is more likely when the elder has multiple chronic mental and physical health problems and when he or she is dependent on others for food, medical care, and various activities of daily living.

Persons who abuse elders are almost always in a caregiver position or the elders depend on them in some way. Most cases of elder abuse occur when one older spouse is taking care of another. This type of spousal abuse usually happens over many years after a disability renders the abused spouse unable to care for himself or herself. When the abuser is an adult child, it is twice as likely to be a son as a daughter. A psychiatric disorder or a problem with substance abuse also may aggravate abuse of elders (Goldstein, 2005).

Elders are often reluctant to report abuse, even when they can, because the abuse usually involves family members whom the elder wishes to protect. Victims also often fear losing their support and being moved to an institution.

No national estimates of abuse of elders living in institutions are available. However, under a 1978 federal mandate, ombudsmen are allowed to visit nursing homes to check on the care of the elderly. These ombudsmen report that elder abuse is common in institutions (Goldstein, 2005).

Clinical Picture

The victim may have bruises or fractures; may lack needed eyeglasses or hearing aids; may be denied food, fluids, or medications; or may be restrained in a bed or chair. The abuser may use the victim's financial resources for his or her own pleasure while the elder cannot afford food or medications. Abusers may withhold medical care itself from an elder with acute or chronic illness. Self-neglect involves the elder's failure to provide for him or herself.

Assessment

Careful assessment of elderly persons and their caregiving relationships is essential in detecting elder abuse. Often,

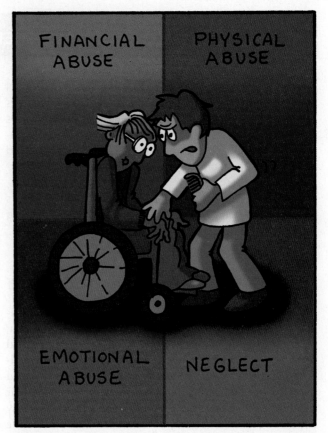

Elder abuse

determining whether the elder's condition results from deterioration associated with a chronic illness or from abuse is difficult. Several potential indicators of abuse require further assessment and careful evaluation (Box 11.4). These indicators by themselves, however, do not necessarily signify abuse or neglect.

The nurse should suspect abuse if injuries have been hidden or untreated or are incompatible with the explanation provided. Such injuries can include cuts, lacerations, puncture wounds, bruises, welts, or burns. Burns can be cigarette burns, scaldings, acid or caustic burns, or friction burns of the wrists or ankles caused from being restrained by ropes, clothing, or chains. Signs of physical neglect include a pervasive smell of urine or feces, dirt, rashes, sores, lice, or inadequate clothing. Dehydration or malnourishment not linked with a specific illness also strongly indicates abuse.

Possible indicators of emotional or psychological abuse include an elder who is hesitant to talk openly to the nurse or who is fearful, withdrawn, depressed, and helpless. The elder also may exhibit anger or agitation for no apparent reason. He or she may deny any problems, even when the facts indicate otherwise.

Possible indicators of self-neglect include inability to manage money (hoarding or squandering while failing to pay bills), inability to perform activities of daily living (personal care, shopping, food preparation, and cleaning), and changes in intellectual function (confusion, disorientation, inappro-

Box 11.4   POSSIBLE INDICATORS OF ELDER ABUSE

PHYSICAL ABUSE INDICATORS

• Frequent, unexplained injuries accompanied by a habit of seeking medical assistance from various locations
• Reluctance to seek medical treatment for injuries or denial of their existence
• Disorientation or grogginess indicating misuse of medications
• Fear or edginess in the presence of family member or caregiver

PSYCHOLOGICAL OR EMOTIONAL ABUSE INDICATORS

• Helplessness
• Hesitance to talk openly
• Anger or agitation
• Withdrawal or depression

FINANCIAL ABUSE INDICATORS

• Unusual or inappropriate activity in bank accounts
• Signatures on checks that differ from the elder's
• Recent changes in will or power of attorney when elder is not capable of making those decisions
• Missing valuable belongings that are not just misplaced
• Lack of television, clothes, or personal items that are easily affordable
• Unusual concern by the caregiver over the expense of the elder's treatment when it is not the caregiver's money being spent

NEGLECT INDICATORS

• Dirt, fecal or urine smell, or other health hazards in the elder's living environment
• Rashes, sores, or lice on the elder
• Elder has an untreated medical condition or is malnourished or dehydrated not related to a known illness
• Inadequate clothing

INDICATORS OF SELF-NEGLECT

• Inability to manage personal finances, such as hoarding, squandering, or giving away money while not paying bills
• Inability to manage activities of daily living, such as personal care, shopping, or housework
• Wandering, refusing needed medical attention, isolation, substance use
• Failure to keep needed medical appointments
• Confusion, memory loss, unresponsiveness
• Lack of toilet facilities, living quarters infested with animals or vermin

WARNING INDICATORS FROM CAREGIVER

• Elder is not given opportunity to speak for self, to have visitors, or to see anyone without the presence of the caregiver
• Attitudes of indifference or anger toward the elder
• Blaming the elder for his or her illness or limitations
• Defensiveness
• Conflicting accounts of elder's abilities, problems, and so forth
• Previous history of abuse or problems with alcohol or drugs

Adapted from the California Registry, Elder Abuse Indicators (2006). http://www.calregistry.com/resources/eldabpag.html

priate responses, and memory loss and isolation). Other indicators of self-neglect include signs of malnutrition or dehydration, rashes or sores on the body, an odor of urine or feces, or failure to keep needed medical appointments. For self-neglect to be diagnosed, the elder must be evaluated as unable to manage day-to-day life and take care of him or herself. Self-neglect cannot be established based solely on family members' beliefs that the elder cannot manage his or her finances. For example, an older adult cannot be considered to have self-neglect just because he or she gives away large sums of money to a group or charity or invests in some venture of which family members disapprove.

Warnings of financial exploitation or abuse may include numerous unpaid bills (when the client has enough money to pay them), unusual activity in bank accounts, checks signed by someone other than the elder, or recent changes in a will or power of attorney when the elder cannot make such decisions. The elder may lack amenities that he or she can afford, such as clothing, personal products, or a television. The elder may report losing valuable possessions and report that he or she has no contact with friends or relatives.

The nurse also may detect possible indicators of abuse from the caregiver. The caregiver may complain about how difficult caring for the elder is, incontinence, difficulties in feeding, or excessive costs of medication. He or she may display anger or indifference toward the elder and try to keep the nurse from talking with the elder alone. Elder abuse is more likely when the caregiver has a history of family violence or alcohol or drug problems.

Some states have mandatory reporting laws for elder abuse; others have only voluntary reporting laws. Nurses should be familiar with the laws or statutes for reporting abuse in their own states. Many cases remain unreported. The local agency on aging can provide procedures for reporting abuse in accordance with state laws. To find a local agency, call the national information center at 1-800-677-1116.

Treatment and Intervention

Elder abuse may develop gradually as the burden of care exceeds the caregiver's physical or emotional resources. Relieving the caregiver's stress and providing additional resources may help to correct the abusive situation and leave the caregiving relationship intact. In other cases, the neglect or abuse is intentional and designed to provide personal gain to the caregiver, such as access to the victim's financial resources. In these situations, removal of the elder or caregiver is necessary.

RAPE AND SEXUAL ASSAULT

Rape is a crime of violence and humiliation of the victim expressed through sexual means. Rape is the perpetration of an act of sexual intercourse with a female against her will and without her consent, whether her will is overcome by force, fear of force, drugs, or intoxicants. It is also considered rape if the woman is incapable of exercising rational judgment because of mental deficiency or when she is younger than the age of consent (which varies among states from 14 to 18 years; van der Kolk, 2005). The crime of rape requires only slight penetration of the outer vulva; full erection and ejaculation are not necessary. Forced acts of fellatio and anal penetration, although they frequently accompany rape, are legally considered sodomy. The woman who is raped also may be physically beaten and injured.

Rape can occur between strangers, acquaintances, married persons, and persons of the same sex, although seven states define domestic violence in a way that excludes same-sex victims. Strangers commit about 50% of rapes, whereas men known to the victims commit the rest. A phenomenon called **date rape (acquaintance rape)** may occur on a first date, on a ride home from a party, or when the two people have known each other for some time. It is

CLINICAL VIGNETTE: ELDER ABUSE

Josephine is an elderly woman who has moved in with her son, daughter-in-law, and two grandchildren after the death of her husband. She lives in a finished basement apartment with her own bath. Friction with her daughter-in-law begins to develop when Josephine tries to help out around the house. She comments on the poor manners and outlandish clothes of her teenaged grandchildren. She adds spices to food her daughter-in-law is cooking on the stove. She comments on how late the children stay out, their friends, and how hard her son works. All this is annoying but harmless.

Josephine's daughter-in-law gets very impatient, telling her husband, "I'm the one who has to deal with your mother all day long." One day, after another criticism from Josephine, the daughter-in-law slaps her. She then tells Josephine to go downstairs to her room and stay out of sight if she wants to have a place to live. A friend of Josephine's calls on the phone and the daughter-in-law lies and tells her Josephine is sleeping.

Josephine spends more time alone in her room, becomes more isolated and depressed, and is eating and sleeping poorly. She is afraid she will be placed in a nursing home if she doesn't get along with her daughter-in-law. Her son seems too busy to notice what is happening, and Josephine is afraid to tell him for fear he won't believe her or will take his wife's side. Her friends don't seem to call much anymore, and she has no one to talk to about how miserable she is. She just stays to herself most of the day.

more prevalent near college and university campuses. The CDC Division of Violence Prevention (2004) reports that the rate of serious injuries associated with dating violence increases with increased consumption of alcohol by either victim or perpetrator.

Rape is a highly underreported crime: Estimates are that only 1 rape is reported for every 4 to 10 rapes that occur. The underreporting is attributed to the victim's feelings of shame and guilt, the fear of further injury, and the belief that she has no recourse in the legal system. Victims of rape can be any age: Reported cases have victims ranging in age from 15 months to 82 years. The highest incidence is in girls and women 16 to 24 years of age. Girls younger than 18 years were the victims in 61% of rapes reported (van der Kolk, 2005).

Rape most commonly occurs in a woman's neighborhood, often inside or near her home. Most rapes are premeditated. Strangers perpetrate 43% of rapes, husbands and boyfriends commit 19%, and other relatives account for 38%. Rape results in pregnancy about 10% of the time (van der Kolk, 2005).

Male rape is a significantly underreported crime. It can occur between gay partners or strangers but is most prevalent in institutions such as prisons or maximum-security hospitals. Estimates are that 2% to 5% of male inmates are sexually assaulted, but the figure may be much higher. This type of rape is particularly violent, and the dynamics of power and control are the same as for heterosexual rape.

Dynamics of Rape

Most men who commit rape are 25 to 44 years of age. In terms of race, 51% are white and tend to rape white victims, and 47% are African American and tend to rape African-American victims; the remaining 2% come from all other races. Alcohol is involved in 34% of cases. Rape often accompanies another crime. Almost 75% of arrested rapists have prior criminal histories, including other rapes, assaults, robberies, and homicides (van der Kolk, 2005).

Recent research (van der Kolk, 2005) has categorized male rapists into four categories:

- Sexual sadists who are aroused by the pain of their victims
- Exploitive predators who impulsively use their victims as objects for gratification
- Inadequate men who believe that no woman would voluntarily have sexual relations with them and who are obsessed with fantasies about sex
- Men for whom rape is a displaced expression of anger and rage

Feminist theory proposes that women have historically served as objects for aggression, dating back to when women (and children) were legally the property of men. In 1982, for the first time, a married man was convicted of raping his wife, signaling the end of the notion that sexual intercourse could not be denied in the context of marriage.

Women who are raped are frequently in life-threatening situations, so their primary motivation is to stay alive. At times, attempts to resist or fight the attacker succeed; in other situations, fighting and yelling result in more severe physical injuries or even death. Degree of submission is higher when the attacker has a weapon such as a gun or knife. In addition to forcible penetration, the more violent rapist may urinate or defecate on the woman or insert foreign objects into her vagina and rectum.

The physical and psychological trauma that rape victims suffer is severe. Related medical problems can include acute injury, sexually transmitted diseases, pregnancy, and lingering medical complaints. A cross-sectional study of medical patients found that women who had been raped rated themselves as significantly less healthy, visited a physician twice as often, and incurred medical costs more than twice as high as women who had not experienced any criminal victimization (American Medical Association, 2004). The level of violence experienced during the assault was found to be a powerful predictor of future use of medical services. Many victims of rape experience fear, helplessness, shock and disbelief, guilt, humiliation, and embarrassment. They also may avoid the place or circumstances of the rape; give up previously pleasurable activities; and experience depression, sexual dysfunction, insomnia, and impaired memory (American Medical Association, 2004).

Until recently, the rights of rape victims often were ignored. For example, when rape victims reported a rape to authorities, they often faced doubt and embarrassing questions from male officers. The courts did not protect the rights of victims; for example, a woman's past sexual behavior was admissible in court—although the past criminal record of her accused attacker was not. Laws to correct these problems have been enacted on a state-by-state basis since the mid-1980s.

Although the treatment of rape victims and the prosecution of rapists have improved in the past two decades, many people still believe that somehow a woman provokes rape by her behavior and that the woman is partially responsible for this crime. Box 11.5 summarizes common myths and misunderstandings about rape.

Assessment

To preserve possible evidence, the physical examination should occur before the woman has showered, brushed her teeth, douched, changed her clothes, or had anything to drink. This may not be possible, because the woman may have done some of these things before seeking care. If there is no report of oral sex, then rinsing the mouth or drinking fluids can be permitted immediately.

To assess the woman's physical status, the nurse asks the victim to describe what happened. If the woman cannot do so, the nurse may ask needed questions gently and with care. Rape kits and rape protocols are available in most emergency room settings and provide the equipment and instructions

Box 11.5   COMMON MYTHS ABOUT RAPE

- When a woman submits to rape, she really wants it to happen.
- Women who dress provocatively are asking for trouble.
- Some women like rough sex but later call it rape.
- Once a man is aroused by a woman, he cannot stop his actions.
- Walking alone at night is an invitation for rape.
- Rape cannot happen between persons who are married.
- Rape is exciting for some women.
- Rape only occurs between heterosexual couples.
- If a woman has an orgasm, it can't be rape.

Box 11.6   WARNING SIGNS OF RELATIONSHIP VIOLENCE

- Emotionally abuses you (insults, makes belittling comments, acts sulky or angry when you initiate an idea or activity)
- Tells you with whom you may be friends or how you should dress, or tries to control other elements of your life
- Talks negatively about women in general
- Gets jealous for no reason
- Drinks heavily, uses drugs, or tries to get you drunk
- Acts in an intimidating way by invading your personal space such as standing too close or touching you when you don't want him to
- Cannot handle sexual or emotional frustration without becoming angry
- Does not view you as an equal: sees himself as smarter or socially superior
- Guards his masculinity by acting tough
- Is angry or threatening to the point that you have changed your life or yourself so you won't anger him
- Goes through extreme highs and lows; is kind one minute, cruel the next
- Berates you for not getting drunk or high, or not wanting to have sex with him
- Is physically aggressive, grabbing and holding you, or pushing and shoving

Adapted from the State University of New York at Buffalo Counseling Center (2006). http://ub-counseling.buffalo.edu/warnings.shtml

needed to collect physical evidence. The physician is primarily responsible for this step of the examination.

Treatment and Intervention

Victims of rape fare best when they receive immediate support and can express fear and rage to family members, nurses, physicians, and law enforcement officials who believe them. Education about rape and the needs of victims is an ongoing requirement for health care professionals, law enforcement officers, and the general public.

Box 11.6 lists warning signs of relationship violence. These signs, used at the State University of New York at

CLINICAL VIGNETTE: RAPE

Cynthia is a 22-year-old college student who spent Saturday afternoon with a group of friends at the football game. Afterward, they were going to attend a few parties to celebrate the victory. Alcohol was served freely at these parties. At one party, Cynthia became separated from her friends but started talking to Ron, whom she recognized from her English Lit course. They spent the rest of the evening together, talking, dancing, and drinking. She had had more drinks then she was used to, as Ron kept bringing her more every time her glass was empty. At the end of the night, Ron asked if she wanted him to drive her home. Her friends were staying longer at the party.

When Ron and Cynthia arrived at her apartment, none of her roommates had returned yet, so she asked Ron to come in. She was feeling a little tipsy, and they began kissing. She could feel Ron really getting excited. He began to try to remove her skirt, but she said, "No" and tried to move away from him. She remembered him saying, "What's the matter with you? Are you a prude or what?" She told him she had had a good time but didn't want to go further. He responded, "Come on, you've been trying to turn me on all night. You want this as much as I do." He forced himself on top of her and held his arm over her neck and raped her.

When her roommates return in about 1 hour, Cynthia is huddled in the corner of her room, seems stunned, and is crying uncontrollably. She feels sick and confused. Did she do something to cause this whole thing? She keeps asking herself whether she might not have gotten into that situation had she not been a little tipsy. She is so confused.

Buffalo (2006) to educate students about date rape, can alert women to the characteristics of men who are likely to commit dating violence. Examples include expressing negativity about women, acting tough, engaging in heavy drinking, exhibiting jealousy, making belittling comments, expressing anger, and using intimidation.

Rape treatment centers (emergency services that coordinate psychiatric, gynecologic, and physical trauma services in one location and work with law enforcement agencies) are most helpful to the victim. In the emergency setting, the nurse is an essential part of the team in providing emotional support to the victim. The nurse should allow the woman to proceed at her own pace and not rush her through any interview or examination procedures.

Giving as much control back to the victim as possible is important. Ways to do so include allowing her to make decisions, when possible, about whom to call, what to do next, what she would like done, and so on. It is the woman's decision about whether or not to file charges and testify against the perpetrator. The victim must sign consent forms before any photographs or hair and nail samples are taken for future evidence.

Prophylactic treatment for sexually transmitted diseases such as chlamydia or gonorrhea is offered. Doing so is cost effective: many victims of rape will not return to get definitive test results for these diseases. HIV testing is strongly encouraged at specified intervals because seroconversion to positive status does not occur immediately. Women are also encouraged to engage in safe-sex practices until the results of HIV testing are available. Prophylaxis with ethinyl estradiol and norgestrel (Ovral) can be offered to prevent pregnancy. Some women may elect to wait to initiate intervention until they have a positive pregnancy test result or miss a menstrual period.

Rape crisis centers, women's advocacy groups, and other local resources often provide a counselor or volunteer to be with the victim from the emergency room through longer-term follow-up. This person provides emotional support, serves as an advocate for the woman throughout the process, and can be totally available to the victim. This type of complete and unconditional support is often crucial to recovery.

Therapy usually is supportive in approach and focuses on restoring the victim's sense of control; relieving feelings of helplessness, dependency, and obsession with the assault that frequently follow rape; regaining trust; improving daily functioning; finding adequate social support; and dealing with feelings of guilt, shame, and anger. Group therapy with other women who have been raped is a particularly effective treatment. Some women attend both individual and group therapies.

It often takes 1 year or more for survivors of rape to regain previous levels of functioning. In some cases, survivors of rape have long-term consequences, such as post-traumatic stress disorder (PTSD), which is discussed later in this chapter.

COMMUNITY VIOLENCE

The CDC (2004), the U.S. Department of Education, the Department of Justice, and the National School Safety Center have been examining homicides and suicides associated with schools. The study examined events on the way to and from school, on school property, and at school-sponsored events and found that 83% of the victims of school homicide or suicide were male and 65% of school-associated violent deaths were students, 11% were teachers or staff, and 23% were community members killed on school property.

The original study was expanded to cover school-associated violent deaths from July 1994 to June 1998. The results showed 173 incidents, most of which were homicides committed with firearms. The total number of events decreased since the 1992–1993 school year, but the number of multiple-victim events during that period increased. This means that fewer events involving one person occurred, but multiple-victim events increased from one per year between 1992 and 1995 to five events per year between August 1995 and July 1998. A person only has to watch the evening news to know that this is the trend.

The CDC has been working with schools to develop curricula that emphasize problem-solving skills, anger management, and social skills development. In addition, parenting programs that promote strong bonding between parents and children and conflict management in the home, as well as mentoring programs for young people, show promise in dealing with school-related violence. A few people responsible for such violence have been diagnosed with a psychiatric disorder, often conduct disorder, which is discussed in Chapter 20. Often, however, this violence seems to occur when alienation, disregard for others, and little regard for self predominate.

Nearly one third of U.S. students report they experience bullying, either as a target or a perpetrator. More than 16% said they'd been bullied occasionally, whereas 8% reported being bullied at least once a week. The frequency of bullying was highest among sixth through eighth graders. Children who were bullied reported more loneliness and difficulty making friends, and those who bullied were more likely to have poor grades and to use alcohol and tobacco. Children with special physical health care needs are bullied more often, and children with a chronic emotional, behavioral, or developmental problem are more likely to be both a bully and a victim of bullying (Van Cleave & Davis, 2006).

Hazing, or initiation rites, is prevalent in both high school and college. Forty-eight percent of high school students reported belonging to groups that involved hazing activities. Forty-three percent reported being subjected to humiliating activities, and 30% reported hazing that involved illegal activities. Seventy-one percent of the students subjected to hazing reported negative consequences such as fighting; being injured; hurting other people; doing poorly in school; difficulty eating, sleeping, or concentrating; and experiencing feelings of anger, confusion, embarrassment, or guilt (Lipkins, 2006).

Exposure to community violence tremendously affects children and young adults. When children witness violence they experience stress-related symptoms that increase with the amount of violence they see. In addition, witnessing violence can lead to future problems with aggression, depression, relationships, achievement, and abuse of drugs and alcohol (Skybo, 2005). Addressing the problem of violence exposure may help to alleviate the cycle of dysfunction and further violence.

On a larger scale, violence such as the terrorist attacks in New York, Washington, and Pennsylvania in 2001 also has far-reaching effects on citizens. In the immediate aftermath, children were afraid to go to school or have their parents leave them for any reason. Adults had difficulty going to work, leaving their homes, using public transportation, and flying. Research is now showing that 1 in 10 New York area residents suffers lingering stress and depression as a result of September 11, and an additional 532,240 cases of PTSD have been reported in the New York City metropolitan area alone (Schlenger et al., 2002). In addition, people are reporting higher relapse rates of depression and anxiety disorders. The study showed no increase of PTSD nationwide as a result of individuals watching the attacks and associated coverage on television, however, which had been an initial concern.

Early intervention and treatment are key to dealing with victims of violence. After several instances of school or workplace shootings, counseling, referrals, and ongoing treatment were instituted immediately to help those involved deal with the horror of their experiences. Since the 2001 terrorist attacks, teams of physicians, therapists, and other health professionals (many associated with universities and medical centers) have been working with survivors, families, and others affected. Despite such efforts, many people will continue to experience long-term difficulties, as described in the next section.

PSYCHIATRIC DISORDERS RELATED TO ABUSE AND VIOLENCE

Posttraumatic Stress Disorder

Posttraumatic stress disorder is a disturbing pattern of behavior demonstrated by someone who has experienced a traumatic event such as a natural disaster, combat, or an assault. The person with PTSD was exposed to an event that posed a threat of death or serious injury and responded with intense fear, helplessness, or terror. Three clusters of symptoms are present: reliving the event, avoiding reminders of the event, and being on guard, or experiencing *hyperarousal*. The person persistently re-experiences the trauma through memories, dreams, flashbacks, or reactions to external cues about the event and therefore avoids stimuli associated with the trauma. The victim feels a numbing of general responsiveness and shows persistent signs of increased arousal such as insomnia, hyperarousal or hypervigilance, irritability, or

angry outbursts. He or she reports losing a sense of connection and control over his or her life. In PTSD, the symptoms occur 3 months or more after the trauma, which distinguishes PTSD from **acute stress disorder**. This diagnosis from the *Diagnostic and Statistical Manual of Mental Disorders, 4th edition, Text Revision (DSM-IV-TR;* American Psychiatric Association [APA], 2000) is appropriate when symptoms appear within the first month after the trauma and do not persist longer than 4 weeks.

PTSD can occur at any age, including during childhood. Estimates are that up to 60% of people at risk, such as combat veterans and victims of violence and natural disasters, develop PTSD. Complete recovery occurs within 3 months for about 50% of people. The severity and duration of the trauma and the proximity of the person to the event are the most important factors affecting the likelihood of developing PTSD (APA, 2000). One-fourth of all victims of physical assault develop PTSD. Victims of rape have one of the highest rates of PTSD—approximately 70 percent (Van der Kolk, 2005).

Dissociative Disorders

Dissociation is a subconscious defense mechanism that helps a person protect his or her emotional self from recognizing the full effects of some horrific or traumatic event by allowing the mind to forget or remove itself from the painful situation or memory. Dissociation can occur both during

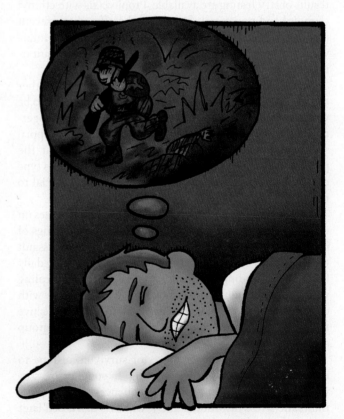

Posttraumatic stress disorder

DSM-IV-TR DIAGNOSTIC CRITERIA:
MAJOR SYMPTOMS OF POSTTRAUMATIC STRESS DISORDER

- Recurrent, intrusive, distressing memories of the event
- Nightmares
- Flashbacks
- Avoidance of thoughts, feelings, or conversations associated with the trauma
- Avoidance of activities, places, or people that arouse memories of the trauma
- Inability to recall important aspect of the trauma
- Marked decrease in interest or participation in significant events
- Feeling detached or estranged from others
- Restricted range of affect
- Sense of foreshortened future
- Difficulty falling or staying asleep
- Irritability or anger outbursts
- Difficulty concentrating
- Hypervigilance
- Exaggerated startle response

Adapted from DSM-IV-TR, 2000.

and after the event. As with any other protective coping mechanism, dissociating becomes easier with repeated use.

Dissociative disorders have the essential feature of a disruption in the usually integrated functions of consciousness, memory, identity, or environmental perception. This often interferes with the person's relationships, ability to function in daily life, and ability to cope with the realities of the abusive or traumatic event. This disturbance varies greatly in intensity in different people, and the onset may be sudden or gradual, transient or chronic. Dissociative symptoms are seen in clients with PTSD.

The *DSM-IV-TR* describes different types of dissociative disorders:

- *Dissociative amnesia:* The client cannot remember important personal information (usually of a traumatic or stressful nature).
- *Dissociative fugue:* The client has episodes of suddenly leaving the home or place of work without any explanation, traveling to another city, and being unable to remember his or her past or identity. He or she may assume a new identity.
- *Dissociative identity disorder* (formerly *multiple personality disorder*): The client displays two or more distinct identities or personality states that recurrently take control of his or her behavior. This is accompanied by the inability to recall important personal information.
- *Depersonalization disorder:* The client has a persistent or recurrent feeling of being detached from his or her mental processes or body. This is accompanied by intact

reality testing; that is, the client is not psychotic or out of touch with reality.

Dissociative disorders, relatively rare in the general population, are much more prevalent among those with histories of childhood physical and sexual abuse. Some believe the recent increase in the diagnosis of dissociative disorders in the United States is the result of more awareness of this disorder by mental health professionals (APA, 2000).

The media has focused much attention on the theory of **repressed memories** in victims of abuse. Many professionals believe that memories of childhood abuse can be buried deeply in the subconscious mind or repressed because they are too painful for the victims to acknowledge and that victims can be helped to recover or remember such painful memories. If a person comes to a mental health professional experiencing serious problems in relationships, symptoms of PTSD, or flashbacks involving abuse, the mental health professional may help the person remember or recover those memories of abuse. Some believe that mental health professionals may be overzealous in helping clients "remember" abuse that really did not happen or encouraging clients to see themselves as having many parts or as having inner children (Piper & Merskey, 2004). This so-called *false memory syndrome* has created problems in families when clients made groundless accusations of abuse. Fears exist, however, that people abused in childhood will be more reluctant to talk about their abuse history because, once again, no one will believe them. Still other therapists argue that people thought to have dissociative identity disorder are suffering anxiety, terror, and intrusive ideas and emotions and therefore need help, and the therapist should remain open-minded about the diagnosis (Middleton et al., 2005).

Treatment and Interventions

Survivors of trauma and abuse who have PTSD or dissociative disorders often are involved in group or individual therapy in the community to address the long-term effects

DSM-IV-TR DIAGNOSTIC CRITERIA:
MAJOR SYMPTOMS OF DISSOCIATIVE IDENTITY DISORDER

- Presence of two or more distinct identities or personality states
- At least two identities recurrently take control of the person's behavior
- Inability to recall important personal information: more extensive than ordinary forgetfulness
- Symptoms are not related to any substance use or medical condition

Adapted from DSM-IV-TR, 2000.

CLINICAL VIGNETTE: POSTTRAUMATIC STRESS DISORDER

Julie sat up in bed. She felt her heart pounding, she was perspiring, and she felt like she couldn't breathe. She was gasping for breath and felt the pressure on her throat! The picture of that dark figure knocking her to the ground and his hands around her throat was vivid in her mind. Her heart was pounding and she was reliving it all over again, the pain and the terror of that night! It had been 2 years since she was attacked and raped in the park while jogging, but sometimes it felt like just yesterday. She had nightmares of panic almost every night. She would never be rid of that night.

Lately, the dread of reliving the nightmare made Julie afraid to fall asleep, and she wasn't getting much sleep. She felt exhausted. She didn't feel much like eating and was losing weight. This ordeal had ruined her life. She was missing work more and more. Even while at work, she often felt an over-whelming sense of dread. Sometimes even in the daytime, the memories of that night and flashbacks would come.

Her friends didn't seem to want to be around her anymore because she was often moody and couldn't seem to enjoy herself. Sure, they were supportive and listened to her for the first 6 months, but now it was 2 years since the rape. Before the rape, she was always ready to go to a party or out to dinner and a movie with friends. Now she just felt like staying home. She was tired of her mother and friends telling her she needed to go out and have some fun. Nobody could understand what she had gone through and how she felt. Julie had had several boyfriends since then, but the relationships just never seemed to work out. She was moody and would often become anxious and depressed for no reason and cancel dates at the last minute. Everyone was getting tired of her moods, but she felt she had no control over them.

of their experiences. Cognitive behavioral therapy is effective in dealing with the thoughts and subsequent feelings and behavior of trauma and abuse survivors. Therapy for clients who dissociate focuses on reassociation, or putting the consciousness back together. Both paroxetine (Paxil) and sertraline (Zoloft) have been used to treat PTSD successfully. Clients with dissociative disorders may be treated symptomatically, that is, with medications for anxiety, depression, or both if these symptoms are predominant.

Clients with PTSD and dissociative disorders are found in all areas of health care, from clinics to primary care offices. The nurse is most likely to encounter these clients in acute care settings when there are concerns for their safety or the safety of others or when acute symptoms have become intense and require stabilization. Treatment in acute care is usually short-term, with the client returning to community-based treatment as quickly as possible.

APPLICATION OF THE NURSING PROCESS
Assessment

BACKGROUND

The health history reveals that the client has a history of trauma or abuse. It may be abuse as a child or in a current or recent relationship. It generally is not necessary or desirable for the client to detail specific events of the abuse or trauma; rather, in-depth discussion of the actual abuse is usually undertaken during individual psychotherapy sessions.

GENERAL APPEARANCE AND MOTOR BEHAVIOR

The nurse assesses the client's overall appearance and motor behavior. The client often appears hyperalert and reacts to even small environmental noises with a startle response. He or she may be very uncomfortable if the nurse is too close physically and may require greater distance or personal space than most people. The client may appear anxious or agitated and may have difficulty sitting still, often needing to pace or move around the room. Sometimes the client may sit very still, seeming to curl up with arms around knees.

MOOD AND AFFECT

In assessing mood and affect, the nurse must remember that a wide range of emotions is possible, from passivity to anger. The client may look frightened or scared or agitated and hostile depending on his or her experience. When the client experiences a flashback, he or she appears terrified and may cry, scream, or attempt to hide or run away. When the client is dissociating, he or she may speak in a different tone of voice or appear numb with a vacant stare. The client may report intense rage or anger or feeling dead inside and unable to identify any feelings or emotions.

THOUGHT PROCESS AND CONTENT

The nurse asks questions about thought process and content. Clients who have been abused or traumatized report reliving the trauma, often through nightmares or flashbacks. Intrusive, persistent thoughts about the trauma interfere with the client's ability to think about other things or to focus on daily living. Some clients report hallucinations or buzzing voices in their heads. Self-destructive thoughts and impulses as well as intermittent suicidal ideation are also common. Some clients report fantasies in which they take revenge on their abusers.

SENSORIUM AND INTELLECTUAL PROCESSES

During assessment of sensorium and intellectual processes, the nurse usually finds that the client is oriented to reality except if the client is experiencing a flashback or dissociative episode. During those experiences, the client may not respond to the nurse or may be unable to communicate at all. The nurse also may find that clients who have been abused or traumatized have *memory gaps,* which are periods for which they have no clear memories. These periods may be short or extensive and are usually related to the time of the abuse or trauma. Intrusive thoughts or ideas of self-harm often impair the client's ability to concentrate or pay attention.

JUDGMENT AND INSIGHT

The client's insight is often related to the duration of his or her problems with dissociation or PTSD. Early in treatment, the client may report little idea about the relationship of past trauma to his or her current symptoms and problems. Other clients may be quite knowledgeable if they have progressed further in treatment. The client's ability to make decisions or solve problems may be impaired.

SELF-CONCEPT

The nurse is likely to find these clients have low self-esteem. They may believe they are bad people who somehow deserve or provoke the abuse. Many clients believe they are unworthy or damaged by their abusive experiences to the point that they will never be worthwhile or valued. Clients may believe they are going crazy and are out of control with no hope of regaining control. Clients may see themselves as helpless, hopeless, and worthless.

ROLES AND RELATIONSHIPS

Clients generally report a great deal of difficulty with all types of relationships. Problems with authority figures often lead to problems at work, such as being unable to take directions from another or have another person monitor his or her performance. Close relationships are difficult or impossible because the client's ability to trust others is severely compromised. Often the client has quit work or has been fired, and he or she may be estranged from family members. Intrusive thoughts, flashbacks, or dissociative episodes may interfere with the client's ability to socialize with family or friends, and the client's avoidant behavior may keep him or her from participating in social or family events.

PHYSIOLOGIC CONSIDERATIONS

Most clients report difficulty sleeping because of nightmares or anxiety over anticipating nightmares. Overeating or lack of appetite is also common. Frequently, these clients use alcohol or other drugs to attempt to sleep or to blot out intrusive thoughts or memories.

Data Analysis

Nursing diagnoses commonly used in the acute care setting when working with clients who dissociate or have PTSD related to trauma or abuse include the following:
- Risk for Self-Mutilation
- Ineffective Coping
- Post-Trauma Response
- Chronic Low Self-Esteem
- Powerlessness

In addition, the following nursing diagnoses may be pertinent for clients over longer periods, although not all diagnoses apply to each client:
- Disturbed Sleep Pattern
- Sexual Dysfunction
- Rape-Trauma Syndrome
- Spiritual Distress
- Social Isolation

Outcome Identification

Treatment outcomes for clients who have survived trauma or abuse may include the following:

1. The client will be physically safe.
2. The client will distinguish between ideas of self-harm and taking action on those ideas.
3. The client will demonstrate healthy, effective ways of dealing with stress.
4. The client will express emotions nondestructively.
5. The client will establish a social support system in the community.

Intervention

PROMOTING THE CLIENT'S SAFETY

The client's safety is a priority. The nurse continually must assess the client's potential for self-harm or suicide and take action accordingly. The nurse and treatment team must provide safety measures when the client cannot do so (see Chapters 10 and 15). To increase the client's sense of personal control, he or she must begin to manage safety needs as soon as possible. The nurse can talk with the client about the difference between having self-harm thoughts and taking action on those thoughts: having the thoughts does not mean the client must act on those thoughts. Gradually, the nurse can help the client to find ways to tolerate the thoughts until they diminish in intensity.

The nurse can help the client learn to go to a safe place during destructive thoughts and impulses so that he or she can calm down and wait until they pass. Initially, this may mean just sitting with the nurse or around others. Later, the client can find a safe place at home, often a closet or small room, where he or she feels safe. The client may want to keep a blanket or pillows there for comfort and pictures or a tape recording to serve as reminders of the present.

HELPING THE CLIENT COPE WITH STRESS AND EMOTIONS

Grounding techniques are helpful to use with the client who is dissociating or experiencing a flashback. Grounding techniques remind the client that he or she is in the present, is an adult, and is safe. Validating what the client is feeling during these experiences is important: "I know this is frightening, but you are safe now." In addition, the nurse can increase contact with reality and diminish the dissociative experience by helping the client focus on what he or she is currently experiencing through the senses:

- "What are you feeling?"
- "Are you hearing something?"
- "What are you touching?"
- "Can you see me and the room we're in?"
- "Do you feel your feet on the floor?"
- "Do you feel your arm on the chair?"
- "Do you feel the watch on your wrist?"

For the client experiencing dissociative symptoms, the nurse can use grounding techniques to focus the client on the present. For example, the nurse approaches the client and speaks in a calm reassuring tone. First, the nurse calls the client by name and then introduces him or herself by name and role. If the area is dark, the nurse turns on the lights. He or she can reorient the client by saying the following:

"Janet, I'm here with you. My name is Sheila. I'm the nurse working with you today. Today is Thursday, February 8, 2007. You're here in the hospital. This is your room at the hospital. Can you open your eyes and look at me? Janet, my name is Sheila."

The nurse repeats this reorienting information as needed. Asking the client to look around the room encourages the client to move his or her eyes and avoid being locked in a daze or flashback.

As soon as possible, the nurse encourages the client to change positions. Often during a flashback, the client curls up in a defensive posture. Getting the client to stand and walk around helps to dispel the dissociative or flashback experience. At this time, the client can focus on his or her feet moving on the floor or the swinging movements of his or her arms. The nurse must not grab the client or attempt to force him or her to stand up or move. The client experiencing a flashback may respond to such attempts aggressively or defensively, even striking out at the nurse. Ideally, the nurse asks the client how he or she responds to touch when dissociating or experiencing a flashback before one occurs; then the nurse knows if using touch is beneficial for that client. Also, the nurse may ask the client to touch the nurse's arm. If the client does so, then supportive touch is beneficial for this client.

Many clients have difficulty identifying or gauging the intensity of their emotions. They also may report that extreme emotions appear out of nowhere with no warning. The nurse can help clients to get in touch with their feelings by using a log or journal. Initially, clients may use a "feelings list" so they can select the feeling that most closely matches their experience. The nurse encourages the client to write down feelings throughout the day at specified intervals, for example, every 30 minutes. Once clients have identified their feelings, they can gauge the intensity of those feelings, for example, rating each feeling on a scale of 1 to 10. Using this process, clients have a greater awareness of their feelings and the different intensities; this step is important in managing and expressing those feelings.

After identifying feelings and their intensities, clients can begin to find triggers, or feelings that precede the flashbacks or dissociative episodes. Clients can then begin to use grounding techniques to diminish or avoid these episodes. They can use deep breathing and relaxation, focus on sensory information or stimuli in the environment, or engage in positive distractions until the feelings subside. Such distractions may include physical exercise, listening to music, talking to others, or engaging in a hobby or activity. Clients must find which distractions work for them; they should then write them down and keep the list and the necessary materials for the activities close at hand. When clients begin to experience intense feelings, they can look at the list and pick up a book, listen to a tape, or draw a picture, for instance.

HELPING TO PROMOTE THE CLIENT'S SELF-ESTEEM

Often it is useful to view the client as a **survivor** of trauma or abuse rather than as a victim. For these clients, who believe they are worthless and have no power over the situation, it helps to refocus their view of themselves from being victims to being survivors. Defining themselves as survivors allows them to see themselves as strong enough to survive their ordeal. It is a more empowering image than seeing oneself as a victim.

ESTABLISHING SOCIAL SUPPORT

The client needs to find support people or activities in the community. The nurse can help the client to prepare a list of support people. Problem-solving skills are difficult for these clients when under stress, so having a prepared list eliminates confusion or stress. This list should include a local crisis hotline to call when the client experiences self-harm thoughts or urges and friends or family to call when the client is feeling lonely or depressed. The client can also identify local activities or groups that provide a diversion and a chance to get out of the house. The client needs to establish community supports to reduce dependency on health care professionals.

Local support groups can be located by calling the county mental health services or the Department of Health and Human Services. A variety of support groups, both online and in person, can be found on the Internet.

Evaluation

Long-term treatment outcomes for clients who have survived trauma or abuse may take years to achieve. These clients

NURSING INTERVENTIONS

Promote Client's Safety

- Discuss self-harm thoughts.
- Help client develop plan for going to safe place when having destructive thoughts or impulses.

Help Client Cope with Stress and Emotions

- Use grounding techniques to help client who is dissociating or experiencing flashbacks.
- Validate client's feelings of fear, but try to increase contact with reality.
- During dissociative experience or flashback, help client change body position but do not grab or force client to stand up or move.
- Use supportive touch if client responds well to it.
- Teach deep breathing and relaxation techniques.
- Use distraction techniques such as participating in physical exercise, listening to music, talking with others, or engaging in a hobby or other enjoyable activity.
- Help to make a list of activities and keep materials on hand to engage client when client's feelings are intense.

Help Promote Client's Self-Esteem

- Refer to client as "survivor" rather than "victim."
- Establish social support system in community.
- Make a list of people and activities in the community for client to contact when he or she needs help.

usually make gradual progress in protecting themselves, learning to manage stress and emotions, and functioning in their daily lives. Although clients learn to manage their feelings and responses, the effects of trauma and abuse can be far-reaching and last a lifetime.

SELF-AWARENESS ISSUES

Nurses sometimes are reluctant to ask women about abuse, partly because they may believe some common myths about abuse. They may believe that questions about abuse will offend the client or fear that incorrect interventions will worsen the situation. Nurses may even believe that a woman who stays in an abusive relationship might deserve or enjoy the abuse or that abuse between husband and wife is private. Some nurses may believe abuse to be a societal or legal, not a health, problem.

Listening to stories of family violence or rape is difficult; the nurse may feel horror or revulsion. Because clients often watch for the nurse's reaction, containing these feelings and focusing on the client's needs are important. The nurse must be prepared to listen to the client's story, no matter how disturbing, and support and validate the client's feelings with comments such as "That must have been terrifying" or "Sounds like you were afraid for your life." The

nurse must convey acceptance and regard for the client as a person with worth and dignity regardless of the circumstances. These clients often have low self-esteem and guilt. They must learn to accept and face what has occurred. If the client believes that the nurse can accept him or her after hearing what has happened, he or she then may gain self-acceptance. Although this acceptance is often painful, it is essential to healing. The nurse must remember that he or she cannot fix or change things; the nurse's role is to listen and convey acceptance and support for the client.

Nurses with a personal history of abuse or trauma must seek professional assistance to deal with these issues before working with survivors of trauma or abuse. Such nurses can be very effective and supportive of other survivors but only after engaging in therapeutic work and accepting and understanding their own trauma.

Points to Consider When Working With Abused or Traumatized Clients

- These clients have many strengths they may not realize. The nurse can help them move from being victims to being survivors.
- Nurses should ask all women about abuse. Some will be offended and angry, but it is more important not to miss

(text continues on p. 210)

Nursing Care Plan *for a Client With PTSD*

Nursing Diagnosis

PTSD: *Sustained maladaptive response to a traumatic, overwhelming event.*

ASSESSMENT DATA

- Flashbacks or re-experiencing the traumatic event(s)
- Nightmares or recurrent dreams of the event or other trauma
- Sleep disturbances (e.g., insomnia, early awakening, crying out in sleep)
- Depression
- Denial of feelings or emotional numbness
- Projection of feelings
- Difficulty in expressing feelings
- Anger (may not be overt)
- Guilt or remorse
- Low self-esteem
- Frustration and irritability
- Anxiety, panic, or separation anxiety
- Fears—may be displaced or generalized (as in fear of men in rape victims)
- Decreased concentration
- Difficulty expressing love or empathy
- Difficulty experiencing pleasure
- Difficulty with interpersonal relationships, marital problems, divorce
- Abuse in relationships
- Sexual problems
- Substance use
- Employment problems
- Physical symptoms

EXPECTED OUTCOMES

Immediate
The client will
- Identify the traumatic event
- Demonstrate decreased physical symptoms
- Verbalize need to grieve loss(es)
- Establish an adequate balance of rest, sleep, and activity
- Demonstrate decreased anxiety, fear, guilt, and so forth
- Participate in treatment program

Stabilization
The client will
- Begin the grieving process
- Express feelings directly and openly in non-destructive ways
- Identify strengths and weaknesses realistically
- Demonstrate an increased ability to cope with stress
- Eliminate substance use
- Verbalize knowledge of illness, treatment plan, or safe use of medications, if any

Community
The client will
- Demonstrate initial integration of the traumatic experience into his or her life outside the hospital
- Identify support systems in the community
- Implement plans for follow-up or ongoing therapy, if indicated

IMPLEMENTATION

Nursing Interventions *denotes collaborative interventions

When you approach the client, be nonthreatening and professional.

Initially, assign the same staff members to the client if possible; try to respect the client's fears and feelings. Gradually increase the number and variety of staff members interacting with the client.

Rationale

The client's fears may be triggered by authority figures of other characteristics (e.g., gender, ethnicity).

Limiting the number of staff members who interact with the client at first will facilitate familiarity and trust. The client may have strong feelings of fear or mistrust about working with staff members with certain characteristics. These feelings may have been reinforced in previous encounters with professionals and may interfere with the therapeutic relationship.

continued ···▷

Nursing Care Plan: for a Client With PTSD, cont.

IMPLEMENTATION

Nursing Interventions *denotes collaborative interventions	**Rationale**
*Educate yourself and other staff members about the client's experience and about posttraumatic behavior.	Learning about the client's experience will help prepare you for the client's feelings and the details of his or her experience.
Examine and remain aware of your own feelings regarding both the client's traumatic experience and his or her feelings and behavior. Talk with other staff members to ventilate and work through your feelings.	Traumatic events engender strong feelings in others and may be quite threatening. You may be reminded of a related experience or of your own vulnerability, or issues related to sexuality, morality, safety, or well-being. It is essential that you remain aware of your feelings so that you do not unconsciously project feelings, avoid issues, or be otherwise nontherapeutic with the client.
Remain nonjudgmental in your interactions with the client.	It is important not to reinforce blame that the client may have internalized related to the experience.
Be consistent with the client; convey acceptance of him or her as a person while setting and maintaining limits regarding behaviors.	The client may test limits or the therapeutic relationship. Problems with acceptance, trust, or authority often occur with posttraumatic behavior.
*Assess the client's history of substance use (information from significant others might be helpful).	Client often use substances to help repress (or release) emotions.
Be aware of the client's use or abuse of substances. Set limits and consequences for this behavior; it may be helpful to allow the client or group to have input into these decisions.	Substance use undermines therapy and may endanger the client's health. Allowing input from the client or group may minimize power struggles.
*If substance use is a major problem, refer the client to a substance dependence treatment program.	Substance use must be dealt with because it may affect all other areas of the client's life.
Encourage the client to talk about his or her experience(s); be accepting and nonjudgmental of the client's accounts and perceptions.	Retelling the experience can help the client to identify the reality of what has happened and help to identify and work through related feelings.
Encourage the client to express his or her feelings through talking, writing, crying, or other ways in which the client is comfortable.	Identification and expression of feelings are central to the grieving process.
Especially encourage the expression of anger, guilt, and rage.	These feelings often occur in clients who have experienced trauma. The client may feel survivor's guilt that he or she survived when others did not or guilt about the behavior he or she undertook to survive (killing others in combat, enduring a rape, not saving others).
*Teach the client and the family or significant others about posttraumatic behavior and treatment.	Knowledge about posttraumatic behavior may help alleviate anxiety or guilt and may increase hope for recovery.
*As tolerated, encourage the client to share his or her feelings and experiences in group therapy, in a support group related to posttrauma, or with other clients informally.	The client needs to know that his or her feelings are acceptable to others and can be shared. Peer or support groups can offer understanding, support, and the opportunity for sharing experiences.
Give the client positive feedback for expressing feelings and sharing experiences. Remain nonjudgmental toward the client.	The client may feel that he or she is burdening others with his or her problems. It is important not to reinforce the client's internalized blame.

continued ⋯⇢

Nursing Care Plan: for a Client With PTSD, cont.

IMPLEMENTATION

Nursing Interventions *denotes collaborative interventions	Rationale
*If the client has a religious or spiritual orientation, referral to a member of the clergy or a chaplain may be appropriate.	Guilt and forgiveness often are religious or spiritual issues for the client.
Encourage the client to make realistic plans for the future, integrating his or her traumatic experience.	Integrating traumatic experiences and making future plans are important resolution steps in the grief process.
Help the client learn and practice stress management and relaxation techniques, assertiveness or self-defense training, or other skills as appropriate.	The client's traumatic experience may have resulted in a loss or decrease in self-confidence, sense of safety, or ability to deal with stress.
*Provide social skills and leisure time counseling, or refer the client to a recreational therapist as appropriate.	Social isolation and lack of interest in recreational activities are common problems following trauma.
*Talk with the client about employment, job-related stress, and so forth. Refer the client to vocational services as needed.	Problems with employment frequently occur in clients with posttraumatic behavior.
*Help the client arrange for follow-up therapy as needed.	Recovering from trauma may be a long-term process. Follow-up therapy can offer continuing support in the client's recovery.

Adapted from Schultz, J. M. & Videbeck, S. L. (2005). Lippincott's manual of psychiatric nursing care plans (7th ed.). Philadelphia: Lippincott Williams & Wilkins.

the opportunity of helping the woman who replies, "Yes. Can you help me?"

- The nurse should help the client focus on the present rather than dwell on horrific things in the past.
- Usually, a nurse works best with either the survivors of abuse or the abusers themselves. Most find it too difficult emotionally to work with both groups.

Critical Thinking Questions

1. Is spanking a child an acceptable form of discipline, or is it abusive? What determines the appropriateness of discipline? Who should make these decisions, and why?
2. How can the nurse continue to have a positive relationship with the client who returns to an abusive relationship? What should the nurse say to the client who has decided to return to an abusive relationship?
3. A client has just told the nurse that in the past he has lost his temper and has beaten his child. How should the nurse respond? What factors would affect the nurse's response?

KEY POINTS

- The U.S. Department of Health and Human Services has identified violence and abusive behavior as national health concerns.
- Women and children are the most likely victims of abuse and violence.
- Characteristics of violent families include an intergenerational transmission process, social isolation, power and control, and the use of alcohol and other drugs.
- Spousal abuse can be emotional, physical, sexual, or all three.
- Women have difficulty leaving abusive relationships because of financial and emotional dependence on the abusers and the risk for suffering increased violence or death.
- Nurses in various settings can uncover abuse by asking women about their safety in relationships. Many hospitals and clinics now ask women about safety issues as an integral part of the intake interview or health history.
- Rape is a crime of violence and humiliation through sexual means. Half of reported cases are perpetrated by someone the victim knows.

INTERNET 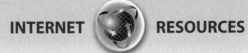 RESOURCES

RESOURCE*	INTERNET ADDRESS
Administration on Aging	http://www.aoa.dhhs.gov
American Bar Association Commission on Domestic Violence	http://www.abanet.org/domviol/home.html
American Medical Association	http://www.ama-assn.org
Centers for Disease Control and Prevention	http://www.cdc.gov
Domestic Violence Notepad: Resources for Victims	http://www.womenlawyers.com/domestic.htm
National Clearinghouse on Child Abuse and Neglect Information	http://nccanch.acf.hhs.gov
Trauma Anonymous (PTSD support group)	http://www.bein.com/trauma

*All of these Web sites have multiple links to other sites on the topic.

- Child abuse includes neglect and physical, emotional, and sexual abuse. It affects 3 million children in the United States.
- Elder abuse may include physical and sexual abuse, psychological abuse, neglect, exploitation, and medical abuse.
- Survivors of abuse and trauma often experience guilt and shame, low self-esteem, substance abuse, depression, PTSD, and dissociative disorders.
- PTSD is a response to a traumatic event. It can include flashbacks, nightmares, insomnia, mistrust, avoidance behaviors, and intense psychological distress.
- Dissociation is a defense mechanism that protects the emotional self from the full reality of abusive or traumatic events during and after those events.
- Dissociative disorders have the essential feature of disruption in the usually integrated functions of consciousness, memory, identity, and environmental perception. The four types are dissociative amnesia, dissociative fugue, dissociative identity disorder, and depersonalization disorder.
- Survivors of trauma and abuse may be admitted to the hospital for safety concerns or stabilization of intense symptoms such as flashbacks or dissociative episodes.
- The nurse can help the client to minimize dissociative episodes or flashbacks through grounding techniques and reality orientation.
- Important nursing interventions for survivors of abuse and trauma include protecting the client's safety, helping the client learn to manage stress and emotions, and working with the client to build a network of community support.
- Important self-awareness issues for the nurse include managing his or her own feelings and reactions about abuse, being willing to ask about abuse, and recognizing and dealing with any abuse issues he or she may have experienced personally.

REFERENCES

American Medical Association. (2004). Available: http://www.ama-assn.org/.

American Psychiatric Association. (2000). *Diagnostic and statistical manual of mental disorders* (4th ed., Text Revision). Washington, DC: American Psychiatric Association.

Bacchus, L., Mezey, G., & Bewley, S. (2006). A qualitative exploration of the nature of domestic violence in pregnancy. *Violence Against Women, 12*(6), 558–604.

Basile, K. C., Swahn, M. H., Chen, J., & Saltzman, L. E. (2006). Stalking in the United States: Recent national prevalence rates. *American Journal of Preventative Medicine, 31*(2), 172–175.

Bernet, W. (2005). Child maltreatment. In B. J. Sadock & V. A. Sadock (Eds.), *Comprehensive textbook of psychiatry* (Vol. 2, 8th ed., pp. 3412–3424). Philadelphia: Lippincott Williams & Wilkins.

Bureau of Justice Statistics. (2006). Available: http://www.ojp.usdoj.gov/bjs.

Centers for Disease Control and Prevention. (2004). Available: http://www.cdc.gov/cdc.html.

Dube, S. R., Anda, R. F., Whitfield, C. L., et al. (2005). Long-term consequences of childhood sexual abuse by gender of victim. *American Journal of Preventative Medicine, 28*(5), 430–438.

Goldstein, M. Z. (2005). Elder abuse, neglect, and exploitation. In B. J. Sadock & V. A. Sadock (Eds.), *Comprehensive textbook of psychiatry* (Vol. 2, 8th ed., pp. 3828–3834). Philadelphia: Lippincott Williams & Wilkins.

Koepsell, J. K., Kernic, M. K., & Holt, V. L. (2006). Factors that influence battered women to leave their abusive relationships. *Violence and Victims, 21*(2), 131–147.

Lipkins, S. (2006). *How parents, teachers, and coaches can stop the violence, harassment, and humiliation.* San Francisco: Guilford Press.

Marin Institute. Alcohol and violence. Retrieved December 31, 2006: http://www.marininstitute.org/print/alcohol_policy/violence.htm.

McCloskey, L. A., Lichter, E., Williams, C., et al. (2006). Assessing intimate partner violence in health care settings leads to women's receipt of interventions and improved health. *Public Health Reports, 121*(14), 435–444.

Middleton, W., Cromer, L. M., & Freyd, J. (2005). Remembering the past, anticipating a future. *Australasian Psychiatry 13*(3), 223–233.

Muehlbauer, M., & Crane, P. A. (2006). Elder abuse and neglect. *Journal of Psychosocial Nursing, 44*(11), 43–48.

National Institutes of Health. Child abuse and neglect. Retrieved December 15, 2006: http://www.nlm.nih.gov/medlineplus/childabuse.htm.

Piper, A., & Merskey, H. (2004). The persistence of folly: Critical examination of dissociative identity disorder. II. The defence and decline of multiple personality or dissociative identity disorder. *Canadian Journal of Psychiatry, 49*(10), 678–683.

Ryan, B. A. (2003). Do you suspect child abuse? *RN, 66*(9), 73–74, 76–79.

Schlenger, W. E., Caddell, J. M., Ebert, L., et al. (2002). Psychological reactions to terrorist attacks: Findings from the national study of Americans' reactions. *Journal of the American Medical Association, 288*(5), 581–588.

Skybo, T. (2005). Witnessing violence: Biopsychosocial impact on children. *Pediatric Nursing, 31*(4), 263–270.

State University of New York at Buffalo, Counseling Center. (2006) Available: http://ub-counseling.buffalo.edu/warnings.shtml.

Van Cleave, J., & Davis M. M. (2006). Bullying and peer victimization among children with special health care needs. *Pediatrics, 118*(4), e1212–1219.

van der Kolk, B. A. (2005). Physical and sexual abuse of adults. In B. J. Sadock & V. A. Sadock (Eds.), *Comprehensive textbook of psychiatry* (Vol. 2, 8th ed., pp. 2393–2398). Philadelphia: Lippincott Williams & Wilkins.

ADDITIONAL READINGS

Johnson, D. M., & Zlotnick, C. (2006). A cognitive-behavioral treatment for battered women with PTSD in shelters: Findings from a pilot study. *Journal of Traumatic Stress, 19*(4), 559–564.

Lyznicki, J. M., McCaffree, M. A., & Robonowitz, C. B. (2004). Childhood bullying: Implications for physicians. *American Family Physician, 70*(9), 1723–1728.

McCabe, M. P., & Wauchope, M. (2005). Behavioral characteristics of men accused of rape: Evidence for different types of rapists. *Archives of Sexual Behavior, 34*(2), 241–253.

Sheehan, K., Kim, L. E., & Galvin, J. P., Jr. (2004). Urban children's perceptions of violence. *Archives of Pediatric & Adolescent Medicine, 158*(1), 74–77.

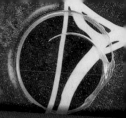

Chapter Study Guide

MULTIPLE-CHOICE QUESTIONS

Select the best answer for each of the following questions.

1. Which of the following is the best action for the nurse to take when assessing a child who might be abused?
   A. Confront the parents with the facts and ask them what happened.
   B. Consult with a professional member of the health team about making a report.
   C. Ask the child which of his parents caused this injury.
   D. Say or do nothing; the nurse has only suspicions, not evidence.

2. Which of the following interventions would be most helpful for a client with dissociative disorder having difficulty expressing feelings?
   A. Distraction
   B. Reality orientation
   C. Journaling
   D. Grounding techniques

3. Which of the following is true about touching a client who is experiencing a flashback?
   A. The nurse should stand in front of the client before touching.
   B. The nurse should never touch a client who is having a flashback.
   C. The nurse should touch the client only after receiving permission to do so.
   D. The nurse should touch the client to increase feelings of security.

4. Which of the following is true about domestic violence between same-sex partners?
   A. Such violence is less common than that between heterosexual partners.
   B. The frequency and intensity of violence are greater than between heterosexual partners.
   C. Rates of violence are about the same as between heterosexual partners.
   D. None of the above.

5. The nurse working with a client during a flashback says, "I know you're scared, but you're in a safe place. Do you see the bed in your room? Do you feel the chair you're sitting on?" The nurse is using which of the following techniques?
   A. Distraction
   B. Reality orientation
   C. Relaxation
   D. Grounding

6. Which of the following assessment findings might indicate elder self-neglect?
   A. Hesitancy to talk openly with nurse
   B. Inability to manage personal finances
   C. Missing valuables that are not misplaced
   D. Unusual explanations for injuries

7. Which type of child abuse can be most difficult to treat effectively?
   A. Emotional
   B. Neglect
   C. Physical
   D. Sexual

8. Women in battering relationships often remain in those relationships as a result of faulty or incorrect beliefs. Which of the following beliefs is valid?
   A. If she tried to leave, she would be at increased risk for violence.
   B. If she would do a better job of meeting his needs, the violence would stop.
   C. No one else would put up with her dependent clinging behavior.
   D. She often does things that provoke the violent episodes.

FILL-IN-THE-BLANK QUESTIONS

Identify the type of abuse described in the following situations.

_____   A parent does not see a doctor or give medicine to a 3-month-old with a fever of 103° F.

_____   An elderly woman's utilities are cut off for non-payment of bills, yet she has three uncashed Social Security checks in her possession.

_____   An adult daughter tells her elderly mother, "I'll send you to a nursing home if you don't give me your Social Security check!"

_____   A parent repeatedly tells a child, "You're stupid. You'll never amount to anything!"

SHORT-ANSWER QUESTIONS

Explain and give an example to illustrate each of the following concepts:

• Cycle of violence or abuse

• Blaming the victim of abuse or rape

• Survivor's guilt

• Intergenerational transmission process in violent families

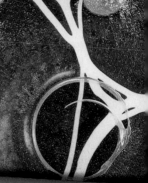

Chapter
12

Grief and Loss

Key Terms

- acculturation
- adaptive denial
- anticipatory grieving
- attachment behaviors
- attentive presence
- bereavement
- complicated grieving
- disenfranchised grief
- dysfunctional grieving
- grief
- grieving
- homeostasis
- mourning
- phase of disorganization and despair
- phase of numbing
- phase of reorganization
- phase of yearning and searching
- spirituality

Learning Objectives

After reading this chapter, you should be able to

1. Identify the types of losses for which people may grieve.
2. Discuss various theories related to understanding the grief process.
3. Describe the five dimensions of grieving.
4. Discuss universal and culturally specific mourning rituals.
5. Discuss disenfranchised grief and the vulnerability of nurses who experience it.
6. Identify factors that increase a person's susceptibility to complications related to grieving.
7. Discuss factors that are critical to integrating loss into life.
8. Apply the nursing process to facilitate grieving for clients and families.

Visit thePoint. http://thePoint.lww.com for
NCLEX-style questions, journal articles, and more!

Experiences of loss are normal and essential in human life. Letting go, relinquishing, and moving on are unavoidable passages as a person moves through the stages of growth and development. People frequently say goodbye to places, people, dreams, and familiar objects. Examples of necessary losses accompanying growth include abandoning a favorite blanket or toy, leaving a first-grade teacher, and giving up the adolescent hope of becoming a famous rock star. Loss allows a person to change, develop, and fulfill innate human potential. It may be planned, expected, or sudden. Although it can be difficult, loss sometimes is beneficial. Other times, it is devastating and debilitating.

Grief refers to the subjective emotions and affect that are a normal response to the experience of loss. **Grieving**, also known as **bereavement**, refers to the process by which a person experiences the grief. It involves not only the content (*what* a person thinks, says, and feels) but also the process (*how* a person thinks, says, and feels). All people grieve when they experience life's changes and losses. Often, grieving is one of the most difficult and challenging processes of human existence; rarely is it comfortable or pleasant. **Anticipatory grieving** is when people facing an imminent loss begin to grapple with the very real possibility of the loss or death in the near future (Ziemba & Lynch-Sauer, 2005). **Mourning** is the outward expression of grief. Rituals of mourning include having a wake, sitting Shiva, holding religious ceremonies, and arranging funerals.

This chapter examines the human experience of loss and the process by which a person moves through bereavement and integrates loss into his or her life. To support and care for the grieving client, the nurse must understand these phases as well as cultural responses to loss. At times, grief is the focus of treatment. The nursing process section outlines the nurse's role in grieving and gives guidelines for offering support and for teaching coping skills to clients. The chapter also outlines the importance of the nurse's self-awareness and competency in helping clients and families during bereavement.

TYPES OF LOSSES

A helpful way to examine different types of losses is to use Abraham Maslow's hierarchy of human needs. According to Maslow (1954), a hierarchy of needs motivates human actions. The hierarchy begins with physiologic needs (food, air, water, sleep), safety needs (a safe place to live and work), and security and belonging needs (satisfying relationships). The next set of needs includes self-esteem needs, which lead to feelings of adequacy and confidence. The last and final need is self-actualization, the ability to realize one's full innate potential. When these human needs are taken away or not met for some reason, a person experiences loss. Examples of losses related to specific human needs in Maslow's hierarchy are as follows:

- *Physiologic loss:* Examples include amputation of a limb, loss of adequate air exchange, or decrease in pancreatic functioning.

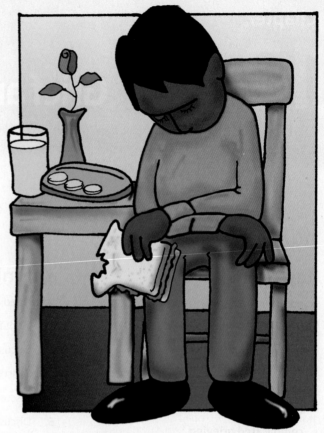

Grief

- *Safety loss:* Loss of a safe environment is evident in domestic or public violence. A person may perceive a breach of confidentiality in a professional relationship as a loss of psychological safety secondary to broken trust of self and the care provider.
- *Loss of security and a sense of belonging:* The loss of a loved one affects the need to love and be loved. Loss accompanies changes in relationships, such as birth, marriage, divorce, illness, and death; as the meaning of a relationship changes, a person may lose roles within a family or group.
- *Loss of self-esteem:* Any change in how a person is valued at work or in relationships can threaten his or her self-esteem needs. A change in self-perception can challenge sense of self-worth. A loss of role function and the self-perception and worth tied to that role may accompany the death of a loved one.
- *Loss related to self-actualization:* An external or internal crisis that blocks or inhibits strivings toward fulfillment may threaten personal goals and individual potential. A change in goals or direction will precipitate an inevitable period of grief as the person gives up a creative thought to make room for new ideas and directions. Examples include having to give up plans to attend graduate school or losing the hope of marriage and family.

The fulfillment of human needs requires dynamic movement throughout the various levels in the hierarchy. The simultaneous maintenance of needs in the areas of physiologic integrity, safety, security and sense of belonging, self-esteem, and self-actualization is challenging and demands flexibility and focus. At times, a focus on protection may take priority over professional or self-actualization goals. Likewise, human losses demand a grieving process that simultaneously challenges each level of need. Specific examples include the loss of a pregnancy or loss of sight or hearing.

THE GRIEVING PROCESS

Nurses interact with clients responding to myriad losses along the continuum of health and illness. Regardless of the type of loss, nurses must have a basic understanding of what is involved to meet the challenge that grief brings to clients. By understanding the phenomena that clients experience as they deal with the discomfort of loss, nurses may promote the expression and release of emotional as well as physical pain during grieving. Supporting this process means ministering to psychological—and physical—needs.

The therapeutic relationship and therapeutic communication skills such as active listening are paramount when assisting grieving clients (see Chapters 5 and 6). Recognizing the verbal and nonverbal communication content of the various stages of grieving can help nurses to select interventions that meet the client's psychological and physical needs.

Theories of the Grieving Process

KUBLER-ROSS'S STAGES OF GRIEVING

Elisabeth Kubler-Ross (1969) established a basis for understanding how loss affects human life. As she attended to clients with terminal illnesses, a process of dying became apparent to her. Through her observations and work with dying clients and their families, Kubler-Ross developed a model of five stages to explain what people experience as they grieve and mourn:

1. *Denial* is shock and disbelief regarding the loss.
2. *Anger* may be expressed toward God, relatives, friends, or health care providers.
3. *Bargaining* occurs when the person asks God or fate for more time to delay the inevitable loss.
4. *Depression* results when awareness of the loss becomes acute.
5. *Acceptance* occurs when the person shows evidence of coming to terms with death.

This model became a prototype for care providers as they looked for ways to understand and assist their clients in the grieving process.

BOWLBY'S THEORY OF ATTACHMENT BEHAVIORS

John Bowlby, a British psychoanalyst, proposed a theory that humans instinctively attain and retain affectional bonds with significant others through **attachment behaviors.** These attachment behaviors are crucial to the development of a sense of security and survival. Examples of attachment behaviors include following, clinging, calling out, and crying. Bowlby saw that human beings modified these attachment behaviors as they matured from childhood into adulthood, but he also noticed that patterns of attachment behavior formed early in life endure throughout the life cycle. People experience the most intense emotions when *forming* a bond such as falling in love, *maintaining* a bond such as loving someone, *disrupting* a bond such as in a divorce, and *renewing* an attachment such as resolving a conflict or renewing a relationship (Bowlby, 1980).

An attachment that is maintained is a source of security; an attachment that is renewed is a source of joy. When a bond is threatened or broken, however, the person responds with anxiety, protest, and anger. Actual loss leads to sorrow. According to Bowlby, these emotions reflect affectional bonds. Loss strongly activates or arouses attachment behaviors. Thus, the clinical picture of increased anxiety, sorrow, anger, looking for the lost person or object, calling out, crying, and protesting is an attempt to restore the lost affectional bond.

PHASES OF THE GRIEVING PROCESS

Although other theories are described, Bowlby's understanding of grieving serves as the predominant framework for this chapter. Bowlby described the grieving process as having four phases:

1. Experiencing numbness and denying the loss
2. Emotionally yearning for the lost loved one and protesting the permanence of the loss
3. Experiencing cognitive disorganization and emotional despair with difficulty functioning in the everyday world
4. Reorganizing and reintegrating the sense of self to pull life back together

Another theorist, John Harvey (1998), described similar phases of grieving:

1. Shock, outcry, and denial
2. Intrusion of thoughts, distractions, and obsessive review of the loss
3. Confiding in others as a way to emote and to cognitively restructure an account of the loss

Rodebaugh and colleagues (1999) viewed the process of grief as a journey through four stages:

1. *Reeling:* The person feels shock, disbelief, or denial.
2. *Feeling:* The person experiences anguish, guilt, profound sadness, anger, lack of concentration, sleep disturbances, appetite changes, fatigue, and general physical discomfort.

3. *Dealing*: The person begins to adapt to the loss by engaging in support groups, grief therapy, reading, and spiritual guidance.
4. *Healing*: The person integrates the loss as part of life. Acute anguish lessens. Healing does not imply, however, that the person has forgotten or accepted the loss.

Table 12.1 compares the theories of grieving.

Nurses should not expect all clients to follow predictable steps in the grieving process. Indeed, such an expectation may put added pressure or stress on a client when he or she most needs acceptance, reflection, and support from care providers. Interventions that nurses can use to facilitate the grieving process are discussed later in this chapter.

Tasks of the Grieving Process

Rando (1984) described tasks inherent to grieving:
- Undoing psychosocial bonds to the loved one and eventually creating new ties
- Adding new roles, skills, and behaviors and revising old ones into a "new identity and sense of self"
- Pursuing a healthy lifestyle that includes people and activities
- Integrating the loss into life, which does not mean ending the grieving but accommodating the reality of the loss

The accompanying *Clinical Vignette: Grief* gives an example of integrating loss into life. Margaret has come to view James's death and the painful period of grief as a profound and poignant "search for meaning in life." The sense of his presence remains with her as she pursues her life without him, and she often pictures him before he became ill. Viewing the grieving process more positively, she believes that his death in some way has encouraged her to become more independent and to participate in new opportunities.

DIMENSIONS OF GRIEVING

People have many and varied responses to loss. They express their bereavement in their thoughts, words, feelings, and actions as well as through their physiologic responses. Therefore, nurses must use a holistic model of grieving that encompasses cognitive, emotional, spiritual, behavioral, and physiologic dimensions (Lobb et al., 2006).

Cognitive Responses to Grief

In some respects, the pain that accompanies grieving results from a disturbance in the person's beliefs. The loss disrupts, if not shatters, basic assumptions about life's meaning and purpose. Grieving often causes a person to change beliefs about self and the world, such as perceptions of the world's benevolence, the meaning of life as related to justice, and a sense of destiny or life path. Other changes in thinking and attitude include reviewing and ranking val-

Table 12.1	THEORETICAL UNDERSTANDING OF THE GRIEVING PROCESS			
Theorist/Clinician	Phase I	Phase II	Phase III	Phase IV
Kubler-Ross (1969)	Stage I: denial	Stage II: anger Stage III: bargaining	Stage IV: depression	Stage V: acceptance
Bowlby (1980)	Numbness; denial	Emotional yearning for the loved one; protesting permanence of the loss	Cognitive disorganization; emotional despair; difficulty functioning	Cognitive reorganization; reintegrating sense of self
Harvey (1998)	Shock; outcry; denial	Intrusion of thoughts, distractions; obsessive reviewing of the loss	Confiding in others to emote and to cognitively restructure account of loss	
Rodebaugh, Schwindt, & Valentine (1999)	Reeling: shock, disbelief, or denial	Feeling: anguish, guilt, sadness, anger, lack of concentration, sleep disturbances, appetite changes, fatigue, general discomfort	Dealing: adapting to the loss	Healing: integration of loss; acute anguish dissipated; loss may or may not be forgotten or accepted

CLINICAL VIGNETTE: GRIEF

"If I had known what the grief process was like, I would never have married, or I would have prayed every day of my married life that I would be the first to die," reflects Margaret, 9 years after the death of her husband.

She recalls her initial thought, denying and acknowledging reality simultaneously, when James was diagnosed with multiple myeloma in October 1987: "It's a mistake . . . but I know it isn't."

For 2½ years, Margaret and James diligently followed his regimen of treatment while taking time for work and play, making the most of their life together in the moment. "We were not melodramatic people. We told ourselves, 'This is what's happening; we'll deal with it.'"

For Margaret, it was a shock to realize that some friends who had been so readily present for social gatherings were no longer available. She waited alone in the wee hours of the night when James had emergency surgery. Again, she was shocked when she told a priest who came into the room, "My husband is having surgery," and his reply was "Oh, sorry to bother you; I'm looking for the paper."

Margaret began to undergo a shift in her thinking: "You begin to evaluate your perceptions of others. I asked myself, 'Who is there for me?' Friends, *are* they *really*? It can be painful to find out they really aren't. It frees you later, though. You can let them go."

When James died, Margaret remained "level-headed and composed" until one day shortly after the funeral when she suddenly became aware of her exhaustion. While shopping, she found herself in protest of the emotional pain and wanting to shout, "Doesn't anybody know that I have just lost my husband?"

Surprised with how overwhelmed she felt, one of her hardest moments was putting her sister on the plane and going home to "an empty house." It was at this time that she began to feel the initial shock of her loss. Her body felt like it was "wired with electricity." She felt as though she was "just going through the motions," doing routine chores like grocery shopping and putting gas in the car, all the while feeling numb.

Crying spells lasted 6 months. She became "tired of mourning" and would ask herself, "When is this going to be relieved?" She also felt anger. "I was upset with James, wondering why he didn't go for his complete physical. Maybe James's death might not have happened so soon."

After a few months and well into the grief process, Margaret knew she needed to "do something constructive." She did. She attended support groups, traveled, and became involved with church activities.

Her faith in God was a plus. Exercising this faith, she trusted that eventually her emotions would catch up with the intellectual understanding of all that had transpired in James's dying. She developed an "inner knowing that God is all-seeing, all-knowing." This belief gave her spiritual strength and empowered her as she grieved.

Nearly a decade after James's death, Margaret views the grief process as a profound and poignant "search for meaning in life. If he had not gone, I would not have come to where I am in life. I am content, confident, and happy with how authentic life is."

Even so, a sense of James's presence remains with her as she pictures the way he was before he became ill. She states, "This is good for me."

---

ues, becoming wiser, shedding illusions about immortality, viewing the world more realistically, and reevaluating religious or spiritual beliefs (Zisook & Zisook, 2005).

QUESTIONING AND TRYING TO MAKE SENSE OF THE LOSS

The grieving person needs to make sense of the loss. He or she undergoes self-examination and questions accepted ways of thinking. The loss challenges old assumptions about life. For example, when a loved one dies prematurely, the grieving person often questions the belief that "life is fair" or that "one has control over life or destiny." He or she searches for answers to why the trauma occurred. The goal of the search is to give meaning and purpose to the loss. The nurse might hear the following questions:

- "Why did this have to happen? He took such good care of himself!"
- "Why did such a young person have to die?"

- "He was such a good person! Why did this happen to him?"

Questioning may help the person accept the reality of why someone died. For example, perhaps the death is related to the person's health practices—maybe he did not take good care of himself and have regular checkups. Questioning may result in realizing that loss and death are realities that everyone must face one day. Others may discover explanations and meaning and even gain comfort from a religious or spiritual perspective such as believing that the dead person is with God and at peace (Neimeyer et al., 2006).

ATTEMPTING TO KEEP THE LOST ONE PRESENT

Belief in an afterlife and the idea that the lost one has become a personal guide are cognitive responses that serve to keep the lost one present. Carrying on an internal dialogue with the loved one while doing an activity is an example: "John,

I wonder what you would do in this situation. I wish you were here to show me. Let's see, I think you would probably. . . ." This method of keeping the lost one present helps soften the effects of the loss while assimilating its reality.

Emotional Responses to Grief

Anger, sadness, and anxiety are the predominant emotional responses to loss. The grieving person may direct anger and resentment toward the dead person and his or her health practices, family members, or health care providers or institutions. Common reactions the nurse might hear are as follows:

- "He should have stopped smoking years ago."
- "If I had taken her to the doctor earlier, this might not have happened."
- "It took you too long to diagnose his illness."

Guilt over things not done or said in the lost relationship is another painful emotion. Feelings of hatred and revenge are common when death has resulted from extreme circumstances such as suicide, murder, or war (Zisook & Zisook, 2005). In addition to despair and anger, some people may also experience feelings of loss of control in their lives, uncharacteristic feelings of dependency on others, and even anxiety about their own death.

Emotional responses are evident in all phases of Bowlby's grief process. During the **phase of numbing**, the common first response to the news of a loss is to be stunned, as though not perceiving reality. Emotions vacillate in frequency and intensity. Contrasting emotions are common, such as experiencing an impulsive outburst of anger toward the deceased, oneself, or others at one moment and then feeling unexpected elation at a sense of union with the deceased the next (Bowlby, 1980). The person may function automatically in a state of calm and then suddenly become overwhelmed with panic. In the clinical vignette, Margaret discusses having felt "numbness" while going through routine functions immediately after her husband's death and then one day finding herself in a department store overwhelmed with frustration and wanting to shout, "Doesn't anyone realize I've just lost my husband?"

In the second **phase of yearning and searching**, reality begins to set in. The grieving person exhibits anger, profound sorrow, and crying. He or she often reverts to the attachment behaviors of childhood by acting similar to a child who loses his or her mother in a store or park. The grieving person may express irritability, bitterness, and hostility toward clergy, medical providers, relatives, comforters, and even the dead person. The hopeless yet intense desire to restore the bond with the lost person compels the bereaved to search for and recover him or her. The grieving person interprets sounds, sights, and smells associated with the lost one as signs of the deceased's presence, which may intermittently provide comfort and ignite hope for a reunion. For example, the ring of the telephone at a time in the day when the deceased regularly called will trigger the excitement of hearing his or her voice. Or the scent of the deceased's perfume will spur her late husband to scan the room for her smiling face. As hopes for the lost one's return diminish, sadness and loneliness become constant.

In the vignette, Margaret became angry with her husband for not having his physical examination sooner and upset with friends who seemed to disappear after James became critically ill. Such emotional tumult may last several months and seems necessary for the person to begin to acknowledge the true permanence of the loss.

During the **phase of disorganization and despair**, the bereaved person begins to understand the loss's permanence. He or she recognizes that patterns of thinking, feeling, and acting attached to life with the deceased must change. As the person relinquishes all hope of recovering the lost one, he or she inevitably experiences moments of depression, apathy, or despair. Night is a time of acute loneliness during this phase.

In the final phase, the **phase of reorganization**, the bereaved person begins to reestablish a sense of personal identity, direction, and purpose for living. He or she gains independence and confidence (Bowlby, 1980). By experimenting with and accomplishing newly defined roles and functions, the bereaved becomes personally empowered. This emotional and affective experience is associated closely with the inherent cognitive recognition that life without the loved one is a reality and therefore must be different. In this phase, the person still misses the deceased, but thinking of him or her no longer evokes painful feelings. In the vignette, hearing Spanish music, which Margaret associated with James's love and her sense of being loved, was unbearable for many months. Spanish music now inspires warm memories of their love for each other and comforts Margaret.

Spiritual Responses to Grief

Closely associated with the cognitive and emotional dimensions of grief are the deeply embedded personal values that give meaning and purpose to life. These values and the belief systems that sustain them are central components of **spirituality** and the spiritual response to grief. During loss, it is within the spiritual dimension of human experience that a person may be most comforted, challenged, or devastated. The grieving person may become disillusioned and angry with God or other religious figures such as the priest who, in Margaret's situation, seemed more concerned about getting a paper than being aware of her loneliness in the waiting room. The anguish of abandonment, loss of hope, or loss of meaning can cause deep spiritual suffering.

Ministering to the spiritual needs of those grieving is an essential aspect of nursing care. The client's emotional and spiritual responses become intertwined as he or she grapples with pain. With an astute awareness of such suffering, nurses can promote a sense of well-being. Providing opportunities for clients to share their suffering assists in the psychological and spiritual transformation that can evolve through grieving. Finding explanations and meaning through religious or spiritual beliefs, the client may begin to identify positive aspects of grieving. The grieving person also can experience loss as significant to his or her own growth and development. In the vignette, although Margaret was "disillusioned" with aspects of her religious support system, she eventually finds much comfort, hope, and strength in her spiritual beliefs. She begins to see that her husband's death gave her life new direction and empowered her to act in new ways. She states, "If he hadn't gone, I wouldn't be the person I am today. I'm very content and peaceful about who I am and what I am doing." Through her volunteer work, she comforts others who have terminal illness.

Behavioral Responses to Grief

Behavioral responses to grief are often the easiest to observe. By recognizing behaviors common to grieving, the nurse can provide supportive guidance for the client's journey of emotionally and cognitively rough terrain. To promote the process, the nurse must provide a context of acceptance in which the client can explore his or her behavior. For example, observing the grieving person as functioning "automatically" or routinely without much thought can indicate that the person is in the phase of numbness—the reality of the loss has not set in. Tearfully sobbing, crying uncontrollably, showing great restlessness, and searching are evidence of yearning and seeking. The person actually may call out for the deceased or visually scan the room for him or her. Irritability and hostility toward others reveal anger and frustration in the process. Seeking out as well as avoiding places or activities once shared with the deceased, and keeping or wanting to discard valuables and belongings of the deceased, illustrate fluctuating emotions and perceptions of hope for a reconnection.

During the phase of disorganization, the cognitive act of redefining self-identity is essential but difficult. Although superficial at first, efforts made in social or work activities are behavioral means to support the person's cognitive and emotional shifts. Drug or alcohol abuse indicates a maladaptive behavioral response to the emotional and spiritual despair. Suicide and homicide attempts may be extreme responses if the bereaved person cannot move through the grieving process.

In the phase of reorganization, the bereaved person participates in activities and reflection that are personally meaningful and satisfying. After finding creative outlets and building her personal growth, Margaret states, "I'm happy with who I am and what I do. My life is more authentic."

Physiologic Responses to Grief

Physiologic symptoms and problems associated with grief responses are often a source of anxiety and concern for the grieving person as well as for friends or caregivers. Those grieving may complain of insomnia, headaches, impaired

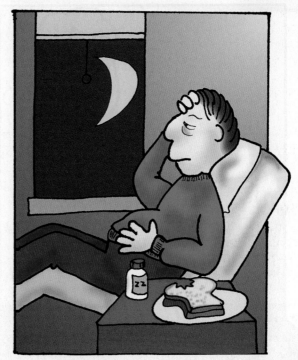

Physiologic symptoms

appetite, weight loss, lack of energy, palpitations, indigestion, and changes in the immune and endocrine systems. Sleep disturbances are among the most frequent and persistent bereavement-associated symptoms (Zisook & Zisook, 2005).

CULTURAL CONSIDERATIONS

Universal Reactions to Loss

Although all people grieve for lost loved ones, rituals and habits surrounding death vary among cultures. Each culture defines the context in which grieving, mourning, and integrating loss into life are given meaningful expression. The context for expression is consistent with beliefs about life, death, and an afterlife. Certain aspects of the experience are more important than other aspects for each culture (Kemp, 2005; Ng, 2005).

Universal reactions include the initial response of shock and social disorientation, attempts to continue a relationship with the deceased, anger with those perceived as responsible for the death, and a time for mourning. Each culture, however, defines specific acceptable ways to exhibit shock and sadness, display anger, and mourn (Bowlby, 1980). Cultural awareness of rituals for mourning can help nurses understand an individual's or a family's behavior.

Culture-Specific Rituals

As people immigrate to the United States and Canada, they may lose rich ethnic and cultural roots during the adjustment of **acculturation** (altering cultural values or behaviors

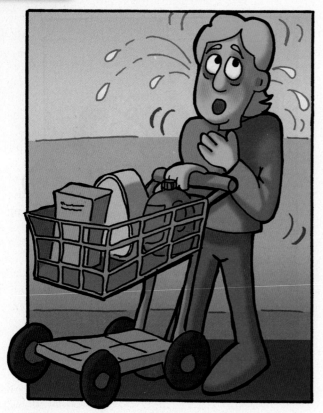

Panic attack

as a way to adapt to another culture). For example, funeral directors may discourage specific rites of passage that celebrate or mourn the loss of loved ones, or they may be reluctant to allow behavioral expressions they perceive as disruptive. Many such expressions are culturally related, and health care providers must be aware of such instances. For example, the Hmong (people of a mountainous region of Southeast Asia) believe that the deceased person enters the next world appearing as she or he did at the time of death. This may lead to a request for removal of needles, tubes, or other "foreign objects" before death.

Because cultural bereavement rituals have roots in several of the world's major religions (i.e., Buddhism, Christianity, Hinduism, Islam, Judaism), religious or spiritual beliefs and practices regarding death frequently guide the client's mourning. In the United States, various mourning rituals and practices exist. A few of the major ones are summarized next.

AFRICAN AMERICANS

Most ancestors of today's African Americans came to the United States as slaves and lived under the influence of European-American and Christian religious practices. Therefore, many mourning rituals are tied to religious traditions. In Catholic and Episcopalian services, hymns may be sung, poetry read, and a eulogy spoken; less formal Baptist and Holiness traditions may involve singing, speaking in tongues, and liturgical dancing. Typically, the deceased is viewed in church before being buried in a cemetery. Mourning also may be expressed through public prayers, black clothing, and decreased social activities. The mourning period may last a few weeks to several years.

MUSLIM AMERICANS

Islam does not permit cremation. It is important to follow the five steps of the burial procedure, which specify washing, dressing, and positioning of the body. The first step is traditional washing of the body by a Muslim of the same gender (Yasien-Esmael & Rubin, 2005).

HAITIAN AMERICANS

Some Haitian Americans practice *vodun* (voodoo), also called "root medicine." Derived from Roman Catholic rituals and cultural practices of western Africa (Benin and Togo) and Sudan, vodun is the practice of calling on a group of spirits with whom one periodically makes peace during specific events in life. The death of a loved one may be such a time. This practice can be found in several states (Alabama, Louisiana, Florida, North Carolina, South Carolina, and Virginia) and in some communities within New York City.

CHINESE AMERICANS

The largest Asian population in the United States, the Chinese have strict norms for announcing death, preparing the body, arranging the funeral and burial, and mourning after burial. Burning incense and reading scripture are ways to assist the spirit of the deceased in the afterlife journey. If the deceased and family are Buddhists, meditating before a shrine in the room is important. For 1 year after death, the family may place bowls of food on a table for the spirit.

JAPANESE AMERICANS

Buddhist Japanese Americans view death as a life passage. Close family members may bathe the deceased with warm water and dress the body in a white kimono after purification rites. For 2 days, family and friends bearing gifts may visit or offer money for the deceased while saying prayers and burning incense.

FILIPINO AMERICANS

Most Filipino Americans are Catholic, and, depending on how close one was to the deceased, wearing black clothing or armbands is customary during mourning. Family and friends place wreaths on the casket and drape a broad black cloth on the home of the deceased. Family members commonly place announcements in local newspapers asking for prayers and blessings on the soul of the deceased.

VIETNAMESE AMERICANS

Vietnamese Americans are predominately Buddhists, who bathe the deceased and dress him or her in black clothes. They may put a few grains of rice in the mouth and place money with the deceased so that he or she can buy a drink as the spirit moves on in the afterlife. The body may be displayed for viewing in the home before burial. When friends enter, music is played as a way to warn the deceased of the arrival.

HISPANIC AMERICANS

Hispanic or Latino Americans have their origins in Spain, Mexico, Cuba, Puerto Rico, and the Dominican Republic. They are predominately Roman Catholic. They may pray for the soul of the deceased during a novena (9-day devotion) and a rosary (devotional prayer). They manifest *luto* (mourning) by wearing black or black and white while keeping a subdued manner. Respect for the deceased may include not watching TV, going to the movies, listening to the radio, or attending dances or other social events for some time. Friends and relatives bring flowers and crosses to decorate the grave.

Guatemalan Americans may include a marimba band in the funeral procession and services. Lighting candles and blessing the deceased during a wake in the home are common practices.

NATIVE AMERICANS

Ancient beliefs and practices influence the more than 500 Native American tribes in the United States even though many are now Christian. A tribe's medicine man or priestly healer, who assists the friends and family of the deceased to regain their spiritual equilibrium, is an essential spiritual guide. Ceremonies of baptism for the spirit of the deceased seem to help ward off depression of the bereaved. Perceptions about the meaning of death and its effects on family and friends are as varied as the number of tribal communities.

Death may be viewed as a state of unconditional love in which the spirit of the deceased remains present, comforts the tribe, and encourages movement toward life's purpose of being happy and living in harmony with nature and others. Belief in and fear of ghosts and believing death signifies the end of all that is good are other views. Yet another view is the belief in a happy afterlife called the "land of the spirits"; proper mourning is essential not only for the soul of the deceased but also for the protection of community members. To designate the end of mourning, a ceremony at the burial grounds is held during which the grave is covered with a blanket or cloth for making clothes. Later, the cloth is given to a tribe member. A dinner during which singing, speech-making, and money is given away completes the ceremony.

ORTHODOX JEWISH AMERICANS

An Orthodox Jewish custom is for a relative to stay with a dying person so that the soul does not leave the body while the person is alone. To leave the body alone after death is disrespectful. The family of the deceased may request to cover the body with a sheet. The eyes of the deceased should be closed, and the body should remain covered and untouched until family, a rabbi, or a Jewish undertaker can begin rites. Although organ donation is permitted, autopsy is not; burial must occur within 24 hours unless delayed by the Sabbath (Weinstein, 2003).

Nurse's Role

The diverse cultural environment of the United States offers the sensitive nurse many opportunities to individualize care when working with grieving clients. In extended families, varying expressions and responses to loss can exist depending on the degree of acculturation to the dominant culture of society. Rather than assuming that he or she understands a particular culture's grieving behaviors, the nurse must encourage clients to discover and use what is effective and meaningful for them. For example, the nurse could ask a Hispanic or Latino client who also is a practicing Catholic if he or she would like to pray for the deceased. If an Orthodox Jew has just died, the nurse could offer to stay with the body while the client notifies relatives.

As the insensitive or inflexible pressures of acculturation have caused people to lose, minimize, or modify specific culture-related rituals, they have consciously put others aside. Many Americans, however, have experienced a renewed and deepened awareness for meaningful mourning through ritual. An example of such awareness is the creation of the AIDS quilt. The planting of a flag in the chaotic debris at Ground Zero during the immediate aftermath of the terrorist attack on the World Trade Center in September 2001 signaled the beginnings of such a ritual. As bodies were recovered and removed, the caring diligence and attentive presence of those facilitating their transport continued this meaningful rite of passage. Through the media, the United States and much of the world became companions in grief. In April 2000, a memorial was dedicated for the 168 persons who died in the bombing of the Alfred P. Murrah Federal Building in Oklahoma City. During the ceremony, a police chaplain delivered a message to grieving family and friends to "live in the present, dream of the future." Memorials and public services play an important role in the healing process.

DISENFRANCHISED GRIEF

Disenfranchised grief is grief over a loss that is not or cannot be acknowledged openly, mourned publicly, or supported socially. Three categories of circumstances can result in disenfranchised grief:

• A relationship has no legitimacy.
• The loss itself is not recognized.
• The griever is not recognized.

In each situation, there was an attachment followed by a loss that leads to grief. The grief process is more complex because the usual supports that facilitate grieving and healing are absent (Schultz & Videbeck, 2005).

In our culture, kin-based relationships receive the most attention in cases of death. Relationships between lovers, friends, neighbors, foster parents, colleagues, and caregivers may be long-lasting and intense, but people suffering loss in these relationships may not be able to mourn publicly with the social support and recognition given to family members. In addition, some relationships are not always recognized publicly or sanctioned socially. Possible examples include same-sex relationships (Smolinski & Colon, 2006), cohabitation without marriage, and extramarital affairs.

Other losses are not recognized or seen as socially significant; thus, accompanying grief is not legitimized, expected, or supported. Examples in this category include prenatal death, abortion, relinquishing a child for adoption, death of a pet (Kaufman & Kaufman, 2006), or other losses not involving death, such as job loss, separation, divorce, and children leaving home. Though these losses can lead to intense grief for the bereaved, other people may perceive them as minor (Schultz & Videbeck, 2005).

Some people who experience a loss may not be recognized or fully supported as grievers. For example, older adults and children experience limited social recognition for their losses and the need to mourn. As people grow older, they "should expect" others their age to die. Adults sometimes view children as "not understanding or comprehending" the loss and may assume wrongly that their children's grief is minimal. Children may experience the loss of a "nurturing parental figure" from death, divorce, or family dysfunction such as alcoholism or abuse. These losses are very significant, yet they may not be recognized.

Nurses may experience disenfranchised grief when their need to grieve is not recognized. For example, nurses who work in areas involving organ donation or transplantation are involved intimately with the death of clients who may donate organs to another person. The daily intensity of relationships between nurses and clients/families creates strong bonds among them. The emotional effects of loss are significant for these nurses; however, there is seldom a socially ordained place or time to grieve. The solitude in which the grieving occurs usually provides little or no comfort (Doka, 2006).

COMPLICATED GRIEVING

Some believe **complicated grieving** to be a response outside the norm, occurring when a person is void of emotion, grieves for prolonged periods, or has expressions of grief that seem disproportionate to the event. People may suppress emotional responses to the loss or become obsessively preoccupied with the deceased person or lost object. Others actually may suffer from clinical depression when they cannot make progress in the grief process (Zhang et al., 2006). Figure 12.1 depicts an overview of complicated grieving.

Previously existing psychiatric disorders also may complicate the grief process, so nurses must be particularly alert to clients with psychiatric disorders who also are grieving. Grief can precipitate major depression in a person with a history of the disorder. These clients also can experience

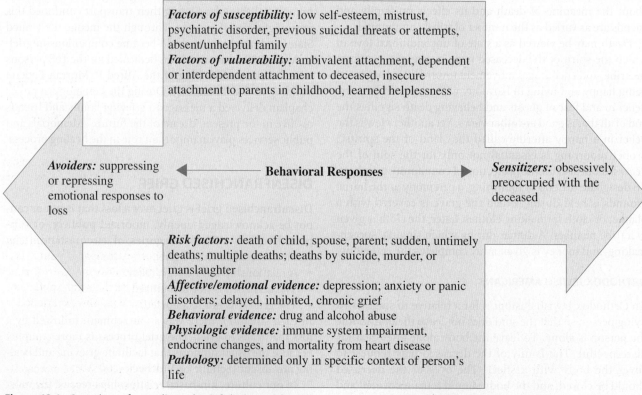

Figure 12.1. Overview of complicated grief. (Adapted from Groot et al., 2006; Zhang et al., 2006; Zisook & Zisook, 2005.)

grief and a sense of loss when they encounter changes in treatment settings, routine, environment, or even staff.

Although nurses must recognize that complications may arise in the grief process, the process remains unique and dynamic for each person. Immense variety exists in terms of the cultural determinants in communicating the experience and the individual differences in emotional reactions, depth of pain, and time needed to acknowledge and grasp the personal meaning or assimilate the loss. Box 12.1 discusses styles of grieving.

Characteristics of Susceptibility

For some, the effects of grief are particularly devastating because their personalities, emotional states, or situations make them susceptible to complications during the process. People who are vulnerable to complicated grieving include those with the following characteristics:

- Low self-esteem
- Low trust in others
- A previous psychiatric disorder
- Previous suicide threats or attempts
- Absent or unhelpful family members
- An ambivalent, dependent, or insecure attachment to the deceased person
  - In an *ambivalent attachment,* at least one partner is unclear about how the couple loves or does not love each other. For example, when a woman is uncertain about and feels pressure from others to have an abortion, she is experiencing ambivalence about her unborn child.

Box 12.1   STYLES OF GRIEVING

When determining whether a person may be experiencing a complicated grieving process, the nurse should consider viewing the person's behavior as a unique style of grieving. Silver and Wortman (1980) suggested three styles of grieving:

- The bereaved vacillates from high to low distress over time.
- The bereaved shows no distress either as an immediate response to loss or subsequently.
- The bereaved remains in a high state of distress for a period beyond what others would consider appropriate.

Silver, R. L., & Wortman, C. B. (1980). Coping with undesirable life events. In J. Garber & M. E. P. Seligman (Eds.), Human helplessness: Theory and applications (pp. 279–340). New York: Academic Press.

- In a *dependent attachment,* one partner relies on the other to provide for his or her needs without necessarily meeting the partner's needs.
- An *insecure attachment* usually forms during childhood, especially if a child has learned fear and helplessness (i.e., through intimidation, abuse, or control by parents).

A person's perception is another factor contributing to vulnerability: Perception, or how a person thinks or feels about a situation, is not always reality. After the death of a loved one, a person may believe that he or she really cannot continue and is at a great disadvantage. He or she may become increasingly sad and depressed, not eat or sleep, and perhaps entertain suicidal thoughts.

Risk Factors Leading to Vulnerability

Zhang, El-Jawahri, and Prigerson (2006) and Zisook and Zisook (2005) identified experiences that increase the risk for complicated grieving for the vulnerable parties previously mentioned. These experiences are related to trauma or individual perceptions of vulnerability and include the following:

- Death of a spouse or child
- Death of a parent (particularly in early childhood or adolescence)
- Sudden, unexpected, and untimely death
- Multiple deaths
- Death by suicide or murder

Based on the experiences previously identified, those most intimately affected by the terrorist attacks on September 11, 2001 could be considered at increased risk for complicated grieving.

Complicated Grieving as a Unique and Varied Experience

The person with complicated grieving also can experience physiologic and emotional reactions. Physical reactions can include an impaired immune system, increased adrenocortical activity, increased levels of serum prolactin and growth hormone, psychosomatic disorders, and increased mortality from heart disease. Characteristic emotional responses include depression, anxiety or panic disorders, delayed or inhibited grief, and chronic grief (Zisook & Zisook, 2005).

Because the grieving process is unique to each person, the nurse must assess the degree of impairment within the context of the client's life and experiences—for example, by examining current coping responses compared with previous experiences and assessing whether or not the client is engaging in maladaptive behaviors such as drug and alcohol abuse as a means to deal with the painful experience.

APPLICATION OF THE NURSING PROCESS

Because the strong emotional attachment created in a significant relationship is not released easily, the loss of that relationship is a major crisis with momentous consequences.

Aquilera and Messick (1982) developed a broad approach to assessment and intervention in their work on crisis intervention. The state of disequilibrium that a crisis produces causes great consternation, compelling the person to return to **homeostasis**, a state of equilibrium or balance. Factors that influence the grieving person's return to homeostasis are adequate perception of the situation, adequate situational support, and adequate coping. These factors help the person to regain balance and return to previous functioning or even to use the crisis as an opportunity to grow. Because any loss may be perceived as a personal crisis, it seems appropriate for the nurse to link understanding of crisis theory with the nursing process.

For the nurse to support and facilitate the grief process for clients, he or she must observe and listen for cognitive, emotional, spiritual, behavioral, and physiologic cues. Although the nurse must be familiar with the phases, tasks, and dimensions of human response to loss, he or she must realize that each client's experience is unique. Skillful communication is key to performing assessment and providing interventions.

To meet clients' needs effectively, the nurse must examine his or her own personal attitudes, maintain an attentive presence, and provide a psychologically safe environment for deeply intimate sharing. Awareness of one's own beliefs and attitudes is essential so that the nurse can avoid imposing them on the client. **Attentive presence** is being with the client and focusing intently on communicating with and understanding him or her. The nurse can maintain attentive presence by using open body language such as standing or sitting with arms down, facing the client, and maintaining moderate eye contact, especially as the client speaks. Creating a psychologically safe environment includes ensuring the client of confidentiality, refraining from judging or giving specific advice, and allowing the client to share thoughts and feelings freely (Larson, 2005).

Assessment

Effective assessment involves observing all dimensions of human response: what the person is thinking (cognitive), how the person is feeling (emotional), what the person's values and beliefs are (spiritual), how the person is acting (behavioral), and what is happening in the person's body (physiologic) (Box 12.2). Effective communication skills during assessment can lead the client toward understanding his or her experience. Thus, assessment facilitates the client's grief process.

While observing for client responses in the dimensions of grieving, the nurse explores three critical components in assessment:
- Adequate perception regarding the loss
- Adequate support while grieving for the loss
- Adequate coping behaviors during the process

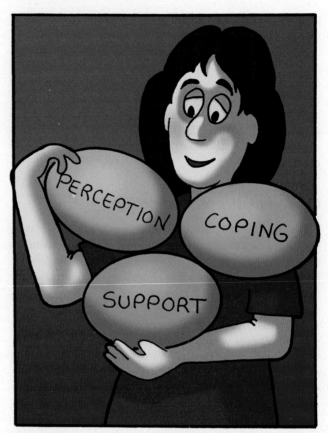

Three major areas to explore to facilitate a grieving client

PERCEPTION OF THE LOSS

Assessment begins with exploration of the client's perception of the loss. What does the loss mean to the client? For the woman who has spontaneously lost her first unborn child and the woman who has elected to abort a pregnancy, this question could have similar or different answers. Nevertheless, the question is valuable for beginning to facilitate the grief process.

Other questions that assess perception and encourage the client's movement through the grief process include the following:
- What does the client think and feel about the loss?
- How is the loss going to affect the client's life?
- What information does the nurse need to clarify or share with the client?

Assessing the client's "need to know" in plain and simple language invites the client to verbalize perceptions that may need clarification. This is especially true for the person who is anticipating a loss, such as one facing a life-ending illness or the loss of a body part. The nurse uses open-ended questions and helps to clarify any misperceptions.

Consider the following. The doctor has just informed Ms. Morrison that the lump on her breast is cancerous and that she is scheduled for a mastectomy in 2 days. The nurse visits the client after rounds and finds her quietly watching television.

Box 12.2   DIMENSIONS (RESPONSES) AND SYMPTOMS OF THE GRIEVING CLIENT

Cognitive responses
- Disruption of assumptions and beliefs
- Questioning and trying to make sense of the loss
- Attempting to keep the lost one present
- Believing in an afterlife and as though the lost one is a guide

Emotional responses
- Anger, sadness, anxiety
- Resentment
- Guilt
- Feeling numb
- Vacillating emotions
- Profound sorrow, loneliness
- Intense desire to restore bond with lost one or object
- Depression, apathy, despair during phase of disorganization
- Sense of independence and confidence as phase of reorganization evolves

Spiritual responses
- Disillusioned and angry with God
- Anguish of abandonment or perceived abandonment
- Hopelessness; meaninglessness

Behavioral responses
- Functioning "automatically"
- Tearful sobbing; uncontrollable crying
- Great restlessness; searching behaviors
- Irritability and hostility
- Seeking and avoiding places and activities shared with lost one
- Keeping valuables of lost one while wanting to discard them
- Possibly abusing drugs or alcohol
- Possible suicidal or homicidal gestures or attempts
- Seeking activity and personal reflection during phase of reorganization

Physiologic responses
- Headaches, insomnia
- Impaired appetite, weight loss
- Lack of energy
- Palpitations, indigestion
- Changes in immune and endocrine systems

Nurse: *"How are you?"* (offering presence; giving a broad opening)

Client: *"Oh, I'm fine. Really, I am."*

Nurse: *"The doctor was just here. Tell me, what is your understanding of what he said?"* (using open-ended questions for description of perception)

Client: *"Well, I think he said that I will have to have surgery on my breast."*

Nurse: *"How do you feel about that news?"* (using open-ended question for what it means to the client)

Exploring what the person believes about the grieving process is another important assessment. Does the client have preconceived ideas about when or how grieving should

happen? The nurse can help the client realize that grieving is very personal and unique: each person grieves in his or her own way.

Later in the shift, the nurse finds Ms. Morrison hitting her pillow and crying. She has eaten little food and has refused visitors.

Nurse: *"Ms. Morrison, I see that you are upset. Tell me, what is happening right now?"* (sharing observation; encouraging description)

Client: *"Oh, I'm so disgusted with myself. I'm sorry you had to see me act this way. I should be able to handle this. Other people have lost their breasts to cancer, and they are doing OK."*

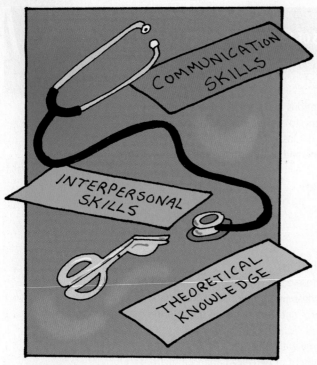

Nurses' tools

Nurse: *"You're pretty upset with yourself, thinking you should feel differently."* (using reflection)

Client: *"Yes, exactly. Don't you think so?"*

Nurse: *"You've had to deal with quite a shock today. Sounds to me like you are expecting quite a bit of yourself. What do you think?"* (using reflection; sharing perceptions; seeking validation)

Client: *"I don't know, maybe. How long is this going to go on? I'm a wreck emotionally."*

Nurse: *"You are grieving, and there is no fixed timetable for what you are dealing with. Everyone has a unique time and way of doing this work."* (informing; validating experience)

SUPPORT

Purposeful assessment of support systems provides the grieving client with an awareness of those who can meet his or her emotional and spiritual needs for security and love. The nurse can help the client to identify his or her support systems and reach out and accept what they can offer.

Nurse: *"Who in your life should or would really want to know what you've just heard from the doctor?"* (seeking information about situational support)

Client: *"Oh, I'm really alone. I'm not married and don't have any relatives in town."*

Nurse: *"There's no one who would care about this news?"* (voicing doubt)

Client: *"Oh, maybe a friend I talk with on the phone now and then."*

COPING BEHAVIORS

The client's behavior is likely to give the nurse the easiest and most concrete information about coping skills. The nurse must be careful to observe the client's behavior throughout the grief process and never assume that a client is at a particular phase. The nurse must use effective communication skills to assess how the client's behavior reflects coping as well as emotions and thoughts.

The following day, the nurse has heard in report that Ms. Morrison had a restless night. She enters Ms. Morrison's room and sees her crying with a full tray of food untouched.

Nurse: *"I wonder if you are upset about your upcoming surgery."* (making an observation, assuming client was crying as an expected behavior of loss and grief)

Client: *"I'm not having surgery. You have me mistaken for someone else."* (using denial to cope)

The nurse also must consider several other questions when assessing the client's coping. How has the person dealt with loss previously? How is the person currently impaired? How does the current experience compare with previous experiences? What does the client perceive as a problem? Is it related to unrealistic ideas about what he or she should feel or do?. The interaction of the dimensions of human response is fluid and dynamic. What a person thinks about during grieving affects his or her feelings, and those feelings influence his or her behavior. The critical factors of perception, support, and coping are interrelated as well and provide a framework for assessing and assisting the client.

Data Analysis and Planning

The nurse must base nursing diagnoses for the person experiencing loss on subjective and objective assessment data. Nursing diagnoses used for clients experiencing grief include the following:

- Grieving, related to actual or perceived loss such as a physiologic loss (e.g., loss of a limb). Loss of security and sense of belonging (e.g., loss of a loved one) is defined as a normal process in the human experience of loss.
- Anticipatory Grieving, related to the intellectual and emotional responses and behaviors by which individuals, families, and communities work through the process of modifying self-concept based on the perception of potential loss.
- **Dysfunctional Grieving** (NANDA diagnosis for complicated grieving), related to the extended unsuccessful use of intellectual and emotional responses by which individuals, families, and communities attempt to work through the process of modifying self-concept based on the perception of loss.

Outcome Identification

Examples of outcomes for the three nursing diagnoses are as follows:

- Grieving: The client will
  - Identify the effects of his or her loss.
  - Seek adequate support.
  - Apply effective coping strategies while expressing and assimilating all dimensions of human response to loss in his or her life.
- Anticipatory Grieving: The client will
  - Identify the meaning of the expected loss in his or her life.
  - Seek adequate support while expressing grief.
  - Develop a plan for coping with the loss as it becomes a reality.
- Dysfunctional Grieving: The client will
  - Identify the meaning of his or her loss.
  - Recognize the negative effects of the loss on his or her life.
  - Seek or accept professional assistance to promote the grieving process.

Interventions

The nurse's guidance helps the client examine and make changes. Changes imply movement as the client progresses through the grief process. Sometimes the client takes one painful step at a time. Sometimes he or she may seem to go over the same ground repeatedly.

INTERVENTIONS REGARDING THE PERCEPTION OF LOSS

Cognitive responses are connected significantly with the intense emotional turmoil that accompanies grieving. For example, in the vignette, Margaret's disillusionment with those friends unavailable after her husband's death added great pain to her loss. She had counted on them to be there as she dealt with James's death. A cognitive shift occurred when she realized they would not be there, meaning she was alone and they no longer cared. She felt abandoned. She then had two immediate losses: James's death and realizing that people she had counted on were unavailable.

Exploring the client's perception and meaning of the loss is a first step that can help alleviate the pain of what some would call the initial emotional overload in grieving. Using the example of Margaret, the nurse could ask what being alone means to her and explore the possibility of others being supportive. Further exploration could focus on her perception that those who had abandoned her no longer cared. Perhaps Margaret would then discover that others could meet her need to be cared for. She may begin to believe that it was fear or discomfort about death that kept former friends away. In fact, it was in just this way that she could accept the caring of some friends and release the importance of those who would not or could not be there for her. In this situation, exploring perceptions and the mean-ing of the loss helped the bereaved to make cognitive shifts that valuably influenced her emotional experience.

When loss occurs, especially if it is sudden and without warning, the cognitive defense mechanism of denial acts as a cushion to soften the effects. Typical verbal responses are, "I can't believe this has happened," "It can't be true," and "There's been a mistake."

Adaptive denial, in which the client gradually adjusts to the reality of the loss, can help the client let go of previous (before the loss) perceptions while creating new ways of thinking about himself or herself, others, and the world. For example, Margaret had to face the reality that although she believed that a priest (because he was a priest) would care about her being alone in the surgery waiting room, he actually was concerned only about getting a paper. Gradually, she was able to relinquish this assumption.

Effective communication skills can be useful in helping the client in adaptive denial move toward acceptance. Note the intervention the nurse makes in the scenario with Ms. Morrison. The nurse enters Ms. Morrison's room and sees her crying with a full tray of food untouched.

Nurse: "You must be quite upset about the news you received from your doctor about your surgery." (using reflection, assuming the client was crying as an expected response of grief; focusing on the surgery is an indirect approach regarding the subject of cancer)

Client: "I'm not having surgery. You have me mistaken for someone else." (using denial)

Nurse: "I saw you crying and wonder what is upsetting you. I'm interested in how you are feeling." (focusing on behavior and sharing observation while indicating concern and accepting the client's denial)

Client: "I'm just not hungry. I don't have an appetite and I'm not clear about what the doctor said." (focusing on physiologic response; nonresponsive to nurse's encouragement to talk about feelings; acknowledging doctor's visit but unsure of what he said—beginning to adjust cognitively to reality of condition)

Nurse: "I wonder if not wanting to eat may be related to what you are feeling. Are there times when you don't have an appetite and you feel upset about something?" (suggesting a connection between physiologic response and feelings; promoting adaptive denial)

Client: "Well, as a matter of fact, yes. But I can't think what I would be upset about." (acknowledging a connection between behavior and feeling; continuing to deny reality)

Nurse: "You said you were unclear about what the doctor said. I wonder if things didn't seem clear because it may have upset you to hear what he had to say. And now, tonight, you don't have an appetite." (using client's experience to make connection between doctor's news and client's physiologic response and behavior)

Client: "What did he say, do you know?" (requesting information; demonstrating a readiness to hear it again while continuing to adjust to reality)

In this example, the nurse gently but persistently guides the client toward acknowledging the reality of her impending loss.

INTERVENTIONS REGARDING SUPPORT

The nurse can help the client to reach out and accept what others want to give in support of his or her grieving process. Note the assessment is developed into a plan for support.

> **Nurse:** *"Who in your life would really want to know what you've just heard from the doctor?"* (seeking information about situational support for the client)
>
> **Client:** *"Oh, I'm really alone. I'm not married."*
>
> **Nurse:** *"There's no one who would care about this news?"* (voicing doubt)
>
> **Client:** *"Oh, maybe a friend I talk with on the phone now and then."*
>
> **Nurse:** *"Why don't I get the phone book for you and you can call her right now?"* (continuing to offer presence; suggesting an immediate source of support; developing a plan of action providing further support)

Many Internet resources are available to nurses who want to help a client find information, support groups, and activities related to the grieving process. Using the search words "bereavement" and "hospice," the nurse can link to numerous organizations that provide support and education throughout the United States. If a client does not have Internet access, most public libraries can help to locate groups and activities that would serve his or her needs. Depending on the state in which a person lives, specific groups exist for those who have lost a child, spouse, or other loved one to suicide, murder, motor vehicle crash, or cancer.

INTERVENTIONS REGARDING COPING BEHAVIORS

When attempting to focus Ms. Morrison on the reality of her surgery, the nurse was helping her shift from an unconscious mechanism of denial to conscious coping with reality. The nurse used communication skills to encourage Ms. Morrison to examine her experience and behavior as possible ways in which she might be coping with the news of loss. Margaret and James's logical approach to life allowed them to cope by continuing to have fun together while attending to medical regimens as they faced the reality of his impending death.

Intervention involves giving the client the opportunity to compare and contrast ways in which he or she has coped with significant loss in the past and helping him or her to review strengths and renew a sense of personal power. Remembering and practicing old behaviors in a new situation may lead to experimentation with new methods and self-discovery. Having a historical perspective helps the person's grief work by allowing shifts in thinking about himself or herself, the loss, and perhaps the meaning of the loss. Margaret's religious practices of prayer and spiritual reading helped her to discover new depths of meaning and purpose in her life.

Encouraging the client to care for himself or herself is another intervention that helps the client cope. The nurse can offer food without pressuring the client to eat. Being careful to eat, sleep well, exercise, and take time for comforting activities are ways that the client can nourish himself or herself. Just as the tired hiker needs to stop, rest, and replenish himself or herself, so must the bereaved person take a break from the exhausting process of grieving. Going back to a routine of work or focusing on other members of the family may provide that respite. Volunteer activities—volunteering at a hospice or botanical garden, taking part in church activities, or speaking to bereavement education groups, for example—can affirm the client's talents and abilities and can renew feelings of self-worth.

Communication and interpersonal skills are tools of the effective nurse, just like a stethoscope, scissors, and gloves. The client trusts that the nurse will have what it takes to assist him or her in grieving. In addition to previously mentioned skills, these tools include the following:

- Using simple nonjudgmental statements to acknowledge loss: "I want you to know I'm thinking of you."
- Referring to a loved one or object of loss by name (if acceptable in the client's culture)
- Remembering words are not always necessary; a light touch on the elbow, shoulder, or hand or just being there indicates caring
- Respecting the client's unique process of grieving
- Respecting the client's personal beliefs
- Being honest, dependable, consistent, and worthy of the client's trust

A welcoming smile and eye contact from the client during intimate conversations indicate the nurse's trustworthiness.

Evaluation

Evaluation of progress depends on the goals established for the client. A review of the tasks and phases of grieving (discussed earlier in the chapter) can be useful in making a statement about the client's status at any given moment. We could say that although Margaret, in the vignette, still misses James, she is in the reorganization phase of grieving. She has a sense of independence and confidence and has accomplished several tasks of grieving: creating new ties, developing a new sense of self, pursuing new activities, and integrating the loss into her life.

SELF-AWARENESS ISSUES

Clients who are grieving need more than someone who is equipped with skills and basic knowledge; they need the support of someone they can trust with their emotions and thoughts. For clients to see nurses as trustworthy, nurses must be willing to examine their personal attitudes about loss and the grieving process.

NURSING INTERVENTIONS FOR GRIEF

Explore client's perception and meaning of his or her loss.

Allow adaptive denial.

Encourage or assist client to reach out for and accept support.

Encourage client to examine patterns of coping in past and present situation of loss.

Encourage client to review personal strengths and personal power.

Encourage client to care for himself or herself.

Offer client food without pressure to eat.

Use effective communication:

- Offer presence and give broad openings.
- Use open-ended questions.
- Encourage description.
- Share observations.
- Use reflection.
- Seek validation of perceptions.
- Provide information.
- Voice doubt.
- Use focusing.
- Attempt to translate into feelings or verbalize the implied.

Establish rapport and maintain interpersonal skills such as

- Attentive presence
- Respect for client's unique grieving process
- Respect for client's personal beliefs
- Being trustworthy: honest, dependable, consistent
- Periodic self-inventory of attitudes and issues related to loss

Points to Consider When Working With Clients With Grief and Loss

Taking a self-awareness inventory means periodic reflection on questions, such as the following:

- What are the losses in my life, and how do they affect me?
- Am I currently grieving for a significant loss? How does my loss affect my ability to be present to my client?
- Who is there for me as I grieve?
- How am I coping with my loss?
- Is the pain of my personal grief spilling over as I listen and watch for cues of the client's grieving?
- Am I making assumptions about the client's experience based on my own process?
- Can I keep appropriate nurse–client boundaries as I attend to the client's needs?
- Do I have the strength to be present and to facilitate the client's grief?

- What does my supervisor or a trusted colleague observe about my current ability to support a client in the grief process?

Ongoing self-examination is an effective method of keeping the therapeutic relationship goal-directed and acutely attentive to the client's needs.

Critical Thinking Questions

1. Although grieving is explained in terms of a process of stages, the client experiences a myriad of emotions and thoughts. What phenomena of the grieving process give the nurse concrete information about the client's progress? Of these phenomena, which is easiest to observe? How must the nurse investigate the meaning of this phenomenon?

2. What issues of loss does the nurse deal with every day? What are the nurse's most valuable tools for dealing with these losses? How might the nurse use these tools across health care settings?

3. A client in the psychiatric setting has recently lost his mother. How will the nurse differentiate between the client's psychiatric illness and a normal response to grief? How will the nurse determine the risk for complicated grief for this client?

4. How might the nurse maintain his or her professional responsibility toward the therapeutic relationship with those who are grieving for a loss? What components of trustworthiness must the nurse cultivate in relation to the client who is grieving?

KEY POINTS

- Grief refers to the subjective emotions and affect that are normal responses to the experience of loss.
- Grieving is the process through which a person travels as he or she experiences grief.
- Types of losses can be identified as unfulfilled or unmet human needs. Maslow's hierarchy of human needs is a useful model by which to understand loss as it relates to unfulfilled human needs.
- Grief work is one of life's most difficult challenges. The challenge of integrating a loss requires all that the person can give of mind, body, and spirit.
- Because the nurse constantly interacts with clients at various points on the health–illness continuum, he or she must understand loss and the process of grieving.
- Loss of a significant other activates attachment behaviors that range from quiet glances toward the significant other to following, clinging to, searching for, and calling out for the other, to wails of protest when the significant other or object is gone.

- The process of grieving has been described in terms of dynamically interrelated phases: numbness and denial, yearning and protesting, cognitive disorganization and emotional despair, and reorganization and reintegration.
- Dimensions of human response include cognitive, emotional, spiritual, behavioral, and physiologic. People may be experiencing more than one phase of the grieving process.
- Culturally bound reactions to loss are often lost in the acculturation to dominant societal norms. Both universal and culture-specific rituals facilitate grieving.
- Nurses and other health care providers who are constantly interacting with dying clients are vulnerable to disenfranchised grief.
- Complicated grieving is a response that lies outside the norm. The person may be void of emotion, grieve for a prolonged period, or express feelings that seem out of proportion. With so many variables in the grieving process, what may appear to be complicated grieving may be only the person's unique style of grieving.
- Low self-esteem, distrust of others, a psychiatric disorder, previous suicide threats or attempts, and absent or unhelpful family members increase the risk for complicated grieving.

- Situations considered risk factors for complicated grief in those already vulnerable include death of a spouse or child, a sudden unexpected death, and murder.
- During assessment, the nurse observes and listens for cues in what the person thinks and feels and how he or she behaves and then uses these relevant data to guide the client in the grieving process.
- Crisis theory can be used to help the nurse working with a grieving client. Adequate perception, adequate support, and adequate coping are critical factors.
- Effective communication skills are the key to successful assessment and interventions.
- Interventions focused on the perception of loss include exploring the meaning of the loss and allowing adaptive denial, which is the process of gradually adjusting to the reality of a loss.
- Being there to help the client while assisting him or her to seek other sources of support is an essential intervention.
- Encouraging the client to care for himself or herself promotes adequate coping.
- To earn the client's trust, the nurse must examine his or her own attitudes about loss and periodically take a self-awareness inventory.

Nursing Care Plan *Grief*

Nursing Diagnosis

Grieving: *A normal response in the human experience of loss.*

ASSESSMENT DATA

Cognitive Responses
- Questioning and trying to make sense of the loss
- Experiencing disillusionment
- Attempting to make sense of the loss

Emotional Responses
- Feeling numb
- Experiencing sorrow, loneliness
- Crying, sobbing
- Having vacillating emotions including anger
- Experiencing hopelessness
- Feeling helpless, powerless

Behavioral Responses
- Experiencing great restlessness; searching for the deceased
- Seeking and avoiding places and activities once shared with the lost one
- Functioning "automatically"

EXPECTED OUTCOMES

The client will
- Identify the loss and its meaning for self (adequate perception)
- Express feelings, verbally and nonverbally
- Establish and maintain adequate nutrition, hydration, and elimination (adequate coping)
- Establish and maintain an adequate balance of rest, sleep, and activity (adequate coping)
- Establish and maintain an adequate support system
- Verbalize knowledge of the grief process
- Demonstrate initial integration of loss into his or her life (adequate coping)
- Verbalize realistic future plans integrating loss (adequate perception)

Nursing Care Plan: Grief, cont.

ASSESSMENT DATA

Physiologic Responses
- Headaches
- Insomnia
- Lack of energy

Critical Component of Perception—questions to explore and listen for while talking with the client:
- What is the meaning of the loss for the client?
- What is the client's understanding of his or her current experience in grieving?
- Are the client's perceptions adequate? (Do the client's perceptions reflect the process of grieving?)

Critical Component of Support—questions to explore with the client:
- Who in the client's life needs to be present to offer adequate support for the client?
- How can resources be established to offer optimum support for the client?

Critical Component of Coping—questions to keep in mind during planning and implementation of care:
- How has the client handled past crises?
- How can the client use skills that have helped in the past for this current situation?
- Considering the phase of his or her grieving process, how is the client's current experience a reflection of adequate coping?

IMPLEMENTATION

Nursing Interventions *denotes collaborative interventions	**Rationale**
After establishing rapport with the client, bring up the loss in a supportive manner; if the client refuses to discuss it, withdraw and state your intention to return. ("I can understand that you may not want to talk with me about this now. I will come to talk with you again at 11:00. Maybe we can talk about it then.") Return at the stated time, then continue to be as supportive as possible rather than confronting the client.	Your presence demonstrates interest and caring. Telling the client you will return conveys your support. The client may need emotional support to face and express uncomfortable or painful feelings. Confronting the client or pushing him or her to express feelings may increase anxiety and lead to further denial or avoidance.
Talk with the client realistically about his or her loss; discuss concrete changes that the client must now begin to make as a result of the loss.	Discussing the loss on this level may help to make it more real for the client.
Encourage the expression of feelings in ways the client is comfortable—for example, talking, writing, drawing, crying, wailing, or yelling. Convey your acceptance of these feelings and means of expression. Offer the client verbal support for attempts to express feelings.	Expression of feelings can help the client to identify, accept, and work through his or her feelings even if these are painful or otherwise uncomfortable for the client.

continued ⇢

Nursing Care Plan: Grief, cont.

IMPLEMENTATION

Nursing Interventions *denotes collaborative interventions

Rationale

Nursing Interventions	Rationale
Encourage the client to recall experiences, talk about what was involved in his or her relationship with the lost person or object, and so forth. Discuss with the client the changes in his or her feelings toward self, others, and the lost person or object as a result of the loss and grief process.	Discussing the lost object or person can help the client to identify and express the loss, what the loss means to him or her, and his or her emotional response.
Encourage appropriate (that is, safe) expression of all feelings that the client has toward the lost person or object and convey acceptance. Assure the client that even "negative" feelings like anger and resentment are normal and healthy in grieving.	Feelings are not inherently bad or good. Giving the client support for expressing feelings may help the client to accept uncomfortable feelings.
Convey to the client that although feelings may be uncomfortable, they are natural and necessary to this process, that he or she can withstand having these feelings, and that the feelings will not harm him or her.	The client may fear the intensity of his or her feelings.
Discourage rumination if the client is dwelling on his or her guilt or worthlessness. After listening to the client's feelings, tell the client you will talk about other aspects of grief and feelings.	The client needs to identify and express the feelings that underlie the rumination and to proceed through the grief process.
Referral to the facility chaplain, clergy, or other spiritual resource person may be indicated. Encourage a connection with those in his or her life who may be a source of support.	The client may be more comfortable discussing spiritual issues with an advisor who shares his or her belief system.
Provide opportunities for the release of tension, anger, guilt, and so forth through physical activities. Promote regular exercise as a healthy means of dealing with stress and tension.	Physical activity provides a way to relieve tension in a healthy, nondestructive manner.
Limit times and frequency of therapeutic interactions with the client. Encourage independent, spontaneous expression of feelings (writing, initiating interactions with other clients or with other staff members, getting involved in a physical activity). Plan staff-initiated interactions at times that allow the client to fulfill responsibilities (activities, unit duties) and maintain personal care (sleeping, eating, hygiene).	The client needs to develop independent skills of communicating feelings and to integrate the loss into his or her daily life, while meeting his or her own basic needs.
Encourage the client to talk with others, individually and in small groups (larger as tolerated), about the loss in terms of his or her own and others' feelings and about experiences and changes resulting from the loss.	The client needs to develop independent skills of communicating feelings and expressing grief to others.
Promote sharing, communicating, expressing feelings, and support among clients. Use larger groups (such as open report) for a general discussion of loss and grief (with or without focusing on this client's loss). Also help the client to realize that there are limits to sharing grief in a social context.	Sharing grief and experiences with others can help the client to identify and express feelings and to feel normal in grieving. Dwelling on grief in social interactions, however, can result in other people's discomfort with their own feelings and may lead to friends and significant others avoiding the client.
Point out to the client that a major aspect of loss is a real physical stress. Encourage good nutrition, hydration, and elimination as well as adequate rest and daily physical exercise (such as walking, running, swim-	The client may be unaware of the physical stress of the loss or may lack interest in activities of daily living. Physical exercise can relieve tension or pent-up feelings in a healthy, nondestructive manner.

Nursing Care Plan: Grief, cont.

IMPLEMENTATION

Nursing Interventions *denotes collaborative interventions	**Rationale**
ming, or cycling) in the hospital and after discharge.	These people may have little or no knowledge of grief or the process involved in recovery.
Teach the client (and his or her family or significant others) about the grief process.	The grief process allows the client to adjust to a change in his or her life and to begin to move toward future opportunities.
Point out to the client that time spent grieving can be nurturing, that it is a time of learning and growth from which to gather the strength to go forward.	

Adapted from Schultz, J. M., & Videbeck, S. L. (2005). Lippincott's manual of psychiatric nursing care plans (7th ed.). Philadelphia: Lippincott Williams & Wilkins.

INTERNET RESOURCES

RESOURCE	**INTERNET ADDRESS**
• Grief support groups	http://www.griefshare.org
• Death and dying	http://www.dying.about.com
• Hospice	http://www.hospicenet.org

REFERENCES

Aquilera, D. C., & Messick, J. M. (1982). *Crisis intervention: Theory and methodology.* St. Louis: C. V. Mosby.

Bowlby, J. (1980). *Attachment and loss, Vol. 3: Loss, sadness, and depression.* New York: Basic Books.

Doka, K. J. (2006). Grief: The constant companion of illness. *Anesthesiology Clinics, 24*(1), 205–212.

Groot, M. H., Keijser, J., & Neeleman, J. (2006). Grief shortly after suicide and natural death: A comparative study among spouses and first-degree relatives. *Suicide & Life-threatening Behavior, 36*(4), 418–431.

Harvey, J. H., & Miller, E. D. (1998). Toward a psychology of loss. *Psychological Science, 9*(6), 429.

Kaufman, K. R., & Kaufman, N. D. (2006). And then the dog died. *Death Studies, 30*(1), 61–76.

Kemp, C. (2005). Cultural issues in palliative care. *Seminars in Oncology Nursing, 21*(1), 44–52.

Kubler-Ross, E. (1969). *On death and dying.* New York: Macmillan.

Larson, D. G. (2005). Becky's legacy: More lessons. *Death Studies, 29*(8), 745–757.

Lobb, E. A., Clayton, J. M., & Price, M. A. (2006). Suffering, loss and grief in palliative care. *Australian Family Physician, 35*(10), 772–775.

Maslow, A. H. (1954). *Motivation and personality.* New York: Harper.

Neimeyer, R. A., Baldwin, S. A., & Gillies, J. (2006) Continuing bonds and reconstructing meaning: Mitigating complications in bereavement. *Death Studies, 30*(8), 715–738.

Ng, B. Y. (2005). Grief revisited. *Annals of the Academy of Medicine, Singapore, 34*(5), 352–355.

Rando, T. A. (1984). *Grief, dying, and death: Clinical interventions for caregivers.* Champaign, IL: Research Press.

Rodebaugh, L. S., Schwindt, R. G., & Valentine, F. M. (1999). How to handle grief with wisdom. *Nursing, 29,* 52.

Schultz, J. M., & Videbeck, S. L. (2005). *Lippincott's manual of psychiatric nursing care plans* (7th ed.). Philadelphia: Lippincott Williams & Wilkins.

Smolinski, K. M., & Colon, Y. (2006). Silent voices and invisible walls: Exploring end of life care with lesbians and gay men. *Journal of Psychosocial Oncology, 24*(1), 51–64.

Weinstein, L. B. (2003). Bereaved orthodox Jewish families and their community: A cross-cultural perspective. *Journal of Community Health Nursing, 20*(4), 233–243.

Yasien-Esmael, H., & Rubin, S. S. (2005). The meaning structures of Muslim bereavements in Israel: Religious traditions, mourning practices, and human experience. *Death Studies, 29*(6), 495–518.

Zhang, B., El-Jawahri, A., & Prigerson, H. G. (2006). Update on bereavement research: Evidence-based guidelines for the diagnosis and treatment of complicated bereavement. *Journal of Palliative Medicine, 9*(5), 1188–1203.

Ziemba, R. A., Lynch-Sauer, J. M. (2005). Preparedness for taking care of elderly parents: "First, you get ready to cry." *Journal of Women & Aging, 17*(1–2), 99–113.

Zisook, S., & Zisook, S. A. (2005). Death, dying, and bereavement. In B. J. Sadock & V. A. Sadock (Eds.), *Comprehensive Textbook of Psychiatry* (Vol. 2, 8th ed., pp. 2367–2393). Philadelphia: Lippincott Williams & Wilkins.

ADDITIONAL READINGS

Fahey-McCarthy, E. (2003). Exploring theories of grief: Personal reflection. *British Journal of Midwifery, 11*(10), 595–612.

Stroebe, M. S., Folkman, S., Hansson, R. O., & Schut, H. (2006). The prediction of bereavement outcome: Development of an integrative risk factor framework. *Social Science & Medicine, 63*(9), 2440–2451.

Summers, J., Zisook, S., Sciolla, A. D., et al. (2004). Gender, AIDS, and bereavement: A comparison of women and men living with HIV. *Death Studies, 28*(3), 225–241.

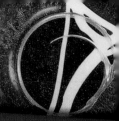

Chapter Study Guide

MULTIPLE-CHOICE QUESTIONS

Select the best answer for each of the following questions.

1. Which of the following accurately lists Bowlby's phases of the grieving process?
   A. Denial, anger, depression, bargaining, acceptance
   B. Shock, outcry, and denial; intrusion of thought, distractions, and obsessive reviewing of the loss; confiding in others to emote and cognitively restructure an account of the loss
   C. Numbness and denial of the loss, emotional yearning for the loved one and protesting permanence of the loss, cognitive disorganization and emotional despair, reorganizing and reintegrating a sense of self
   D. Reeling, feeling, dealing, healing

2. Which of the following give cues to the nurse that a client may be grieving for a loss?
   A. Sad affect, anger, anxiety, and sudden changes in mood
   B. Thoughts, feelings, behavior, and physiologic complaints
   C. Hallucinations, panic level of anxiety, and sense of impending doom
   D. Complaints of abdominal pain, diarrhea, and loss of appetite

3. Situations that are considered risk factors for complicated grief are
   A. Inadequate support and old age
   B. Childbirth, marriage, and divorce
   C. Death of a spouse or child, death by suicide, and sudden and unexpected death
   D. Inadequate perception of the grieving crisis

4. Physiologic responses of complicated grieving include
   A. Tearfulness when recalling significant memories of the lost one
   B. Impaired appetite, weight loss, lack of energy, palpitations
   C. Depression, panic disorders, chronic grief
   D. Impaired immune system, increased serum prolactin level, increased mortality rate from heart disease

5. Critical factors for successful integration of loss during the grieving process are
   A. The client's adequate perception, adequate support, and adequate coping
   B. The nurse's trustworthiness and healthy attitudes about grief
   C. Accurate assessment and intervention by the nurse or helping person
   D. The client's predictable and steady movement from one stage of the process to the next

FILL-IN-THE-BLANK QUESTIONS

Identify the dimension of grieving for each of the following client expressions or behaviors.

_____ "I have this insatiable yearning to be with him."

_____ Irritability and hostility toward others

_____ "I thought a priest would certainly understand my need for support at this time. Why didn't he ask how I was feeling when I told him my husband was having surgery?"

_____ "Why has God done this to me?"

_____ "I've lost my appetite, and I just can't seem to get to sleep at night when I go to bed."

SHORT-ANSWER QUESTIONS

1. Give an example of each of the following:

Styles of grieving

Critical factor of adequate support

Emotional response during phase of numbing in the grieving process

2. For each of the following client statements, write a response that the nurse might make and the rationale for the nurse's response:

"This is unbearable. I can't believe she's gone."

"No one will want to hire me at this age."

"There's nowhere for me to turn."

"Get out of here! Leave me alone! I don't need your help."

Unit 4

Nursing Practice for Psychiatric Disorders

Chapter

13

Anxiety and Stress-Related Illness

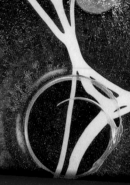

Key Terms

- agoraphobia
- anxiety
- anxiety disorders
- assertiveness training
- automatisms
- avoidance behavior
- compulsions
- decatastrophizing
- defense mechanisms
- depersonalization
- derealization
- exposure
- fear
- flooding
- mild anxiety
- moderate anxiety
- obsessions
- panic anxiety
- panic attack
- panic disorder
- phobia
- positive reframing
- primary gain
- response prevention
- secondary gain
- severe anxiety
- stress
- systematic desensitization

Learning Objectives

After reading this chapter, you should be able to

1. Describe anxiety as a response to stress.

2. Describe the levels of anxiety with behavioral changes related to each level.

3. Discuss the use of defense mechanisms by people with anxiety disorders.

4. Describe the current theories regarding the etiologies of major anxiety disorders.

5. Evaluate the effectiveness of treatment including medications for clients with anxiety disorders.

6. Apply the nursing process to the care of clients with anxiety and anxiety disorders.

7. Provide teaching to clients, families, caregivers, and communities to increase understanding of anxiety and stress-related disorders.

8. Examine your feelings, beliefs, and attitudes regarding clients with anxiety disorders.

Anxiety is a vague feeling of dread or apprehension; it is a response to external or internal stimuli that can have behavioral, emotional, cognitive, and physical symptoms. Anxiety is distinguished from **fear**, which is feeling afraid or threatened by a clearly identifiable external stimulus that represents danger to the person. Anxiety is unavoidable in life and can serve many positive functions such as motivating the person to take action to solve a problem or to resolve a crisis. It is considered normal when it is appropriate to the situation and dissipates when the situation has been resolved.

Anxiety disorders comprise a group of conditions that share a key feature of excessive anxiety with ensuing behavioral, emotional, cognitive, and physiologic responses. Clients suffering from anxiety disorders can demonstrate unusual behaviors such as panic without reason, unwarranted fear of objects or life conditions, uncontrollable repetitive actions, re-experiencing of traumatic events, or unexplainable or overwhelming worry. They experience significant distress over time, and the disorder significantly impairs their daily routines, social lives, and occupational functioning.

This chapter discusses anxiety as an expected response to stress. It also explores anxiety disorders, with particular emphasis on panic disorder and obsessive-compulsive disorder (OCD).

ANXIETY AS A RESPONSE TO STRESS

Stress is the wear and tear that life causes on the body (Selye, 1956). It occurs when a person has difficulty dealing with life situations, problems, and goals. Each person handles stress differently: One person can thrive in a situation that creates great distress for another. For example, many people view public speaking as scary, but for teachers and actors, it is an everyday, enjoyable experience. Marriage, children, airplanes, snakes, a new job, a new school, and leaving home are examples of stress-causing events.

Hans Selye (1956, 1974), an endocrinologist, identified the physiologic aspects of stress, which he labeled the *general adaptation syndrome*. He used laboratory animals to assess biologic system changes; the stages of the body's physical responses to pain, heat, toxins, and restraint; and, later, the mind's emotional responses to real or perceived stressors. He determined three stages of reaction to stress:

- In the *alarm reaction stage,* stress stimulates the body to send messages from the hypothalamus to the glands (such as the adrenal gland, to send out adrenaline and norepinephrine for fuel) and organs (such as the liver, to reconvert glycogen stores to glucose for food) to prepare for potential defense needs.
- In the *resistance stage,* the digestive system reduces function to shunt blood to areas needed for defense. The lungs take in more air, and the heart beats faster and harder so it can circulate this highly oxygenated and highly nourished blood to the muscles to defend the

body by fight, flight, or freeze behaviors. If the person adapts to the stress, the body responses relax, and the gland, organ, and systemic responses abate.

- The *exhaustion stage* occurs when the person has responded negatively to anxiety and stress: body stores are depleted or the emotional components are not resolved, resulting in continual arousal of the physiologic responses and little reserve capacity.

Autonomic nervous system responses to fear and anxiety generate the involuntary activities of the body that are involved in self-preservation. Sympathetic nerve fibers "charge up" the vital signs at any hint of danger to prepare the body's defenses. The adrenal glands release adrenalin (epinephrine), which causes the body to take in more oxygen, dilate the pupils, and increase arterial pressure and heart rate while constricting the peripheral vessels and shunting blood from the gastrointestinal and reproductive systems and increasing glycogenolysis to free glucose for fuel for the heart, muscles, and central nervous system. When the danger has passed, parasympathetic nerve fibers reverse this process and return the body to normal operating conditions until the next sign of threat reactivates the sympathetic responses.

Anxiety causes uncomfortable cognitive, psychomotor, and physiologic responses such as difficulty with logical thought, increasingly agitated motor activity, and elevated vital signs. To reduce these uncomfortable feelings, the person tries to reduce the level of discomfort by implementing new adaptive behaviors or defense mechanisms. Adaptive behaviors can be positive and help the person to learn, for

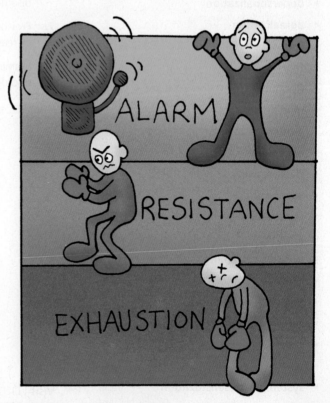

Three reactions or stages of stress

example, using imagery techniques to refocus attention on a pleasant scene, practicing sequential relaxation of the body from head to toe, and breathing slowly and steadily to reduce muscle tension and vital signs. Negative responses to anxiety can result in maladaptive behaviors such as tension headaches, pain syndromes, and stress-related responses that reduce the efficiency of the immune system.

People can communicate anxiety to others both verbally and nonverbally. If someone yells "fire," others around them can become anxious as they picture a fire and the possible threat that represents. Viewing a distraught mother searching for her lost child in a shopping mall can cause anxiety in others as they imagine the panic she is experiencing. They can convey anxiety nonverbally through empathy, which is the sense of walking in another person's shoes for a moment in time (Sullivan, 1952). Examples of nonverbal empathetic communication are when the family of a client undergoing surgery can tell from the physician's body language that their loved one has died, when the nurse reads a plea for help in a client's eyes, or when a person feels the tension in a room where two people have been arguing and are now not speaking to each other.

Levels of Anxiety

Anxiety has both healthy and harmful aspects depending on its degree and duration as well as on how well the person

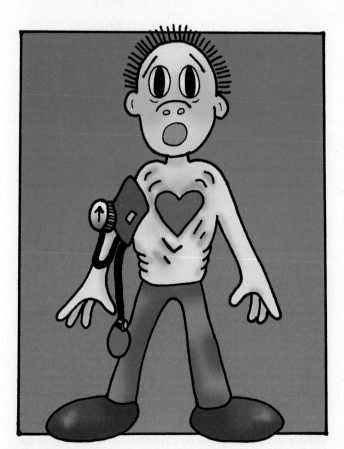

Physiologic response

copes with it. Anxiety has four levels: mild, moderate, severe, and panic (Table 13.1). Each level causes both physiologic and emotional changes in the person.

Mild anxiety is a sensation that something is different and warrants special attention. Sensory stimulation increases and helps the person focus attention to learn, solve problems, think, act, feel, and protect himself or herself. Mild anxiety often motivates people to make changes or to engage in goal-directed activity. For example, it helps students to focus on studying for an examination.

Moderate anxiety is the disturbing feeling that something is definitely wrong; the person becomes nervous or agitated. In moderate anxiety, the person can still process information, solve problems, and learn new things with assistance from others. He or she has difficulty concentrating independently but can be redirected to the topic. For example, the nurse might be giving preoperative instructions to a client who is anxious about the upcoming surgical procedure. As the nurse is teaching, the client's attention wanders but the nurse can regain the client's attention and direct him or her back to the task at hand.

As the person progresses to **severe anxiety** and panic, more primitive survival skills take over, defensive responses ensue, and cognitive skills decrease significantly. A person with severe anxiety has trouble thinking and reasoning. Muscles tighten and vital signs increase. The person paces; is restless, irritable, and angry; or uses other similar emotional-psychomotor means to release tension. In panic, the emotional-psychomotor realm predominates with accompanying fight, flight, or freeze responses. Adrenaline surge greatly increases vital signs. Pupils enlarge to let in more light, and the only cognitive process focuses on the person's defense.

Working With Anxious Clients

Nurses encounter anxious clients and families in a wide variety of situations such as before surgery and in emergency departments, intensive care units, offices, and clinics. First and foremost, the nurse must assess the person's anxiety level because that determines what interventions are likely to be effective.

Mild anxiety is an asset to the client and requires no direct intervention. People with mild anxiety can learn and solve problems and are even eager for information. Teaching can be very effective when the client is mildly anxious.

In moderate anxiety, the nurse must be certain that the client is following what the nurse is saying. The client's attention can wander, and he or she may have some difficulty concentrating over time. Speaking in short, simple, and easy-to-understand sentences is effective; the nurse must stop to ensure that the client is still taking in information correctly. The nurse may need to redirect the client back to the topic if the client goes off on an unrelated tangent.

When anxiety becomes severe, the client no longer can pay attention or take in information. The nurse's goal must be to lower the person's anxiety level to moderate or mild

Table 13.1   LEVELS OF ANXIETY

Anxiety Level	Psychological Responses	Physiologic Responses
Mild	Wide perceptual field Sharpened senses Increased motivation Effective problem solving Increased learning ability Irritability	Restlessness Fidgeting GI "butterflies" Difficulty sleeping Hypersensitivity to noise
Moderate	Perceptual field narrowed to immediate task Selectively attentive Cannot connect thoughts or events independently Increased use of automatisms	Muscle tension Diaphoresis Pounding pulse Headache Dry mouth High voice pitch Faster rate of speech GI upset Frequent urination
Severe	Perceptual field reduced to one detail or scattered details Cannot complete tasks Cannot solve problems or learn effectively Behavior geared toward anxiety relief and is usually ineffective Doesn't respond to redirection Feels awe, dread, or horror Cries Ritualistic behavior	Severe headache Nausea, vomiting, and diarrhea Trembling Rigid stance Vertigo Pale Tachycardia Chest pain
Panic	Perceptual field reduced to focus on self Cannot process any environmental stimuli Distorted perceptions Loss of rational thought Doesn't recognize potential danger Can't communicate verbally Possible delusions and hallucination May be suicidal	May bolt and run OR Totally immobile and mute Dilated pupils Increased blood pressure and pulse Flight, fight, or freeze

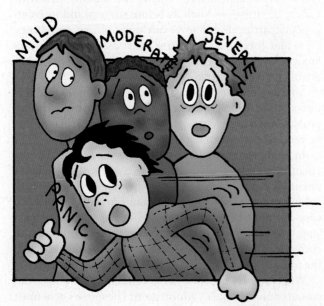

Levels of anxiety

before proceeding with anything else. It is also essential to remain with the person because anxiety is likely to worsen if he or she is left alone. Talking to the client in a low, calm, and soothing voice can help. If the person cannot sit still, walking with him or her while talking can be effective. What the nurse talks about matters less than how he or she says the words. Helping the person to take deep even breaths can help lower anxiety.

During panic-level anxiety, the person's safety is the primary concern. He or she cannot perceive potential harm and may have no capacity for rational thought. The nurse must keep talking to the person in a comforting manner, even though the client cannot process what the nurse is saying. Going to a small, quiet, and nonstimulating environment may help to reduce anxiety. The nurse can reassure the person that this is anxiety, that it will pass, and that he or she is in a safe place. The nurse should remain with the client until the panic recedes. Panic-level anxiety is not sustained indefinitely but can last from 5 to 30 minutes.

When working with an anxious person, the nurse must be aware of his or her own anxiety level. It is easy for the nurse to become increasingly anxious. Remaining calm and in control is essential if the nurse is going to work effectively with the client.

Short-term anxiety can be treated with anxiolytic medications (Table 13.2). Most of these drugs are benzodiazepines, which are commonly prescribed for anxiety. Benzodiazepines have a high potential for abuse and dependence, however, so their use should be short-term, ideally no longer than 4 to 6 weeks. These drugs are designed to relieve anxiety so that the person can deal more effectively with whatever crisis or situation is causing stress. Unfortunately, many people see these drugs as a "cure" for anxiety and continue to use them instead of learning more effective coping skills or making needed changes. Chapter 2 contains additional information about anxiolytic drugs.

Overview of Anxiety Disorders

Anxiety disorders are diagnosed when anxiety no longer functions as a signal of danger or a motivation for needed change but becomes chronic and permeates major portions of the person's life, resulting in maladaptive behaviors and emotional disability. Anxiety disorders have many manifestations, but anxiety is the key feature of each (American Psychiatric Association [APA], 2000). Types of anxiety disorders include the following:

- Agoraphobia with or without panic disorder
- Panic disorder
- Specific phobia
- Social phobia
- OCD
- Generalized anxiety disorder (GAD)
- Acute stress disorder
- Posttraumatic stress disorder

Panic disorder and OCD are the most common and are the focus of this chapter. Posttraumatic stress disorder is addressed in Chapter 11.

INCIDENCE

Anxiety disorders have the highest prevalence rates of all mental disorders in the United States. Nearly one in four adults in the United States is affected, and the magnitude of anxiety disorders in young people is similar (Merikangas, 2005). Anxiety disorders are more prevalent in women, people younger than age 45 years, people who are divorced or separated, and people of lower socioeconomic status. The exception is OCD, which is equally prevalent in men and women but is more common among boys than girls.

ONSET AND CLINICAL COURSE

The onset and clinical course of anxiety disorders are extremely variable depending on the specific disorder. These aspects are discussed later in this chapter within the context of each disorder.

Table 13.2 ANXIOLYTIC DRUGS

Generic (Trade) Name	Speed of Onset	Side Effects	Nursing Implications
Benzodiazepines			
Diazepam (Valium)	Very fast	Dizziness, clumsiness, sedation, headache, fatigue, sexual dysfunction, blurred vision, dry throat and mouth, constipation, high potential for abuse and dependence	Avoid other CNS depressants such as antihistamines and alcohol.
Chlorazepate (Tranxene)	Fast		Avoid caffeine.
Alprazolam (Xanax)	Intermediate		Take care with potentially hazardous activities such as driving.
Chlordiazepoxide (Librium)	Intermediate		Rise slowly from lying or sitting position.
Clonazepam (Klonopin)	Intermediate		Use sugar-free beverages or hard candy.
			Drink adequate fluids.
			Take only as prescribed.
			Do not stop taking the drug abruptly.
Lorazepam (Ativan)	Moderately slow		
Oxazepam (Serax)	Moderately slow		
Nonbenzodiazepines			
Buspirone (BuSpar)	Very slow	Dizziness, restlessness, agitation, drowsiness, headache, weakness, nausea, vomiting, paradoxical excitement or euphoria	Rise slowly from sitting position.
Meprobamate (Miltown, Equanil)	Rapid		Take care with potentially hazardous activities such as driving.
			Take with food.
			Report persistent restlessness, agitation, excitement, or euphoria to physician.

Disorder	Symptoms
Agoraphobia is anxiety about or avoidance of places or situations from which escape might be difficult or help might be unavailable.	Avoids being outside alone or at home alone; avoids traveling in vehicles; impaired ability to work; difficulty meeting daily responsibilities (e.g., grocery shopping, going to appointments); knows response is extreme
Panic disorder is characterized by recurrent, unexpected panic attacks that cause constant concern. **Panic attack** is the sudden onset of intense apprehension, fearfulness, or terror associated with feelings of impending doom.	A discrete episode of panic lasting 15 to 30 minutes with four or more of the following: palpitations, sweating, trembling or shaking, shortness of breath, choking or smothering sensation, chest pain or discomfort, nausea, derealization or depersonalization, fear of dying or going crazy, paresthesias, chills or hot flashes
Specific phobia is characterized by significant anxiety provoked by a specific feared object or situation, which often leads to avoidance behavior.	Marked anxiety response to the object or situation; avoidance or suffered endurance of object or situation; significant distress or impairment of daily routine, occupation, or social functioning; adolescents and adults recognize their fear as excessive or unreasonable.
Social phobia is characterized by anxiety provoked by certain types of social or performance situations, which often leads to avoidance behavior.	Fear of embarrassment or inability to perform; avoidance or dreaded endurance of behavior or situation; recognition that response is irrational or excessive; belief that others are judging him or her negatively; significant distress or impairment in relationships, work, or social life; anxiety can be severe or panic level.
Obsessive-compulsive disorder involves obsessions (thoughts, impulses, or images) that cause marked anxiety and/or compulsions (repetitive behaviors or mental acts) that attempt to neutralize anxiety.	Recurrent, persistent, unwanted, intrusive thoughts, impulses, or images beyond worrying about realistic life problems; attempts to ignore, suppress, or neutralize obsessions with compulsions that are mostly ineffective; adults and adolescents recognize that obsessions and compulsions are excessive and unreasonable.
Generalized anxiety disorder is characterized by at least 6 months of persistent and excessive worry and anxiety.	Apprehensive expectations more days than not for 6 months or more about several events or activities; uncontrollable worrying; significant distress or impaired social or occupational functioning; three of the following symptoms: restlessness, easily fatigued, difficulty concentrating or mind going blank, irritability, muscle tension, sleep disturbance
Acute stress disorder is the development of anxiety, dissociation, and other symptoms within 1 month of exposure to an extremely traumatic stressor; it lasts 2 days to 4 weeks.	Exposure to traumatic event causing intense fear, helplessness, or horror; marked anxiety symptoms or increased arousal; significant distress or impaired functioning; persistent re-experiencing of the event; three of the following symptoms: sense of emotional numbing or detachment, feeling dazed, derealization, depersonalization, dissociative amnesia (inability to recall important aspect of the event)
Posttraumatic stress disorder is characterized by the re-experiencing of an extremely traumatic event, avoidance of stimuli associated with the event, numbing of responsiveness, and persistent increased arousal; it begins within 3 months to years after the event and may last a few months or years.	Exposure to traumatic event involving intense fear, helplessness or horror; re-experiencing (intrusive recollections or dreams, flashbacks, physical and psychological distress over reminders of the event); avoidance of memory-provoking stimuli and numbing of general responsiveness (avoidance of thoughts, feelings, conversations, people, places, amnesia, diminished interest or participation in life events, feeling detached or estranged from others, restricted affect, sense of foreboding); increased arousal (sleep disturbance, irritability or angry outbursts, difficulty concentrating, hypervigilance, exaggerated startle response); significant distress or impairment

Adapted from American Psychiatric Association. (2000). DSM-IV-TR: Diagnostic and statistical manual of mental disorders (4th ed., text revision). Washington DC: Author.

Nursing Care Plan

Anxious Behavior

Nursing Diagnosis

Anxiety: *Vague uneasy feeling of discomfort or dread accompanied by an autonomic response (the source often nonspecific or unknown to the individual); a feeling of apprehension caused by anticipation of danger. It is an alerting signal that warns of impending danger and enables the individual to take measures to deal with the threat.*

ASSESSMENT DATA

- Decreased attention span
- Restlessness, irritability
- Poor impulse control
- Feelings of discomfort, apprehension, or helplessness
- Hyperactivity, pacing
- Wringing hands
- Perceptual field deficits
- Decreased ability to communicate verbally

In addition, in panic anxiety

- Inability to discriminate harmful stimuli or situations
- Disorganized thought processes
- Delusions

EXPECTED OUTCOMES

Immediate

The client will

- Be free from injury
- Discuss feelings of dread, anxiety, and so forth
- Respond to relaxation techniques with a decreased anxiety level

Stabilization

The client will

- Demonstrate the ability to perform relaxation techniques
- Reduce own anxiety level

Community

The client will

- Be free from anxiety attacks
- Manage the anxiety response to stress effectively

IMPLEMENTATION

Nursing Interventions *denotes collaborative interventions	**Rationale**
Remain with the client at all times when levels of anxiety are high (severe or panic).	The client's safety is a priority. A highly anxious client should not be left alone—his or her anxiety will escalate.
Move the client to a quiet area with minimal or decreased stimuli such as a small room or seclusion area.	Anxious behavior can be escalated by external stimuli. In a large area, the client can feel lost and panicked, but a smaller room can enhance a sense of security.
Remain calm in your approach to the client.	The client will feel more secure if you are calm and if the client feels you are in control of the situation.
Use short, simple, and clear statements.	The client's ability to deal with abstractions or complexity is impaired.
Avoid asking or forcing the client to make choices.	The client may not make sound decisions or may be unable to make decisions or solve problems.
PRN medications may be indicated for high levels of anxiety, delusions, disorganized thoughts, and so forth.	Medication may be necessary to decrease anxiety to a level at which the client can feel safe.
Be aware of your own feelings and level of discomfort.	Anxiety is communicated interpersonally. Being with an anxious client can raise your own anxiety level.

continued ⋯⟡

Nursing Care Plan: Anxious Behavior, cont.

IMPLEMENTATION

Nursing Interventions *denotes collaborative interventions	**Rationale**
Encourage the client's participation in relaxation exercises such as deep breathing, progressive muscle relaxation, meditation, and imagining being in a quiet, peaceful place.	Relaxation exercises are effective, nonchemical ways to reduce anxiety.
Teach the client to use relaxation techniques independently.	Using relaxation techniques can give the client confidence in having control over anxiety.
Help the client see that mild anxiety can be a positive catalyst for change and does not need to be avoided.	The client may feel that all anxiety is bad and not useful.

Adapted from Schultz, J. M., & Videbeck, S. L. (2005). Lippincott's manual of psychiatric care plans (7th ed.). Philadelphia: Lippincott Williams & Wilkins.

RELATED DISORDERS

Anxiety disorder due to a general medical condition is diagnosed when the prominent symptoms of anxiety are judged to result directly from a physiologic condition. The person may have panic attacks, generalized anxiety, or obsessions or compulsions. Medical conditions causing this disorder can include endocrine dysfunction, chronic obstructive pulmonary disease, congestive heart failure, and neurologic conditions.

Substance-induced anxiety disorder is anxiety directly caused by drug abuse, a medication, or exposure to a toxin. Symptoms include prominent anxiety, panic attacks, phobias, obsessions, or compulsions.

Separation anxiety disorder is excessive anxiety concerning separation from home or from persons, parents, or caregivers to whom the client is attached. It occurs when it is no longer developmentally appropriate and before 18 years of age.

Adjustment disorder is an emotional response to a stressful event, such as one involving financial issues, medical illness, or a relationship problem, that results in clinically significant symptoms such as marked distress or impaired functioning.

ETIOLOGY

Biologic Theories

GENETIC THEORIES

Anxiety may have an inherited component because first-degree relatives of clients with increased anxiety have higher rates of developing anxiety. *Heritability* refers to the proportion of a disorder that can be attributed to genetic factors:

• High heritabilities are greater than 0.6 and indicate that genetic influences dominate.

• Moderate heritabilities are 0.3 to 0.5 and suggest an even greater influence of genetic and nongenetic factors.
• Heritabilities less than 0.3 mean that genetics are negligible as a primary cause of the disorder.

Panic disorder and social and specific phobias, including agoraphobia, have moderate heritability. GAD and OCD tend to be more common in families, indicating a strong genetic component, but still require further in-depth study (McMahon & Kassem, 2005). At this point, current research indicates a clear genetic susceptibility to or vulnerability for anxiety disorders; however, additional factors are necessary for these disorders to actually develop.

NEUROCHEMICAL THEORIES

Gamma-aminobutyric acid (γ-aminobutyric acid; GABA) is the amino acid neurotransmitter believed to be dysfunctional in anxiety disorders. GABA, an inhibitory neurotransmitter, functions as the body's natural antianxiety agent by reducing cell excitability, thus decreasing the rate of neuronal firing. It is available in one third of the nerve synapses, especially those in the limbic system and in the locus ceruleus, the area where the neurotransmitter norepinephrine, which excites cellular function, is produced. Because GABA reduces anxiety and norepinephrine increases it, researchers believe that a problem with the regulation of these neurotransmitters occurs in anxiety disorders.

Serotonin, the indolamine neurotransmitter usually implicated in psychosis and mood disorders, has many subtypes. 5-Hydroxytryptamine type 1a plays a role in anxiety, and it also affects aggression and mood. Serotonin is believed to play a distinct role in OCD, panic disorder, and GAD. An excess of norepinephrine is suspected in panic disorder, GAD, and posttraumatic stress disorder (Neumeister et al., 2005).

Psychodynamic Theories

INTRAPSYCHIC/PSYCHOANALYTIC THEORIES

Freud (1936) saw a person's innate anxiety as the stimulus for behavior. He described defense mechanisms as the human's attempt to control awareness of and to reduce anxiety (see Chapter 3). **Defense mechanisms** are cognitive distortions that a person uses unconsciously to maintain a sense of being in control of a situation, to lessen discomfort, and to deal with stress. Because defense mechanisms arise from the unconscious, the person is unaware of using them. Some people overuse defense mechanisms, which stops them from learning a variety of appropriate methods to resolve anxiety-producing situations. The dependence on one or two defense mechanisms also can inhibit emotional growth, lead to poor problem-solving skills, and create difficulty with relationships.

INTERPERSONAL THEORY

Harry Stack Sullivan (1952) viewed anxiety as being generated from problems in interpersonal relationships. Caregivers can communicate anxiety to infants or children through inadequate nurturing, agitation when holding or handling the child, and distorted messages. Such communicated anxiety can result in dysfunction such as failure to achieve age-appropriate developmental tasks. In adults, anxiety arises from the person's need to conform to the norms and values of his or her cultural group. The higher the level of anxiety, the lower the ability to communicate and to solve problems and the greater chance for anxiety disorders to develop.

Hildegard Peplau (1952) understood that humans exist in interpersonal and physiologic realms; thus, the nurse can better help the client to achieve health by attending to both areas. She identified the four levels of anxiety and developed nursing interventions and interpersonal communication techniques based on Sullivan's interpersonal view of anxiety. Nurses today use Peplau's interpersonal therapeutic communication techniques to develop and to nurture the nurse–client relationship and to apply the nursing process.

BEHAVIORAL THEORY

Behavioral theorists view anxiety as being learned through experiences. Conversely, people can change or "unlearn" behaviors through new experiences. Behaviorists believe that people can modify maladaptive behaviors without gaining insight into the causes for them. They contend that disturbing behaviors that develop and interfere with a person's life can be extinguished or unlearned by repeated experiences guided by a trained therapist.

CULTURAL CONSIDERATIONS

Each culture has rules governing the appropriate ways to express and deal with anxiety. Culturally competent nurses should be aware of them while being careful not to stereotype clients.

People from Asian cultures often express anxiety through somatic symptoms such as headaches, backaches, fatigue, dizziness, and stomach problems. One intense anxiety reaction is *koro,* or a man's profound fear that his penis will retract into the abdomen and he will then die. Accepted forms of treatment include having the person firmly hold his penis until the fear passes, often with assistance from family members or friends, and clamping the penis to a wooden box. In women, *koro* is the fear that the vulva and nipples will disappear (Spector, 2004).

Susto is diagnosed in some Hispanics (Peruvians, Bolivians, Colombians, and Central and South American Indians) during cases of high anxiety, sadness, agitation, weight loss, weakness, and heart rate changes. The symptoms are believed to occur because supernatural spirits or bad air from dangerous places and cemeteries invades the body.

TREATMENT

Treatment for anxiety disorders usually involves medication and therapy. This combination produces better results than either one alone (Charney, 2005). Drugs used to treat anxiety disorders are listed in Table 13.3. Antidepressants are discussed in detail in Chapter 15. Cognitive-behavioral therapy is used successfully to treat anxiety disorders. **Positive reframing** means turning negative messages into positive messages. The therapist teaches the person to create positive messages for use during panic episodes. For example, instead of thinking, "My heart is pounding. I think I'm going to die!" the client thinks, "I can stand this. This is just anxiety. It will go away." The client can write down these messages and keep them readily accessible such as in an address book, calendar, or wallet.

Decatastrophizing involves the therapist's use of questions to more realistically appraise the situation. The therapist may ask, "What is the worst thing that could happen? Is that likely? Could you survive that? Is that as bad as you imagine?" The client uses thought-stopping and distraction techniques to jolt him or herself from focusing on negative thoughts. Splashing the face with cold water, snapping a rubber band worn on the wrist, or shouting are all techniques that can break the cycle of negative thoughts.

Assertiveness training helps the person take more control over life situations. Techniques help the person negotiate interpersonal situations and foster self-assurance. They involve using "I" statements to identify feelings and to communicate concerns or needs to others. Examples include "I feel angry when you turn your back while I'm talking," "I want to have 5 minutes of your time for an uninterrupted conversation about something important," and "I would like to have about 30 minutes in the evening to relax without interruption."

Table 13.3 DRUGS USED TO TREAT ANXIETY DISORDERS

Drug Name Generic (Trade)	Classification	Used to Treat
Alprazolam (Xanax)	Benzodiazepine	Anxiety, panic disorder, OCD, social phobia, agoraphobia
Buspirone (BuSpar)	Nonbenzodiazepine anxiolytic	Anxiety, OCD, social phobia, GAD
Chlorazepate (Tranxene)	Benzodiazepine	Anxiety
Chlordiazepoxide (Librium)	Benzodiazepine	Anxiety
Clomipramine (Anafranil)	Tricyclic antidepressant	OCD
Clonazepam (Klonopin)	Benzodiazepine	Anxiety, panic disorder, OCD
Clonidine (Catapres)	Beta-blocker	Anxiety, panic disorder
Diazepam (Valium)	Benzodiazepine	Anxiety, panic disorder
Fluoxetine (Prozac)	SSRI antidepressant	Panic disorder, OCD, GAD
Fluvoxamine (Luvox)	SSRI antidepressant	OCD
Hydroxyzine (Vistaril, Atarax)	Antihistamine	Anxiety
Imipramine (Tofranil)	Tricyclic antidepressant	Anxiety, panic disorder, agoraphobia
Meprobamate (Miltown, Equanil)	Nonbenzodiazepine anxiolytic	Anxiety
Oxazepam (Serax)	Benzodiazepine	Anxiety
Paroxetine (Paxil)	SSRI antidepressant	Social phobia, GAD
Propranolol (Inderal)	Alpha-adrenergic agonist	Anxiety, panic disorder, GAD
Sertraline (Zoloft)	SSRI antidepressant	Panic disorder, OCD, social phobia, GAD

GAD, generalized anxiety disorder; OCD, obsessive-compulsive disorder; SSRI, selective serotonin reuptake inhibitor

ELDER CONSIDERATIONS

Anxiety that starts for the first time in late life is frequently associated with another condition such as depression, dementia, physical illness, or medication toxicity or withdrawal. Phobias, particularly agoraphobia, and GAD are the most common late-life anxiety disorders. Most people with late-onset agoraphobia attribute the start of the disorder to the abrupt onset of a physical illness or as a response to a traumatic event such as a fall or mugging. Late-onset GAD is usually associated with depression. Though less common, panic attacks can occur in later life and are often related to depression or a physical illness such as cardiovascular, gastrointestinal, or chronic pulmonary diseases. Ruminative thoughts are common in late-life depression and can take the form of obsessions such as contamination fears, pathologic doubt, or fear of harming others. The treatment of choice for anxiety disorders in the elderly is selective serotonin reuptake inhibitor (SSRI) antidepressants. Initial treatment involves doses lower than the usual starting doses for adults to ensure the elderly client can tolerate the medication: if started on too high a dose, SSRIs can exacerbate anxiety symptoms in elderly clients (Flint, 2004).

COMMUNITY-BASED CARE

Nurses encounter many people with anxiety disorders in community settings rather than in inpatient settings. Formal treatment for these clients usually occurs in community mental health clinics and in the offices of physicians, psychiatric clinical specialists, psychologists, or other mental health counselors. Because the person with an anxiety disorder often believes the sporadic symptoms are related to medical problems, the family practitioner or advanced practice nurse can be the first health care professional to evaluate him or her.

Knowledge of community resources helps the nurse guide the client to appropriate referrals for assessment, diagnosis, and treatment. The nurse can refer the client to a psychiatrist or to an advanced practice psychiatric nurse for diagnosis, therapy, and medication. Other community resources such as anxiety disorder groups or self-help groups can provide support and help the client feel less isolated and lonely.

MENTAL HEALTH PROMOTION

Too often, anxiety is viewed negatively as something to avoid at all costs. Actually, for many people, anxiety is a warning they are not dealing with stress effectively. Learning to heed this warning and to make needed changes is a healthy way to deal with the stress of daily events.

Stress and resulting anxiety are not associated exclusively with life problems. Events that are "positive" or desired, such as going away to college, getting a first job, getting married, and having children, are stressful and cause anxiety. Managing the effects of stress and anxiety in one's life is important to being healthy. Tips for managing stress include the following:

- Keep a positive attitude and believe in yourself.
- Accept there are events you cannot control.
- Communicate assertively with others.

- Talk about your feelings to others.
- Express your feelings through laughing, crying, and so forth.
- Learn to relax.
- Exercise regularly.
- Eat well-balanced meals.
- Limit intake of caffeine and alcohol.
- Get enough rest and sleep.
- Set realistic goals and expectations.
  - Find an activity that is personally meaningful.
- Learn stress management techniques such as relaxation, guided imagery, and meditation; practice them as part of your daily routine.

For people with anxiety disorders, it is important to emphasize that the goal is effective management of stress and anxiety, not the total elimination of anxiety. Although medication is important to relieve excessive anxiety, it does not solve or eliminate the problem entirely. Learning anxiety management techniques and effective methods for coping with life and its stresses is essential for overall improvement in life quality.

PANIC DISORDER

Panic disorder is composed of discrete episodes of **panic attacks,** that is, 15 to 30 minutes of rapid, intense, escalating anxiety in which the person experiences great emotional fear as well as physiologic discomfort. During a panic attack, the person has overwhelmingly intense anxiety and displays four or more of the following symptoms: palpitations, sweating, tremors, shortness of breath, sense of suffocation, chest pain, nausea, abdominal distress, dizziness, paresthesias, chills, or hot flashes.

Panic disorder is diagnosed when the person has recurrent, unexpected panic attacks followed by at least 1 month of persistent concern or worry about future attacks or their meaning or a significant behavioral change related to them. Slightly more than 75% of people with panic disorder have spontaneous initial attacks with no environmental trigger. Half of those with panic disorder have accompanying agoraphobia. Panic disorder is more common in people who have not graduated from college and are not married. The risk increases by 18% in people with depression (Merikangas, 2005).

Clinical Course

The onset of panic disorder peaks in late adolescence and the mid-30s. Although **panic anxiety** might be normal in someone experiencing a life-threatening situation, a person with panic disorder experiences these emotional and physiologic responses without this stimulus. The memory of the panic attack coupled with the fear of having more can lead to **avoidance behavior.** In some cases, the person becomes homebound or stays in a limited area near home such as on the block or within town limits. This behavior is known as **agoraphobia** ("fear of the marketplace" or fear of being

outside). Some people with agoraphobia fear stepping outside the front door because a panic attack may occur as soon as they leave the house. Others can leave the house but feel safe from the anticipatory fear of having a panic attack only within a limited area. Agoraphobia also can occur alone without panic attacks.

The behavior patterns of people with agoraphobia clearly demonstrate the concepts of primary and secondary gain associated with many anxiety disorders. **Primary gain** is the relief of anxiety achieved by performing the specific anxiety-driven behavior such as staying in the house to avoid the anxiety of leaving a safe place. **Secondary gain** is the attention received from others as a result of these behaviors. For instance, the person with agoraphobia may receive attention and caring concern from family members, who also assume all the responsibilities of family life outside the home (e.g., work, shopping). Essentially, these compassionate significant others become enablers of the self-imprisonment of the person with agoraphobia.

Treatment

Panic disorder is treated with cognitive-behavioral techniques, deep breathing and relaxation, and medications such as benzodiazepines, SSRI antidepressants, tricyclic antidepressants, and antihypertensives such as clonidine (Catapres) and propranolol (Inderal).

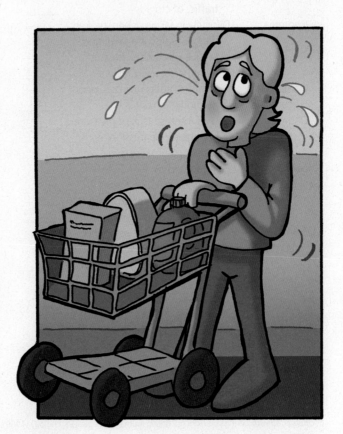

Panic attack

APPLICATION OF THE NURSING PROCESS: PANIC DISORDER

Assessment

Box 13.1 presents the Hamilton Rating Scale for Anxiety. The nurse can use this tool along with the following detailed discussion to guide his or her assessment of the client with panic disorder.

HISTORY

The client usually seeks treatment for panic disorder after he or she has experienced several panic attacks. The client

---

Box 13.1 HAMILTON RATING SCALE FOR ANXIETY

Instructions: This checklist is to assist the physician or psychiatrist in evaluating each patient as to his or her degree of anxiety and pathological condition. Please fill in the appropriate rating:

NONE = 0   MILD = 1   MODERATE = 2   SEVERE = 3   SEVERE, GROSSLY DISABLING = 4

Item		Rating	Item		Rating
Anxious mood	Worries, anticipation of the worst, fearful anticipation, irritability	_____	Cardiovascular symptoms	Tachycardia, palpitations, pain in chest, throbbing of vessels, fainting feelings, missing beat	_____
Tension	Feelings of tension, fatigability, startle response, moved to tears easily, trembling, feelings of restlessness, inability to relax	_____	Respiratory symptoms	Pressure or constriction in chest, choking feelings, sighing, dyspnea	_____
Fears	Of dark, of strangers, of being left alone, of animals, of traffic, of crowds	_____	Gastrointestinal symptoms	Difficulty in swallowing, wind, abdominal pain, burning sensations, abdominal fullness, nausea, vomiting, borborygmi, looseness of bowels, loss of weight, constipation	_____
Insomnia	Difficulty in falling asleep, broken sleep, unsatisfying sleep and fatigue on waking, dreams, nightmares, night terrors	_____	Genitourinary symptoms	Frequency of micturition, urgency of micturition, amenorrhea, menorrhagia, development of frigidity, premature ejaculation, loss of libido, impotence	
Intellectual (cognitive)	Difficulty in concentration, poor memory	_____			_____
Depressed mood	Loss of interest, lack of pleasure in hobbies, depression, early waking, diurnal swing	_____			
Somatic (muscular)	Pains and aches, twitching, stiffness, myoclonic jerks, grinding of teeth, unsteady voice, increased muscular tone	_____	Autonomic symptoms	Dry mouth, flushing, pallor, tendency to sweat, giddiness, tension headache, raising of hair	_____
Somatic (sensory)	Tinnitus, blurring of vision, hot and cold flushes, feelings of weakness, picking sensation	_____	Behavior at interview	Fidgeting, restlessness or pacing, tremor of hands, furrowed brow, strained face, sighing or rapid respiration, facial pallor, swallowing, belching, brisk tendon jerks, dilated pupils, exophthalmos	_____

Additional Comments:

Investigator's Signature:

_____

CLINICAL VIGNETTE: PANIC DISORDER

Nancy spent as much time in her friend Jen's condo as she did in her own home. It was at Jen's place that Nancy had her first panic attack. For no reason at all, she felt the walls closing in on her, no air to breathe, and her heart pounding out of her chest. She needed to get out—Hurry! Run!—so she could live. While a small, still-rational part of her mind assured her there was no reason to run, the need to flee was overwhelming. She ran out of the apartment and down the hall, repeatedly smashing the elevator button with the heel of her hand in hopes of instant response. "What if the elevator doesn't come?" Where were the stairs she so desperately wanted but couldn't find?

The elevator door slid open. Scurrying into the elevator and not realizing she had been holding her breath, Nancy exhaled with momentary relief. She had the faint perception of someone following her to ask, "What's wrong?" She couldn't answer! She still couldn't breathe. She held onto the rail on the wall of the elevator because it was the only way to keep herself from falling. "Breathe," she told herself as she forced herself to inhale. She searched for the right button to push, the one for the ground floor. She couldn't make a mistake, couldn't push the wrong button, couldn't have the elevator take more time, because she might not make it. Heart pounding, no air, run, run!!! When the elevator doors opened, she ran outside and then bent forward, her hands on her knees. It took 5 minutes for her to realize she was safe and would be all right. Sliding onto a bench, breathing more easily, she sat there long enough for her heart rate to decrease. Exhausted and scared, she wondered, "Am I having a heart attack? Am I going crazy? What's happening to me?"

Instead of returning to Jen's, Nancy walked across the street to her own apartment. She couldn't face going into Jen's place until she recovered. She sincerely hoped she would never have this happen to her again; in fact, it might not be a good idea to go to Jen's for a few days. As she sat in her apartment, she thought about what had happened to her that afternoon and how to prevent it from ever happening again.

may report, "I feel like I'm going crazy. I thought I was having a heart attack, but the doctor says it's anxiety." Usually, the client cannot identify any trigger for these events.

GENERAL APPEARANCE AND MOTOR BEHAVIOR

The nurse assesses the client's general appearance and motor behavior. The client may appear entirely "normal" or may have signs of anxiety if he or she is apprehensive about having a panic attack in the next few moments. If the client is anxious, speech may increase in rate, pitch, and volume, and he or she may have difficulty sitting in a chair. **Automatisms**, which are automatic, unconscious mannerisms, may be apparent. Examples include tapping fingers, jingling keys, or twisting hair. Automatisms are geared toward anxiety relief and increase in frequency and intensity with the client's anxiety level.

MOOD AND AFFECT

Assessment of mood and affect may reveal that the client is anxious, worried, tense, depressed, serious, or sad. When discussing the panic attacks, the client may be tearful. He or she may express anger at himself or herself for being "unable to control myself." Most clients are distressed about the intrusion of anxiety attacks in their lives. During a panic attack, the client may describe feelings of being disconnected from himself or herself (**depersonalization**) or sensing that things are not real (**derealization**).

THOUGHT PROCESSES AND CONTENT

During a panic attack, the client is overwhelmed, believing that he or she is dying, losing control, or "going insane."

The client may even consider suicide. Thoughts are disorganized, and the client loses the ability to think rationally. At other times, the client may be consumed with worry about when the next panic attack will occur or how to deal with it.

SENSORIUM AND INTELLECTUAL PROCESSES

During a panic attack, the client may become confused and disoriented. He or she cannot take in environmental cues and respond appropriately. These functions are restored to normal after the panic attack subsides.

JUDGMENT AND INSIGHT

Judgment is suspended during panic attacks; in an effort to escape, the person can run out of a building and into the street in front of a speeding car before the ability to assess safety has returned. Insight into panic disorder occurs only after the client has been educated about the disorder. Even then, clients initially believe they are helpless and have no control over their anxiety attacks.

SELF-CONCEPT

It is important for the nurse to assess self-concept in clients with panic disorder. These clients often make self-blaming statements such as "I can't believe I'm so weak and out of control" or "I used to be a happy, well-adjusted person." They may evaluate themselves negatively in all aspects of their lives. They may find themselves consumed with worry about impending attacks and unable to do many things they did before having panic attacks.

ROLES AND RELATIONSHIPS

Because of the intense anticipation of having another panic attack, the person may report alterations in his or her social, occupational, or family life. The person typically avoids people, places, and events associated with previous panic attacks. For example, the person may no longer ride the bus if he or she has had a panic attack on a bus. Although avoiding these objects does not stop the panic attacks, the person's sense of helplessness is so great that he or she may take even more restrictive measures to avoid them, such as quitting work and remaining at home.

PHYSIOLOGIC AND SELF-CARE CONCERNS

The client often reports problems with sleeping and eating. The anxiety of apprehension between panic attacks may interfere with adequate, restful sleep even though the person may spend hours in bed. Clients may experience loss of appetite or eat constantly in an attempt to ease the anxiety.

Data Analysis

The following nursing diagnoses may apply to the client with panic disorder:
- Risk for Injury
- Anxiety
- Situational Low Self-Esteem (panic attacks)
- Ineffective Coping
- Powerlessness
- Ineffective Role Performance
- Disturbed Sleep Pattern

Outcome Identification

Outcomes for clients with panic disorders include the following:
- The client will be free from injury.
- The client will verbalize feelings.
- The client will demonstrate use of effective coping mechanisms.
- The client will demonstrate effective use of methods to manage anxiety response.
- The client will verbalize a sense of personal control.
- The client will reestablish adequate nutritional intake.
- The client will sleep at least 6 hours per night.

Intervention

PROMOTING SAFETY AND COMFORT

During a panic attack, the nurse's first concern is to provide a safe environment and to ensure the client's privacy. If the environment is overstimulating, the client should move to a less stimulating place. A quiet place reduces anxiety and provides privacy for the client.

NURSING INTERVENTIONS FOR PANIC DISORDER

- Provide a safe environment and ensure client's privacy during a panic attack.
- Remain with the client during a panic attack.
- Help client to focus on deep breathing.
- Talk to client in a calm, reassuring voice.
- Teach client to use relaxation techniques.
- Help client to use cognitive restructuring techniques.
- Engage client to explore how to decrease stressors and anxiety-provoking situations.

The nurse remains with the client to help calm him or her down and to assess client behaviors and concerns. After getting the client's attention, the nurse uses a soothing, calm voice and gives brief directions to assure the client that he or she is safe:

"John, look around. It's safe, and I'm here with you. Nothing is going to happen. Take a deep breath."

Reassurances and a calm demeanor can help to reduce anxiety. When the client feels out of control, the nurse can let the client know that the nurse is in control until the client regains self-control.

USING THERAPEUTIC COMMUNICATION

Clients with anxiety disorders can collaborate with the nurse in the assessment and planning of their care; thus, rapport between nurse and client is important. Communication should be simple and calm because the client with severe anxiety cannot pay attention to lengthy messages and may pace to release energy. The nurse can walk with the client who feels unable to sit and talk. The nurse should evaluate carefully the use of touch because clients with high anxiety may interpret touch by a stranger as a threat and pull away abruptly.

As the client's anxiety diminishes, cognition begins to return. When anxiety has subsided to a manageable level, the nurse uses open-ended communication techniques to discuss the experience:

Nurse: *"It seems your anxiety is subsiding. Is that correct?" or "Can you share with me what it was like a few minutes ago?"*

At this point, the client can discuss his or her emotional responses to physiologic processes and behaviors and can try to regain a sense of control.

MANAGING ANXIETY

The nurse can teach the client relaxation techniques to use when he or she is experiencing stress or anxiety. Deep breathing is simple; anyone can do it. Guided imagery and progressive relaxation are methods to relax taut muscles: Guided imagery involves imagining a safe, enjoyable place to relax. In progressive relaxation, the person progressively tightens, holds, and then relaxes muscle groups while letting tension flow from the body through rhythmic breathing. Cognitive restructuring techniques (discussed earlier) also may help the client to manage his or her anxiety response.

For any of these techniques, it is important for the client to learn and to practice them when he or she is relatively calm. When adept at these techniques, the client is more likely to use them successfully during panic attacks or periods of increased anxiety. Clients are likely to believe that self-control is returning when using these techniques helps them to manage anxiety. When clients believe they can manage the panic attack, they spend less time worrying about and anticipating the next one, which reduces their overall anxiety level.

PROVIDING CLIENT AND FAMILY EDUCATION

Client and family education is of primary importance when working with clients who have anxiety disorders. The client learns ways to manage stress and to cope with reactions to stress and stress-provoking situations. With education about the efficacy of combined psychotherapy and medication and the effects of the prescribed medication, the client can become the chief treatment manager of the anxiety disorder. It is important for the nurse to educate the client and family members about the physiology of anxiety and the merits of using combined psychotherapy and drug management. Such a combined treatment approach along with stress-reduction techniques can help the client to manage these drastic reactions and allow him or her to gain a sense of self-control. The nurse should help the client to understand that these therapies and drugs do not "cure" the disorder but are methods to help him or her to control and manage it. Client and family education regarding medications should include the recommended dosage and dosage regimen, expected effects, side effects and how to handle them, and substances that have a synergistic or antagonistic effect with the drug.

The nurse encourages the client to exercise regularly. Routine exercise helps to metabolize adrenaline, reduces panic reactions, and increases production of endorphins; all these activities increase feelings of well-being.

Evaluation

Evaluation of the plan of care must be individualized. Ongoing assessment provides data to determine whether the client's outcomes were achieved. The client's perception of the success of treatment also plays a part in eval-uation. Even if all outcomes are achieved, the nurse must ask if the client is comfortable or satisfied with the quality of life.

Evaluation of the treatment of panic disorder is based on the following:
- Does the client understand the prescribed medication regimen, and is he or she committed to adhering to it?
- Have the client's episodes of anxiety decreased in frequency or intensity?
- Does the client understand various coping methods and when to use them?
- Does the client believe that his or her quality of life is satisfactory?

PHOBIAS

A **phobia** is an illogical, intense, persistent fear of a specific object or a social situation that causes extreme distress and interferes with normal functioning. Phobias usually do not result from past negative experiences. In fact, the person may never have had contact with the object of the phobia. People with phobias understand that their fear is unusual and irrational and may even joke about how "silly" it is. Nevertheless, they feel powerless to stop it (Andreasen & Black, 2006).

People with phobias develop anticipatory anxiety even when thinking about possibly encountering the dreaded phobic object or situation. They engage in avoidance behavior that often severely limits their lives. Such avoidance behavior usually does not relieve the anticipatory anxiety for long.

There are three categories of phobias:
- Agoraphobia (discussed earlier)
- Specific phobia, which is an irrational fear of an object or situation
- Social phobia, which is anxiety provoked by certain social or performance situations

---

CLIENT/FAMILY EDUCATION FOR PANIC DISORDER

- Review breathing control and relaxation techniques.
- Discuss positive coping strategies.
- Encourage regular exercise.
- Emphasize the importance of maintaining prescribed medication regimen and regular follow-up.
- Describe time management techniques such as creating "to do" lists with realistic estimated deadlines for each activity, crossing off completed items for a sense of accomplishment, and saying "no."
- Stress the importance of maintaining contact with community and participating in supportive organizations.

Many people express "phobias" about snakes, spiders, rats, or similar objects. These fears are very specific, easy to avoid, and cause no anxiety or worry. The diagnosis of a phobic disorder is made only when the phobic behavior significantly interferes with the person's life by creating marked distress or difficulty in interpersonal or occupational functioning.

Specific phobias are subdivided into the following categories:

- Natural environmental phobias: fear of storms, water, heights, or other natural phenomena
- Blood-injection phobias: fear of seeing one's own or others' blood, traumatic injury, or an invasive medical procedure such as an injection
- Situational phobias: fear of being in a specific situation such as on a bridge or in a tunnel, elevator, small room, hospital, or airplane
- Animal phobia: fear of animals or insects (usually a specific type). Often this fear develops in childhood and can continue through adulthood in both men and women. Cats and dogs are the most common phobic objects.
- Other types of specific phobias: for example, fear of getting lost while driving if not able to make all right (and no left) turns to get to one's destination

In *social phobia*, also known as *social anxiety disorder*, the person becomes severely anxious to the point of panic or incapacitation when confronting situations involving people. Examples include making a speech, attending a social engagement alone, interacting with the opposite sex or with strangers, and making complaints. The fear is rooted in low self-esteem and concern about others' judgments. The person fears looking socially inept, appearing anxious, or doing something embarrassing such as burping or spilling food. Other social phobias include fear of eating in public, using public bathrooms, writing in public, or becoming the center of attention. A person may have one or several social phobias; the latter is known as generalized social phobia (Culpepper, 2006).

Onset and Clinical Course

Specific phobias usually occur in childhood or adolescence. In some cases, merely thinking about or handling a plastic model of the dreaded object can create fear. Specific phobias that persist into adulthood are lifelong 80% of the time.

The peak age of onset for social phobia is middle adolescence; it sometimes emerges in a person who was shy as a child. The course of social phobia is often continuous, although the disorder may become less severe during adulthood. Severity of impairment fluctuates with life stress and demands.

Treatment

Behavioral therapy works well. Behavioral therapists initially focus on teaching what anxiety is, helping the client to identify anxiety responses, teaching relaxation techniques, setting goals, discussing methods to achieve those goals, and helping the client to visualize phobic situations. Therapies that help the client to develop self-esteem and self-control are common and include positive reframing and assertiveness training (explained earlier).

One behavioral therapy often used to treat phobias is **systematic** (serial) **desensitization,** in which the therapist progressively exposes the client to the threatening object in a safe setting until the client's anxiety decreases. During each exposure, the complexity and intensity of exposure gradually increase, but the client's anxiety decreases. The reduced anxiety serves as a positive reinforcement until the anxiety is ultimately eliminated. For example, for the client who fears flying, the therapist would encourage the client to hold a small model airplane while talking about his or her experiences; later, the client would hold a larger model airplane and talk about flying. Even later exposures might include walking past an airport, sitting in a parked airplane, and, finally, taking a short ride in a plane. Each session's challenge is based on the success achieved in previous sessions (Andreasen & Black, 2006).

Flooding is a form of rapid desensitization in which a behavioral therapist confronts the client with the phobic object (either a picture or the actual object) until it no longer produces anxiety. Because the client's worst fear has been realized and the client did not die, there is little rea-

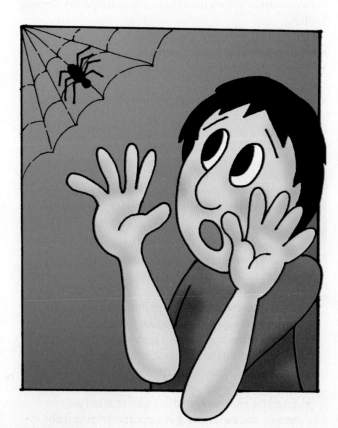

Specific phobias

son to fear the situation anymore. The goal is to rid the client of the phobia in one or two sessions. This method is highly anxiety producing and should be conducted only by a trained psychotherapist under controlled circumstances and with the client's consent.

Drugs used to treat phobias are listed in Table 13.3.

OBSESSIVE-COMPULSIVE DISORDER

Obsessions are recurrent, persistent, intrusive, and unwanted thoughts, images, or impulses that cause marked anxiety and interfere with interpersonal, social, or occupational function. The person knows these thoughts are excessive or unreasonable but believes he or she has no control over them. **Compulsions** are ritualistic or repetitive behaviors or mental acts that a person carries out continuously in an attempt to neutralize anxiety. Usually, the theme of the ritual is associated with that of the obsession, such as repetitive hand-washing when someone is obsessed with contamination or repeated prayers or confession for someone obsessed with blasphemous thoughts. Common compulsions include the following:

- Checking rituals (repeatedly making sure the door is locked or the coffee pot is turned off)
- Counting rituals (each step taken, ceiling tiles, concrete blocks, desks in a classroom)
- Washing and scrubbing until the skin is raw
- Praying or chanting
- Touching, rubbing, or tapping (feeling the texture of each material in a clothing store; touching people, doors, walls, or oneself)
- Hoarding items (for fear of throwing away something important)
- Ordering (arranging and rearranging furniture or items on a desk or shelf into perfect order; vacuuming the rug pile in one direction)
- Exhibiting rigid performance (getting dressed in an unvarying pattern)
- Having aggressive urges (for instance, to throw one's child against a wall)

Obsessive-compulsive disorder (OCD) is diagnosed only when these thoughts, images, and impulses consume the person or he or she is compelled to act out the behaviors to a point at which they interfere with personal, social, and occupational function. Examples include a man who can no longer work because he spends most of his day aligning and realigning all items in his apartment or a woman who feels compelled to wash her hands after touching any object or person.

OCD can be manifested through many behaviors, all of which are repetitive, meaningless, and difficult to conquer. The person understands that these rituals are unusual and unreasonable but feels forced to perform them to alleviate anxiety or to prevent terrible thoughts. Obsessions and compulsions are a source of distress and shame to the person, who may go to great lengths to keep them secret.

Onset and Clinical Course

OCD can start in childhood, especially in males. In females, it more commonly begins in the twenties. Overall, distribution between the sexes is equal. Onset is usually gradual, although there have been cases of acute onset with periods of waxing and waning symptoms. Exacerbation of symptoms may be related to stress. Eighty percent of those treated with behavior therapy and medication report success in managing obsessions and compulsions, whereas 15% show progressive deterioration in occupational and social functioning (APA, 2000).

Treatment

Like other anxiety disorders, optimal treatment for OCD combines medication and behavior therapy. Table 13.3 lists drugs used to treat OCD. Behavior therapy specifically includes exposure and response prevention: **Exposure** involves assisting the client to deliberately confront the situations and stimuli that he or she usually avoids. **Response prevention** focuses on delaying or avoiding performance of rituals. The person learns to tolerate the anxiety and to recognize that it will recede without the disastrous imagined consequences. Other techniques discussed previously, such as deep breathing and relaxation, also can assist the person to tolerate and eventually manage the anxiety (Geffken et al., 2004).

APPLICATION OF THE NURSING PROCESS: OBSESSIVE-COMPULSIVE DISORDER

Assessment

Box 13.2 presents the Yale-Brown Obsessive-Compulsive Scale. The nurse can use this tool along with the following detailed discussion to guide his or her assessment of the client with OCD.

HISTORY

The client usually seeks treatment only when obsessions become too overwhelming, when compulsions interfere with daily life (e.g., going to work, cooking meals, participating in leisure activities with family or friends), or both. Clients are hospitalized only when they have become completely unable to carry out their daily routines. Most treatment is outpatient. The client often reports that rituals began many years before; some begin as early as childhood. The more responsibility the client has as he or she gets older, the more the rituals interfere with the ability to fulfill those responsibilities.

GENERAL APPEARANCE AND MOTOR BEHAVIOR

The nurse assesses the client's appearance and behavior. Clients with OCD often seem tense, anxious, worried, and

Box 13.2   YALE-BROWN OBSESSIVE-COMPULSIVE SCALE

For each item circle the number identifying the response which best characterizes the patient.

1. Time occupied by obsessive thoughts
   How much of your time is occupied by obsessive thoughts?
   How frequently do the obsessive thoughts occur?
   0 None
   1 Mild (less than 1 h/day) or occasional (intrusion occurring no more than 8 times a day)
   2 Moderate (1–3 h/day) or frequent (intrusion occurring more than 8 times a day, but most of the hours of the day are free of obsessions)
   3 Severe (greater than 3 and up to 8 h/day) or very frequent (intrusion occurring more than 8 times a day and occurring during most of the hours of the day)
   4 Extreme (greater than 8 h/day) or near consistent intrusion (too numerous to count and an hour rarely passes without several obsessions occurring)

2. Interference due to obsessive thoughts
   How much do your obsessive thoughts interfere with your social or work (or role) functioning?
   Is there anything that you don't do because of them?
   0 None
   1 Mild, slight interference with social or occupational activities, but overall performance not impaired
   2 Moderate, definite interference with social or occupational performance but still manageable
   3 Severe, causes substantial impairment in social or occupational performance
   4 Extreme, incapacitating

3. Distress associated with obsessive thoughts
   How much distress do your obsessive thoughts cause you?
   0 None
   1 Mild, infrequent, and not too disturbing
   2 Moderate, frequent, and disturbing but still manageable
   3 Severe, very frequent, and very disturbing
   4 Extreme, near constant, and disabling distress

4. Resistance against obsessions
   How much of an effort do you make to resist the obsessive thoughts?
   How often do you try to disregard or turn your attention away from these thoughts as they enter your mind?
   0 Makes an effort to always resist, or symptoms so minimal doesn't need to actively resist
   1 Tries to resist most of the time
   2 Makes some effort to resist
   3 Yields to all obsessions without attempting to control them, but does so with some reluctance

   4 Completely and willingly yields to all obsessions

5. Degree of control over obsessive thoughts
   How much control do you have over your obsessive thoughts?
   How successful are you in stopping or diverting your obsessive thinking?
   0 Complete control
   1 Much control, usually able to stop or divert obsessions with some effort and concentration
   2 Moderate control, sometimes able to stop or divert obsessions
   3 Little control, rarely successful in stopping obsessions
   4 No control, experienced as completely involuntary, rarely able to even momentarily divert thinking

6. Time spent performing compulsive behaviors
   How much time do you spend performing compulsive behaviors?
   How frequently do you perform compulsions?
   0 None
   1 Mild (less than 1 h/day performing compulsions) or occasional (performance of compulsions occurring no more than 8 times a day)
   2 Moderate (1–3 h/day performing compulsions) or frequent (performance of compulsions occurring more than 8 times a day, but most of the hours of the day are free of compulsive behaviors)
   3 Severe (greater than 3 and up to 8 h/day performing compulsions) or very frequent (performance of compulsions occurring more than 8 times a day and occurring during most of the hours of the day)
   4 Extreme (greater than 8 h/day performing compulsions) or near consistent performance of compulsions (too numerous to count and an hour rarely passes without several compulsions being performed)

7. Interference due to compulsive behaviors
   How much do your compulsive behaviors interfere with your social or work (or role) functioning? Is there anything that you don't do because of the compulsions?
   0 None
   1 Mild, slight interference with social or occupational activities, but overall performance not impaired
   2 Moderate, definite interference with social or occupational performance but still manageable
   3 Severe, causes substantial impairment in social or occupational performance
   4 Extreme, incapacitating

Box 13.2: Yale-Brown Obsessive-Compulsive Scale, cont.

8. Distress associated with compulsive behavior
   How would you feel if prevented from performing your compulsions?
   How anxious would you become? How anxious do you get while performing compulsions until you are satisfied they are completed?
   0 None
   1 Mild, only slightly anxious if compulsions prevented or only slightly anxious during performance of compulsions
   2 Moderate, reports that anxiety would mount but remain manageable if compulsions prevented or that anxiety increases but remains manageable during performance of compulsions
   3 Severe, prominent and very disturbing increase in anxiety if compulsions interrupted or prominent and very disturbing increases in anxiety during performance of compulsions
   4 Extreme, incapacitating anxiety from any intervention aimed at modifying activity or incapacitating anxiety develops during performance of compulsions

9. Resistance against compulsions
   How much of an effort do you make to resist the compulsions?
   0 Makes an effort to always resist, or symptoms so minimal doesn't need to actively resist
   1 Tries to resist most of the time
   2 Makes some effort to resist
   3 Yields to all compulsions without attempting to control them but does so with some reluctance
   4 Completely and willingly yields to all compulsions

10. Degree of control over compulsive behavior
    0 Complete control
    1 Much control, experiences pressure to perform the behavior but usually able to exercise voluntary control over it
    2 Moderate control, strong pressure to perform behavior, can control it only with difficulty
    3 Little control, very strong drive to perform behavior, must be carried to completion, can only delay with difficulty
    4 No control, drive to perform behavior experienced as completely involuntary

Reprinted with permission from Goodman, W. K., Price, L. H., Rasmussen, S. A., et al. (1989). The Yale-Brown Obsessive-Compulsive Scale, I: Development, use, and reliability. Arch Gen Psychiatry, 46, *1006.*

fretful. They may have difficulty relating symptoms because of embarrassment. Their overall appearance is unremarkable, that is, nothing observable seems to be "out of the ordinary." The exception is the client who is almost immobilized by her or his thoughts and the resulting anxiety.

MOOD AND AFFECT

During assessment of mood and affect, clients report ongoing, overwhelming feelings of anxiety in response to the obsessive thoughts, images, or urges. They may look sad and anxious.

THOUGHT PROCESSES AND CONTENT

The nurse explores the client's thought processes and content. Many clients describe the obsessions as arising from nowhere during the middle of normal activities. The harder the client tries to stop the thought or image, the more intense it becomes. The client describes how these obsessions are not what he or she wants to think about and that he or she would never willingly have such ideas or images.

Assessment reveals intact intellectual functioning. The client may describe difficulty concentrating or paying atten-

CLINICAL VIGNETTE: OCD

Sam had just returned home from work. He immediately got undressed and entered the shower. As he showered, he soaped and resoaped his washcloth and rubbed it vigorously over every inch of his body. "I can't miss anything! I must get off all the germs," he kept repeating to himself. He spent 30 minutes scrubbing and scrubbing. As he stepped out of the shower, Sam was very careful to step on the clean, white bath towel on the floor. He dried himself thoroughly, making sure his towel didn't touch the floor or sink. He had intended to put on clean clothes after his shower and fix something to eat. But now he wasn't sure he had gotten clean. He couldn't get dressed if he wasn't clean. Slowly, Sam turned around, got back in the shower, and started all over again.

tion when obsessions are strong. There is no impairment of memory or sensory functioning.

JUDGMENT AND INSIGHT

The nurse examines the client's judgment and insight. The client recognizes that the obsessions are irrational, but he or she cannot stop them. He or she can make sound judgments (e.g., "I know the house is safe") but cannot act on them. The client still engages in ritualistic behavior when the anxiety becomes overwhelming.

SELF-CONCEPT

During exploration of self-concept, the client voices concern that he or she is "going crazy." Feelings of powerlessness to control the obsessions or compulsions contribute to low self-esteem. The client may believe that if he or she were "stronger" or had more will power, he or she could possibly control these thoughts and behaviors.

ROLES AND RELATIONSHIPS

It is important for the nurse to assess the effects of OCD on the client's roles and relationships. As the time spent performing rituals increases, the client's ability to fulfill life roles successfully decreases. Relationships also suffer as family and friends tire of the repetitive behavior, and the client is less available to them as he or she is more consumed with anxiety and ritualistic behavior.

PHYSIOLOGIC AND SELF-CARE CONSIDERATIONS

The nurse examines the effects of OCD on physiology and self-care. As with other anxiety disorders, clients with OCD may have trouble sleeping. Performing rituals may take time away from sleep, or anxiety may interfere with the ability to go to sleep and wake refreshed. Clients also may report a loss of appetite or unwanted weight loss. In severe cases, personal hygiene may suffer because the client cannot complete needed tasks.

Data Analysis

Depending on the particular obsession and its accompanying compulsions, clients have varying symptoms. Nursing diagnoses can include the following:

- Anxiety
- Ineffective Coping
- Fatigue
- Situational Low Self-Esteem
- Impaired Skin Integrity (if scrubbing or washing rituals)

Outcome Identification

Outcomes for clients with OCD include the following:

- The client will complete daily routine activities within a realistic time frame.

- The client will demonstrate effective use of relaxation techniques.
- The client will discuss feelings with another person.
- The client will demonstrate effective use of behavior therapy techniques.
- The client will spend less time performing rituals.

Intervention

USING THERAPEUTIC COMMUNICATION

Offering support and encouragement to the client is important to help him or her manage anxiety responses. The nurse can validate the overwhelming feelings the client experiences while indicating the belief that the client can make needed changes and regain a sense of control. The nurse encourages the client to talk about the feelings and to describe them in as much detail as the client can tolerate. Because many clients try to hide their rituals and to keep obsessions secret, discussing these thoughts, behaviors, and resulting feelings with the nurse is an important step. Doing so can begin to relieve some of the "burden" the client has been keeping to himself or herself.

TEACHING RELAXATION AND BEHAVIORAL TECHNIQUES

The nurse can teach the client about relaxation techniques such as deep breathing, progressive muscle relaxation, and guided imagery. This intervention should take place when the client's anxiety is low so he or she can learn more effectively. Initially, the nurse can demonstrate and practice the techniques with the client. Then, the nurse encourages the client to practice these techniques until he or she is comfortable doing them alone. When the client has mastered relaxation techniques, he or she can begin to use them when anxiety increases. In addition to decreasing anxiety, the client gains an increased sense of control that can lead to improved self-esteem.

To manage anxiety and ritualistic behaviors, a baseline of frequency and duration is necessary. The client can keep a diary to chronicle situations that trigger obsessions, the intensity of the anxiety, the time spent performing rituals, and the avoidance behaviors. This record provides a clear picture for both client and nurse. The client then can begin to use exposure and response prevention behavioral techniques. Initially, the client can decrease the time he or she spends performing the ritual or delay performing the ritual while experiencing anxiety. Eventually, the client can eliminate the ritualistic response or decrease it significantly to the point that interference with daily life is minimal. Clients can use relaxation techniques to assist them in managing and tolerating the anxiety they are experiencing.

It is important to note that the client must be willing to engage in exposure and response prevention. These are not techniques that can be forced on the client.

NURSING INTERVENTIONS FOR OCD

- Offer encouragement, support, and compassion.
- Be clear with the client that you believe he or she can change.
- Encourage the client to talk about feelings, obsessions, and rituals in detail.
- Gradually decrease time for the client to carry out ritualistic behaviors.
- Assist client to use exposure and response prevention behavioral techniques.
- Encourage client to use techniques to manage and tolerate anxiety responses.
- Assist client to complete daily routine and activities within agreed-on time limits.
- Encourage the client to develop and follow a written schedule with specified times and activities.

CLIENT/FAMILY EDUCATION FOR OCD

- Teach about OCD.
- Review the importance of talking openly about obsessions, compulsions, and anxiety.
- Emphasize medication compliance as an important part of treatment.
- Discuss necessary behavioral techniques for managing anxiety and decreasing prominence of obsessions.

COMPLETING A DAILY ROUTINE

To accomplish tasks efficiently, the client initially may need additional time to allow for rituals. For example, if breakfast is at 8:00 AM and the client has a 45-minute ritual before eating, the nurse must plan that time into the client's schedule. It is important for the nurse not to interrupt or to attempt to stop the ritual because doing so will escalate the client's anxiety dramatically. Again, the client must be willing to make changes in his or her behavior. The nurse and client can agree on a plan to limit the time spent performing rituals. They may decide to limit the morning ritual to 40 minutes, then to 35 minutes, and so forth, taking care to decrease this time gradually at a rate the client can tolerate. When the client has completed the ritual or the time allotted has passed, the client then must engage in the expected activity. This may cause anxiety and is a time when the client can use relaxation and stress reduction techniques. At home, the client can continue to follow a daily routine or written schedule that helps him or her to stay on tasks and accomplish activities and responsibilities.

PROVIDING CLIENT AND FAMILY EDUCATION

It is important for both the client and family to learn about OCD. They often are relieved to find the client is not "going crazy" and that the obsessions are unwanted, rather than a reflection of any "dark side" to the client's personality. Helping the client and family to talk openly about the obsessions, anxiety, and rituals eliminates the client's need to keep these things secret and to carry the guilty burden alone. Family members also can better give the client needed emotional support when they are fully informed.

Teaching about the importance of medication compliance to combat OCD is essential. The client may need to try different medications until his or her response is satisfactory. The chances for improved OCD symptoms are enhanced when the client takes medication and uses behavioral techniques.

Evaluation

Treatment has been effective when OCD symptoms no longer interfere with the client's ability to carry out responsibilities. When obsessions occur, the client manages resulting anxiety without engaging in complicated or time-consuming rituals. He or she reports regained control over his or her life and the ability to tolerate and manage anxiety with minimal disruption.

GENERALIZED ANXIETY DISORDER

A person with generalized anxiety disorder (GAD) worries excessively and feels highly anxious at least 50% of the time for 6 months or more. Unable to control this focus on worry, the person has three or more of the following symptoms: uneasiness, irritability, muscle tension, fatigue, difficulty thinking, and sleep alterations. More people with this chronic disorder are seen by family physicians than psychiatrists. The quality of life is diminished greatly in older adults with GAD. Buspirone (BuSpar) and SSRI antidepressants are the most effective treatments (Starcevic, 2006).

POSTTRAUMATIC STRESS DISORDER

Posttraumatic stress disorder can occur in a person who has witnessed an extraordinarily terrifying and potentially deadly event. After the traumatic event, the person re-experiences all or some of it through dreams or waking recollections and responds defensively to these flashbacks. New behaviors develop related to the trauma, such as sleep difficulties, hypervigilance, thinking difficulties, severe startle response, and agitation (APA, 2000; see Chapter 11).

ACUTE STRESS DISORDER

Acute stress disorder is similar to posttraumatic stress disorder in that the person has experienced a traumatic situation but the response is more dissociative. The person has a sense that the event was unreal, believes he or she is unreal, and forgets some aspects of the event through amnesia, emotional detachment, and muddled obliviousness to the environment (APA, 2000).

SELF-AWARENESS ISSUES

Working with people who have anxiety disorders is a different kind of challenge for the nurse. These clients are usually average people in other respects who know that their symptoms are unusual but feel unable to stop them. They experience much frustration and feelings of helplessness and failure. Their lives are out of their control, and they live in fear of the next episode. They go to extreme measures to try to prevent episodes by avoiding people and places where previous events occurred.

It may be difficult for nurses and others to understand why the person cannot simply stop performing the bizarre behaviors interfering with his or her life. Why does the hand-washer who has scrubbed himself raw keep washing his poor sore hands every hour on the hour? Nurses must understand what and how anxiety behaviors work, not just for client care but to help understand the role anxiety plays in performing nursing responsibilities. Nurses are expected to function at a high level and to avoid allowing their own feelings and needs to hinder the care of their clients. But as emotional beings, nurses are just as vulnerable to stress and anxiety as others, and they have needs of their own.

Points to Consider When Working With Clients With Anxiety and Stress-Related Illness

- Remember that everyone occasionally suffers from stress and anxiety that can interfere with daily life and work.
- Avoid falling into the pitfall of trying to "fix" the client's problems.
- Discuss any uncomfortable feelings with a more experienced nurse for suggestions on how to deal with your feelings toward these clients.
- Remember to practice techniques to manage stress and anxiety in your own life.

Critical Thinking Questions

1. Because all people occasionally have anxiety, it is important for nurses to be aware of their own coping mechanisms. Do a self-assessment: What causes you anxiety? What physical, emotional, and cognitive responses occur when you are anxious? What coping mechanisms do you use? Are they healthy?
2. Some clients take benzodiazepine anxiolytics for months or even years even though these medications are designed for short-term use. Why does this happen? What, if anything, should be done for these clients? How would you approach the situation?

KEY POINTS

- Anxiety is a vague feeling of dread or apprehension. It is a response to external or internal stimuli that can have behavioral, emotional, cognitive, and physical symptoms.
- Anxiety has positive and negative side effects. The positive effects produce growth and adaptive change. The negative effects produce poor self-esteem, fear, inhibition, and anxiety disorders (in addition to other disorders).
- The four levels of anxiety are mild anxiety (helps people learn, grow, and change); moderate anxiety (increases focus on the alarm; learning is still possible); severe anxiety (greatly decreases cognitive function, increases preparation for physical responses, increases space needs); and panic (fight, flight, or freeze response; no learning is possible; the person is attempting to free him or herself from the discomfort of this high stage of anxiety).
- Defense mechanisms are intrapsychic distortions that a person uses to feel more in control. It is believed that these defense mechanisms are overused when a person develops an anxiety disorder.
- Current etiologic theories and studies of anxiety disorders have shown a familial incidence and have implicated the neurotransmitters GABA, norepinephrine, and serotonin.
- Treatment for anxiety disorders involves medication (anxiolytics, SSRI and tricyclic antidepressants, and clonidine and propranolol) and therapy.
- Cognitive-behavioral techniques include positive reframing, decatastrophizing, thought stopping, and distraction. Behavioral techniques for OCD include exposure and response prevention.
- In a panic attack, the person feels as if he or she is dying. Symptoms can include palpitations, sweating, tremors, shortness of breath, a sense of suffocation, chest pain, nausea, abdominal distress, dizziness, paresthesias, and vasomotor lability. The person has a fight, flight, or freeze response.
- Phobias are excessive anxiety about being in public or open places (agoraphobia), a specific object, or social situations.
- OCD involves recurrent, persistent, intrusive, and unwanted thoughts, images, or impulses (obsessions) and ritualistic or repetitive behaviors or mental acts (com-

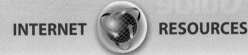

INTERNET RESOURCES

RESOURCE	INTERNET ADDRESS
• Anxiety Disorders Association of America	http://www.adaa.org
• Obsessive–Compulsive Foundation	http://www.ocfoundation.org
• OCD Online Home Page	http://www.ocdonline.com
• Panic Anxiety Disorders Help and Support	http://www.panicdisorder.about.com
• Phobia List	http://www.phobialist.com
• Social Anxiety Network Home Page	http://www.social-anxiety-network.com
• Social Phobia/Social Anxiety Association	http://www.socialphobia.org

pulsions) carried out to eliminate the obsessions or to neutralize anxiety.

- Self-awareness about one's anxiety and responses to it greatly improves both personal and professional relationships.

REFERENCES

American Psychiatric Association. (2000). *DSM-IV-TR: Diagnostic and statistical manual of mental disorders* (4th ed., text revision). Washington, DC: American Psychiatric Association.

Andreasen, N. C., & Black, D. W. (2006). *Introductory textbook of psychiatry* (4th ed.). Washington DC: American Psychiatric Publishing.

Charney, D. S. (2005). Anxiety disorders: Introduction and overview. In B. J. Sadock & V. A. Sadock (Eds.), *Comprehensive textbook of psychiatry* (Vol. 1, 8th ed., pp. 1718–1719). Philadelphia: Lippincott Williams & Wilkins.

Culpepper, L. (2006). Social anxiety disorder in the primary care setting. *Journal of Clinical Psychiatry, 67*(Suppl 12), 31–37.

Flint, A. J. (2004). Anxiety disorders. In J. Sadavoy, L. F. Jarvik, G. T. Grossberg, et al. (Eds.), *Comprehensive textbook of geriatric psychiatry* (3rd ed., pp. 687–699). New York: W. W. Norton and Company.

Freud, S. (1936). *The problem of anxiety.* New York: W. W. Norton.

Geffken, G. R., Storch, E. A., Gelfand, K. M., Adkins, J. W., & Goodman, W. K. (2004). Cognitive-behavioral therapy for obsessive-compulsive disorder: Review of treatment techniques. *Journal of Psychosocial Nursing, 42*(12), 44–51.

McMahon, F. J., & Kassem, L. (2005). Anxiety disorders: Genetics. In B. J. Sadock & V. A. Sadock (Eds.), *Comprehensive textbook of psychiatry* (Vol. 1., 8th ed., pp. 1759–1762). Philadelphia: Lippincott Williams & Wilkins.

Merikangas, K. R. (2005). Anxiety disorders: Epidemiology. In B. J. Sadock & V. A. Sadock (Eds.), *Comprehensive textbook of psychiatry* (Vol. 1, 8th ed., pp. 1720–1728). Philadelphia: Lippincott Williams & Wilkins.

Neumeister, A., Bonne, O., & Charney, D. S. (2005). Anxiety disorders: Neurochemical aspects. In B. J. Sadock & V. A. Sadock (Eds.), *Comprehensive textbook of psychiatry* (Vol. 1, 8th ed., pp. 1739–1748). Philadelphia: Lippincott Williams & Wilkins.

Peplau, H. (1952). *Interpersonal relations.* New York: Putnam.

Schultz, J. M., & Videbeck, S. L. (2005). *Lippincott's manual of psychiatric nursing care plans* (7th ed.). Philadelphia: Lippincott Williams & Wilkins.

Selye, H. (1956). *The stress life.* St. Louis: McGraw-Hill.

Selye, H. (1974). *Stress without distress.* Philadelphia: J. B. Lippincott.

Spector, R. E. (2004). *Cultural diversity in health and illness* (6th ed.). Upper Saddle River, NJ: Prentice-Hall Health.

Starcevic, V. (2006). Anxiety states: A review of conceptual and treatment issues. *Current Opinion in Psychiatry, 19*(1), 79–83.

Sullivan, H. S. (1952). *Interpersonal theory of psychiatry.* New York: W. W. Norton.

ADDITIONAL READINGS

Iancu, I. et. al. (2006). Social phobia symptoms: Prevalence, sociodemographic correlates, and overlap with specific phobia symptoms. *Comprehensive Psychiatry, 47*(5), 399–405.

Mataix-Cois, D., do Rosario-Campos, M. C., & Leckman, J. F. (2005). A multidimensional model of obsessive-compulsive disorder. *American Journal of Psychiatry, 162*(2), 228–238.

Uhlenhuth, E. H., Leon, A. C., & Matuzas, W. (2006). Psychopathology of panic attacks in panic disorder. *Journal of Affective Disorders, 92*(1), 55–62.

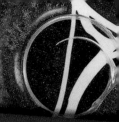

Chapter Study Guide

MULTIPLE-CHOICE QUESTIONS

Select the best answer for each of the following questions.

1. The nurse observes a client who is becoming increasingly upset. He is rapidly pacing, hyperventilating, clenching his jaw, wringing his hands, and trembling. His speech is high-pitched and random; he seems preoccupied with his thoughts. He is pounding his fist into his other hand. The nurse identifies his anxiety level as
   A. Mild
   B. Moderate
   C. Severe
   D. Panic

2. When assessing a client with anxiety, the nurse's questions should be
   A. Avoided until the anxiety is gone
   B. Open ended
   C. Postponed until the client volunteers information
   D. Specific and direct

3. During the assessment, the client tells the nurse that she cannot stop worrying about her appearance and that she often removes "old" makeup and applies fresh makeup every hour or two throughout the day. The nurse identifies this behavior as indicative of a(n)
   A. Acute stress disorder
   B. Generalized anxiety disorder
   C. Panic disorder
   D. Obsessive-compulsive disorder

4. The best goal for a client learning a relaxation technique is that the client will
   A. Confront the source of anxiety directly
   B. Experience anxiety without feeling overwhelmed
   C. Report no episodes of anxiety
   D. Suppress anxious feelings

5. Which of the four classes of medications used for panic disorder is considered the safest because of low incidence of side effects and lack of physiologic dependence?
   A. Benzodiazepines
   B. Tricyclics
   C. Monoamine oxidase inhibitors
   D. Selective serotonin reuptake inhibitors

6. Which of the following would be the best intervention for a client having a panic attack?
   A. Involve the client in a physical activity.
   B. Offer a distraction such as music.
   C. Remain with the client.
   D. Teach the client a relaxation technique.

7. A client with generalized anxiety disorder states, "I have learned that the best thing I can do is to forget my worries." How would the nurse evaluate this statement?
   A. The client is developing insight.
   B. The client's coping skills have improved.
   C. The client needs encouragement to verbalize feelings.
   D. The client's treatment has been successful.

8. A client with anxiety is beginning treatment with lorazepam (Ativan). It is most important for the nurse to assess the client's
   A. Motivation for treatment
   B. Family and social support
   C. Use of coping mechanisms
   D. Use of alcohol

FILL-IN-THE-BLANK QUESTIONS

Identify the level of anxiety represented by the following descriptions.

_____ 1. Severe muscle tension, limited perceptual field, frantic

_____ 2. Attentive, impatient, optimal learning level

_____ 3. Flight, fight, or freeze; out of control; irrational

_____ 4. Selective inattention, voice changes, decreased perceptual field

SHORT-ANSWER QUESTIONS

1. Discuss the concepts of primary and secondary gain; give an example of each.

2. Describe systematic desensitization.

CLINICAL EXAMPLE

Mr. Noe has discussed in detail with the community health nurse how his wife cannot be expected to walk 2 to 3 miles a day after her triple-bypass operation because she is afraid to leave the house. He has been taking care of her for the past 13 years, during which time she has rarely left the house and then only with great distress and only accompanied by him. His wife says she gets so anxious she wants to scream and run back in the door if she tries to walk out of it. She believes something terrible will happen to her. She knows this is true because the last time she left the house to go to the doctor, she had to have triple-bypass surgery the next day. Mr. Noe takes care of necessary chores outside the house, attends parents' weekends at their children's colleges, does the grocery shopping, and so forth.

Mrs. Noe has asked the nurse to "figure out how I can get outside and walk every day," but for each suggestion the nurse makes, Mrs. Noe finds some reason it will not work. The nurse is getting frustrated with Mrs. Noe's constant rejection of her suggestions and sternly says, "If you aren't going to try any of my suggestions, then I guess we're wasting our time."

1. Rather than giving Mrs. Noe suggestions to get her outside, what might be a better plan?

2. How is Mr. Noe's behavior affecting Mrs. Noe's agoraphobia? What does the nurse need to explain and to recommend to Mr. Noe about his response to her behavior?

3. What other treatments are available for Mrs. Noe?

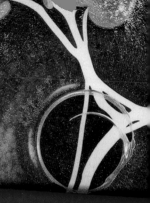

Chapter

14

Schizophrenia

Key Terms

- Abnormal Involuntary Movement Scale (AIMS)
- akathisia
- alogia
- anhedonia
- blunted affect
- catatonia
- command hallucinations
- delusions
- depersonalization
- dystonic reactions
- echolalia
- echopraxia
- extrapyramidal side effects
- flat affect
- hallucination
- ideas of reference
- latency of response
- neuroleptic malignant syndrome (NMS)
- neuroleptics
- polydipsia
- pseudoparkinsonism
- psychomotor retardation

- psychosis
- tardive dyskinesia
- thought blocking
- thought broadcasting

- thought insertion
- thought withdrawal
- waxy flexibility
- word salad

Learning Objectives

After reading this chapter, you should be able to

1. Discuss various theories of the etiology of schizophrenia.

2. Describe the positive and negative symptoms of schizophrenia.

3. Describe a functional and mental status assessment for a client with schizophrenia.

4. Apply the nursing process to the care of a client with schizophrenia.

5. Evaluate the effectiveness of antipsychotic medications for clients with schizophrenia.

6. Provide teaching to clients, families, caregivers, and community members to increase knowledge and understanding of schizophrenia.

7. Describe the supportive and rehabilitative needs of clients with schizophrenia who live in the community.

8. Evaluate your own feelings, beliefs, and attitudes regarding clients with schizophrenia.

Schizophrenia causes distorted and bizarre thoughts, perceptions, emotions, movements, and behavior. It cannot be defined as a single illness; rather, schizophrenia is thought of as a syndrome or disease process with many different varieties and symptoms, much like the varieties of cancer. For decades, the public vastly misunderstood schizophrenia, fearing it as dangerous and uncontrollable and causing wild disturbances and violent outbursts. Many people believed that those with schizophrenia needed to be locked away from society and institutionalized. Only recently has the mental health industry come to learn and educate the community at large that schizophrenia has many different symptoms and presentations and is an illness that medication can control. Thanks to the increased effectiveness of newer atypical antipsychotic drugs and advances in community-based treatment, many clients with schizophrenia live successfully in the community. Clients whose illness is medically supervised and whose treatment is maintained often continue to live and sometimes work in the community with family and outside support.

Schizophrenia usually is diagnosed in late adolescence or early adulthood. Rarely does it manifest in childhood. The peak incidence of onset is 15 to 25 years of age for men and 25 to 35 years of age for women (American Psychiatric Association [APA], 2000). The prevalence of schizophrenia is estimated at about 1% of the total population. In the United States, that translates to nearly 3 million people who are, have been, or will be affected by the disease. The incidence and the lifetime prevalence are roughly the same throughout the world (Buchanan & Carpenter, 2005).

The symptoms of schizophrenia are divided into two major categories: *positive* or *hard symptoms/signs,* which include delusions, hallucinations, and grossly disorganized thinking, speech, and behavior; and *negative* or *soft symptoms/ signs,* which include flat affect, lack of volition, and social withdrawal or discomfort. For *Diagnostic and Statistical Manual of Mental Disorders, 4th edition, Text Revision (DSM-IV-TR;* APA, 2000) diagnostic criteria for schizophrenia, please refer to the box below. Medication can control the positive symptoms, but frequently the negative symptoms persist after positive symptoms have abated. The persistence of these negative symptoms over time presents a major barrier to recovery and improved functioning in the client's daily life.

The following are the types of schizophrenia according to the *DSM-IV-TR* (APA, 2000). The diagnosis is made according to the client's predominant symptoms:

- *Schizophrenia, paranoid type:* characterized by persecutory (feeling victimized or spied on) or grandiose delusions, hallucinations, and, occasionally, excessive religiosity (delusional religious focus) or hostile and aggressive behavior
- *Schizophrenia, disorganized type:* characterized by grossly inappropriate or flat affect, incoherence, loose associations, and extremely disorganized.behavior
- *Schizophrenia, catatonic type:* characterized by marked psychomotor disturbance, either motionless or excessive motor activity. Motor immobility may be manifested by

catalepsy (waxy flexibility) or stupor. Excessive motor activity is apparently purposeless and is not influenced by external stimuli. Other features include extreme negativism, mutism, peculiarities of voluntary movement, echolalia, and echopraxia.
- *Schizophrenia, undifferentiated type:* characterized by mixed schizophrenic symptoms (of other types) along with disturbances of thought, affect, and behavior
- *Schizophrenia, residual type:* characterized by at least one previous, though not a current, episode; social withdrawal; flat affect; and looseness of associations

CLINICAL COURSE

Although the symptoms of schizophrenia are always severe, the long-term course does not always involve progressive deterioration. The clinical course varies among clients.

Onset

Onset may be abrupt or insidious, but most clients slowly and gradually develop signs and symptoms such as social withdrawal, unusual behavior, loss of interest in school or work, and neglected hygiene. The diagnosis of schizophrenia usually is made when the person begins to display more actively positive symptoms of delusions, hallucinations, and disordered thinking (psychosis). Regardless of when and how the illness begins and the type of schizophrenia, consequences for most clients and their families are substantial and enduring.

When and how the illness develops seems to affect the outcome. Age at onset appears to be an important factor in how well the client fares: Those who develop the illness earlier show worse outcomes than those who develop it later. Younger clients display a poorer premorbid adjustment, more prominent negative signs, and greater cognitive impairment than do older clients. Those who experience a gradual onset of the disease (about 50%) tend to have both a poorer immediate and long-term course than those who experience an acute and sudden onset (Buchanan & Carpenter, 2005). Approximately one third of clients with schizophrenia relapse within 1 year of an acute episode (Ucok et al., 2006).

Immediate Course

In the years immediately after the onset of psychotic symptoms, two typical clinical patterns emerge. In one pattern, the client experiences ongoing psychosis and never fully recovers, although symptoms may shift in severity over time. In another pattern, the client experiences episodes of psychotic symptoms that alternate with episodes of relatively complete recovery from the psychosis.

Long-Term Course

The intensity of psychosis tends to diminish with age. Many clients with long-term impairment regain some degree of

DSM-IV-TR DIAGNOSTIC CRITERIA: POSITIVE AND NEGATIVE SYMPTOMS OF SCHIZOPHRENIA

Positive or Hard Symptoms

Ambivalence: Holding seemingly contradictory beliefs or feelings about the same person, event, or situation

Associative looseness: Fragmented or poorly related thoughts and ideas

Delusions: Fixed false beliefs that have no basis in reality

Echopraxia: Imitation of the movements and gestures of another person whom the client is observing

Flight of ideas: Continuous flow of verbalization in which the person jumps rapidly from one topic to another

Hallucinations: False sensory perceptions or perceptual experiences that do not exist in reality

Ideas of reference: False impressions that external events have special meaning for the person

Perseveration: Persistent adherence to a single idea or topic; verbal repetition of a sentence, word, or phrase; resisting attempts to change the topic

Negative or Soft Symptoms

Alogia: Tendency to speak very little or to convey little substance of meaning (poverty of content)

Anhedonia: Feeling no joy or pleasure from life or any activities or relationships

Apathy: Feelings of indifference toward people, activities, and events

Blunted affect: Restricted range of emotional feeling, tone, or mood

Catatonia: Psychologically induced immobility occasionally marked by periods of agitation or excitement; the client seems motionless, as if in a trance

Flat affect: Absence of any facial expression that would indicate emotions or mood

Lack of volition: Absence of will, ambition, or drive to take action or accomplish tasks

Adapted from DSM-IV-TR, 2000.

CLINICAL VIGNETTE: SCHIZOPHRENIA

Ricky was staying with his father for a few weeks on a visit. During the first week, things had gone pretty well, but Ricky forgot to take his medication for a few days. His father knew Ricky wasn't sleeping well at night, and he could hear Ricky talking to himself in the next room.

One day while his father was at work, Ricky began to hear some voices outside the apartment. The voices grew louder, saying "You're no good; you can't do anything right. You can't take care of yourself or protect your dad. We're going to get you both." Ricky grew more frightened and went to the closet where his dad kept his tools. He grabbed a hammer and ran outside. When his father came home from work early, Ricky wasn't in the apartment though his coat and wallet were still there. Ricky's father called a neighbor, and they drove around the apartment complex looking for Ricky. They finally found Ricky crouched behind some bushes. Although it was 45°F (7°C), he was wearing only a T-shirt and shorts and no

shoes. Ricky's neighbor called emergency services. Meanwhile Ricky's father tried to coax Ricky into the car, but Ricky wouldn't come. The voices had grown louder, and Ricky was convinced that the devil had kidnapped his father and was coming for him too. He saw someone else in the car with his dad. The voices said they would crash the car if he got in. They were laughing at him! He couldn't get into the car; it was only a trap. His dad had tried his best, but he was trapped, too. The voices told Ricky to use the hammer and to destroy the car to kill the devil. He began to swing the hammer into the windshield, but someone held him back.

The emergency services staff arrived and spoke quietly and firmly as they removed the hammer from Ricky's hands. They told Ricky they were taking him to the hospital where he and his father would be safe. They gently put him on a stretcher with restraints, and his father rode in the emergency van with him to the hospital.

social and occupational functioning. Over time, the disease becomes less disruptive to the person's life and easier to manage, but rarely can the client overcome the effects of many years of dysfunction (Buchanan & Carpenter, 2005). In later life, these clients may live independently or in a structured family-type setting and may succeed at jobs with stable expectations and a supportive work environment. However, most clients with schizophrenia have difficulty functioning in the community, and few lead fully independent lives (Carter, 2006). This is primarily due to persistent negative symptoms, impaired cognition, or treatment-refractory positive symptoms.

Antipsychotic medications play a crucial role in the course of the disease and individual outcomes. They do not cure the disorder; however, they are crucial to its successful management. The more effective the client's response and adherence to his or her medication regimen, the better the client's outcome. Marshall and Rathbone (2006) found that early detection and aggressive treatment of the first psychotic episode were associated with improved outcomes.

RELATED DISORDERS

Other disorders are related to but distinguished from schizophrenia in terms of presenting symptoms and the duration or magnitude of impairment. The *DSM-IV-TR* (APA, 2000) categorizes these disorders as follows:

- *Schizophreniform disorder:* The client exhibits the symptoms of schizophrenia but for less than the 6 months necessary to meet the diagnostic criteria for schizophrenia. Social or occupational functioning may or may not be impaired.
- *Schizoaffective disorder:* The client exhibits the symptoms of psychosis and, at the same time, all the features of a mood disorder, either depression or mania.
- *Delusional disorder:* The client has one or more nonbizarre delusions—that is, the focus of the delusion is believable. Psychosocial functioning is not markedly impaired, and behavior is not obviously odd or bizarre.
- *Brief psychotic disorder:* The client experiences the sudden onset of at least one psychotic symptom, such as delusions, hallucinations, or disorganized speech or behavior, which lasts from 1 day to 1 month. The episode may or may not have an identifiable stressor or may follow childbirth.
- *Shared psychotic disorder* (folie à deux): Two people share a similar delusion. The person with this diagnosis develops this delusion in the context of a close relationship with someone who has psychotic delusions.

Two other diagnoses, schizoid personality disorder and schizotypal personality disorder, are not psychotic disorders and should not be confused with schizophrenia even though the names sound similar. These two diagnoses are covered in Chapter 16.

ETIOLOGY

Whether schizophrenia is an organic disease with underlying physical brain pathology has been an important question for researchers and clinicians for as long as they have studied the illness. In the first half of the 20th century, studies focused on trying to find a particular pathologic structure associated with the disease, largely through autopsy. Such a site was not discovered. In the 1950s and 1960s, the emphasis shifted to examination of psychological and social causes. Interpersonal theorists suggested that schizophrenia resulted from dysfunctional relationships in early life and adolescence. None of the interpersonal theories has been proved, and newer scientific studies are finding more evidence to support neurologic/neurochemical causes. However, some therapists still believe that schizophrenia results from dysfunctional parenting or family dynamics. For parents or family members of persons diagnosed with schizophrenia, such beliefs cause agony over what they did "wrong" or what they could have done to help prevent it.

Newer scientific studies began to demonstrate that schizophrenia results from a type of brain dysfunction. In the 1970s, studies began to focus on possible neurochemical causes, which remain the primary focus of research and theory today. These neurochemical/neurologic theories are supported by the effects of antipsychotic medications, which help to control psychotic symptoms, and neuroimaging tools such as computed tomography, which have shown that the brain of people with schizophrenia differs in structure and function from the brain of control subjects.

Biologic Theories

The biologic theories of schizophrenia focus on genetic factors, neuroanatomic and neurochemical factors (structure and function of the brain), and immunovirology (the body's response to exposure to a virus).

GENETIC FACTORS

Most genetic studies have focused on immediate families (i.e., parents, siblings, offspring) to examine whether schizophrenia is genetically transmitted or inherited. Few have focused on more distant relatives. The most important studies have centered on twins; these findings have demonstrated that identical twins have a 50% risk for schizophrenia; that is, if one twin has schizophrenia, the other has a 50% chance of developing it as well. Fraternal twins have only a 15% risk (Kirkpatrick & Tek, 2005). This finding indicates that schizophrenia is at least partially inherited.

Other important studies have shown that children with one biologic parent with schizophrenia have a 15% risk; the risk rises to 35% if both biologic parents have schizophrenia. Children adopted at birth into a family with no history of schizophrenia but whose biologic parents have a history of schizophrenia still reflect the genetic risk of their biologic parents. All these studies have indicated a genetic risk or

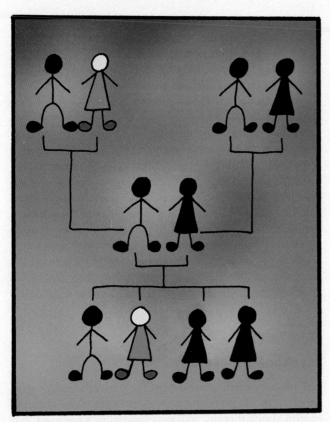

Genetics plays a role in mental illness

tendency for schizophrenia, but genetics cannot be the only factor: identical twins have only a 50% risk even though their genes are 100% identical (Riley & Kendler, 2005).

NEUROANATOMIC AND NEUROCHEMICAL FACTORS

With the development of noninvasive imaging techniques such as computed tomography, magnetic resonance imaging, and positron emission tomography in the past 25 years, scientists have been able to study the brain structure (neuroanatomy) and activity (neurochemical) of people with schizophrenia. Findings have demonstrated that people with schizophrenia have relatively less brain tissue and cerebrospinal fluid than people who do not have schizophrenia (Schneider-Axmann et al., 2006); this could represent a failure in development or a subsequent loss of tissue. Computed tomography scans have shown enlarged ventricles in the brain and cortical atrophy. Positron emission tomography studies suggest that glucose metabolism and oxygen are diminished in the frontal cortical structures of the brain. The research consistently shows decreased brain volume and abnormal brain function in the frontal and temporal areas of persons with schizophrenia. This pathology correlates with the positive signs of schizophrenia (temporal lobe), such as psychosis, and the negative signs of schizophrenia (frontal lobe), such as lack of volition or motivation and anhedonia. It is unknown whether these changes in the frontal and temporal lobes are the result of

a failure of these areas to develop properly or if a virus, trauma, or immune response has damaged them. Intrauterine influences such as poor nutrition, tobacco, alcohol and other drugs, and stress also are being studied as possible causes of the brain pathology found in people with schizophrenia (Buchanan & Carpenter, 2005).

Neurochemical studies have consistently demonstrated alterations in the neurotransmitter systems of the brain in people with schizophrenia. The neuronal networks that transmit information by electrical signals from a nerve cell through its axon and across synapses to postsynaptic receptors on other nerve cells seem to malfunction. The transmission of the signal across the synapse requires a complex series of biochemical events. Studies have implicated the actions of dopamine, serotonin, norepinephrine, acetylcholine, glutamate, and several neuromodulary peptides.

Currently, the most prominent neurochemical theories involve dopamine and serotonin. One prominent theory suggests excess dopamine as a cause. This theory was developed based on two observations: First, drugs that increase activity in the dopaminergic system, such as amphetamine and levodopa, sometimes induce a paranoid psychotic reaction similar to schizophrenia. Second, drugs blocking postsynaptic dopamine receptors reduce psychotic symptoms; in fact, the greater the ability of the drug to block dopamine receptors, the more effective it is in decreasing symptoms of schizophrenia (Buchanan & Carpenter, 2005).

More recently, serotonin has been included among the leading neurochemical factors affecting schizophrenia. The theory regarding serotonin suggests that serotonin modulates and helps to control excess dopamine. Some believe that excess serotonin itself contributes to the development of schizophrenia. Newer atypical antipsychotics such as clozapine (Clozaril) are both dopamine and serotonin antagonists. Drug studies have shown that clozapine can dramatically reduce psychotic symptoms and ameliorate the negative signs of schizophrenia (Kane & Marder, 2005).

Researchers also are exploring the possibility that schizophrenia may have three separate symptom complexes or syndromes: hallucinations/delusions, disorganization of thought and behavior, and negative symptoms (Buchanan & Carpenter, 2005). Investigations show that the three syndromes relate to neurobiologic differences in the brain. It is postulated that schizophrenia has (these three) subgroups, which may be homogeneous relative to course, pathophysiology, and, therefore, treatment.

IMMUNOVIROLOGIC FACTORS

Popular theories have emerged stating that exposure to a virus or the body's immune response to a virus could alter the brain physiology of people with schizophrenia. Although scientists continue to study these possibilities, few findings have validated them.

Cytokines are chemical messengers between immune cells, mediating inflammatory and immune responses. Specific cytokines also play a role in signaling the brain to produce behavioral and neurochemical changes needed in the face of physical or psychological stress to maintain homeostasis. It is believed that cytokines may have a role in the development of major psychiatric disorders such as schizophrenia (Brown et al., 2005).

Recently, researchers have been focusing on infections in pregnant women as a possible origin for schizophrenia. Waves of schizophrenia in England, Wales, Denmark, Finland, and other countries have occurred a generation after influenza epidemics. Also, there are higher rates of schizophrenia among children born in crowded areas in cold weather, conditions that are hospitable to respiratory ailments (Brown et al., 2005).

CULTURAL CONSIDERATIONS

Awareness of cultural differences is important when assessing for symptoms of schizophrenia. Ideas that are considered delusional in one culture, such as beliefs in sorcery or witchcraft, may be commonly accepted by other cultures. Also, auditory or visual hallucinations, such as seeing the Virgin Mary or hearing God's voice, may be a normal part of religious experiences in some cultures. The assessment of affect requires sensitivity to differences in eye contact, body language, and acceptable emotional expression; these vary across cultures (APA, 2000).

Psychotic behavior observed in countries other than the United States or among particular ethnic groups has been identified as a "culture-bound" syndrome. Although these episodes exist primarily in certain countries, they may be seen in other places as people visit or immigrate to other countries or areas. Mojtabai (2005) summarized some of these psychotic behaviors:

- *Bouffée délirante*, a syndrome found in West Africa and Haiti, involves a sudden outburst of agitated and aggressive behavior, marked confusion, and psychomotor excitement. It is sometimes accompanied by visual and auditory hallucinations or paranoid ideation.
- *Ghost sickness* is preoccupation with death and the deceased frequently observed among members of some Native American tribes. Symptoms include bad dreams, weakness, feelings of danger, loss of appetite, fainting, dizziness, fear, anxiety, hallucinations, loss of consciousness, confusion, feelings of futility, and a sense of suffocation.
- *Locura* refers to a chronic psychosis experienced by Latinos in the United States and Latin America. Symptoms include incoherence, agitation, visual and auditory hallucinations, inability to follow social rules, unpredictability, and, possibly, violent behavior.
- *Qi-gong* psychotic reaction is an acute, time-limited episode characterized by dissociative, paranoid, or other psychotic symptoms that occur after participating in the Chinese folk health-enhancing practice of *qi-gong*. Especially vulnerable are those who become overly involved in the practice.

- *Zar*, an experience of spirits possessing a person, is seen in Ethiopia, Somalia, Egypt, Sudan, Iran, and other North African and Middle Eastern societies. The afflicted person may laugh, shout, wail, bang her or his head on a wall, or be apathetic and withdrawn, refusing to eat or carry out daily tasks. Locally, such behavior is not considered pathologic.

Ethnicity also may be a factor in the way a person responds to psychotropic medications. This difference in response is probably the result of the person's genetic makeup. Some people metabolize certain drugs more slowly, so the drug level in the bloodstream is higher than desired. African Americans, white Americans, and Hispanic Americans appear to require comparable therapeutic doses of antipsychotic medications. Asian clients, however, need lower doses of drugs such as haloperidol (Haldol) to obtain the same effects; therefore, they would be likely to experience more severe side effects if given the traditional or usual doses.

TREATMENT

Psychopharmacology

The primary medical treatment for schizophrenia is psychopharmacology. In the past, electroconvulsive therapy, insulin shock therapy, and psychosurgery were used, but since the creation of chlorpromazine (Thorazine) in 1952, other treatment modalities have become all but obsolete. Antipsychotic medications, also known as neuroleptics, are prescribed primarily for their efficacy in decreasing psychotic symptoms. They do not cure schizophrenia; rather, they are used to manage the symptoms of the disease.

The older, or conventional, antipsychotic medications are dopamine antagonists. The newer, or atypical, antipsychotic medications are both dopamine and serotonin antagonists (see Chapter 2). These medications, usual daily dosages, and common side effects are listed in Table 14.1. The conventional antipsychotics target the positive signs of schizophrenia, such as delusions, hallucinations, disturbed thinking, and other psychotic symptoms, but have no observable effect on the negative signs. The atypical antipsychotics not only diminish positive symptoms but also, for many clients, lessen the negative signs of lack of volition and motivation, social withdrawal, and anhedonia.

MAINTENANCE THERAPY

Two antipsychotics are available in depot injection forms for maintenance therapy: fluphenazine (Prolixin) in decanoate and enanthate preparations and haloperidol (Haldol) in decanoate. The vehicle for depot injections is sesame oil; therefore, the medications are absorbed slowly over time into the client's system. The effects of the medications last 2 to 4 weeks, eliminating the need for daily oral antipsychotic medication (see Chapter 2). The duration of action is 7 to 28 days for fluphenazine and 4 weeks for haloperidol. It may take several weeks of oral therapy with these medications to

Table 14.1 ANTIPSYCHOTIC DRUGS, USUAL DAILY DOSAGES, AND INCIDENCE OF SIDE EFFECTS

Generic (Trade) Name	Usual Daily Dosage* (mg)	Sedation	Hypotension	EPS	Anticholinergic
Conventional Antipsychotics					
Chlorpromazine (Thorazine)	200–1,600	++++	+++	++	+++
Perphenazine (Trilafon)	16–32	++	++++	+	+
Fluphenazine (Prolixin)	2.5–20	+	+	++++	+
Thioridazine (Mellaril)	200–600	++++	+++	+	+++
Mesoridazine (Serentil)	75–300	++++	++	+	++
Thiothixene (Navane)	6–30	+	+	++++	+
Haloperidol (Haldol)	2–20	+	+	++++	+/0
Loxapine (Loxitane)	60–100	+++	++	+++	++
Molindone (Moban)	50–100	+	+/0	+	++
Perphenazine (Etrafon)	16–32	++	++	+++	+
Trifluoperazine (Stelazine)	6–50	+	+	++++	+
Atypical Antipsychotics					
Clozapine (Clozaril)	150–500	++++	++	+/0	++
Risperidone (Risperdal)	2–8	+++	++	++	+
Olanzapine (Zyprexa)	5–20	++++	+++	+	++
Quetiapine (Seroquel)	150–500	+/0	++++	+	+
Ziprasidone (Geodon)	40–160 mg	++	+/0	+	+
Paliperidone (Invega)	6 mg	++	++	++	+
Aripiprazole (Abilify)	10–40 mg	+	++	+	+++

*Oral dosage only

EPS, extrapyramidal side effects

++++, very significant; +++, significant; ++, moderate; +, mild; +/0, rare or absent

reach a stable dosing level before the transition to depot injections can be made. Therefore, these preparations are not suitable for the management of acute episodes of psychosis. They are, however, very useful for clients requiring supervised medication compliance over an extended period.

SIDE EFFECTS

The side effects of antipsychotic medications are significant and can range from mild discomfort to permanent movement disorders (Kane & Marder, 2005). Because many of these side effects are frightening and upsetting to clients, they are frequently cited as the primary reason that clients discontinue or reduce the dosage of their medications. Serious neurologic side effects include **extrapyramidal side effects** (acute dystonic reactions, akathisia, and parkinsonism), tardive dyskinesia, seizures, and neuroleptic malignant syndrome (NMS; discussion to follow). Nonneurologic side effects include weight gain, sedation, photosensitivity, and anticholinergic symptoms such as dry mouth, blurred vision, constipation, urinary retention, and orthostatic hypotension. Table 14.2 lists the side effects of antipsychotic medications and appropriate nursing interventions.

Extrapyramidal Side Effects. Extrapyramidal side effects are reversible movement disorders induced by neuroleptic medication. They include dystonic reactions, parkinsonism, and akathisia.

Dystonic reactions to antipsychotic medications appear early in the course of treatment and are characterized by spasms in discrete muscle groups such as the neck muscles (torticollis) or eye muscles (oculogyric crisis). These spasms also may be accompanied by protrusion of the tongue, dysphagia, and laryngeal and pharyngeal spasms that can compromise the client's airway, causing a medical emergency. Dystonic reactions are extremely frightening and painful for the client. Acute treatment consists of diphenhydramine (Benadryl) given either intramuscularly or intravenously or benztropine (Cogentin) given intramuscularly.

Pseudoparkinsonism, or neuroleptic-induced parkinsonism, includes a shuffling gait, mask-like facies, muscle stiffness (continuous) or cogwheeling rigidity (ratchet-like movements of joints), drooling, and akinesia (slowness and difficulty initiating movement). These symptoms usually appear in the first few days after starting or increasing the dosage of an antipsychotic medication. Treatment of pseudoparkinsonism and prevention of further dystonic reactions are achieved with the medications listed in Table 14.3.

Akathisia is characterized by restless movement, pacing, inability to remain still, and the client's report of inner restlessness. Akathisia usually develops when the antipsychotic is started or when the dose is increased. Clients are very uncomfortable with these sensations and may stop taking the antipsychotic medication to avoid these side

Table 14.2   SIDE EFFECTS OF ANTIPSYCHOTIC MEDICATIONS AND NURSING INTERVENTIONS

Side Effect	Nursing Intervention
Dystonic reactions	Administer medications as ordered; assess for effectiveness; reassure client if he or she is frightened.
Tardive dyskinesia	Assess using tool such as AIMS; report occurrence or score increase to physician.
Neuroleptic malignant syndrome	Stop all antipsychotic medications; notify physician immediately.
Akathisia	Administer medications as ordered; assess for effectiveness.
Extrapyramidal side effects or neuroleptic-induced parkinsonism	Administer medications as ordered; assess for effectiveness.
Seizures	Stop medication; notify physician; protect client from injury during seizure; provide reassurance and privacy for client after seizure.
Sedation	Caution about activities requiring client to be fully alert, such as driving a car.
Photosensitivity	Caution client to avoid sun exposure; advise client when in the sun to wear protective clothing and sun-blocking lotion.
Weight gain	Encourage balanced diet with controlled portions and regular exercise; focus on minimizing gain.
Anticholinergic symptoms	
Dry mouth	Use ice chips or hard candy for relief.
Blurred vision	Assess side effect, which should improve with time; report to physician if no improvement.
Constipation	Increase fluid and dietary fiber intake; client may need a stool softener if unrelieved.
Urinary retention	Instruct client to report any frequency or burning with urination; report to physician if no improvement over time.
Orthostatic hypotension	Instruct client to rise slowly from sitting or lying position; wait to ambulate until no longer dizzy or light-headed.

Table 14.3   EFFICACY OF DRUGS USED TO TREAT EXTRAPYRAMIDAL SIDE EFFECTS AND NURSING INTERVENTIONS

Generic (Trade) Name	Akathisia	Dystonia	Rigidity	Tremor	Nursing Interventions
Benztropine (Cogentin)	2	2	3	2	Increase fluid and fiber intake to avoid constipation; use ice chips or hard candy for dry mouth; assess for memory impairment (another side effect).
Trihexyphenidyl (Artane)	2	3	3	3	
Biperiden (Akineton)	1	3	3	3	
Procyclidine (Kemadrin)	1	3	3	3	
Amantadine (Symmetrel)	3	2	3	2	Use ice chips or hard candy for dry mouth; assess for worsening psychosis (an occasional side effect).
Diphenhydramine (Benadryl)	2	2–3	1	2	Use ice chips or hard candy for dry mouth; observe for sedation.
Diazepam (Valium)	2	1–2	1–2	0–1	Observe for sedation; potential for misuse or abuse.
Lorazepam (Ativan)	2	1–2	1–2	0–1	Observe for sedation; potential for misuse or abuse.
Propranolol (Inderal)	3	0	0	1–2	Assess for palpitations, dizziness, cold hands and feet.

effects. Beta-blockers such as propranolol have been most effective in treating akathisia, whereas benzodiazepines have provided some success as well.

The early detection and successful treatment of extrapyramidal side effects is very important in promoting the client's compliance with medication. The nurse is most often the person who observes these symptoms or the person to whom the client reports symptoms. To provide consistency in assessment among nurses working with the client, a standardized rating scale for extrapyramidal symptoms is useful. The Simpson-Angus scale for extrapyramidal side effects is one tool that can be used.

Tardive Dyskinesia. Tardive dyskinesia, a late-appearing side effect of antipsychotic medications, is characterized by abnormal, involuntary movements such as lip smacking, tongue protrusion, chewing, blinking, grimacing, and choreiform movements of the limbs and feet. These involuntary movements are embarrassing for clients and may cause them to become more socially isolated. Tardive dyskinesia is irreversible once it has appeared, but decreasing or discontinuing the medication can arrest the progression. Clozapine (Clozaril), an atypical antipsychotic drug, has not been found to cause this side effect, so it often is recommended for clients who have experienced tardive dyskinesia while taking conventional antipsychotic drugs.

Screening clients for late-appearing movement disorders such as tardive dyskinesia is important. The Abnormal Involuntary Movement Scale (AIMS) is used to screen for symptoms of movement disorders. The client is observed in several positions, and the severity of symptoms is rated from 0 to 4. The AIMS can be administered every 3 to 6 months. If the nurse detects an increased score on the AIMS, indicating increased symptoms of tardive dyskinesia, he or she should notify the physician so that the client's dosage or drug can be changed to prevent advancement of tardive dyskinesia. The AIMS examination procedure is presented in Box 14.1.

Seizures. Seizures are an infrequent side effect associated with antipsychotic medications. The incidence is 1% of people taking antipsychotics. The notable exception is clozapine, which has an incidence of 5%. Seizures may be associated with high doses of the medication. Treatment is a lowered dosage or a different antipsychotic medication.

Neuroleptic Malignant Syndrome. NMS is a serious and frequently fatal condition seen in those being treated with antipsychotic medications. It is characterized by muscle rigidity, high fever, increased muscle enzymes (particularly creatine phosphokinase), and leukocytosis (increased leukocytes). It is estimated that 0.1% to 1% of all clients taking antipsychotics develop NMS. Any of the antipsychotic medications can cause NMS, which is treated by stopping the medication. The client's ability to tolerate other antipsychotic medications after NMS varies, but use of another antipsychotic appears possible in most instances.

Agranulocytosis. Clozapine has the potentially fatal side effect of agranulocytosis (failure of the bone marrow to produce adequate white blood cells). Agranulocytosis develops suddenly and is characterized by fever, malaise, ulcerative sore throat, and leukopenia. This side effect may not be manifested immediately but can occur as long as 18 to 24 weeks after the initiation of therapy. The drug must be discontinued immediately. Clients taking this antipsychotic must have weekly white blood cell counts for the first 6 months of clozapine therapy and every 2 weeks thereafter. Clozapine is dispensed every 7 or 14 days only, and evidence of a white cell count above 3500 cells/mm^3 is required before a refill is furnished.

Psychosocial Treatment

In addition to pharmacologic treatment, many other modes of treatment can help the person with schizophrenia. Individual and group therapies, family therapy, family education, and social skills training can be instituted for clients in both inpatient and community settings.

Individual and group therapy sessions are often supportive in nature, giving the client an opportunity for social contact and meaningful relationships with other people. Groups that focus on topics of concern such as medication management, use of community supports, and family concerns also have been beneficial to clients with schizophrenia (Pfammatter et al., 2006).

Clients with schizophrenia can improve their social competence with social skill training, which translates into more effective functioning in the community. Basic social skill training involves breaking complex social behavior into simpler steps, practicing through role-playing, and applying the concepts in the community or real-world setting. Cognitive adaptation training using environmental supports is designed to improve adaptive functioning in the home setting. Individually tailored environmental supports such as signs, calendars, hygiene supplies, and pill containers, cue the client to perform associated tasks (Velligan et al., 2006). Moriana, Alarcon, and Herruzo (2006) found that psychosocial skill training was more effective when carried out during in-home visits in the client's own environment rather than in an outpatient setting.

A new therapy, cognitive enhancement therapy (CET), combines computer-based cognitive training with group sessions that allow clients to practice and develop social skills. This approach is designed to remediate or improve the clients' social and neurocognitive deficits, such as attention, memory, and information processing. The experiential exercises help the client to take the perspective of another person, rather than focus entirely on self. Positive results of CET include increased mental stamina, active rather than passive information processing, and spontaneous and appropriate negotiation of unrehearsed social challenges (Hogarty et al., 2006).

Family education and therapy are known to diminish the negative effects of schizophrenia and reduce the relapse rate (Penn et al., 2005). Although inclusion of the family is a factor that improves outcomes for the client, family

Box 14.1   ABNORMAL INVOLUNTARY MOVEMENT SCALE (AIMS) EXAMINATION PROCEDURE

Client identification: _____   Date: _____

Rated by: _____

Either before or after completing the examination procedure, observe the client unobtrusively at rest (e.g., in waiting room). The chair to be used in this examination should be a hard, firm one without arms.

After observing the client, he or she may be rated on a scale of 0 (none), 1 (minimal), 2 (mild), 3 (moderate), and 4 (severe) according to the severity of symptoms.

Ask the client if there is anything in his/her mouth (i.e., gum, candy, etc.) and, if there is, to remove it.

Ask client about the current condition of his/her teeth. Ask client if he/she wears dentures. Do teeth or dentures bother client now?

Ask client whether he/she notices any movement in mouth, face, hands, or feet. If yes, ask to describe and to what extent the movements currently bother patient or interfere with his/her activities.

0 1 2 3 4	Have client sit in chair with hands on knees, legs slightly apart, and feet flat on floor. (Look at entire body for movements while in this position.)
0 1 2 3 4	Ask client to sit with hands hanging unsupported. If male, hands between legs; if female and wearing a dress, hands hanging over knees. (Observe hands and other body areas.)
0 1 2 3 4	Ask client to open mouth. (Observe tongue at rest within mouth.) Do this twice.
0 1 2 3 4	Ask client to protrude tongue. (Observe abnormalities of tongue movement.) Do this twice.
0 1 2 3 4	Ask client to tap thumb with each finger as rapidly as possible for 10–15 seconds; separately with right hand, then with left hand. (Observe facial and leg movements.)
0 1 2 3 4	Flex and extend client's left and right arms. (One at a time.)
0 1 2 3 4	Ask client to stand up. (Observe in profile. Observe all body areas again, hips included.)
0 1 2 3 4	*Ask client to extend both arms outstretched in front with palms down. (Observe trunk, legs, and mouth.)
0 1 2 3 4	*Have client walk a few paces, turn, and walk back to chair. (Observe hands and gait.) Do this twice.

*Activated movements.

involvement often is neglected by health care professionals. Families often have a difficult time coping with the complexities and ramifications of the client's illness. This creates stress among family members that is not beneficial for the client or family members. Family education helps to make family members part of the treatment team. See Chapter 3 for a discussion of the National Alliance for the Mentally Ill Family to Family Education course.

In addition, family members can benefit from a supportive environment that helps them cope with the many difficulties presented when a loved one has schizophrenia. These concerns include continuing as a caregiver for the child who is now an adult; worrying about who will care for the client when the parents are gone; dealing with the social stigma of mental illness; and possibly facing financial problems, marital discord, and social isolation. Such support is available through the National Alliance for the Mentally Ill and local support groups. The client's health care provider can make referrals to meet specific family needs.

APPLICATION OF THE NURSING PROCESS

Assessment

Schizophrenia affects thought processes and content, perception, emotion, behavior, and social functioning; however, it affects each individual differently. The degree of impairment in both the acute or psychotic phase and the chronic or long-term phase varies greatly; thus, so do the needs of and the nursing interventions for each affected client. The nurse must not make assumptions about the client's abilities or limitations based solely on the medical diagnosis of schizophrenia.

For example, the nurse may care for a client in an acute inpatient setting. The client may appear frightened, hear voices (hallucinate), make no eye contact, and mumble constantly. The nurse would deal with the positive, or psychotic, signs of the disease. Another nurse may encounter a client with schizophrenia in a community setting who is not experiencing psychotic symptoms; rather, this client lacks energy for daily tasks and has feelings of loneliness and isolation (negative signs of schizophrenia). Although both clients have the same medical diagnosis, the approach and interventions that each nurse takes would be very different.

HISTORY

The nurse first elicits information about the client's previous history with schizophrenia to establish baseline data. He or she asks questions about how the client functioned before the crisis developed, such as "How do you usually spend your time?" and "Can you describe what you do each day?"

The nurse assesses the age at onset of schizophrenia, knowing that poorer outcomes are associated with an earlier age at onset. Learning the client's previous history of hospital admissions and response to hospitalization also is important.

The nurse also assesses the client for previous suicide attempts. Ten percent of all people with schizophrenia eventually commit suicide. The nurse might ask, "Have you ever attempted suicide?" or "Have you ever heard voices telling you to hurt yourself?" Likewise, it is important to elicit information about any history of violence or aggression because a history of aggressive behavior is a strong predictor of future aggression. The nurse might ask, "What do you do when you are angry, frustrated, upset, or scared?"

The nurse assesses whether the client has been using current support systems by asking the client or significant others the following questions:

- Has the client kept in contact with family or friends?
- Has the client been to scheduled groups or therapy appointments?
- Does the client seem to run out of money between paychecks?
- Have the client's living arrangements changed recently?

Finally, the nurse assesses the client's perception of his or her current situation—that is, what the client believes to be significant present events or stressors. The nurse can gather such information by asking, "What do you see as the primary problem now?" or "What do you need help managing now?"

GENERAL APPEARANCE, MOTOR BEHAVIOR, AND SPEECH

Appearance may vary widely among different clients with schizophrenia. Some appear normal in terms of being dressed appropriately, sitting in a chair conversing with the nurse, and exhibiting no strange or unusual postures or gestures. Others exhibit odd or bizarre behavior. They may appear disheveled and unkempt with no obvious concern for their hygiene, or they may wear strange or inappropriate clothing (for instance, a heavy wool coat and stocking cap in hot weather).

Overall motor behavior also may appear odd. The client may be restless and unable to sit still, exhibit agitation and pacing, or appear unmoving (catatonia). He or she also may demonstrate seemingly purposeless gestures (stereotypic behavior) and odd facial expressions such as grimacing. The client may imitate the movements and gestures of someone whom he or she is observing (echopraxia). Rambling speech that may or may not make sense to the listener is likely to accompany these behaviors.

Conversely, the client may exhibit psychomotor retardation (a general slowing of all movements). Sometimes the client may be almost immobile, curled into a ball (fetal position). Clients with the catatonic type of schizophrenia can exhibit waxy flexibility: they maintain any position in which they are placed, even if the position is awkward or uncomfortable.

The client may exhibit an unusual speech pattern. Two typical patterns are word salad (jumbled words and phrases that are disconnected or incoherent and make no sense to the listener) and echolalia (repetition or imitation of what someone else says). Speech may be slowed or accelerated in rate and volume: the client may speak in whispers or hushed tones or may talk loudly or yell. Latency of response refers to hesitation before the client responds to questions. This latency or hesitation may last 30 or 45 seconds and usually indicates the client's difficulty with cognition or thought processes. Box 14.2 lists and gives examples of these unusual speech patterns.

MOOD AND AFFECT

Clients with schizophrenia report and demonstrate wide variances in mood and affect. They often are described as having flat affect (no facial expression) or blunted affect (few observable facial expressions). The typical facial expression often is described as mask-like. The affect also may be described as silly, characterized by giddy laughter for no apparent reason. The client may exhibit an inappropriate expression or emotions incongruent with the context of the situation. This incongruence ranges from mild or subtle to grossly inappropriate. For example, the client may laugh and grin while describing the death of a family member or weep while talking about the weather.

Box 14.2   UNUSUAL SPEECH PATTERNS OF CLIENTS WITH SCHIZOPHRENIA

Clang associations are ideas that are related to one another based on sound or rhyming rather than meaning.
   Example: "I will take a pill if I go up the hill but not if my name is Jill, I don't want to kill."
Neologisms are words invented by the client.
   Example: "I'm afraid of grittiz. If there are any grittiz here, I will have to leave. Are you a grittiz?"
Verbigeration is the stereotyped repetition of words or phrases that may or may not have meaning to the listener.
   Example: "I want to go home, go home, go home, go home."
Echolalia is the client's imitation or repetition of what the nurse says.
   Example: *Nurse:* "Can you tell me how you're feeling?" *Client:* "Can you tell me how you're feeling, how you're feeling?"
Stilted language is use of words or phrases that are flowery, excessive, and pompous.
   Example: "Would you be so kind, as a representative of Florence Nightingale, as to do me the honor of providing just a wee bit of refreshment, perhaps in the form of some clear spring water?"
Perseveration is the persistent adherence to a single idea or topic and verbal repetition of a sentence, phrase, or word, even when another person attempts to change the topic.
   Example: *Nurse:* "How have you been sleeping lately?" *Client:* "I think people have been following me." *Nurse:* "Where do you live?" *Client:* "At my place people have been following me." *Nurse:* "What do you like to do in your free time?" *Client:* "Nothing because people are following me."
Word salad is a combination of jumbled words and phrases that are disconnected or incoherent and make no sense to the listener.
   Example: "Corn, potatoes, jump up, play games, grass, cupboard."

The client may report feeling depressed and having no pleasure or joy in life (anhedonia). Conversely, he or she may report feeling all-knowing, all-powerful, and not at all concerned with the circumstance or situation. It is more common for the client to report exaggerated feelings of well-being during episodes of psychotic or delusional thinking and a lack of energy or pleasurable feelings during the chronic, or long-term, phase of the illness.

THOUGHT PROCESS AND CONTENT

Schizophrenia often is referred to as a thought disorder because that is the primary feature of the disease: thought processes become disordered, and the continuity of thoughts and information processing is disrupted. The nurse can assess thought process by inferring from what the client says. He or she can assess thought content by evaluating what the client actually says. For example, clients may suddenly stop talking in the middle of a sentence and remain silent for several seconds to 1 minute (thought blocking). They also may state that they believe others can hear their thoughts (thought broadcasting), that others are taking their thoughts (**thought withdrawal**), or that others are placing thoughts in their mind against their will (**thought insertion**).

Clients also may exhibit tangential thinking, which is veering onto unrelated topics and never answering the original question:

Nurse: "How have you been sleeping lately?"
   Client: "Oh, I try to sleep at night. I like to listen to music to help me sleep. I really like country-western music best. What do you like? Can I have something to eat pretty soon? I'm hungry."
Nurse: "Can you tell me how you've been sleeping?"

Circumstantiality may be evidenced if the client gives unnecessary details or strays from the topic but eventually provides the requested information:

Nurse: "How have you been sleeping lately?"
   Client: "Oh, I go to bed early, so I can get plenty of rest. I like to listen to music or read before bed. Right now I'm reading a good mystery. Maybe I'll write a mystery someday. But it isn't helping, reading I mean. I have been getting only 2 or 3 hours of sleep at night."

Poverty of content (**alogia**) describes the lack of any real meaning or substance in what the client says:

Nurse: "How have you been sleeping lately?"
   Client: "Well, I guess, I don't know, hard to tell."

DELUSIONS

Clients with schizophrenia usually experience **delusions** (fixed, false beliefs with no basis in reality) in the psychotic phase of the illness. A common characteristic of schizophrenic delusions is the direct, immediate, and total certainty with which the client holds these beliefs. Because the client believes the delusion, he or she therefore acts accordingly. For example, the client with delusions of persecution is probably suspicious, mistrustful, and guarded about disclosing personal information; he or she may examine the room periodically or speak in hushed, secretive tones.

The theme or content of the delusions may vary. Box 14.3 describes and provides examples of the various types of delusions. External contradictory information or facts cannot alter these delusional beliefs. If asked why he or she believes such an unlikely idea, the client often replies, "I just know it."

Initially, the nurse assesses the content and depth of the delusion to know what behaviors to expect and to try to establish reality for the client. When eliciting information about the client's delusional beliefs, the nurse must be careful not to support or challenge them. The nurse might ask the client to explain what he or she believes by saying "Please explain that to me" or "Tell me what you're thinking about that."

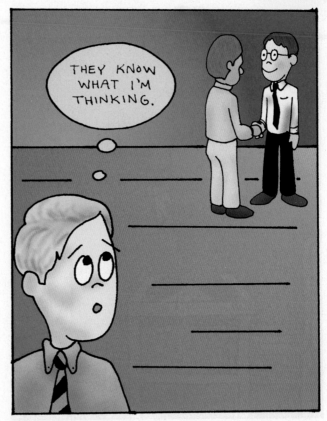

Thought broadcasting

Box 14.3 TYPES OF DELUSIONS

Persecutory/paranoid delusions involve the client's belief that "others" are planning to harm the client or are spying, following, ridiculing, or belittling the client in some way. Sometimes the client cannot define who these "others" are.
Examples: The client may think that food has been poisoned or that rooms are bugged with listening devices. Sometimes the "persecutor" is the government, FBI, or other powerful organization. Occasionally, specific individuals, even family members, may be named as the "persecutor."

Grandiose delusions are characterized by the client's claim to association with famous people or celebrities, or the client's belief that he or she is famous or capable of great feats.
Examples: The client may claim to be engaged to a famous movie star or related to some public figure, such as claiming to be the daughter of the president of the United States, or he or she may claim to have found a cure for cancer.

Religious delusions often center around the second coming of Christ or another significant religious figure or prophet. These religious delusions appear suddenly as part of the client's psychosis and are not part of his or her religious faith or that of others.
Examples: Client claims to be the Messiah or some prophet sent from God; believes that God communicates directly to him or her, or that he or she has a "special" religious mission in life or special religious powers.

Somatic delusions are generally vague and unrealistic beliefs about the client's health or bodily functions. Factual information or diagnostic testing does not change these beliefs.
Examples: A male client may say that he is pregnant, or a client may report decaying intestines or worms in the brain.

Referential delusions or ideas of reference involve the client's belief that television broadcasts, music, or newspaper articles have special meaning for him or her.
Examples: The client may report that the president was speaking directly to him on a news broadcast or that special messages are sent through newspaper articles.

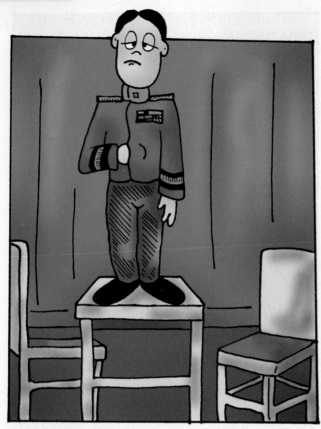

Delusions of grandeur

SENSORIUM AND INTELLECTUAL PROCESSES

One hallmark symptom of schizophrenic psychosis is **hallucinations** (false sensory perceptions, or perceptual experiences that do not exist in reality). Hallucinations can involve the five senses and bodily sensations. They can be threatening and frightening for the client; less frequently, clients report hallucinations as pleasant. Initially, the client perceives hallucinations as real, but later in the illness, he or she may recognize them as hallucinations.

Hallucinations are distinguished from *illusions*, which are misperceptions of actual environmental stimuli. For example, while walking through the woods, a person believes he sees a snake at the side of the path. On closer examination, however, he discovers it is only a curved stick. Reality or factual information corrected this illusion. Hallucinations, however, have no such basis in reality.

The following are the various types of hallucinations (Kirkpatrick & Tek, 2005):

- *Auditory hallucinations,* the most common type, involve hearing sounds, most often voices, talking to or about the client. There may be one or multiple voices; a familiar or unfamiliar person's voice may be speaking. **Command hallucinations** are voices demanding that the client take action, often to harm self or others, and are considered dangerous.
- *Visual hallucinations* involve seeing images that do not exist at all, such as lights or a dead person, or distortions such as seeing a frightening monster instead of the nurse. They are the second most common type of hallucination.
- *Olfactory hallucinations* involve smells or odors. They may be a specific scent such as urine or feces or a more general scent such as a rotten or rancid odor. In addition to clients with schizophrenia, this type of hallucination often occurs with dementia, seizures, or cerebrovascular accidents.
- *Tactile hallucinations* refer to sensations such as electricity running through the body or bugs crawling on the skin. Tactile hallucinations are found most often in clients undergoing alcohol withdrawal; they rarely occur in clients with schizophrenia.
- *Gustatory hallucinations* involve a taste lingering in the mouth or the sense that food tastes like something else. The taste may be metallic or bitter or may be represented as a specific taste.
- *Cenesthetic hallucinations* involve the client's report that he or she feels bodily functions that are usually undetectable. Examples would be the sensation of urine forming or impulses being transmitted through the brain.
- *Kinesthetic hallucinations* occur when the client is motionless but reports the sensation of bodily movement. Occasionally, the bodily movement is something unusual, such as floating above the ground.

During episodes of psychosis, clients are commonly disoriented to time and sometimes place. The most extreme form of disorientation is **depersonalization**, in which the client feels detached from her or his behavior. Although the client can state her or his name correctly, she or he feels as if her or his body belongs to someone else or that her or his spirit is detached from the body.

Assessing the intellectual processes of a client with schizophrenia is difficult if he or she is experiencing psychosis. The client usually demonstrates poor intellectual functioning as a result of disordered thoughts. Nevertheless, the nurse should not assume that the client has limited intellectual capacity based on impaired thought processes. It may be that the client cannot focus, concentrate, or pay adequate attention to demonstrate his or her intellectual abilities accurately. The nurse is more likely to obtain accurate assessments of the client's intellectual abilities when the client's thought processes are clearer.

Clients often have difficulty with abstract thinking and may respond in a very literal way to other people and the environment. For example, when asked to interpret the proverb, "A stitch in time saves nine," the client may explain it by saying, "I need to sew up my clothes." The client may not understand what is being said and can easily misinterpret instructions. This can pose serious problems during medication administration. For example, the nurse may tell the client, "It is always important to take all your medications." The client may misinterpret the nurse's statement and take the entire supply of medication at one time.

JUDGMENT AND INSIGHT

Judgment is frequently impaired in the client with schizophrenia. Because judgment is based on the ability to interpret the environment correctly, it follows that the client with disordered thought processes and environmental misinterpretations will have great difficulty with judgment. At times, lack of judgment is so severe that clients cannot meet their needs for safety and protection and place themselves in harm's way. This difficulty may range from failing to wear warm clothing in cold weather to failing to seek medical care even when desperately ill. The client also may fail to recognize needs for sleep or food.

Insight also can be severely impaired, especially early in the illness, when the client, family, and friends do not understand what is happening. Over time, some clients can learn about the illness, anticipate problems, and seek appropriate assistance as needed. However, chronic difficulties result in clients who fail to understand schizophrenia as a long-term health problem requiring consistent management.

SELF-CONCEPT

Deterioration of the concept of self is a major problem in schizophrenia. The phrase *loss of ego boundaries* describes the client's lack of a clear sense of where his or her own body, mind, and influence end and where those aspects of other animate and inanimate objects begin. This lack of ego boundaries is evidenced by depersonalization, derealization (environmental objects become smaller or larger or seem unfamiliar), and **ideas of reference**. Clients may believe they are fused with another person or object, may not recognize body parts as their own, or may fail to know whether they are male or female. These difficulties are the source of many bizarre behaviors such as public undressing or masturbating, speaking about oneself in the third person, or physically clinging to objects in the environment. Body image distortion also may occur.

ROLES AND RELATIONSHIPS

Social isolation is prevalent in clients with schizophrenia, partly as a result of positive signs such as delusions, hallucinations, and loss of ego boundaries. Relating to others is difficult when one's self-concept is not clear. Clients also have problems with trust and intimacy, which interfere with the ability to establish satisfactory relationships. Low self-esteem, one of the negative signs of schizophrenia, further complicates the client's ability to interact with others and the environment. These clients lack confidence, feel strange or different from other people, and do not believe they are worthwhile. The result is avoidance of other people.

The client may experience great frustration in attempting to fulfill roles in the family and community. Success in school or at work can be severely compromised because the client has difficulty thinking clearly, remembering, paying attention, and concentrating. Subsequently, he or she lacks motivation. Clients who develop schizophrenia at young ages have more difficulties than those whose illness developed later in life because they did not have the opportunity to succeed in these areas before the illness.

Fulfilling family roles, such as that of son or daughter or sibling, is difficult for these clients. Often, their erratic or unpredictable behavior frightens or embarrasses family members, who become unsure what to expect next. Families also may feel guilty or responsible, believing they somehow failed to provide a loving supportive home life. These clients also may believe they have disappointed their families because they cannot become independent or successful.

PHYSIOLOGIC AND SELF-CARE CONSIDERATIONS

Clients with schizophrenia may have significant self-care deficits. Inattention to hygiene and grooming needs is common, especially during psychotic episodes. The client can become so preoccupied with delusions or hallucinations that he or she fails to perform even basic activities of daily living.

Clients also may fail to recognize sensations such as hunger or thirst, and food or fluid intake may be inadequate. This can result in malnourishment and constipation. Constipation is also a common side effect of antipsychotic medications, compounding the problem. Paranoia or excessive fears that food and fluids have been poisoned are common and may interfere with eating. If the client is agitated and pacing, he or she may be unable to sit down long enough to eat.

Occasionally, clients develop **polydipsia** (excessive water intake), which leads to water intoxication. Serum sodium levels can become dangerously low, leading to seizures. Polydipsia usually is seen in clients who have had severe and persistent mental illness for many years as well as long-term therapy with antipsychotic medications. Polydipsia may be caused by the behavioral state itself or may be precipitated by the use of antidepressant or antipsychotic medications (Reynolds et al., 2004).

Sleep problems are common. Hallucinations may stimulate clients, resulting in insomnia. Other times, clients are suspicious and believe harm will come to them if they sleep. As in other self-care areas, the client may not correctly perceive or acknowledge physical cues such as fatigue.

To assist the client with community living, the nurse assesses daily living skills and functional abilities. Such skills—having a bank account and paying bills, buying food and preparing meals, and using public transportation—are often difficult tasks for the client with schizophrenia. He or she might never have learned such skills or may be unable to accomplish them consistently.

Data Analysis

The nurse must analyze assessment data for clients with schizophrenia to determine priorities and establish an effective plan of care. Not all clients have the same problems and needs, nor is it likely that any individual client has all the problems that can accompany schizophrenia. Levels of family and community support and available services also vary, all of which influence the client's care and outcomes.

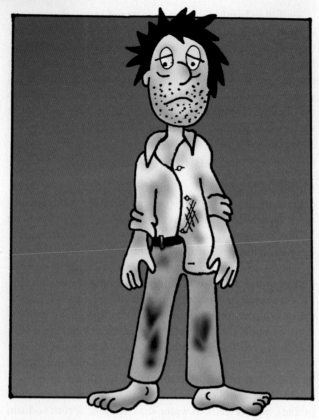

Self-care deficits

The analysis of assessment data generally falls into two main categories: data associated with the positive signs of the disease and data associated with the negative signs. The North American Nursing Diagnosis Association's nursing diagnoses commonly established based on the assessment of psychotic symptoms or positive signs are as follows:

• Risk for Other-Directed Violence
• Risk for Suicide
• Disturbed Thought Processes
• Disturbed Sensory Perception
• Disturbed Personal Identity
• Impaired Verbal Communication

The North American Nursing Diagnosis Association's nursing diagnoses based on the assessment of negative signs and functional abilities include the following:

• Self-Care Deficits
• Social Isolation
• Deficient Diversional Activity
• Ineffective Health Maintenance
• Ineffective Therapeutic Regimen Management

Outcome Identification

It is likely that the client with an acute psychotic episode of schizophrenia will receive treatment in an intensive setting such as an inpatient hospital unit. During this phase, the focus of care is stabilizing the client's thought processes

and reality orientation as well as ensuring safety. This is also the time to evaluate resources, make referrals, and begin planning for the client's rehabilitation and return to the community.

Examples of outcomes appropriate to the acute, psychotic phase of treatment are as follows:

1. The client will not injure self or others.
2. The client will establish contact with reality.
3. The client will interact with others in the environment.
4. The client will express thoughts and feelings in a safe and socially acceptable manner.
5. The client will participate in prescribed therapeutic interventions.

Once the crisis or the acute, psychotic symptoms have been stabilized, the focus is on developing the client's ability to live as independently and successfully as possible in the community. This usually requires continued follow-up care and participation of the client's family in community support services. Prevention and early recognition and treatment of relapse symptoms are important parts of successful rehabilitation. Dealing with the negative signs of schizophrenia, which medication generally does not affect, is a major challenge for the client and caregivers. Examples of treatment outcomes for continued care after the stabilization of acute symptoms are as follows:

1. The client will participate in the prescribed regimen (including medications and follow-up appointments).
2. The client will maintain adequate routines for sleeping and food and fluid intake.
3. The client will demonstrate independence in self-care activities.
4. The client will communicate effectively with others in the community to meet his or her needs.
5. The client will seek or accept assistance to meet his or her needs when indicated.

The nurse must appreciate the severity of schizophrenia and the profound and sometimes devastating effects it has on the lives of clients and their families. It is equally important to avoid treating the client as a "hopeless case," someone who no longer is capable of having a meaningful and satisfying life. It is not helpful to expect either too much or too little from the client. Careful ongoing assessment is necessary so that appropriate treatment and interventions address the client's needs and difficulties while helping the client to reach his or her optimal level of functioning.

Intervention

PROMOTING THE SAFETY OF CLIENT AND OTHERS

Safety for both the client and the nurse is the priority when providing care for the client with schizophrenia. The client may be paranoid and suspicious of the nurse and the environment and may feel threatened and intimidated. Although the client's behavior may be threatening to the nurse, the client also is feeling unsafe and may believe his or her well-being to be in jeopardy. Therefore, the nurse must approach the client in a nonthreatening manner. Making demands or being authoritative only increases the client's fears. Giving the client ample personal space usually enhances his or her sense of security.

A fearful or agitated client has the potential to harm self or others. The nurse must observe for signs of building agitation or escalating behavior such as increased intensity of pacing, loud talking or yelling, and hitting or kicking objects. The nurse must institute interventions to protect the client, nurse, and others in the environment. This may involve administering medication, moving the client to a quiet, less-stimulating environment, and, in extreme situations, temporarily using seclusion or restraints. See Chapter 10 for a discussion of how to deal with anger and hostility and Chapter 15 for how to deal with clients who are suicidal.

ESTABLISHING A THERAPEUTIC RELATIONSHIP

Establishing trust between the client and nurse also helps to allay the fears of a frightened client. Initially, the client may tolerate only 5 or 10 minutes of contact at one time. Establishing a therapeutic relationship takes time, and the nurse must be patient. The nurse provides explanations that are clear, direct, and easy to understand. Body language should include eye contact but not staring, a relaxed body posture, and facial expressions that convey genuine interest and concern. Telling the client one's name and calling the client by name are helpful in establishing trust as well as reality orientation.

The nurse must assess carefully the client's response to the use of touch. Sometimes gentle touch conveys caring and concern. At other times, the client may misinterpret the nurse's touch as threatening and therefore undesirable. As the nurse sits near the client, does he or she move or look away? Is the client frightened or wary of the nurse's presence? If so, that client may not be reassured by touch but frightened or threatened by it.

USING THERAPEUTIC COMMUNICATION

Communicating with clients experiencing psychotic symptoms can be difficult and frustrating. The nurse tries to understand and make sense of what the client is saying, but this can be difficult if the client is hallucinating, withdrawn from reality, or relatively mute. The nurse must maintain nonverbal communication with the client, especially when verbal communication is not very successful. This involves spending time with the client, perhaps through fairly lengthy periods of silence. The presence of the nurse is a contact with reality for the client and also can demonstrate the nurse's genuine interest and caring to the client. Calling the client by name, making references to the day and time, and commenting on the environment are all helpful ways to continue to make contact with a client who is having problems with reality orientation and verbal communication.

Clients who are left alone for long periods become more deeply involved in their psychosis, so frequent contact and time spent with a client are important even if the nurse is unsure that the client is aware of the nurse's presence.

Active listening is an important skill for the nurse trying to communicate with a client whose verbalizations are disorganized or nonsensical. Rather than dismissing what the client says because it is not clear, the nurse must make efforts to determine the meaning the client is trying to convey. Listening for themes or recurrent statements, asking clarifying questions, and exploring the meaning of the client's statements are all useful techniques to increase understanding.

The nurse must let the client know when his or her meaning is not clear. It is never useful to pretend to understand or just to agree or go along with what the client is saying: this is dishonest and violates trust between client and nurse.

> **Nurse:** *"How are you feeling today?"* (using a broad opening statement)
>> **Client:** *"Invisible."*
>> **Nurse:** *"Can you explain that to me?"* (seeking clarification)
> **Client:** *"Oh, it doesn't matter."*
> **Nurse:** *"I'm interested in how you feel; I'm just not sure I understand."* (offering self/seeking clarification)
> **Client:** *"It doesn't mean much."*
> **Nurse:** *"Let me see if I can understand. Do you feel like you're being ignored, that no one is really listening?"* (verbalizing the implied)

IMPLEMENTING INTERVENTIONS FOR DELUSIONAL THOUGHTS

The client experiencing delusions utterly believes them and cannot be convinced they are false or untrue. Such delusions powerfully influence the client's behavior. For example, if the client's delusion is that he or she is being poisoned, he or she will be suspicious, mistrustful, and probably resistant to providing information and taking medications.

The nurse must avoid openly confronting the delusion or arguing with the client about it. The nurse also must avoid reinforcing the delusional belief by "playing along" with what the client says. It is the nurse's responsibility to present and maintain reality by making simple statements such as

> *"I have seen no evidence of that"* (presenting reality)
>
> or
>
> *"It doesn't seem that way to me"* (casting doubt).

As antipsychotic medications begin to have a therapeutic effect, it will be possible for the nurse to discuss the delusional ideas with the client and identify ways in which the delusions interfere with the client's daily life.

The nurse also can help the client minimize the effects of delusional thinking. Distraction techniques, such as listening to music, watching television, writing, or talking to friends, are useful. Direct action, such as engaging in positive self-talk and positive thinking and ignoring the delusional thoughts, may be beneficial as well.

IMPLEMENTING INTERVENTIONS FOR HALLUCINATIONS

Intervening when the client experiences hallucinations requires the nurse to focus on what is real and to help shift the client's response toward reality. Initially, the nurse must determine what the client is experiencing—that is, what the voices are saying or what the client is seeing. Doing so increases the nurse's understanding of the nature of the client's feelings and behavior. In command hallucinations, the client hears voices directing him or her to do something, often to hurt self or someone else. For this reason, the nurse must elicit a description of the content of the hallucination so that health care personnel can take precautions to protect the client and others as necessary. The nurse might say,

"I don't hear any voices; what are you hearing?" (presenting reality/seeking clarification).

This also can help the nurse understand how to relieve the client's fears or paranoia. For example, the client might be seeing ghosts or monster-like images, and the nurse could respond,

"I don't see anything, but you must be frightened. You are safe here in the hospital" (presenting reality/ translating into feelings).

This acknowledges the client's fear but reassures the client that no harm will come to him or her.

Clients do not always report or identify hallucinations. At times, the nurse must infer from the client's behavior that hallucinations are occurring. Examples of behavior that indicate hallucinations include alternately listening and then talking when no one else is present, laughing inappropriately for no observable reason, and mumbling or mouthing words with no audible sound.

A helpful strategy for intervening with hallucinations is to engage the client in a reality-based activity such as playing cards, participating in occupational therapy, or listening to music. It is difficult for the client to pay attention to hallucinations and reality-based activity at the same time, so this technique of distracting the client is often useful.

It also may be useful to work with the client to identify certain situations or a particular frame of mind that may precede or trigger auditory hallucinations. Intensity of hallucinations often is related to anxiety levels; therefore, monitoring and intervening to lower a client's anxiety may decrease the intensity of hallucinations. Clients who recognize that certain moods or patterns of thinking precede the onset of voices may eventually be able to manage or control the hallucinations by learning to manage or avoid particular states of mind. This may involve learning to relax when voices occur, engaging in diversions, correcting negative self-talk, and seeking out or avoiding social interaction.

Teaching the client to talk back to the voices forcefully also may help him or her manage auditory hallucinations. The client should do this in a relatively private place rather than in public. There is an international self-help movement of "voice-hearer groups," developed to assist people to manage auditory hallucinations. One group devised the strategy of carrying a cell phone (fake or real) to cope with voices when in public places. With cell phones, members can carry on conversations with their voices in the street—and tell them to shut up—while avoiding ridicule by looking like a normal part of the street scene (Hagen & Mitchell, 2001). Being able to verbalize resistance can help the client feel empowered and capable of dealing with the hallucinations.

COPING WITH SOCIALLY INAPPROPRIATE BEHAVIORS

Clients with schizophrenia often experience a loss of ego boundaries, which poses difficulties for themselves and others in their environment and community. Potentially bizarre or strange behaviors include touching others without warning or invitation, intruding into others' living spaces, talking to or caressing inanimate objects, and engaging in such socially inappropriate behaviors as undressing, masturbating, or urinating in public. Clients may approach others and make provocative, insulting, or sexual statements. The nurse must consider the needs of others as well as the needs of clients in these situations.

Protecting the client is a primary nursing responsibility and includes protecting the client from retaliation by others who experience the client's intrusions and socially unacceptable behavior. Redirecting the client away from situations or others can interrupt the undesirable behavior and keep the client from further intrusive behaviors. The nurse also must try to protect the client's right to privacy and dignity. Taking the client to his or her room or to a quiet area with less stimulation and fewer people often helps. Engaging the client in appropriate activities also is indicated. For example, if the client is undressing in front of others, the nurse might say,

"Let's go to your room and you can put your clothes back on" (encouraging collaboration/redirecting to appropriate activity).

If the client is making verbal statements to others, the nurse might ask the client to go for a walk or move to another area to listen to music. The nurse should deal with socially inappropriate behavior nonjudgmentally and matter-of-factly. This means making factual statements with no overtones of scolding and not talking to the client as if he or she were a naughty child.

Some behaviors may be so offensive or threatening that others respond by yelling at, ridiculing, or even taking aggressive action against the client. Although providing physical protection for the client is the nurse's first consideration, helping others affected by the client's behavior also is important. Usually, the nurse can offer simple and factual statements to others that do not violate the client's confidentiality. The nurse might make statements such as

"You didn't do anything to provoke that behavior. Sometimes people's illnesses cause them to act in strange and uncomfortable ways. It is important not to laugh at behaviors that are part of someone's illness" (presenting reality/giving information).

The nurse reassures the client's family that these behaviors are part of the client's illness and not personally directed at them. Such situations present an opportunity to educate family members about schizophrenia and to help allay their feelings of guilt, shame, or responsibility.

Reintegrating the client into the treatment milieu as soon as possible is essential. The client should not feel shunned or punished for inappropriate behavior. Health care personnel should introduce limited stimulation gradually. For example, when the client is comfortable and demonstrating appropriate behavior with the nurse, one or two other people can be engaged in a somewhat structured activity with the client. The client's involvement is gradually increased to small groups and then to larger, less structured groups as he or she can tolerate the increased level of stimulation without decompensating (regressing to previous, less effective coping behaviors).

TEACHING CLIENT AND FAMILY

Coping with schizophrenia is a major adjustment for both the clients and their families. Understanding the illness, the need for continuing medication and follow-up, and the uncertainty of the prognosis or recovery are key issues. Clients and families need help to cope with the emotional upheaval that schizophrenia causes. See Client/Family Education for Schizophrenia for education points.

Identifying and managing one's own health needs are primary concerns for everyone, but this is a particular challenge for clients with schizophrenia because their health needs can be complex and their ability to manage them may be impaired. The nurse helps the client to manage his or her illness and health needs as independently as possible. This can be accomplished only through education and ongoing support.

Teaching the client and family members to prevent or manage relapse is an essential part of a comprehensive plan of care. This includes providing facts about schizophrenia, identifying the early signs of relapse, and teaching health practices to promote physical and psychological well-being. Early identification of these relapse signs (Box 14.4) has been found to reduce the frequency of relapse; when relapse cannot be prevented, early identification provides the foundation for interventions to manage the relapse. For example, if the nurse finds that the client is fatigued or lacks adequate sleep or proper nutrition, interventions to promote rest and nutrition may prevent a relapse or minimize its intensity and duration.

The nurse can use the list of relapse risk factors in several ways. He or she can include these risk factors in discharge teaching before the client leaves the inpatient setting so that the client and family know what to watch for and when to seek assistance. The nurse also can use the list when assessing the client in an outpatient or clinic setting or when working with clients in a community support program. The nurse also can provide teaching to ancillary personnel who may work with the client so they know when to contact a mental health professional. Taking medications as prescribed, keeping regular follow-up appointments, and avoiding alcohol and other drugs have been associated with fewer and shorter hospital stays. In addition, clients who can identify and avoid stressful situations are less likely to suffer frequent relapses. Using a list of relapse risk factors is one way to assess the client's progress in the community.

Families experience a wide variety of responses to the illness of their loved one. Some family members might be ashamed or embarrassed or frightened of the client's strange or threatening behaviors. They worry about a relapse. They may feel guilty for having these feelings or fear for their own mental health or well-being. If the client experiences repeated and profound problems with schizophrenia, the family members may become emotionally exhausted or even alienated from the client, feeling they can no longer deal with the situation. Family members need ongoing support and education, including reassurance that they are not the cause of schizophrenia. Participating in organizations such as the Alliance for the Mentally Ill may help families with their ongoing needs.

Teaching Self-Care and Proper Nutrition. Because of apathy or lack of energy over the course of the illness, poor personal hygiene can be a problem for clients who are experiencing psychotic symptoms as well as for all clients with schizophrenia. When the client is psychotic, he or she may pay little attention to hygiene or may be unable to sustain the attention or concentration required to complete grooming tasks. The nurse may need to direct the client through the necessary steps for bathing, shampooing, dressing, and so forth. The nurse gives directions in short, clear statements to enhance the client's ability to complete the tasks. The nurse allows ample time for grooming and performing hygiene and does not attempt to rush or hurry the client. In this way, the nurse encourages the client to become more independent as soon as possible—that is, when he or she is better oriented to reality and better able to sustain the concentration and attention needed for these tasks.

If the client has deficits in hygiene and grooming resulting from apathy or lack of energy for tasks, the nurse may vary the approach used to promote the client's independence

Nursing Care Plan *Client with Delusions*

Nursing Diagnosis

Disturbed Thought Processes: *Disruption in cognitive operations and activities*

ASSESSMENT DATA

- Thinking not based in reality
- Disorientation
- Labile affect
- Short attention span
- Impaired judgment
- Distractibility

EXPECTED OUTCOMES

Immediate
The client will
- Be free of injury
- Demonstrate decreased anxiety level
- Respond to reality-based interactions initiated by others

Stabilization
The client will
- Interact on reality-based topics
- Sustain attention and concentration to complete tasks or activities

Community
The client will
- Verbalize recognition of delusional thoughts if they persist
- Be free from delusions or demonstrate the ability to function without responding to persistent delusional thoughts

IMPLEMENTATION

Nursing Interventions *denotes collaborative interventions	**Rationale**
Be sincere and honest when communicating with the client. Avoid vague or evasive remarks.	Delusional clients are extremely sensitive about others and can recognize insincerity. Evasive comments or hesitation reinforces mistrust or delusions.
Be consistent in setting expectations, enforcing rules, and so forth.	Clear, consistent limits provide a secure structure for the client.
Do not make promises that you cannot keep.	Broken promises reinforce the client's mistrust of others.
Encourage the client to talk with you, but do not pry for information.	Probing increases the client's suspicion and interferes with the therapeutic relationship.
Explain procedures, and try to be sure the client understands the procedures before carrying them out.	When the client has full knowledge of procedures, he or she is less likely to feel tricked by the staff.
Give positive feedback for the client's successes.	Positive feedback for genuine success enhances the client's sense of well-being and helps to make nondelusional reality a more positive situation for the client.
Recognize the client's delusions as the client's perception of the environment.	Recognizing the client's perceptions can help you understand the feelings he or she is experiencing.
Initially, do not argue with the client or try to convince the client that the delusions are false or unreal.	Logical argument does not dispel delusional ideas and can interfere with the development of trust.

Nursing Care Plan: Client with Delusions, cont.

IMPLEMENTATION

Interact with the client on the basis of real things; do not dwell on the delusional material.	Interacting about reality is healthy for the client.
Engage the client in one-to-one activities at first, then activities in small groups, and gradually activities in larger groups.	A distrustful client can best deal with one person initially. Gradual introduction of others as the client tolerates is less threatening.
Recognize and support the client's accomplishments (projects completed, responsibilities fulfilled, interactions initiated).	Recognizing the client's accomplishments can lessen anxiety and the need for delusions as a source of self-esteem.
Show empathy regarding the client's feelings; reassure the client of your presence and acceptance.	The client's delusions can be distressing. Empathy conveys your caring, interest and acceptance of the client.
Do not be judgmental or belittle or joke about the client's beliefs.	The client's delusions and feelings are not funny to him or her. The client may not understand or may feel rejected by attempts at humor.
Never convey to the client that you accept the delusions as reality.	Indicating belief in the delusions reinforces the delusion (and the client's illness).
Directly interject doubt regarding delusions as soon as the client seems ready to accept this (e.g., "I find that hard to believe."). Do not argue but present a factual account of the situation as you see it.	As the client begins to trust you, he or she may become willing to doubt the delusion if you express your doubt.
Ask the client if he or she can see that the delusions interfere with or cause problems in his or her life.	Discussion of the problems caused by the delusions is a focus on the present and is reality based.

Adapted from Schultz, J. M., & Videbeck, S. L. (2005). Lippincott's manual of psychiatric nursing care plans (7th ed.). Philadelphia: Lippincott Williams & Wilkins.

in these areas. The client is most likely to perform tasks of hygiene and grooming if they become a part of his or her daily routine. The client who has an established structure that incorporates his or her preferences has a greater chance for success than the client who waits to decide about hygiene tasks or performs them randomly. For example, the client may prefer to shower and shampoo on Monday, Wednesday, and Friday upon getting up in the morning. This nurse can assist the client to incorporate this plan into the client's daily routine, which leads to it becoming a habit. The client thus avoids making daily decisions about whether or not to shower or whether he or she feels like showering on a particular day.

Adequate nutrition and fluids are essential to the client's physical and emotional well-being. Careful assessment of the client's eating patterns and preferences allows the nurse to determine whether the client needs assistance in these areas. As with any type of self-care deficit, the nurse provides assistance as long as needed and then gradually promotes the client's independence as soon as the client is capable.

When the client is in the community, factors other than the client's illness may contribute to inadequate nutritional intake. Examples include lack of money to buy food, lack of knowledge about a nutritious diet, inadequate transportation, or limited abilities to prepare food. A thorough assessment of the client's functional abilities for community living helps the nurse to plan appropriate interventions. See the section to come, Community-Based Care.

Teaching Social Skills. Clients may be isolated from others for a variety of reasons. The bizarre behavior or statements of the client who is delusional or hallucinating may frighten or embarrass family or community members. Clients who are suspicious or mistrustful may avoid contact with others. Other times, clients may lack the social or conversation skills they need to make and maintain relationships with others. Also, a stigma remains attached to mental illness, particularly for clients for whom medication fails to relieve the positive signs of the illness.

The nurse can help the client develop social skills through education, role modeling, and practice. The client may not discriminate between the topics suitable for sharing with the nurse and those suitable for using to initiate a conversation on a bus. The nurse can help the client learn neutral social topics appropriate to any conversation, such as the weather or local events. The client also can benefit from learning that he or she should share certain details of

Box 14.4   EARLY SIGNS OF RELAPSE

- Impaired cause-and-effect reasoning
- Impaired information processing
- Poor nutrition
- Lack of sleep
- Lack of exercise
- Fatigue
- Poor social skills, social isolation, loneliness
- Interpersonal difficulties
- Lack of control, irritability
- Mood swings
- Ineffective medication management
- Low self-concept
- Looks and acts different
- Hopeless feelings
- Loss of motivation
- Anxiety and worry
- Disinhibition
- Increased negativity
- Neglecting appearance
- Forgetfulness

CLIENT/FAMILY EDUCATION FOR SCHIZOPHRENIA

- How to manage illness and symptoms
- Recognizing early signs of relapse
- Developing a plan to address relapse signs
- Importance of maintaining prescribed medication regimen and regular follow-up
- Avoiding alcohol and other drugs
- Self-care and proper nutrition
- Teaching social skills through education, role modeling, and practice
- Seeking assistance to avoid or manage stressful situations
- Counseling and education of family/significant others about the biologic causes and clinical course of schizophrenia and the need for ongoing support
- Importance of maintaining contact with community and participating in supportive organizations and care

his or her illness, such as the content of delusions or hallucinations, only with a health care provider.

Modeling and practicing social skills with the client can help him or her experience greater success in social interactions. Specific skills such as eye contact, attentive listening, and taking turns talking can increase the client's abilities and confidence in socializing.

Medication Management. Maintaining the medication regimen is vital to a successful outcome for clients with schizophrenia. Failing to take medications as prescribed is one of the most frequent reasons for recurrence of psychotic symptoms and hospital admission (Kane & Marder, 2005). Clients who respond well to and maintain an antipsychotic medication regimen may lead relatively normal lives with only an occasional relapse. Those who do not respond well to antipsychotic agents may face a lifetime of dealing with delusional ideas and hallucinations, negative signs, and marked impairment. Many clients find themselves somewhere between these two extremes. See Client Education for Medication Management: Antipsychotics.

There are many reasons why clients may not maintain the medication regimen. The nurse must determine the barriers to compliance for each client. Sometimes clients intend to take their medications as prescribed but have difficulty remembering when and if they did so. They may find it difficult to adhere to a routine schedule for medications. Several methods are available to help clients remember when to take medications. One is using a pill box with

compartments for days of the week and times of the day. After the box has been filled, perhaps with assistance from the nurse or case manager, the client often has no more difficulties. It is also helpful to make a chart of all administration times so that the client can cross off each time he or she has taken the medications.

Clients may have practical barriers to medication compliance, such as inadequate funds to obtain expensive medications, lack of transportation or knowledge about how to obtain refills for prescriptions, or inability to plan ahead to get new prescriptions before current supplies run out. Clients usually can overcome all these obstacles once they have been identified.

Sometimes clients decide to decrease or discontinue their medications because of uncomfortable or embarrassing side effects. Unwanted side effects are frequently reported as the reason clients stop taking medications (Kane & Marder, 2005). Interventions, such as eating a proper diet and drinking enough fluids, using a stool softener to avoid constipation, sucking on hard candy to minimize dry mouth, or using sunscreen to avoid sunburn, can help to control some of these uncomfortable side effects (see Table 13.2). Some side effects, such as dry mouth and blurred vision, improve with time or with lower doses of medication. Medication may be warranted to combat common neurologic side effects such as extrapyramidal side effects or akathisia.

Some side effects, such as those affecting sexual functioning, are embarrassing for the client to report, and the client may confirm these side effects only if the nurse directly inquires about them. This may require a call to the client's physician or primary provider to obtain a prescription for a different type of antipsychotic.

CLIENT EDUCATION FOR MEDICATION MANAGEMENT: ANTIPSYCHOTICS

- Drink sugar-free fluids and eat sugar-free hard candy to ease the anticholinergic effects of dry mouth.
- Avoid calorie-laden beverages and candy because they promote dental caries, contribute to weight gain, and do little to relieve dry mouth.
- Constipation can be prevented or relieved by increasing intake of water and bulk-forming foods in the diet and by exercising.
- Stool softeners are permissible, but laxatives should be avoided.
- Use sunscreen to prevent burning. Avoid long periods of time in the sun, and wear protective clothing. Photosensitivity can cause you to burn easily.
- Rising slowly from a lying or sitting position prevents falls from orthostatic hypotension or dizziness due to a drop in blood pressure. Wait until any dizziness has subsided before you walk.
- Monitor the amount of sleepiness or drowsiness you experience. Avoid driving a car or performing other potentially dangerous activities until your response time and reflexes seem normal.
- If you forget a dose of antipsychotic medication, take it if the dose is only 3 to 4 hours late. If the missed dose is more than 4 hours late or the next dose is due, omit the forgotten dose.
- If you have difficulty remembering your medication, use a chart to record doses when taken, or use a pill box labeled with dosage times and/or days of the week to help you remember when to take medication.

Sometimes a client discontinues medications because he or she dislikes taking them or believes he or she does not need them. The client may have been willing to take the medications when experiencing psychotic symptoms but may believe that medication is unnecessary when he or she feels well. By refusing to take the medications, the client may be denying the existence or severity of schizophrenia. These issues of noncompliance are much more difficult to resolve. The nurse can teach the client about schizophrenia, the nature of chronic illness, and the importance of medications in managing symptoms and preventing recurrence. For example, the nurse could say, "This medication helps you think more clearly" or "Taking this medication will make it less likely that you'll hear troubling voices in your mind again."

Even after education, some clients continue to refuse to take medication; they may understand the connection between medication and prevention of relapse only after experiencing a return of psychotic symptoms. A few clients still do not understand the importance of consistently taking medication and, even after numerous relapses, continue to experience psychosis and hospital admission fairly frequently.

Evaluation

The nurse must consider evaluation of the plan of care in the context of each client and family. Ongoing assessment provides data to determine whether the client's individual outcomes were achieved. The client's perception of the success of treatment also plays a part in evaluation. Even if all outcomes are achieved, the nurse must ask if the client is comfortable or satisfied with the quality of life.

In a global sense, evaluation of the treatment of schizophrenia is based on the following:
- Have the client's psychotic symptoms disappeared? If not, can the client carry out his or her daily life despite the persistence of some psychotic symptoms?
- Does the client understand the prescribed medication regimen? Is he or she committed to adherence to the regimen?
- Does the client possess the necessary functional abilities for community living?
- Are community resources adequate to help the client live successfully in the community?
- Is there a sufficient after-care or crisis plan in place to deal with recurrence of symptoms or difficulties encountered in the community?
- Are the client and family adequately knowledgeable about schizophrenia?
- Does the client believe that he or she has a satisfactory quality of life?

ELDER CONSIDERATIONS

Late-onset schizophrenia refers to development of the disease after age 45; schizophrenia is not initially diagnosed in elder clients. Psychotic symptoms that appear in later life are usually associated with depression or dementia, not schizophrenia. People with schizophrenia do survive into old age, with a variety of long-term outcomes. Jeste, Dunn, and Lindamer (2004) reported that about 20% to 30% of the clients experienced dementia, resulting in a steady, deteriorating decline in health; 20% to 30% actually had a reduction in positive symptoms, somewhat like a remission; and

NURSING INTERVENTIONS FOR CLIENTS WITH SCHIZOPHRENIA

- Promoting safety of client and others and right to privacy and dignity
- Establishing therapeutic relationship by establishing trust
- Using therapeutic communication (clarifying feelings and statements when speech and thoughts are disorganized or confused)
- Interventions for delusions:
  - Do not openly confront the delusion or argue with the client.
  - Establish and maintain reality for the client.
  - Use distracting techniques.
  - Teach the client positive self-talk, positive thinking, and to ignore delusional beliefs.
- Interventions for hallucinations:
  - Help present and maintain reality by frequent contact and communication with client.
  - Elicit description of hallucination to protect client and others. The nurse's understanding of the hallucination helps him or her know how to calm or reassure the client.
  - Engage client in reality-based activities such as card playing, occupational therapy, or listening to music.
- Coping with socially inappropriate behaviors:
  - Redirect client away from problem situations.
  - Deal with inappropriate behaviors in a non-judgmental and matter-of-fact manner; give factual statements; do not scold.
  - Reassure others that the client's inappropriate behaviors or comments are not his or her fault (without violating client confidentiality).
  - Try to reintegrate the client into the treatment milieu as soon as possible.
  - Do not make the client feel punished or shunned for inappropriate behaviors.
  - Teach social skills through education, role modeling, and practice.
- Client and family teaching (see the display)
- Establishing community support systems and care

schizophrenia remained mostly unchanged in the remaining clients.

COMMUNITY-BASED CARE

Clients with schizophrenia are no longer hospitalized for long periods. Most return to live in the community with assistance provided by family and support services. Clients may live with family members, independently, or in a res-

idential program such as a group home where they can receive needed services without being admitted to the hospital. Assertive community treatment programs have shown success in reducing the rate of hospital admissions by managing symptoms and medications; assisting clients with social, recreational, and vocational needs; and providing support to clients and their families. The psychiatric nurse is a member of the multidisciplinary team that works with clients in assertive community treatment programs, focusing on the management of medications and their side effects and the promotion of health and wellness. Behavioral home health care also is expanding, with nurses providing care to persons with schizophrenia (as well as other mental illnesses) using the holistic approach to integrate clients into the community. Although much has been done to give these clients the support they need to live in the community, there is still a need to increase services to homeless persons and those in prison with schizophrenia.

Community support programs often are an important link in helping persons with schizophrenia and their families. A case manager may be assigned to the client to provide assistance in handling the wide variety of challenges that the client in community settings faces. The client who has had schizophrenia for some time may have a case manager in the community. Other clients may need assistance to obtain a case manager. Depending on the type of funding and agencies available in a particular community, the nurse may refer the client to a social worker or may directly refer the client to case management services.

Case management services often include helping the client with housing and transportation, money management, and keeping appointments as well as with socialization and recreation. Frequent face-to-face and telephone contact with clients in the community helps address clients' immediate concerns and avoid relapse and rehospitalization. Common concerns of clients include difficulties with treatment and after-care, dealing with psychiatric symptoms, environmental stresses, and financial issues. Although the support of professionals in the community is vital, the nurse must not overlook the client's need for autonomy and potential abilities to manage his or her own health.

MENTAL HEALTH PROMOTION

Psychiatric rehabilitation has the goal of recovery for clients with major mental illness that goes beyond symptom control and medication management (see Chapter 4). Working with clients to manage their own lives, make effective treatment decisions, and have an improved quality of life—from the client's point of view—are central components of such programs. Mental health promotion involves strengthening the client's ability to bounce back from adversity and to manage the inevitable obstacles encountered in life. Strategies include fostering self-efficacy and empowering the client to have control over his or her life; improving the client's resiliency, or ability to bounce back emotionally from stressful events; and improving the client's ability to cope with the problems, stress, and strains of everyday living. See Chapter 7 for a full discussion of resiliency and self-efficacy.

Early intervention in schizophrenia is an emerging goal of research investigating the earliest signs of the illness that occur predominately in adolescence and young adulthood (Borgmann-Winter et al., 2006). Accurate identification of individuals at greatest risk is the key to early intervention. An initiative of early detection, intervention, and prevention of psychosis has been established in Portland, Oregon (Korn, 2001). This project works with primary care providers to recognize prodromal signs that are predictive of later psychotic episodes, such as sleep difficulties, change in appetite, loss of energy and interest, odd speech, hearing voices, peculiar behavior, inappropriate expression of feelings, paucity of speech, ideas of reference, and feelings of unreality. After these high-risk individuals are identified, individualized intervention is implemented that may include education, stress management, or neuroleptic medication or a combination of these. Treatment also includes family involvement, individual and vocational counseling, and coping strategies to enhance self-mastery. Interventions are intensive, using home visits and daily sessions if needed.

Studies in Switzerland (Simon et al., 2006) focused on identifying at-risk individuals demonstrating a core deficit of prodromal symptoms, including cognitive impairment, affective symptoms, social isolation, and a decline in social functioning. In Germany, comprehensive cognitive-behavioral therapy has been developed for patients in the early initial prodromal phase, whereas those in the late initial prodromal phase receive low-dose antipsychotic medication along with cognitive behavioral therapy (Bechdolf et al., 2006b; Hafner & Maurer, 2006). These early interventions implemented in Germany, Australia, and the United Kingdom have resulted in improvement of prodromal symptoms, prevention of social stagnation or decline, and prevention or delay of progression to psychosis (Bechdorf et al., 2006a).

SELF-AWARENESS ISSUES

Working with clients with schizophrenia can present many challenges for the nurse. Clients have many experiences that are difficult for the nurse to relate to, such as delusions and hallucinations. Suspicious or paranoid behavior on the client's part may make the nurse feel as though he or she is not trustworthy or that his or her integrity is being questioned. The nurse must recognize this type of behavior as part of the illness and not interpret or respond to it as a personal affront. Taking the client's statements or behavior as a personal accusation only causes the nurse to respond defensively, which is counterproductive to the establishment of a therapeutic relationship.

The nurse also may be genuinely frightened or threatened if the client's behavior is hostile or aggressive. The nurse must acknowledge these feelings and take measures to ensure his or her safety. This may involve talking to the client in an open area rather than in a more isolated location or having an additional staff person present rather than being alone with the client. If the nurse pretends to be unafraid, the client may sense the fear anyway and feel less secure, leading to a greater potential for the client to lose personal control.

As with many chronic illnesses, the nurse may become frustrated if the client does not follow the medication regimen, fails to keep needed appointments, or experiences repeated relapses. The nurse may feel as though a great deal of hard work has been wasted or that the situation is futile or hopeless. Schizophrenia is a chronic illness, and clients may suffer numerous relapses and hospital admissions. The nurse must not take responsibility for the success or failure of treatment efforts or view the client's status as a personal success or failure. Nurses should look to their colleagues for helpful support and discussion of these self-awareness issues.

Points to Consider When Working With Clients With Schizophrenia

- Remember that although these clients often suffer numerous relapses and return for repeated hospital stays, they do return to living and functioning in the community. Focusing on the amount of time the client is outside the hospital setting may help decrease the frustration that can result when working with clients with a chronic illness.
- Visualize the client not at his or her worst but as he or she gets better and symptoms become less severe.
- Remember that the client's remarks are not directed at you personally but are a byproduct of the disordered and confused thinking that schizophrenia causes.
- Discuss these issues with a more experienced nurse for suggestions on how to deal with your feelings and actions toward these clients. You are not expected to have all the answers.

Critical Thinking Questions

1. Clients who fail to take medications regularly are often admitted to the hospital repeatedly, and this can become quite expensive. How do you reconcile the client's rights (to refuse treatment or medications) with the need to curtail avoidable health care costs?
2. What is the quality of life for the client with schizophrenia who has a minimal response to antipsychotic medications and therefore poor treatment outcomes?
3. If a client with schizophrenia who experiences frequent relapses has a young child, should the child remain with the parent? What factors influence this decision? Who should be able to make such a decision?
4. How does the nurse maintain a positive but honest relationship with a client's family if the client does not respond well to antipsychotic medications?

KEY POINTS

- Schizophrenia is a chronic illness requiring long-term management strategies and coping skills. Schizophrenia is a disease of the brain, a clinical syndrome that involves a person's thoughts, perceptions, emotions, movements, and behaviors.
- The effects of schizophrenia on the client may be profound, involving all aspects of the client's life: social interactions, emotional health, and ability to work and function in the community.
- Schizophrenia is conceptualized in terms of positive signs such as delusions, hallucinations, and disordered thought processes as well as negative signs such as social isolation, apathy, anhedonia, and lack of motivation and volition.
- The clinical picture, prognosis, and outcomes for clients with schizophrenia vary widely. Therefore, it is important that each client is carefully and individually assessed, with appropriate needs and interventions determined.
- Careful assessment of each client as an individual is essential to planning an effective plan of care.
- Families of clients with schizophrenia may experience fear, embarrassment, and guilt in response to their family member's illness. Families must be educated about the disorder, the course of the disorder, and how it can be controlled.
- Failure to comply with treatment and the medication regimen and the use of alcohol and other drugs are associated with poorer outcomes in the treatment of schizophrenia.
- For clients with psychotic symptoms, key nursing interventions include helping to protect the client's safety and right to privacy and dignity, dealing with socially inappropriate behaviors in a nonjudgmental and matter-of-fact manner, helping present and maintain reality for the client by frequent contact and communication, and ensuring appropriate medication administration.

- For the client whose condition is stabilized with medication, key nursing interventions include continuing to offer a supportive, nonconfrontational approach, maintaining the therapeutic relationship by establishing trust and trying to clarify the client's feelings and statements when speech and thoughts are disorganized or confused, helping to develop social skills by modeling and practicing, and helping to educate the client and family about schizophrenia and the importance of maintaining a therapeutic regimen and other self-care habits.
- Self-awareness issues for the nurse working with clients with schizophrenia include dealing with psychotic symptoms, fear for personal safety, and frustration as a result of relapses and repeated hospital admissions.

REFERENCES

American Psychiatric Association. (2000). *Diagnostic and statistical manual of mental disorders* (4th ed., text revision). Washington, DC: American Psychiatric Association.

Bechdolf, A., Phillips, L. J., Francey, S. M., et al. (2006a). Recent approaches to psychological interventions for people at risk of psychosis. *European Archives of Psychiatry and Clinical Neuroscience, 256*(3), 159–173.

Bechdolf, A., Ruhrmann, S., Wagner, M., et al. (2006b). Interventions in the prodromal states of psychosis in Germany: Concept and recruitment. *British Journal of Psychiatry, 48*(Suppl.), s45–48.

Borgmann-Winter, K., Calkins, M. E., Kniele, K., & Gur, R. E. (2006). Assessment of adolescents at risk for psychosis. *Current Psychiatry Reports, 8*(4), 313–321.

Brown, A. S., Bresnahan, M., & Susser, E. S. (2005). Schizophrenia: Environmental epidemiology. In B. J. Sadock & V. A. Sadock (Eds.), *Comprehensive textbook of psychiatry* (Vol. 1, 8th ed., pp. 1371–1380). Philadelphia: Lippincott Williams & Wilkins.

Buchanan, R. W., & Carpenter, W. T. (2005). Concept of schizophrenia. In B. J. Sadock & V. A. Sadock (Eds.), *Comprehensive textbook of psychiatry* (Vol. 1, 8th ed., pp. 1329–1345). Philadelphia: Lippincott Williams & Wilkins.

Carter, C. S. (2006). Editorial: Understanding the glass ceiling for functional outcome in schizophrenia. *American Journal of Psychiatry, 163*(3), 356–358.

Hafner, H., & Maurer, K. (2006). Early detection of schizophrenia: Current evidence and future perspectives. *World Psychiatry, 5*(3), 130–138.

Hagen, B. F., & Mitchell, D. L. (2001). Might within the madness: Solution-focused therapy and thought-disordered clients. *Archives of Psychiatric Nursing, 15*(2), 86–93.

INTERNET RESOURCES

RESOURCE	INTERNET ADDRESS
National Alliance for the Mentally Ill	http://www.nami.org
National Schizophrenia Foundation	http://www.nsfoundation.org
Schizophrenia	http://imh.nih.gov/publiccat/schizoph.cfm
Schizophrenia.com	http://www.schizophrenia.com
Schizophrenia Health Web Links	http://www.internet-health-directory.com/Mental_Health_Disorders_Schizophrenia.html
Schizophrenia Society of Canada	http://www.schizophrenia.ca
Schizophrenics Anonymous	http://www.schizophrenia.com/help/Schizanon.html

Hogarty, G. E., Greenwald, D. P., & Eack, S. M. (2006). Durability and mechanism of effects of cognitive enhancement therapy. *Psychiatric Services, 57*(12), 1751–1757.

Jeste, D. V., Dunn, L. B., & Lindamer, L. A. (2004). Psychoses. In J. Sadavoy, L. F. Jarvik, G. T. Grossberg, et al. (Eds.), *Comprehensive textbook of geriatric psychiatry* (3rd ed., pp. 655–685). New York: W. W. Norton.

Kane, J. M., & Marder, S. R. (2005). Schizophrenia: Somatic treatment. In B. J. Sadock & V. A. Sadock (Eds.), *Comprehensive textbook of psychiatry* (Vol. 1, 8th ed., pp. 1467–1476). Philadelphia: Lippincott Williams & Wilkins.

Kirkpatrick, B., & Tek, C. (2005). Schizophrenia: Clinical features and psychopathology concepts. In B. J. Sadock & V. A. Sadock (Eds.), *Comprehensive textbook of psychiatry* (Vol. 1, 8th ed., pp. 1416–1436). Philadelphia: Lippincott Williams & Wilkins.

Korn, M. L. (2001, October 11). Early intervention in schizophrenia. Paper presented at the 53rd Institute on Psychiatric Services. Retrieved May 15, 2002, from http://psychiatry.medscape.com/Medscape/CNO/2001/apaips/Story.cfm?story_id=2520.

Marshall, M., & Rathbone, J. (2006). Early intervention for psychosis. *Cochrane Database of Systematic Review (online), 4*(CD004718).

Mojtabai, R. (2005). Culture-bound syndromes with psychotic features. In B. J. Sadock & V. A. Sadock (Eds.), *Comprehensive textbook of psychiatry* (Vol. 1, 8th ed., pp. 1538–1541). Philadelphia: Lippincott Williams & Wilkins.

Miriana, J. A., Alarcon, E., & Herruzo, J. (2006). In-home psychosocial training for patients with schizophrenia. *Psychiatric Services, 57*(2), 260–262.

Penn, D. L., Wldheter, E. J., Perkins, D. O., Mueser, K. T., & Lieberman, J. A. (2005). Psychosocial treatment for first-episode psychosis: A research update. *American Journal of Psychiatry, 162*(12), 2220–2232.

Pfammatter, M., Junghan, U. M., & Brenner, H. D. (2006). Efficacy of psychological therapy in schizophrenia: Conclusions from meta-analysis. *Schizophrenia Bulletin, 32*(Suppl. 1), S64–S80.

Reynolds, S. A., Schmid, M., & Broome, M. E. (2004). Polydipsia screening tool. *Archives of Psychiatric Nursing, XVIII*(2), 49–59.

Riley, B. P., & Kendler, K. S. (2005). Schizophrenia: Genetics. In B. J. Sadock & V. A. Sadock (Eds.), *Comprehensive textbook of psychiatry* (Vol. 1, 8th ed., pp. 1354–1371). Philadelphia: Lippincott Williams & Wilkins.

Schneider-Axmann, T., Kamer, T., Moroni, M., et al. (2006). Relation between cerebrospinal fluid, gray matter and white matter changes in families with schizophrenia. *Journal of Psychiatric Research, 40*(7), 646–655.

Schultz, J. M., & Videbeck, S. L. (2005). *Lippincott's manual of psychiatric nursing care plans* (7th ed.). Philadelphia: Lippincott Williams & Wilkins.

Simon, A. E., et al. (2006). Defining subjects at risk for psychosis: A comparison of two approaches. *Schizophrenia Research, 81*(1), 83–90.

Ucok, A., Polat, A., Cakir, S., & Genc, A. (2006). One year outcome in first episode schizophrenia: Predictors of relapse. *European Archives of Psychiatry and Neuroscience, 256*(1), 37–43.

Velligan, D. I., et al. (2006). Use of environmental supports among patients with schizophrenia. *Psychiatric Services, 57*(2), 219–224.

ADDITIONAL READINGS

Hunt, I. M., et al. (2006). Suicide in schizophrenia: Findings from a national clinical survey. *Journal of Psychiatric Practice, 12*(3), 139–147.

Kane, J. M. (2006). Utilization of long-acting antipsychotic medication in patient care. *CNS Spectrums, 11*(Suppl. 12):14, 1–8.

Klam, J. McLay, M., & Grabke, D. (2006). Personal empowerment program: Addressing health concerns in people with schizophrenia. *Journal of Psychosocial Nursing, 44*(8), 20–28.

Kopelwicz, A., Liberman, R. P., & Zarate, R. (2006). Recent advances in social skills training for schizophrenia. *Schizophrenia Bulletin, 32*(Suppl. 1), S12–23.

Chapter Study Guide

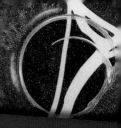

MULTIPLE-CHOICE QUESTIONS

Select the best answer for each of the following questions.

1. Which of the following are considered the positive signs of schizophrenia?
   A. Delusions, anhedonia, ambivalence
   B. Hallucinations, illusions, ambivalence
   C. Delusions, hallucinations, disordered thinking
   D. Disordered thinking, anhedonia, illusions

2. The family of a client with schizophrenia asks the nurse about the difference between conventional and atypical antipsychotic medications. The nurse's answer is based on which of the following?
   A. Atypical antipsychotics are newer medications but act in the same ways as conventional antipsychotics.
   B. Conventional antipsychotics are dopamine antagonists; atypical antipsychotics inhibit the reuptake of serotonin.
   C. Conventional antipsychotics have serious side effects; atypical antipsychotics have virtually no side effects.
   D. Atypical antipsychotics are dopamine and serotonin antagonists; conventional antipsychotics are only dopamine antagonists.

3. The nurse is planning discharge teaching for a client taking clozapine (Clozaril). Which of the following is essential to include?
   A. Caution the client not to be outdoors in the sunshine without protective clothing.
   B. Remind the client to go to the lab to have blood drawn for a white blood cell count.
   C. Instruct the client about dietary restrictions.
   D. Give the client a chart to record a daily pulse rate.

4. The nurse is caring for a client who has been taking fluphenazine (Prolixin) for 2 days. The client suddenly cries out, his neck twists to one side, and his eyes appear to roll back in the sockets. The nurse finds the following PRN medications ordered for the client. Which one should the nurse administer?
   A. Benztropine (Cogentin), 2 mg PO, bid, PRN
   B. Fluphenazine (Prolixin), 2 mg PO, tid, PRN
   C. Haloperidol (Haldol), 5 mg IM, PRN extreme agitation
   D. Diphenhydramine, (Benadryl) 25 mg IM, PRN

5. Which of the following statements would indicate that family teaching about schizophrenia had been effective?
   A. "If our son takes his medication properly, he won't have another psychotic episode."
   B. "I guess we'll have to face the fact that our daughter will eventually be institutionalized."
   C. "It's a relief to find out that we did not cause our son's schizophrenia."
   D. "It is a shame our daughter will never be able to have children."

6. When the client describes fear of leaving his apartment as well as the desire to get out and meet others, it is called
   A. Ambivalence
   B. Anhedonia
   C. Alogia
   D. Avoidance

7. The client who hesitates 30 seconds before responding to any question is described as having
   A. Blunted affect
   B. Latency of response
   C. Paranoid delusions
   D. Poverty of speech

8. The overall goal of psychiatric rehabilitation is for the client to gain
   A. Control of symptoms
   B. Freedom from hospitalization
   C. Management of anxiety
   D. Recovery from the illness

FILL-IN-THE-BLANK QUESTIONS

Identify the type of speech pattern exhibited for each of the following client statements.

_____ 1. "Do you have any phletz here? I like phletz."

_____ 2. "It's time to eat, to eat, to eat."

_____ 3. "Mountains, tigers, pie, singing, spring."

_____ 4. "Is that clock or a sock, can the door lock, tick tock."

SHORT-ANSWER QUESTIONS

Give an example of each of the following.

1. Delusion

2. Hallucination

3. Illusion

For each of the following client statements, write a response the nurse might make and the rationale for the nurse's response.

4. "I can't live in my apartment anymore because it's bugged by the FBI."

5. "Have they told you why I'm here in the hospital?"

6. "I can feel my stomach rotting away."

7. "I must do what God tells me to do."

CLINICAL EXAMPLE

John Jones, 33, has been admitted to the hospital for the third time with a diagnosis of paranoid schizophrenia. John had been taking haloperidol (Haldol) but stopped taking it 2 weeks ago, telling his case manager it was "the poison that is making me sick." Yesterday, John was brought to the hospital after neighbors called the police because he had been up all night yelling loudly in his apartment. Neighbors reported him saying, "I can't do it! They don't deserve to die!" and similar statements.

John appears guarded and suspicious and has very little to say to anyone. His hair is matted, he has a strong body odor, and he is dressed in several layers of heavy clothing even though the temperature is warm. So far, John has been refusing any offers of food or fluids. When the nurse approached John with a dose of haloperidol, he said, "Do you want me to die?"

1. What additional assessment data does the nurse need to plan care for John?

2. Identify the three priorities, nursing diagnoses, and expected outcomes for John's care, with your rationales for the choices.

3. Identify at least two nursing interventions for the three priorities listed above.

4. What community referrals or supports might be beneficial for John when he is discharged?

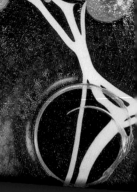

Chapter

15

Mood Disorders

Key Terms

- anergia
- anhedonia
- electroconvulsive therapy (ECT)
- euthymic
- flight of ideas
- hypertensive crisis
- hypomania
- kindling
- labile emotions
- latency of response
- mania
- mood disorders
- pressured speech
- psychomotor agitation
- psychomotor retardation
- ruminate
- seasonal affective disorder (SAD)
- suicidal ideation
- suicide
- suicide precautions

Learning Objectives

After reading this chapter, you should be able to

1. Discuss etiologic theories of depression and bipolar disorder.

2. Describe the risk factors for and characteristics of mood disorders.

3. Apply the nursing process to the care of clients and families with mood disorders.

4. Provide education to clients, families, caregivers, and community members to increase knowledge and understanding of mood disorders.

5. Identify populations at risk for suicide.

6. Apply the nursing process to the care of a suicidal client.

7. Evaluate your feelings, beliefs, and attitudes regarding mood disorders and suicide.

Visit the Point http://thePoint.lww.com for NCLEX-style questions, journal articles, and more!

Everyone occasionally feels sad, low, and tired with the desire to stay in bed and shut out the world. These episodes often are accompanied by **anergia** (lack of energy), exhaustion, agitation, noise intolerance, and slowed thinking processes, all of which make decisions difficult. Work, family, and social responsibilities drive most people to proceed with their daily routines, even when nothing seems to go right and their irritable mood is obvious to all. Such "low periods" pass in a few days, and energy returns. Fluctuations in mood are so common to the human condition that we think nothing of hearing someone say, "I'm depressed because I have too much to do." Everyday use of the word *depressed* doesn't actually mean that the person is clinically depressed but, rather, that the person is just having a bad day. Sadness in mood also can be a response to misfortune: death of a friend or relative, financial problems, or loss of a job may cause a person to grieve (see Chapter 12).

At the other end of the mood spectrum are episodes of exaggeratedly energetic behavior. The person has the sure sense that he or she can take on any task or relationship. In an elated mood, stamina for work, family, and social events is untiring. This feeling of being "on top of the world" also recedes in a few days to a **euthymic** mood (average affect and activity). Happy events stimulate joy and enthusiasm. These mood alterations are normal and do not interfere meaningfully with the person's life.

Mood disorders, also called affective disorders, are pervasive alterations in emotions that are manifested by depression, mania, or both. They interfere with a person's life, plaguing him or her with drastic and long-term sadness, agitation, or elation. Accompanying self-doubt, guilt, and anger alter life activities, especially those that involve self-esteem, occupation, and relationships.

From early history, people have suffered from mood disturbances. Archeologists have found holes drilled into ancient skulls to relieve the "evil humors" of those suffering from sad feelings and strange behaviors. Babylonians and ancient Hebrews believed that overwhelming sadness and extreme behavior were sent to people through the will of God or other divine beings. Biblical notables King Saul, King Nebuchadnezzar, and Moses suffered overwhelming grief of heart, unclean spirits, and bitterness of soul, all of which are symptoms of depression. Abraham Lincoln and Queen Victoria had recurrent episodes of depression. Other famous people with mood disorders were writers Virginia Woolf, Sylvia Plath, and Eugene O'Neill; composer George Frideric Handel; musician Jerry Garcia; artist Vincent Van Gogh; philosopher Frederic Nietzsche; television commentator and host of *60 Minutes* Mike Wallace; and actress Patty Duke.

Until the mid-1950s, no treatment was available to help people with serious depression or mania. These people suffered through their altered moods, thinking they were hopelessly weak to succumb to these devastating symptoms. Family and mental health professionals tended to agree, seeing sufferers as egocentric or viewing life negatively.

Although there are still no cures for mood disorders, effective treatments for both depression and mania are now available.

Mood disorders are the most common psychiatric diagnoses associated with suicide; depression is one of the most important risk factors for it (Sudak, 2005). For that reason, this chapter focuses on major depression, bipolar disorder, and suicide. It is important to note that clients with schizophrenia, substance use disorders, antisocial and borderline personality disorders, and panic disorders also are at increased risk for suicide and suicide attempts.

CATEGORIES OF MOOD DISORDERS

The primary mood disorders are major depressive disorder and bipolar disorder (formerly called manic-depressive illness). A major depressive episode lasts at least 2 weeks, during which the person experiences a depressed mood or loss of pleasure in nearly all activities. In addition, four of the following symptoms are present: changes in appetite or weight, sleep, or psychomotor activity; decreased energy; feelings of worthlessness or guilt; difficulty thinking, concentrating, or making decisions; or recurrent thoughts of

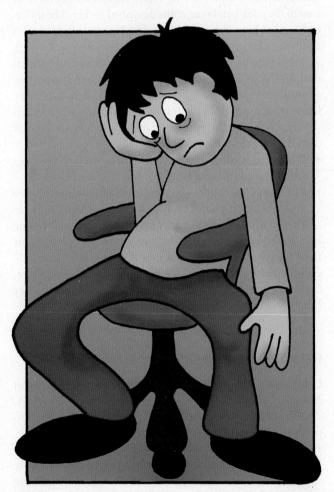

Anergia

death or suicidal ideation, plans, or attempts. These symptoms must be present every day for 2 weeks and result in significant distress or impair social, occupational, or other important areas of functioning (American Psychiatric Association [APA], 2000). Some people also have delusions and hallucinations; the combination is referred to as psychotic depression.

Bipolar disorder is diagnosed when a person's mood cycles between extremes of mania and depression (as described previously). **Mania** is a distinct period during which mood is abnormally and persistently elevated, expansive, or irritable. Typically, this period lasts about 1 week (unless the person is hospitalized and treated sooner), but it may be longer for some individuals. At least three of the following symptoms accompany the manic episode: inflated self-esteem or grandiosity; decreased need for sleep; **pressured speech** (unrelenting, rapid, often loud talking without pauses); **flight of ideas** (racing, often unconnected, thoughts); distractibility; increased involvement in goal-directed activity or psychomotor agitation; and excessive involvement in pleasure-seeking activities with a high potential for painful consequences (APA, 2000). Some people also exhibit delusions and hallucinations during a manic episode. **Hypomania** is a period of abnormally and persistently elevated, expansive, or irritable mood lasting 4 days and including three or four of the additional symptoms described earlier. The difference is that hypomanic episodes do not impair the person's ability to function (in fact, he or she may be quite productive), and there are no psychotic features (delusions and hallucinations). A mixed episode is diagnosed when the person experiences both mania and depression nearly every day for at least 1 week. These mixed episodes often are called rapid cycling. For the purpose of medical diagnosis, bipolar disorders are described as follows:

- Bipolar I disorder—one or more manic or mixed episodes usually accompanied by major depressive episodes
- Bipolar II disorder—one or more major depressive episodes accompanied by at least one hypomanic episode

People with bipolar disorder may experience a euthymic or normal mood and affect between extreme episodes, or they may have a depressed mood swing after a manic episode before returning to a euthymic mood. For some, euthymic periods between extremes are quite short. For others, euthymia lasts months or even years.

RELATED DISORDERS

Other disorders classified in the *Diagnostic and Statistical Manual of Mental Disorders, 4th edition, Text Revision* (APA, 2000) as mood disorders but with symptoms that are less severe or of shorter duration include the following:

- Dysthymic disorder is characterized by at least 2 years of depressed mood for more days than not with some additional, less severe symptoms that do not meet the criteria for a major depressive episode.

- Cyclothymic disorder is characterized by 2 years of numerous periods of both hypomanic symptoms that do not meet the criteria for bipolar disorder.
- Substance-induced mood disorder is characterized by a prominent and persistent disturbance in mood that is judged to be a direct physiologic consequence of ingested substances such as alcohol, other drugs, or toxins.
- Mood disorder due to a general medical condition is characterized by a prominent and persistent disturbance in mood that is judged to be a direct physiologic consequence of a medical condition such as degenerative neurologic conditions, cerebrovascular disease, metabolic or endocrine conditions, autoimmune disorders, human immunodeficiency virus infections, or certain cancers.

Other disorders that involve changes in mood include the following:

- **Seasonal affective disorder (SAD)** has two subtypes. In one, most commonly called winter depression or fall-onset SAD, people experience increased sleep, appetite, and carbohydrate cravings; weight gain; interpersonal conflict; irritability; and heaviness in the extremities beginning in late autumn and abating in spring and summer (Lurie et al., 2006). The other subtype, called spring-onset SAD, is less common, with symptoms of insomnia, weight loss, and poor appetite lasting from late spring or early summer until early fall.
- Postpartum or "maternity" blues are a frequent normal experience after delivery of a baby. They are characterized by labile mood and affect, crying spells, sadness, insomnia, and anxiety. Symptoms begin approximately 1 day after delivery, usually peak in 3 to 7 days, and disappear rapidly with no medical treatment (Sit et al., 2006).
- Postpartum depression meets all the criteria for a major depressive episode, with onset within 4 weeks of delivery.
- Postpartum psychosis is a psychotic episode developing within 3 weeks of delivery and beginning with fatigue, sadness, emotional lability, poor memory, and confusion and progressing to delusions, hallucinations, poor insight and judgment, and loss of contact with reality. This medical emergency requires immediate treatment (Sit et al., 2006).

ETIOLOGY

Various theories for the etiology of mood disorders exist. The most recent research focuses on chemical biologic imbalances as the cause. Nevertheless, psychosocial stressors and interpersonal events appear to trigger certain physiologic and chemical changes in the brain, which significantly alter the balance of neurotransmitters (Akiskal, 2005). Effective treatment addresses both the biologic and psychosocial components of mood disorders. Thus, nurses need a basic knowledge of both perspectives when working with clients experiencing these disorders.

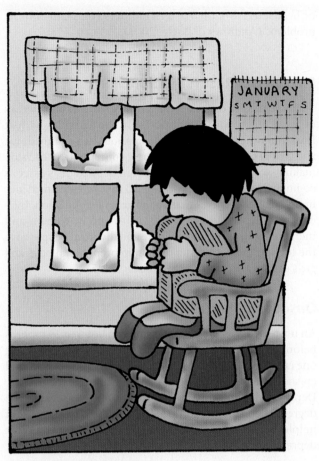

Seasonal affective disorder

Biologic Theories

GENETIC THEORIES

Genetic studies implicate the transmission of major depression in first-degree relatives, who have twice the risk for developing depression compared with the general population (APA, 2000). First-degree relatives of people with bipolar disorder have a 3% to 8% risk for developing bipolar disorder compared with a 1% risk in the general population. For all mood disorders, monozygotic (identical) twins have a concordance rate (both twins having the disorder) two to four times higher than that of dizygotic (fraternal) twins. Although heredity is a significant factor, the concordance rate for monozygotic twins is not 100%, so genetics alone do not account for all mood disorders (Kelsoe, 2005).

Markowitz and Milrod (2005) discussed indications of a genetic overlap between early-onset bipolar disorder and early-onset alcoholism. They noted that people with both problems have a higher rate of mixed and rapid cycling, poorer response to lithium, slower rate of recovery, and more hospital admissions. Mania displayed by these clients involves more agitation than elation; clients may respond better to anticonvulsants than to lithium.

NEUROCHEMICAL THEORIES

Neurochemical influences of neurotransmitters (chemical messengers) focus on serotonin and norepinephrine as the two major biogenic amines implicated in mood disorders. Serotonin has many roles in behavior: mood, activity, aggressiveness and irritability, cognition, pain, biorhythms, and neuroendocrine processes (i.e., growth hormone, cortisol, and prolactin levels are abnormal in depression). Deficits of serotonin, its precursor tryptophan, or a metabolite (5-hydroxyindole acetic acid, or 5-HIAA) of serotonin found in the blood or cerebrospinal fluid occur in people with depression. Positron emission tomography demonstrates reduced metabolism in the prefrontal cortex, which may promote depression (Tecott & Smart, 2005).

Norepinephrine levels may be deficient in depression and increased in mania. This catecholamine energizes the body to mobilize during stress and inhibits kindling. **Kindling** is the process by which seizure activity in a specific area of the brain is initially stimulated by reaching a threshold of the cumulative effects of stress, low amounts of electric impulses, or chemicals such as cocaine that sensitize nerve cells and pathways. These highly sensitized pathways respond by no longer needing the stimulus to induce seizure activity, which now occurs spontaneously. It is theorized that kindling may underlie the cycling of mood disorders as well as addiction. Anticonvulsants inhibit kindling; this may explain their efficacy in the treatment of bipolar disorder (Akiskal, 2005).

Dysregulation of acetylcholine and dopamine also are being studied in relation to mood disorders. Cholinergic drugs alter mood, sleep, neuroendocrine function, and the electroencephalographic pattern; therefore, acetylcholine seems to be implicated in depression and mania. The neurotransmitter problem may not be as simple as underproduction or depletion through overuse during stress. Changes in the sensitivity as well as the number of receptors are being evaluated for their roles in mood disorders (Tecott & Smart, 2005).

NEUROENDOCRINE INFLUENCES

Hormonal fluctuations are being studied in relation to depression. Mood disturbances have been documented in people with endocrine disorders such as those of the thyroid, adrenal, parathyroid, and pituitary. Elevated glucocorticoid activity is associated with the stress response, and evidence of increased cortisol secretion is apparent in about 40% of clients with depression, with the highest rates found among older clients. Postpartum hormone alterations precipitate mood disorders such as postpartum depression and psychosis. About 5% to 10% of people with depression have thyroid dysfunction, notably an elevated thyroid-stimulating hormone. This problem must be corrected with thyroid treatment, or treatment for the mood disorder is affected adversely (Thase, 2005).

Psychodynamic Theories

Many psychodynamic theories about the cause of mood disorders seemed to "blame the victim" and his or her family (Markowitz & Milrod, 2005):

- Freud looked at the self-depreciation of people with depression and attributed that self-reproach to anger turned inward related to either a real or perceived loss. Feeling abandoned by this loss, people became angry while both loving and hating the lost object.
- Bibring believed that one's ego (or self) aspired to be ideal (i.e., good and loving, superior or strong) and that to be loved and worthy, one must achieve these high standards. Depression results when, in reality, the person was not able to achieve these ideals all the time.
- Jacobson compared the state of depression to a situation in which the ego is a powerless, helpless child victimized by the superego, much like a powerful and sadistic mother who takes delight in torturing the child.
- Most psychoanalytical theories of mania view manic episodes as a "defense" against underlying depression, with the id taking over the ego and acting as an undisciplined hedonistic being (child).
- Meyer viewed depression as a reaction to a distressing life experience such as an event with psychic causality.
- Horney believed that children raised by rejecting or unloving parents were prone to feelings of insecurity and loneliness, making them susceptible to depression and helplessness.
- Beck saw depression as resulting from specific cognitive distortions in susceptible people. Early experiences shaped distorted ways of thinking about one's self, the world, and the future; these distortions involve magnification of negative events, traits, and expectations and simultaneous minimization of anything positive.

CULTURAL CONSIDERATIONS

Other behaviors considered age-appropriate can mask depression, which makes the disorder difficult to identify and diagnose in certain age groups. Children with depression often appear cranky. They may have school phobia, hyperactivity, learning disorders, failing grades, and antisocial behaviors. Adolescents with depression may abuse substances, join gangs, engage in risky behavior, be underachievers, or drop out of school. In adults, manifestations of depression can include substance abuse, eating disorders, compulsive behaviors such as workaholism and gambling, and hypochondriasis. Older adults who are cranky and argumentative may actually be depressed.

Many somatic ailments (physiologic ailments) accompany depression. This manifestation varies among cultures and is more apparent in cultures that avoid verbalizing emotions. For example, Asians who are anxious or depressed are more likely to have somatic complaints of headache, backache, or other symptoms. Latin cultures complain of "nerves" or headaches; Middle Eastern cultures complain of heart problems (Andrews & Boyle, 2003).

MAJOR DEPRESSIVE DISORDER

Major depressive disorder typically involves 2 or more weeks of a sad mood or lack of interest in life activities with at least four other symptoms of depression such as anhedonia and changes in weight, sleep, energy, concentration, decision making, self-esteem, and goals. Major depression is twice as common in women and has a 1.5 to 3 times greater incidence in first-degree relatives than in the general population. Incidence of depression decreases with age in women and increases with age in men. Single and divorced people have the highest incidence. Depression in prepubertal boys and girls occurs at an equal rate (Kelsoe, 2005).

Onset and Clinical Course

An untreated episode of depression can last 6 to 24 months before remitting. Fifty percent to 60% of people who have one episode of depression will have another. After a second episode of depression, there is a 70% chance of recurrence. Depressive symptoms can vary from mild to severe. The degree of depression is comparable with the person's sense of helplessness and hopelessness. Some people with severe depression (9%) have psychotic features (APA, 2000).

Treatment and Prognosis

PSYCHOPHARMACOLOGY

Major categories of antidepressants include cyclic antidepressants, monoamine oxidase inhibitors (MAOIs), selective serotonin reuptake inhibitors (SSRIs), and atypical antidepressants. Chapter 2 details biologic treatments. The choice of which antidepressant to use is based on the client's symptoms, age, and physical health needs; drugs that have or have not worked in the past or that have worked for a blood relative with depression; and other medications that the client is taking.

Researchers believe that levels of neurotransmitters, especially norepinephrine and serotonin, are decreased in depression. Usually, presynaptic neurons release these neurotransmitters to allow them to enter synapses and link with postsynaptic receptors. Depression results if too few neurotransmitters are released, if they linger too briefly in synapses, if the releasing presynaptic neurons reabsorb them too quickly, if conditions in synapses do not support linkage with postsynaptic receptors, or if the number of postsynaptic receptors has decreased. The goal is to increase the efficacy of available neurotransmitters and the absorption by postsynaptic receptors. To do so, antidepressants establish a blockade for the reuptake of norepinephrine and serotonin into their specific nerve terminals. This permits them to linger longer in synapses and to be more available to post-

CLINICAL VIGNETTE: DEPRESSION

"Just get out! I am not interested in food," said Chris to her husband, Matt, who had come into their bedroom to invite her to the dinner he and their daughters had prepared. "Can't they leave me alone?" thought Chris to herself as she miserably pulled the covers over her shoulders. Yet she felt guilty about the way she'd snapped at Matt. She knew she'd disparaged her family's efforts to help, but she couldn't stop.

Chris was physically and emotionally exhausted. "I can't remember when I felt well . . . maybe last year sometime, or maybe never," she thought fretfully. She'd always worked hard to get things done; lately, she could not do anything at all except complain. Kathy, her 13-year-old, accused her of hating everything and everybody, including her family. Linda, 11 years old, said, "Everything has to be your way, Mom. You snap at us for every little thing. You never listen anymore." Matt had long ago

withdrawn from her moodiness, acid tongue, and disinterest in sex. One day, she overheard Matt tell his brother that Chris was "crabby, agitated, and self-centered and if it wasn't for the girls, I don't know what I'd do. I've tried to get her to go to a doctor, but she says it's all our fault, then she sulks for days. What is our fault? I don't know what to do for her. I feel as if I am living in a minefield and never know what will set off an explosion. I try to remember the love we had together, but her behavior is getting old."

Chris has lost 12 pounds in the past 2 months, has difficulty sleeping, and is hostile, angry, and guilty about it. She has no desire for any pleasure. "Why bother? There is nothing to enjoy. Life is bleak." She feels stuck, worthless, hopeless, and helpless. Hoping against hope, Chris thinks to herself, "I wish I were dead. I'd never have to do anything again."

synaptic receptors. Antidepressants also increase the sensitivity of the postsynaptic receptor sites (Rush, 2005).

In clients who have acute depression with psychotic features, an antipsychotic is used in combination with an antidepressant. The antipsychotic treats the psychotic features; several weeks into treatment, the client is reassessed to determine whether the antipsychotic can be withdrawn and the antidepressant maintained.

Evidence is increasing that antidepressant therapy should continue for longer than the 3 to 6 months originally believed necessary. Fewer relapses occur in people with depression who receive 18 to 24 months of antidepressant therapy.

DSM-IV-TR DIAGNOSTIC CRITERIA:
SYMPTOMS OF MAJOR DEPRESSIVE DISORDER

- Depressed mood
- Anhedonism (decreased attention to and enjoyment from previously pleasurable activities)
- Unintentional weight change of 5% or more in a month
- Change in sleep pattern
- Agitation or psychomotor retardation
- Tiredness
- Worthlessness or guilt inappropriate to the situation (possibly delusional)
- Difficulty thinking, focusing, or making decisions
- Hopelessness, helplessness, and/or suicidal ideation

Adapted from DSM-IV-TR, 2000.

As a rule, antidepressants should be tapered before being discontinued.

Selective Serotonin Reuptake Inhibitors. SSRIs, the newest category of antidepressants (Table 15.1), are effective for most clients. Their action is specific to serotonin reuptake inhibition; these drugs produce few sedating, anticholinergic, and cardiovascular side effects, which make them safer for use in older adults. Because of their low side effects and relative safety, people using SSRIs are more apt to be compliant with the treatment regimen than clients using more troublesome medications. Insomnia decreases in 3 to 4 days, appetite returns to a more normal state in 5 to 7 days, and energy returns in 4 to 7 days. In 7 to 10 days, mood, concentration, and interest in life improve.

Fluoxetine (Prozac) produces a slightly higher rate of mild agitation and weight loss but less somnolence. It has a half-life of more than 7 days, which differs from the 25-hour half-life of other SSRIs.

Cyclic Antidepressants. Tricyclics, introduced for the treatment of depression in the mid-1950s, are the oldest antidepressants. They relieve symptoms of hopelessness, helplessness, anhedonia, inappropriate guilt, suicidal ideation, and daily mood variations (cranky in the morning and better in the evening). Other indications include panic disorder, obsessive-compulsive disorder, and eating disorders. Each drug has a different degree of efficacy in blocking the activity of norepinephrine and serotonin or increasing the sensitivity of postsynaptic receptor sites. Tricyclic and heterocyclic antidepressants have a lag period of 10 to 14 days before reaching a serum level that begins to alter symptoms; they take 6 weeks to reach full effect. Because they have a long serum half-life, there is a lag period of 1 to 4 weeks before steady plasma levels are reached and the client's symptoms begin to lessen. They

Table 15.1   SELECTIVE SEROTONIN REUPTAKE INHIBITOR (SSRI) ANTIDEPRESSANTS

Generic (Trade) Name	Side Effects	Nursing Implications
Fluoxetine (Prozac)	Headache, nervousness, anxiety, sedation, tremor, sexual dysfunction, anorexia, constipation, nausea, diarrhea, weight loss	Administer in AM (if nervous) or PM (if drowsy). Monitor for hyponatremia. Encourage adequate fluids. Report sexual difficulties to physician.
Sertraline (Zoloft)	Dizziness, sedation, headache, insomnia, tremor, sexual dysfunction, diarrhea, dry mouth and throat, nausea, vomiting, sweating	Administer in PM if client is drowsy. Encourage use of sugar-free beverages or hard candy. Drink adequate fluids. Monitor hyponatremia; report sexual difficulties to physician.
Paroxetine (Paxil)	Dizziness, sedation, headache, insomnia, weakness, fatigue, constipation, dry mouth and throat, nausea, vomiting, diarrhea, sweating	Administer with food. Administer in PM if client is drowsy. Encourage use of sugar-free hard candy or beverages. Encourage adequate fluids.
Citalopram (Celexa)	Drowsiness, sedation, insomnia, nausea, vomiting, weight gain, constipation, diarrhea	Monitor for hyponatremia. Administer with food. Administer dose at 6 PM or later. Promote balanced nutrition and exercise.
Escitalopram (Lexapro)	Drowsiness, dizziness, weight gain, sexual dysfunction, restlessness, dry mouth, headache, nausea, diarrhea	Check orthostatic blood pressure. Assist client to rise slowly from sitting position. Encourage use of sugar-free beverages or hard candy. Administer with food.

cost less primarily because they have been around longer and generic forms are available.

Tricyclic antidepressants are contraindicated in severe impairment of liver function and in myocardial infarction (acute recovery phase). They cannot be given concurrently with MAOIs. Because of their anticholinergic side effects, tricyclic antidepressants must be used cautiously in clients who have glaucoma, benign prostatic hypertrophy, urinary retention or obstruction, diabetes mellitus, hyperthyroidism, cardiovascular disease, renal impairment, or respiratory disorders (Table 15.2).

Overdosage of tricyclic antidepressants occurs over several days and results in confusion, agitation, hallucinations, hyperpyrexia, and increased reflexes. Seizures, coma, and cardiovascular toxicity can occur with ensuing tachycardia, decreased output, depressed contractility, and atrioventricular block. Because many older adults have concomitant health problems, cyclic antidepressants are used less often in the geriatric population than newer types of antidepressants that have fewer side effects and less drug interactions.

Tetracyclic Antidepressants. Amoxapine (Asendin) may cause extrapyramidal symptoms, tardive dyskinesia, and neuroleptic malignant syndrome. It can create tolerance in 1 to 3 months. It increases appetite and causes weight gain and cravings for sweets.

Maprotiline (Ludiomil) carries a risk for seizures (especially in heavy drinkers), severe constipation and urinary retention, stomatitis, and other side effects; this leads to poor compliance. The drug is started and withdrawn gradually. Central nervous system depressants can increase the effects of this drug.

Atypical Antidepressants. Atypical antidepressants are used when the client has an inadequate response to or side effects from SSRIs. Atypical antidepressants include venlafaxine (Effexor), duloxetine (Cymbalta), bupropion (Wellbutrin), nefazodone (Serzone), and mirtazapine (Remeron) (Table 15.3).

Venlafaxine blocks the reuptake of serotonin, norepinephrine, and dopamine (weakly). Bupropion modestly inhibits the reuptake of norepinephrine, weakly inhibits the reuptake of dopamine, and has no effects on serotonin. Bupropion is marketed as Zyban for smoking cessation.

Nefazodone inhibits the reuptake of serotonin and norepinephrine and has few side effects. Its half-life is 4 hours, and it can be used in clients with liver and kidney disease. It increases the action of certain benzodiazepines (alprazolam, estazolam, and triazolam) and the H$_2$ blocker terfenadine. Remeron also inhibits the reuptake of serotonin and norepinephrine, and it has few sexual side effects; however, its use comes with a higher incidence of weight gain, sedation, and anticholinergic side effects (Facts and Comparisons, 2007).

Monoamine Oxidase Inhibitors. This class of antidepressants is used infrequently because of potentially fatal side effects and interactions with numerous drugs, both

Table 15.2   TRICYCLIC ANTIDEPRESSANT MEDICATIONS

Generic (Trade) Name	Side Effects	Nursing Implications
Amitriptyline (Elavil)	Dizziness, orthostatic hypotension, tachycardia, sedation, headache, tremor, blurred vision, constipation, dry mouth and throat, weight gain, urinary hesitancy, sweating	Assist client to rise slowly from sitting position. Administer at bedtime. Encourage use of sugar-free beverages and hard candy. Ensure adequate fluids and balanced nutrition. Encourage exercise. Monitor cardiac function.
Amoxapine (Asendin)	Dizziness, orthostatic hypotension, sedation, insomnia, constipation, dry mouth and throat, rashes	Assist client to rise slowly from sitting position. Administer at bedtime if client is sedated. Ensure adequate fluids. Encourage use of sugar-free beverages and hard candy. Report rashes to physician.
Doxepin (Sinequan)	Dizziness, orthostatic hypotension, tachycardia, sedation, blurred vision, constipation, dry mouth and throat, weight gain, sweating	Assist client to rise slowly from sitting position. Administer at bedtime if client is sedated. Ensure adequate fluids and balanced nutrition. Encourage use of sugar-free beverages and hard candy. Encourage exercise.
Imipramine (Tofranil)	Dizziness, orthostatic hypotension, weakness, fatigue, blurred vision, constipation, dry mouth and throat, weight gain	Assist client to rise slowly from sitting or supine position. Ensure adequate fluids and balanced nutrition. Encourage use of sugar-free beverages and hard candy. Encourage exercise.
Desipramine (Norpramine)	Cardiac dysrhythmias, dizziness, orthostatic hypotension, excitement, insomnia, sexual dysfunction, dry mouth and throat, rashes	Monitor cardiac function. Assist client to rise slowly from sitting position. Administer in AM if client is having insomnia. Encourage sugar-free beverages and hard candy. Report rashes or sexual difficulties to physician.
Nortriptyline (Pamelor)	Cardiac dysrhythmias, tachycardia, confusion, excitement, tremor, constipation, dry mouth and throat	Monitor cardiac function. Administer in AM if stimulated. Ensure adequate fluids. Encourage use of sugar-free beverages and hard candy. Report confusion to physician.

prescription and over-the-counter preparations (Table 15.4). The most serious side effect is **hypertensive crisis**, a life-threatening condition that can result when a client taking MAOIs ingests tyramine-containing foods (see Chapter 2, Box 2-1) and fluids or other medications. Symptoms are occipital headache, hypertension, nausea, vomiting, chills, sweating, restlessness, nuchal rigidity, dilated pupils, fever, and motor agitation. These can lead to hyperpyrexia, cerebral hemorrhage, and death. The MAOI–tyramine interaction produces symptoms within 20 to 60 minutes after ingestion. For hypertensive crisis, transient antihypertensive agents such as phentolamine mesylate are given to dilate blood vessels and decrease vascular resistance (Facts and Comparisons, 2007).

There is a 2- to 4-week lag period before MAOIs reach therapeutic levels. Because of the lag period, adequate wash-out periods of 5 to 6 weeks are recommended between the times that the MAOI is discontinued and another class of antidepressant is started.

OTHER MEDICAL TREATMENTS AND PSYCHOTHERAPY

Electroconvulsive Therapy. Psychiatrists may use **electroconvulsive therapy (ECT)** to treat depression in select groups, such as clients who do not respond to antidepressants or those who experience intolerable side effects at therapeutic doses (particularly true for older adults). In addition, pregnant women can safely have ECT with no harm to the fetus. Clients who are actively suicidal may be given ECT if there is concern for their safety while waiting weeks for the full effects of antidepressant medication.

ECT involves application of electrodes to the head of the client to deliver an electrical impulse to the brain; this

Drug Alert!

Serotonin Syndrome

Serotonin syndrome occurs when there is an inadequate washout period between taking MAOIs and SSRIs or when MAOIs are combined with meperidine. Symptoms of serotonin syndrome include

- Change in mental state: confusion, agitation
- Neuromuscular excitement: muscle rigidity, weakness, sluggish pupils, shivering, tremors, myoclonic jerks, collapse, muscle paralysis
- Autonomic abnormalities: hyperthermia, tachycardia, tachypnea, hypersalivation, diaphoresis

causes a seizure. It is believed that the shock stimulates brain chemistry to correct the chemical imbalance of depression. Historically, clients did not receive any anesthetic or other medication before ECT, and they had full-blown grand mal seizures that often resulted in injuries ranging from biting the tongue to breaking bones. ECT fell into disfavor for a period and was seen as "barbaric." Today, although ECT is administered in a safe and humane way with almost no injuries, there are still critics of the treatment.

Clients usually are given a series of 6 to 15 treatments scheduled three times a week. Generally, a minimum of six treatments is needed to see sustained improvement in depressive symptoms. Maximum benefit is achieved in 12 to 15 treatments.

Preparation of a client for ECT is similar to preparation for any outpatient minor surgical procedure: The client receives nothing by mouth (or, is NPO) after midnight, removes any fingernail polish, and voids just before the procedure. An intravenous line is started for the administration of medication.

Initially, the client receives a short-acting anesthetic so he or she is not awake during the procedure. Next, he or she receives a muscle relaxant/paralytic, usually succinylcholine, that relaxes all muscles to reduce greatly the outward signs of the seizure (e.g., clonic-tonic muscle contractions). Electrodes are placed on the client's head: one on either side (bilateral) or both on one side (unilateral). The electrical stimulation is delivered, which causes seizure activity in the brain that is monitored by an electroencephalogram, or EEG. The client receives oxygen and is assisted to breathe with an Ambu-bag. He or she generally begins to waken after a few minutes. Vital signs are monitored, and the client is assessed for the return of a gag reflex.

After ECT treatment, the client may be mildly confused or briefly disoriented. He or she is very tired and often

Table 15.3   ATYPICAL ANTIDEPRESSANTS

Generic (Trade) Name	Side Effects	Nursing Implications
Venlafaxine (Effexor)	Increased blood pressure and pulse, nausea, vomiting, headache, dizziness, drowsiness, dry mouth, sweating; can alter many lab tests, e.g., AST, ALT, alkaline phosphatase, creatinine, glucose, electrolytes	Administer with food. Ensure adequate fluids. Give in PM. Encourage use of sugar-free beverages or hard candy.
Duloxetine (Cymbalta)	Increased blood pressure and pulse, nausea, vomiting, drowsiness or insomnia, headache, dry mouth, constipation, lowered seizure threshold, sexual dysfunction	Administer with food. Ensure adequate fluids. Encourage use of sugar-free beverages or hard candy.
Bupropion (Wellbutrin)	Nausea, vomiting, lowered seizure threshold, agitation, restlessness, insomnia, may alter taste, blurred vision, weight gain, headache	Give with food. Administer dose in AM. Ensure balanced nutrition and exercise.
Nefazodone (Serzone)	Headache; dizziness; drowsiness; alters results of AST, ALT, LDH, cholesterol, glucose, hematocrit	Administer before meal (food inhibits absorption). Monitor liver and kidney functions.
Mirtazapine (Remeron)	Sedation, dizziness, dry mouth and throat, weight gain, sexual dysfunction, constipation	Administer in PM. Encourage use of sugar-free beverages and hard candy. Ensure adequate fluids and balanced nutrition. Report sexual difficulties to physician.

ALT, alanine aminotransferase; AST, aspartite aminotransferase; LDH, lactate dehydrogenase.

Table 15.4   MONOAMINE OXIDASE INHIBITOR (MAOI) ANTIDEPRESSANTS

Generic (Trade) Name	Side Effects	Nursing Implications
Isocarboxazid (Marplan) Phenelzine (Nardil) Tranylcypromine (Parnate)	Drowsiness, dry mouth, overactivity, insomnia, nausea, anorexia, constipation, urinary retention, orthostatic hypotension	Assist client to rise slowly from sitting position. Administer in AM. Administer with food. Ensure adequate fluids. Perform essential teaching on importance of low tyramine diet.

has a headache. The symptoms are just like those of anyone who has had a grand mal seizure. In addition, the client will have some short-term memory impairment. After a treatment, the client may eat as soon as he or she is hungry and usually sleeps for a period. Headaches are treated symptomatically.

Unilateral ECT results in less memory loss for the client, but more treatments may be needed to see sustained improvement. Bilateral ECT results in more rapid improvement but with increased short-term memory loss.

The literature continues to be divided about the effectiveness of ECT. Some studies report that ECT is as effective as medication for depression, whereas other studies report only short-term improvement. Likewise, some studies report that memory loss side effects of ECT are short-lived, whereas others report they are serious and long-term (Ross, 2006; Fenton et al., 2006).

ECT is also used for relapse prevention in depression. Clients may continue to receive treatments, such as one per month, to maintain their mood improvement. Kellner and colleagues (2006) found that maintenance ECT had limited ability to prevent relapse, whereas other studies found it to be effective in relapse prevention (Frederikse et al., 2006).

Psychotherapy. A combination of psychotherapy and medications is considered the most effective treatment for depressive disorders. There is no one specific type of therapy that is better for the treatment of depression (Rush, 2005). The goals of combined therapy are symptom remission, psychosocial restoration, prevention of relapse or recurrence, reduced secondary consequences such as marital discord or occupational difficulties, and increasing treatment compliance.

Interpersonal therapy focuses on difficulties in relationships, such as grief reactions, role disputes, and role transitions. For example, a person who, as a child, never learned how to make and trust a friend outside the family structure has difficulty establishing friendships as an adult. Interpersonal therapy helps the person to find ways to accomplish this developmental task.

Behavior therapy seeks to increase the frequency of the client's positively reinforcing interactions with the environment and to decrease negative interactions. It also may focus on improving social skills.

Cognitive therapy focuses on how the person thinks about the self, others, and the future and interprets his or her

Drug Alert!

Overdose of MAOI and Cyclic Antidepressants

Both the cyclic compounds and MAOIs are potentially lethal when taken in overdose. To decrease this risk, depressed or impulsive clients who are taking any antidepressants in these two categories may need to have prescriptions and refills in limited amounts.

Drug Alert!

MAOI Drug Interactions

There are numerous drugs that interact with MAOIs. The following drugs cause potentially fatal interactions:

- Amphetamines
- Ephedrine
- Fenfluramine
- Isoproterenol
- Meperidine
- Phenylephrine
- Phenylpropanolamine
- Pseudoephedrine
- SSRI antidepressants
- Tricyclic antidepressants
- Tyramine

experiences. This model focuses on the person's distorted thinking, which, in turn, influences feelings, behavior, and functional abilities. Table 15.5 describes the cognitive distortions that are the focus of cognitive therapy.

Investigational Treatments. Other treatments for depression are being tested. These include transcranial magnetic stimulation (TMS), magnetic seizure therapy, deep brain stimulation, and vagal nerve stimulation. TMS is the closest to approval for clinical use. These novel brain stimulation techniques seem to be safe, but efficacy in relieving depression needs to be established (Eitan & Lerer, 2006).

APPLICATION OF THE NURSING PROCESS: DEPRESSION

Assessment

HISTORY

The nurse can collect assessment data from the client and family or significant others, previous chart information, and others involved in the support or care. It may take several short periods to complete the assessment because clients who are severely depressed feel exhausted and overwhelmed. It can take time for them to process the question asked and to formulate a response. It is important that the nurse does not try to rush clients because doing so leads to frustration and incomplete assessment data.

To assess the client's perception of the problem, the nurse asks about behavioral changes: when they started, what was happening when they began, their duration, and what the client has tried to do about them. Assessing the history is important to determine any previous episodes of depression, treatment, and client's response to treatment. The nurse also asks about family history of mood disorders, suicide, or attempted suicide.

GENERAL APPEARANCE AND MOTOR BEHAVIOR

Many people with depression look sad; sometimes they just look ill. The posture often is slouched with head down, and they make minimal eye contact. They have **psychomotor retardation** (slow body movements, slow cognitive processing, and slow verbal interaction). Responses to questions may be minimal, with only one or two words. **Latency of response** is seen when clients take up to 30 seconds to respond to a question. They may answer some questions with "I don't know" because they are simply too fatigued and overwhelmed to think of an answer or respond in any detail. Clients also may exhibit signs of agitation or anxiety such as wringing their hands and having difficulty sitting still. These clients are said to have **psychomotor agitation** (increased body movements and thoughts), which includes pacing, accelerated thinking, and argumentativeness.

MOOD AND AFFECT

Clients with depression may describe themselves as hopeless, helpless, down, or anxious. They also may say they are a burden on others or are a failure at life, or they may make other similar statements. They are easily frustrated, are angry at themselves, and can be angry at others (APA, 2000). They experience **anhedonia,** losing any sense of pleasure from activities they formerly enjoyed. Clients may be apathetic, that is, not caring about self, activities, or much of anything.

Their affect is sad or depressed or may be flat with no emotional expressions. Typically, depressed clients sit alone, staring into space or lost in thought. When addressed, they interact minimally with a few words or a gesture. They are overwhelmed by noise and people who might make demands on them, so they withdraw from the stimulation of interaction with others.

Table 15.5	DISTORTIONS ADDRESSED BY COGNITIVE THERAPY

Cognitive Distortion	Definition
Absolute, dichotomous thinking	Tendency to view everything in polar categories, i.e., all or none, black or white
Arbitrary inference	Drawing a specific conclusion without sufficient evidence, i.e., jumping to (negative) conclusions
Specific abstraction	Focusing on a single (often minor) detail while ignoring other, more significant aspects of the experience, i.e., concentrating on one small (negative) detail while discounting positive aspects
Overgeneralization	Forming conclusions based on too little or too narrow experience, i.e., if one experience was negative, then all similar experiences will be negative
Magnification and minimization	Over- or undervaluing the significance of a particular event, i.e., one small negative event is the end of the world or a positive experience is totally discounted
Personalization	Tendency to self-reference external events without basis, i.e., believing that events are directly related to one's self, whether they are or not

THOUGHT PROCESS AND CONTENT

Clients with depression experience slowed thinking processes: their thinking seems to occur in slow motion. With severe depression, they may not respond verbally to questions. Clients tend to be negative and pessimistic in their thinking, that is, they believe that they will always feel this bad, things will never get any better, and nothing will help. Clients make self-deprecating remarks, criticizing themselves harshly and focusing only on failures or negative attributes. They tend to **ruminate**, which is repeatedly going over the same thoughts. Those who experience psychotic symptoms have delusions; they often believe they are responsible for all the tragedies and miseries in the world.

Often clients with depression have thoughts of dying or committing suicide. It is important to assess suicidal ideation by asking about it directly. The nurse may ask, "Are you thinking about suicide?" or "What suicidal thoughts are you having?" Most clients readily admit to suicidal thinking. Suicide is discussed more fully later in this chapter.

SENSORIUM AND INTELLECTUAL PROCESSES

Some clients with depression are oriented to person, time, and place; others experience difficulty with orientation, especially if they experience psychotic symptoms or are withdrawn from their environment. Assessing general knowledge is difficult because of their limited ability to respond to questions. Memory impairment is common. Clients have extreme difficulty concentrating or paying attention. If psychotic, clients may hear degrading and belittling voices or they may even have command hallucinations that order them to commit suicide.

JUDGMENT AND INSIGHT

Clients with depression experience impaired judgment because they cannot use their cognitive abilities to solve problems or to make decisions. They often cannot make decisions or choices because of their extreme apathy or their negative belief that it "doesn't matter anyway."

Insight may be intact, especially if clients have been depressed previously. Others have very limited insight and are totally unaware of their behavior, feelings, or even their illness.

SELF-CONCEPT

Sense of self-esteem is greatly reduced; clients often use phrases such as "good for nothing" or "just worthless" to describe themselves. They feel guilty about not being able to function and often personalize events or take responsibility for incidents over which they have no control. They believe that others would be better off without them, a belief which leads to suicidal thoughts.

ROLES AND RELATIONSHIPS

Clients with depression have difficulty fulfilling roles and responsibilities. The more severe the depression, the greater

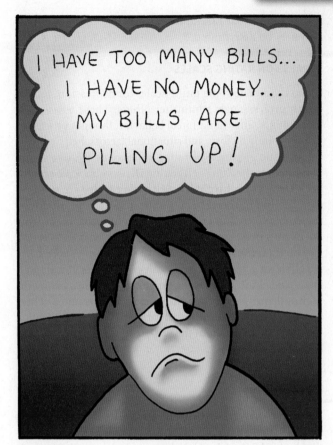

Rumination

the difficulty. They have problems going to work or school; when there, they seem unable to carry out their responsibilities. The same is true with family responsibilities. Clients are less able to cook, clean, or care for children. In addition to the inability to fulfill roles, clients become even more convinced of their "worthlessness" for being unable to meet life responsibilities.

Depression can cause great strain in relationships. Family members who have limited knowledge about depression may believe clients should "just get on with it." Clients often avoid family and social relationships because they feel overwhelmed, experience no pleasure from interactions, and feel unworthy. As clients withdraw from relationships, the strain increases.

PHYSIOLOGIC AND SELF-CARE CONSIDERATIONS

Clients with depression often experience pronounced weight loss because of lack of appetite or disinterest in eating. Sleep disturbances are common: either clients cannot sleep, or they feel exhausted and unrefreshed no matter how much time they spend in bed. They lose interest in sexual activities, and men often experience impotence. Some clients neglect personal hygiene because they lack the interest or energy. Constipation commonly results from decreased food and fluid intake as well as from inactivity. If fluid intake is severely limited, clients also may be dehydrated.

DEPRESSION RATING SCALES

Clients complete some rating scales for depression; mental health professionals administer others. These assessment tools, along with evaluation of behavior, thought processes, history, family history, and situational factors, help to create a diagnostic picture. Self-rating scales of depressive symptoms include the Zung Self-Rating Depression Scale and the Beck Depression Inventory. Self-rating scales are used for case finding in the general public and may be used over the course of treatment to determine improvement from the client's perspective.

The Hamilton Rating Scale for Depression (Table 15.6) is a clinician-rated depression scale used like a clinical interview. The clinician rates the range of the client's behaviors such as depressed mood, guilt, suicide, and insomnia. There is also a section to score diurnal variations, depersonalization (sense of unreality about the self), paranoid symptoms, and obsessions.

Data Analysis

The nurse analyzes assessment data to determine priorities and to establish a plan of care. Nursing diagnoses commonly established for the client with depression include the following:
• Risk for Suicide
• Imbalanced Nutrition: Less Than Body Requirements
• Anxiety
• Ineffective Coping
• Hopelessness
• Ineffective Role Performance
• Self-Care Deficit
• Chronic Low Self-Esteem
• Disturbed Sleep Pattern
• Impaired Social Interaction

Outcome Identification

Outcomes for clients with depression relate to how the depression is manifested—for instance, whether or not the person is slow or agitated, sleeps too much or too little, or eats too much or too little. Examples of outcomes for a client with the psychomotor retardation form of depression include the following:
• The client will not injure himself or herself.
• The client will independently carry out activities of daily living (showering, changing clothing, grooming).
• The client will establish a balance of rest, sleep, and activity.
• The client will establish a balance of adequate nutrition, hydration, and elimination.
• The client will evaluate self-attributes realistically.

• The client will socialize with staff, peers, and family/friends.
• The client will return to occupation or school activities.
• The client will comply with antidepressant regimen.
• The client will verbalize symptoms of a recurrence.

Intervention

PROVIDING FOR SAFETY

The first priority is to determine whether a client with depression is suicidal. If a client has suicidal ideation or hears voices commanding him or her to commit suicide, measures to provide a safe environment are necessary. If the client has a suicide plan, the nurse asks additional questions to determine the lethality of the intent and plan. The nurse reports this information to the treatment team. Health care personnel follow hospital or agency policies and procedures for instituting **suicide precautions** (e.g., removal of harmful items, increased supervision). A thorough discussion is presented later in the chapter.

PROMOTING A THERAPEUTIC RELATIONSHIP

It is important to have meaningful contact with clients who have depression and to begin a therapeutic relationship regardless of the state of depression. Some clients are quite open in describing their feelings of sadness, hopelessness, helplessness, or agitation. Clients may be unable to sustain a long interaction, so several shorter visits help the nurse to assess status and to establish a therapeutic relationship.

The nurse may find it difficult to interact with these clients because he or she empathizes with such sadness and depression. The nurse also may feel unable to "do anything" for clients with limited responses. Clients with psychomotor retardation (slow speech, slow movement, slow thought processes) are very noncommunicative or may even be mute. The nurse can sit with such clients for a few minutes at intervals throughout the day. The nurse's presence conveys genuine interest and caring. It is not necessary for the nurse to talk to clients the entire time; rather, silence can convey that clients are worthwhile even if they are not interacting.

 "My name is Sheila. I'm your nurse today. I'm going to sit with you for a few minutes. If you need anything, or if you would like to talk, please tell me."

After time has elapsed, the nurse would say the following:

 "I'm going now. I will be back in an hour to see you again."

It is also important that the nurse avoids being overly cheerful or trying to "cheer up" clients. It is impossible to coax or to humor clients out of their depression. In fact, an

Table 15.6   HAMILTON RATING SCALE FOR DEPRESSION

For each item select the "cue" that best characterizes the patient.

1: Depressed Mood (sadness, hopeless, helpless, worthless)
   0 Absent
   1 These feeling states indicated only on questioning
   2 These feeling states spontaneously reported verbally
   3 Communicates feeling states nonverbally—i.e., through facial expression, posture, voice, and tendency to weep
   4 Patient reports VIRTUALLY ONLY these feeling states in his spontaneous verbal and nonverbal communication

2: Feelings of guilt
   0 Absent
   1 Self-reproach, feels he has let people down
   2 Ideas of guilt or rumination over past errors or sinful deeds
   3 Present illness is a punishment. Delusions of guilt
   4 Hears accusatory or denunciatory voices and/or experiences threatening visual hallucinations

3: Suicide
   0 Absent
   1 Feels life is not worth living
   2 Wishes he were dead or any thoughts of possible death to self
   3 Suicide ideas or gesture
   4 Attempts at suicide (any serious attempt rates 4)

4: Insomnia early
   0 No difficulty falling asleep
   1 Complains of occasional difficulty falling asleep—i.e., more than 1/4 hour
   2 Complains of nightly difficulty falling asleep

5: Insomnia middle
   0 No difficulty
   1 Patient complains of being restless and disturbed during the night
   2 Waking during the night—any getting out of bed rates 2 (except for purpose of voiding)

6: Insomnia late
   0 No difficulty
   1 Waking in early hours of the morning but goes back to sleep
   2 Unable to fall asleep again if gets out of bed

7: Work and activities
   0 No difficulty
   1 Thoughts and feelings of incapacity, fatigue or weakness related to activities, work, or hobbies
   2 Loss of interest in activity, hobbies, or work—either directly reported by patient, or indirect in listlessness, indecision and vacillation (feels he has to push self to work or activities)
   3 Decrease in actual time spent in activities or decrease in productivity. In hospital, rate 3 if patient does not spend at least 3 hours a day in activities (hospital job or hobbies) exclusive of ward chores
   4 Stopped working because of present illness. In hospital, rate 4 if patient engages in no activities except ward chores, or if patient fails to perform ward chores unassisted

8: Retardation (slowness of thought and speech; impaired ability to concentrate; decreased motor activity)
   0 Normal speech and thought
   1 Slight retardation at interview
   2 Obvious retardation at interview
   3 Interview difficult
   4 Complete stupor

9: Agitation
   0 None
   1 "Playing with" hands, hair, etc.
   2 Hand wringing, nail biting, hair pulling, biting of lips

10: Anxiety psychic
   0 No difficulty
   1 Subjective tension and irritability
   2 Worrying about minor matters
   3 Apprehensive attitude apparent in face or speech
   4 Fears expressed without questioning

11: Anxiety somatic
   0 Absent   Physiologic concomitants of anxiety, such as:
   1 Mild   Gastrointestinal—dry mouth, wind, indigestion, diarrhea, cramps, belching
   2 Moderate   Cardiovascular—palpitations, headaches
   3 Severe   Respiratory—hyperventilation, sighing
   4 Incapacitating   Urinary frequency Sweating

12: Somatic symptoms gastrointestinal
   0 None
   1 Loss of appetite but eating without staff encouragement. Heavy feelings in abdomen.
   2 Difficulty eating without staff urging. Requests or requires laxatives or medication for bowels or medication for GI symptoms

13: Somatic symptoms general
   0 None
   1 Heaviness in limbs, back or head. Backaches, headache, muscle aches. Loss of energy and fatigability
   2 Any clear cut symptom rates 2

14: Genital symptoms
   0 Absent   Symptoms such as:
   1 Mild   Loss of libido
   2 Severe   Menstrual disturbances

15: Hypochondriasis
   0 Not present
   1 Self-absorption (bodily)
   2 Preoccupation with health
   3 Frequent complaints, requests for help, etc.
   4 Hypochondriacal delusions

16: Loss of weight
   A: When rating by history
   0 No weight loss
   1 Probable weight loss associated with present illness
   2 Definite (according to patient) weight loss

(continued)

Table 15.6   HAMILTON RATING SCALE FOR DEPRESSION (*Continued*)

B: On weekly ratings by ward psychiatrist, when actual weight changes are measured

0   Less than 1 lb weight loss in week
1   Greater than 1 lb weight loss in week
2   Greater than 2 lb weight loss in week

17: Insight
0   Acknowledges being depressed and ill
1   Acknowledges illness but attributes cause to bad food, climate, overwork, virus, need for rest, etc.
2   Denies being ill at all

18: Diurnal variation

AM PM
0   0 Absent   If symptoms are worse in the morn-
1   1 Mild   ing or evening, note which it is and
2   2 Severe   rate severity of variation

19: Depersonalization and derealization
0   Absent
1   Mild   Such as:
2   Moderate   Feeling of unreality
3   Severe   Nihilistic ideas
4   Incapacitating

20: Paranoid symptoms
0   None
1
2   Suspiciousness
3   Ideas of reference
4   Delusions of reference and persecution

21: Obsessional and compulsive symptoms
0   Absent
1   Mild
2   Severe

22: Helplessness
0   Not present
1   Subjective feelings that are elicited only by inquiry
2   Patient volunteers his helpless feelings
3   Requires urging, guidance, and reassurance to accomplish ward chores or personal hygiene
4   Requires physical assistance for dress, grooming, eating, bedside tasks, or personal hygiene

23: Hopelessness
0   Not present
1   Intermittently doubts that "things will improve" but can be reassured
2   Consistently feels "hopeless" but accepts reassurances
3   Expresses feelings of discouragement, despair, pessimism about future, which cannot be dispelled
4   Spontaneously and inappropriately perseverates "I'll never get well" or its equivalent

24: Worthlessness (ranges from mild loss of esteem, feelings of inferiority, self-depreciation to delusional notions of worthlessness)
0   Not present
1   Indicates feelings of worthlessness (loss of self-esteem) only on questioning
2   Spontaneously indicates feelings of worthlessness (loss of self-esteem)
3   Different from 2 by degree. Patient volunteers that he is "no good," "inferior," etc.
4   Delusional notions of worthlessness—i.e., "I am a heap of garbage" or its equivalent

Reprinted with permission from Hamilton, M. (1960). A rating scale for depression. *J Neurol Neurosurg Psychiatry, 23,* 56.

NURSING INTERVENTIONS FOR DEPRESSION

- Provide for the safety of the client and others.
- Institute suicide precautions if indicated.
- Begin a therapeutic relationship by spending non-demanding time with the client.
- Promote completion of activities of daily living by assisting the client only as necessary.
- Establish adequate nutrition and hydration.
- Promote sleep and rest.
- Engage the client in activities.
- Encourage the client to verbalize and describe emotions.
- Work with the client to manage medications and side effects.

overly cheerful approach may make clients feel worse or convey a lack of understanding of their despair.

PROMOTING ACTIVITIES OF DAILY LIVING AND PHYSICAL CARE

The ability to perform daily activities is related to the level of psychomotor retardation. To assess ability to perform activities of daily living independently, the nurse first asks the client to perform the global task. For example,

"Martin, it's time to get dressed." (*global task*)

If a client cannot respond to the global request, the nurse breaks the task into smaller segments. Clients with depression can become overwhelmed easily with a task that has several steps. The nurse can use success in small, concrete steps as a basis to increase self-esteem and to build competency for a slightly more complex task the next time.

If clients cannot choose between articles of clothing, the nurse selects the clothing and directs clients to put them on. For example,

"Here are your gray slacks. Put them on."

This still allows clients to participate in dressing. If this is what clients are capable of doing at this point, this activity will reduce dependence on staff. This request is concrete, and if clients cannot do this, the nurse has information about the level of psychomotor retardation.

If a client cannot put on slacks, the nurse assists by saying,

"Let me help you with your slacks, Martin."

The nurse helps clients to dress only when they cannot perform any of the above steps. This allows clients to do as much as possible for themselves and to avoid becoming dependent on the staff. The nurse can carry out this same process with clients when they eat, take a shower, and perform routine self-care activities.

Because abilities change over time, the nurse must assess them on an ongoing basis. This continual assessment takes more time than simply helping clients to dress. Nevertheless, it promotes independence and provides dynamic assessment data about psychomotor abilities.

Often, clients decline to engage in activities because they are too fatigued or have no interest. The nurse can validate these feelings yet still promote participation. For example,

"I know you feel like staying in bed, but it is time to get up for breakfast."

Often, clients may want to stay in bed until they "feel like getting up" or engaging in activities of daily living. The nurse can let clients know they must become more active to feel better rather than waiting passively for improvement. It may be helpful to avoid asking "yes-or-no" questions. Instead of asking, *"Do you want to get up now?"* the nurse would say, *"It is time to get up now."*

Re-establishing balanced nutrition can be challenging when clients have no appetite or don't feel like eating. The nurse can explain that beginning to eat helps stimulate appetite. Food offered frequently and in small amounts can prevent overwhelming clients with a large meal that they feel unable to eat. Sitting quietly with clients during meals can promote eating. Monitoring food and fluid intake may be necessary until clients are consuming adequate amounts.

Promoting sleep may include the short-term use of a sedative or giving medication in the evening if drowsiness or sedation is a side effect. It is also important to encourage clients to remain out of bed and active during the day to facilitate sleeping at night. It is important to monitor the number of hours clients sleep as well as whether they feel refreshed on awakening.

USING THERAPEUTIC COMMUNICATION

Clients with depression are often overwhelmed by the intensity of their emotions. Talking about these feelings can be beneficial. Initially, the nurse encourages clients to describe in detail how they are feeling. Sharing the burden with another person can provide some relief. At these times, the nurse can listen attentively, encourage clients, and validate the intensity of their experience. For example,

Nurse: *"How are you feeling today?"* (broad opening)
    Client: *"I feel so awful . . . terrible."*
    Nurse: *"Tell me more. What is that like for you?"* (using a general lead; encouraging description)
Client: *"I don't feel like myself. I don't know what to do."*
Nurse: *"That must be frightening."* (validating)

It is important at this point that the nurse does not attempt to "fix" the client's difficulties or offer clichés such as "Things will get better" or "But you know your family really needs you." Although the nurse may have good intentions, remarks of this type belittle the client's feelings or make the client feel more guilty and worthless.

As clients begin to improve, the nurse can help them to learn or rediscover more effective coping strategies such as talking to friends, spending leisure time to relax, taking positive steps to deal with stressors, and so forth. Improved coping skills may not prevent depression but may assist clients to deal with the effects of depression more effectively.

MANAGING MEDICATIONS

The increased activity and improved mood that antidepressants produce can provide the energy for suicidal clients to carry out the act. Thus, the nurse must assess suicide risk even when clients are receiving antidepressants. It is also important to ensure that clients ingest the medication and are not saving it in attempt to commit suicide. As clients become ready for discharge, careful assessment of suicide potential is important because they will have a supply of antidepressant medication at home. SSRIs are rarely fatal in overdose, but cyclic and MAOI antidepressants are potentially fatal. Prescriptions may need to be limited to only a 1-week supply at a time if concerns linger about overdose.

An important component of client care is management of side effects. The nurse must make careful observations and ask clients pertinent questions to determine how they are tolerating medications. Tables 15.1 through 15.4 give specific interventions to manage side effects of antidepressant medications.

Clients and family must learn how to manage the medication regimen because clients may need to take these medications for months, years, or even a lifetime. Education promotes compliance. Clients should know how often they need to return for monitoring and diagnostic tests.

PROVIDING CLIENT AND FAMILY TEACHING

Teaching clients and family about depression is important. They must understand that depression is an illness, not a lack of willpower or motivation. Learning about the beginning symptoms of relapse may assist clients to seek treatment early and avoid a lengthy recurrence.

Clients and family should know that treatment outcomes are best when psychotherapy and antidepressants are combined. Psychotherapy helps clients to explore anger, dependence, guilt, hopelessness, helplessness, object loss, interpersonal issues, and irrational beliefs. The goal is to reverse negative views of the future, improve self-image, and help clients gain competence and self-mastery. The nurse can help clients to find a therapist through mental health centers in specific communities.

Support group participation also helps some clients and their families. Clients can receive support and encouragement from others who struggle with depression, and family members can offer support to one another. The National Alliance for the Mentally Ill is an organization

CLIENT/FAMILY EDUCATION FOR DEPRESSION

- Teach about the illness of depression.
- Identify early signs of relapse.
- Discuss the importance of support groups and assist in locating resources.
- Teach the client and family about the benefits of therapy and follow-up appointments.
- Encourage participation in support groups.
- Teach the action, side effects, and special instructions regarding medications.
- Discuss methods to manage side effects of medication.

that can help clients and families connect with local support groups.

Evaluation

Evaluation of the plan of care is based on achievement of individual client outcomes. It is essential that clients feel safe and are not experiencing uncontrollable urges to commit suicide. Participation in therapy and medication compliance produce more favorable outcomes for clients with

---

Nursing Care Plan   *Depression*

Nursing Diagnosis

Ineffective Coping: *Inability to form a valid appraisal of the stressors, inadequate choices of practiced responses, and/or inability to use available resources.*

ASSESSMENT DATA

- Suicidal ideas or behavior
- Slowed mental processes
- Disordered thoughts
- Feelings of despair, hopelessness, and worthlessness
- Guilt
- Anhedonia (inability to experience pleasure)
- Disorientation
- Generalized restlessness or agitation
- Sleep disturbances: early awakening, insomnia, or excessive sleeping
- Anger or hostility (may not be overt)

EXPECTED OUTCOMES

Immediate
The client will
- Be free from self-inflicted harm
- Engage in reality-based interactions
- Be oriented to person, place, and time
- Express anger or hostility outwardly in a safe manner

Stabilization
The client will
- Express feelings directly with congruent verbal and nonverbal messages
- Be free from psychotic symptoms
- Demonstrate functional level of psychomotor activity

Nursing Care Plan: Depression, cont.

ASSESSMENT DATA

- Rumination
- Delusions, hallucinations, or other psychotic symptoms
- Diminished interest in sexual activity
- Fear of intensity of feelings
- Anxiety

EXPECTED OUTCOMES

Community
The client will

- Demonstrate compliance with and knowledge of medications, if any
- Demonstrate an increased ability to cope with anxiety, stress, or frustration
- Verbalize or demonstrate acceptance of loss or change, if any
- Identify a support system in the community

IMPLEMENTATION

Nursing Interventions *denotes collaborative interventions

Provide a safe environment for the client.

Continually assess the client's potential for suicide. Remain aware of this suicide potential at all times.

Observe the client closely, especially under the following circumstances:
After antidepressant medication begins to raise the client's mood.
- Unstructured time on the unit or times when the number of staff on the unit is limited.
- After any dramatic behavioral change (sudden cheerfulness, relief, or giving away personal belongings).

Reorient the client to person, place, and time as indicated (call the client by name, tell the client your name, tell the client where he or she is, and so forth).

Spend time with the client.

If the client is ruminating, tell him or her that you will talk about reality or about the client's feelings, but limit the attention given to repeated expressions of rumination.

Initially assign the same staff members to work with the client whenever possible.

When approaching the client, use a moderate, level tone of voice. Avoid being overly cheerful.

Rationale

Physical safety of the client is a priority. Many common items may be used in a self-destructive manner.

Depressed clients may have a potential for suicide that may or may not be expressed and that may change with time.

You must be aware of the client's activities at all times when there is a potential for suicide or self-injury. Risk for suicide increases as the client's energy level is increased by medication, when the client's time is unstructured, and when observation of the client decreases. These changes may indicate that the client has come to a decision to commit suicide.

Repeated presentation of reality is concrete reinforcement for the client.

Your physical presence is reality.

Minimizing attention may help decrease rumination. Providing reinforcement for reality orientation and expression of feelings will encourage these behaviors.

The client's ability to respond to others may be impaired. Limiting the number of new contacts initially will facilitate familiarity and trust.

However, the number of people interacting with the client should increase as soon as possible to minimize dependency and to facilitate the client's abilities to communicate with a variety of people.

Being overly cheerful may indicate to the client that being cheerful is the goal and that other feelings are not acceptable.

continued ⋯⁛

Nursing Care Plan: Depression, cont.

IMPLEMENTATION

Nursing Interventions *denotes collaborative interventions	**Rationale**
Use silence and active listening when interacting with the client. Let the client know that you are concerned and that you consider the client a worthwhile person.	The client may not communicate if you are talking too much. Your presence and use of active listening will communicate your interest and concern.
When first communicating with the client, use simple, direct sentences; avoid complex sentences or directions.	The client's ability to perceive and respond to complex stimuli is impaired.
Avoid asking the client many questions, especially questions that require only brief answers.	Asking questions and requiring only brief answers may discourage the client from expressing feelings.
Be comfortable sitting with the client in silence. Let the client know you are available to converse, but do not require the client to talk.	Your silence will convey your expectation that the client will communicate and your acceptance of the client's difficulty with communication.
Allow (and encourage) the client to cry. Stay with and support the client if he or she desires. Provide privacy if the client desires and it is safe to do so.	Crying is a healthy way of expressing feelings of sadness, hopelessness, and despair. The client may not feel comfortable crying and may need encouragement or privacy.
Do not cut off interactions with cheerful remarks or platitudes (e.g., "No one really wants to die," or "You'll feel better soon."). Do not belittle the client's feelings. Accept the client's verbalizations of feelings as real, and give support for expressions of emotions, especially those that may be difficult for the client (like anger).	You may be uncomfortable with certain feelings the client expresses. If so, it is important for you to recognize this and discuss it with another staff member rather than directly or indirectly communicating your discomfort to the client. Proclaiming the client's feelings to be inappropriate or belittling them is detrimental.
Encourage the client to ventilate feelings in whatever way is comfortable—verbal and nonverbal. Let the client know you will listen and accept what is being expressed.	Expressing feelings may help relieve despair, hopelessness, and so forth. Feelings are not inherently good or bad. You must remain nonjudgmental about the client's feelings and express this to the client.
Interact with the client on topics with which he or she is comfortable. Do not probe for information.	Topics that are uncomfortable for the client and probing may be threatening and discourage communication. After trust has been established, the client may be able to discuss more difficult topics.
Teach the client about the problem-solving process: explore possible options, examine the consequences of each alternative, select and implement an alternative, and evaluate the results.	The client may be unaware of a systematic method for solving problems. Successful use of the problem-solving process facilitates the client's confidence in the use of coping skills.
Provide positive feedback at each step of the process. If the client is not satisfied with the chosen alternative, assist the client to select another alternative.	Positive feedback at each step will give the client many opportunities for success, encourage him or her to persist in problem solving, and enhance confidence. The client also can learn to "survive" making a mistake.

Adapted from Schultz, J. M., & Videbeck, S. L. (2005). Lippincott's manual of psychiatric nursing care plans (7th ed.). *Philadelphia: Lippincott Williams & Wilkins.*

depression. Being able to identify signs of relapse and to seek treatment immediately can significantly decrease the severity of a depressive episode.

BIPOLAR DISORDER

Bipolar disorder involves extreme mood swings from episodes of mania to episodes of depression. (Bipolar disorder was formerly known as manic-depressive illness.) During manic phases, clients are euphoric, grandiose, energetic, and sleepless. They have poor judgment and rapid thoughts, actions, and speech. During depressed phases, mood, behavior, and thoughts are the same as in people diagnosed with major depression (see previous discussion). In fact, if a person's first episode of bipolar illness is a depressed phase, he or she might be diagnosed with major depression; a diagnosis of bipolar disorder may not be made until the person experiences a manic episode. To increase awareness about bipolar disorder, health care professionals can use tools such as the Mood Disorder Questionnaire (Box 15.1).

Bipolar disorder ranks second only to major depression as a cause of worldwide disability. The lifetime risk for bipolar disorder is at least 1.2%, with a risk of completed suicide for 15%. Young men early in the course of their illness are at highest risk for suicide, especially those with a history of suicide attempts or alcohol abuse as well as those recently discharged from the hospital (Rihmer & Angst, 2005).

Whereas a person with major depression slowly slides into depression that can last for 6 months to 2 years, the person with bipolar disorder cycles between depression and normal behavior (bipolar depressed) or mania and normal behavior (bipolar manic). A person with bipolar mixed episodes alternates between major depressive and manic episodes interspersed with periods of normal behavior. Each mood may last for weeks or months before the pattern begins to descend or ascend once again. Figure 15.1 shows the three categories of bipolar cycles.

Bipolar disorder occurs almost equally among men and women. It is more common in highly educated people. Because some people with bipolar illness deny their mania, prevalence rates may actually be higher than reported.

Onset and Clinical Course

The mean age for a first manic episode is the early twenties, but some people experience onset in adolescence, whereas others start experiencing symptoms when they are older than 50 (APA, 2000). Currently, debate exists about whether or not some children diagnosed with attention deficit hyperactivity disorder actually have a very early onset of bipolar disorder. Manic episodes typically begin suddenly, with rapid escalation of symptoms over a few days, and they last from a few weeks to several months. They tend to be briefer and to end more suddenly than depressive episodes. Adolescents are more likely to have psychotic manifestations.

The diagnosis of a manic episode or mania requires at least 1 week of unusual and incessantly heightened, grandiose, or agitated mood in addition to three or more of the following symptoms: exaggerated self-esteem; sleeplessness; pressured speech; flight of ideas; reduced ability to filter extraneous stimuli; distractibility; increased activities with increased energy; and multiple, grandiose, high-risk activities involving poor judgment and severe consequences, such as spending sprees, sex with strangers, and impulsive investments (APA, 2000).

Clients often do not understand how their illness affects others. They may stop taking medications because they like the euphoria and feel burdened by the side effects, blood tests, and physicians' visits needed to maintain treatment. Family members are concerned and exhausted by their loved ones' behaviors; they often stay up late at night for fear the manic person may do something impulsive and dangerous.

Treatment

PSYCHOPHARMACOLOGY

Treatment for bipolar disorder involves a lifetime regimen of medications: either an antimanic agent called lithium or anticonvulsant medications used as mood stabilizers (see Chapter 2). This is the only psychiatric disorder in which medications can prevent acute cycles of bipolar behavior. Once thought to help reduce manic behavior only, lithium and these anticonvulsants also protect against the effects of bipolar depressive cycles. If a client in the acute stage of mania or depression exhibits psychosis (disordered thinking as seen with delusions, hallucinations, and illusions), an antipsychotic agent is administered in addition to the bipolar medications. Some clients keep taking both bipolar medications and antipsychotics.

Lithium. Lithium is a salt contained in the human body; it is similar to gold, copper, magnesium, manganese, and other trace elements. Once believed to be helpful for bipolar mania only, investigators quickly realized that lithium also could partially or completely mute the cycling toward bipolar depression. The response rate in acute mania to lithium therapy is 70% to 80%. In addition to treating the range of bipolar behaviors, lithium also can stabilize bipolar disorder by reducing the degree and frequency of cycling or eliminating manic episodes (Freeman et al., 2006).

Lithium not only competes for salt receptor sites but also affects calcium, potassium, and magnesium ions as well as glucose metabolism. Its mechanism of action is unknown, but it is thought to work in the synapses to hasten destruction of catecholamines (dopamine, norepinephrine), inhibit neurotransmitter release, and decrease the sensitivity of postsynaptic receptors (Facts and Comparisons, 2006).

Lithium's action peaks in 30 minutes to 4 hours for regular forms and in 4 to 6 hours for the slow-release form.

Box 15.1   MOOD DISORDER QUESTIONNAIRE

The following questionnaire can be used as a starting point to help you recognize the signs/symptoms of bipolar disorder but is not meant to be a substitute for a full medical evaluation. Bipolar disorder is complex and **an accurate, thorough diagnosis can be made through a personal evaluation by your doctor**. However, a positive screening may suggest that you might benefit from seeking such an evaluation from your doctor. Regardless of the questionnaire results, if you or your family has concerns about your mental health, please contact your physician and/or other health care professional.

When completed, you may want to print out your responses.

Instructions: Please answer each question as best you can.

	YES	NO
1. Has there ever been a period of time when you were not your usual self and . . .		
. . . you felt so good or so hyper that other people thought you were not your normal self or you were so hyper that you got into trouble?	☐	☐
. . . you were so irritable that you shouted at people or started fights or arguments?	☐	☐
. . . you felt much more self-confident than usual?	☐	☐
. . . you got much less sleep than usual and found you didn't really miss it?	☐	☐
. . . you were much more talkative or spoke much faster than usual?	☐	☐
. . . thoughts raced through your head or you couldn't slow your mind down?	☐	☐
. . . you were so easily distracted by things around you that you had trouble concentrating or staying on track?	☐	☐
. . . you had much more energy than usual?	☐	☐
. . . you were much more active or did many more things than usual?	☐	☐
. . . you were much more social or outgoing than usual, for example, you telephoned friends in the middle of the night?	☐	☐
. . . you were much more interested in sex than usual?	☐	☐
. . . you did things that were unusual for you or that other people might have thought were excessive, foolish, or risky?	☐	☐
. . . spending money got you or your family into trouble?	☐	☐
2. If you checked YES to more than one of the above, have several of these ever happened during the same period of time?	☐	☐

3. How much of a problem did any of these cause you—like being unable to work; having family, money or legal troubles; getting into arguments or fights? Please select one response only.

[☐] No problem   [☐] Minor problem   [☐] Moderate problem   [☐] Serious problem

	YES	NO
4. Have any of your blood relatives (children, siblings, parents, grandparents, aunts, uncles) had manic-depressive illness or bipolar disorder?	☐	☐
5. Has a health care professional ever told you that you have manic-depressive illness or bipolar disorder?	☐	☐

Hirschfeld, R. M. A., Williams, J. B., Spitzer, R. L., et al. (2000). Development and validation of a screening instrument for bipolar spectrum disorder: The Mood Disorder Questionnaire. American Journal of Psychiatry 157(11), 1873–1875.

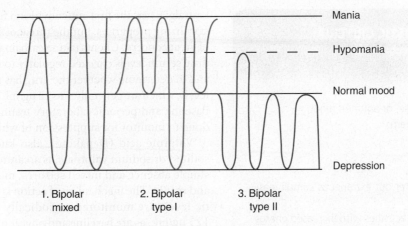

1. Bipolar mixed—Cycles alternate between periods of mania, normal mood, depression, normal mood, mania, and so forth.

2. Bipolar type I—Manic episodes with at least one depressive episode.

3. Bipolar type II—Recurrent depressive episodes with at least one hypomanic episode.

Figure 15.1 Graphic depiction of mood cycles.

It crosses the blood–brain barrier and placenta and is distributed in sweat and breast milk. Lithium use during pregnancy is not recommended because it can lead to first-trimester developmental abnormalities. Onset of action is 5 to 14 days; with this lag period, antipsychotic or antidepressant agents are used carefully in combination with lithium to reduce symptoms in acutely manic or acutely depressed clients. The half-life of lithium is 20 to 27 hours (Facts and Comparisons, 2007).

Anticonvulsant Drugs. Lithium is effective in about 75% of people with bipolar illness. The rest do not respond or have difficulty taking lithium because of side effects, problems with the treatment regimen, drug interactions, or medical conditions such as renal disease that contraindicate use of lithium. Several anticonvulsants traditionally used to treat seizure disorders have proved helpful in stabilizing the moods of people with bipolar illness. These drugs are categorized as miscellaneous anticonvulsants. Their mechanism of action

---

CLINICAL VIGNETTE: MANIC EPISODE

"Everyone is stupid! What is the matter? Have you all taken dumb pills? Dumb pills, rum pills, shlummy shlum lum pills!" Mitch screamed as he waited for his staff to snap to attention and get with the program. He had started the Pickle Barn 10 years ago and now had a money-making business canning and delivering gourmet pickles.

He knew how to do everything in this place and, running from person to person to watch what each was doing, he didn't like what he saw. It was 8 AM, and he'd already fired the supervisor, who had been with him for 5 years.

By 8:02 AM, Mitch had fired six pickle assistants because he did not like the way they looked. Then, Mitch threw pots and paddles at them because they weren't leaving fast enough. Rich, his brother, walked in during this melee and quietly asked everyone to stay, then invited Mitch outside for a walk.

"Are you nuts?" Mitch screamed at his brother. "Everyone here is out of control. I have to do everything." Mitch was trembling, shaking. He hadn't slept in 3 days and didn't need

to. The only time he'd left the building in these 3 days was to have sex with any woman who had agreed. He felt euphoric, supreme, able to leap tall buildings in a single bound. He glared at Rich. "I feel good! What are you bugging me for?" He slammed out the door, shrilly reciting, "Rich and Mitch! Rich and Mitch! Pickle king rich!"

"Rich and Mitch, Rich and Mitch. With dear old auntie, now we're rich." Mitch couldn't stop talking and speed walking. Watching Mitch, Rich gently said, "Aunt Jen called me last night. She says you are manic again. When did you stop taking your lithium?"

"Manic? Who's manic? I'm just feeling good. Who needs that stuff? I like to feel good. It is wonderful, marvelous, stupendous. I am not manic," shrieked Mitch as he swerved around to face his brother. Rich, weary and sad, said, "I am taking you to the emergency psych unit. If you do not agree to go, I will have the police take you. I know you don't see this in yourself, but you are out of control and getting dangerous."

neuralgia, was the first anticonvulsant found to have mood-stabilizing properties, but the threat of agranulocytosis was of great concern. Clients taking carbamazepine need to have drug serum levels checked regularly to monitor for toxicity and to determine whether the drug has reached therapeutic levels, which are generally 4 to 12 µg/mL (Ketter et al., 2006). Baseline and periodic laboratory testing also must also be done to monitor for suppression of white blood cells.

Valproic acid (Depakote), also known as divalproex sodium or sodium valproate, is an anticonvulsant used for simple absence and mixed seizures, migraine prophylaxis, and mania. The mechanism of action is unclear. Therapeutic levels are monitored periodically to remain at 50 to 125 µg/mL, as are baseline and ongoing liver function tests, including serum ammonia levels and platelet and bleeding times (Bowden, 2006).

Gabapentin (Neurontin), lamotrigine (Lamictal), and topiramate (Topamax) are other anticonvulsants sometimes used as mood stabilizers, but they are used less frequently than valproic acid. Value ranges for therapeutic levels are not established.

Clonazepam (Klonopin) is an anticonvulsant and a benzodiazepine (a schedule IV controlled substance) used in simple absence and minor motor seizures, panic disorder, and bipolar disorder. Physiologic dependence can develop with long-term use. This drug may be used in conjunction

is largely unknown, but they may raise the brain's threshold for dealing with stimulation; this prevents the person from being bombarded with external and internal stimuli (Table 15.7).

Carbamazepine (Tegretol), which had been used for grand mal and temporal lobe epilepsy as well as for trigeminal

Table 15.7   ANTICONVULSANTS USED AS MOOD STABILIZERS

Generic (Trade) Name	Side Effects	Nursing Implications
Carbamazepine (Tegretol)	Dizziness, hypotension, ataxia, sedation, blurred vision, leukopenia, rashes	Assist client to rise slowly from sitting position. Monitor gait and assist as necessary. Report rashes to physician.
Divalproex (Depakote)	Ataxia, drowsiness, weakness, fatigue, menstrual changes, dyspepsia, nausea, vomiting, weight gain, hair loss	Monitor gait and assist as necessary. Provide rest periods. Give with food. Establish balanced nutrition.
Gabapentin (Neurontin)	Dizziness, hypotension, ataxia, coordination, sedation, headache, fatigue, nystagmus, nausea, vomiting	Assist client to rise slowly from sitting position. Provide rest periods. Give with food.
Lamotrigine (Lamictal)	Dizziness, hypotension, ataxia, coordination, sedation, headache, weakness, fatigue, menstrual changes, sore throat, flu-like symptoms, blurred or double vision, nausea, vomiting, rashes	Assist client to rise slowly from sitting position. Monitor gait and assist as necessary. Provide rest periods. Monitor physical health. Give with food. Report rashes to physician.
Topiramate (Topamax)	Dizziness, hypotension, anxiety, ataxia, incoordination, confusion, sedation, slurred speech, tremor, weakness, blurred or double vision, anorexia, nausea, vomiting	Assist client to rise slowly from sitting position. Monitor gait and assist as necessary. Orient client. Protect client from potential injury. Give with food.
Oxcarbazepine (Trileptal)	Dizziness, fatigue, ataxia, confusion, nausea, vomiting, anorexia, headache, tremor, confusion, rashes	Assist client to rise slowly from sitting position. Monitor gait and assist as necessary. Give with food. Orient client and protect from injury. Report rashes to physician.

with lithium or other mood stabilizers but is not used alone to manage bipolar disorder.

PSYCHOTHERAPY

Psychotherapy can be useful in the mildly depressive or normal portion of the bipolar cycle. It is not useful during acute manic stages because the person's attention span is brief and he or she can gain little insight during times of accelerated psychomotor activity. Psychotherapy combined with medication can reduce the risk for suicide and injury, provide support to the client and family, and help the client to accept the diagnosis and treatment plan.

APPLICATION OF THE NURSING PROCESS: BIPOLAR DISORDER

The focus of this discussion is on the client experiencing a manic episode of bipolar disorder. The reader should review the Application of the Nursing Process: Depression to examine nursing care of the client experiencing a depressed phase of bipolar disorder.

Assessment

HISTORY

Taking a history with a client in the manic phase often proves difficult. The client may jump from subject to subject, which makes it difficult for the nurse to follow. Obtaining data in several short sessions, as well as talking to family members, may be necessary. The nurse can obtain much information, however, by watching and listening.

GENERAL APPEARANCE AND MOTOR BEHAVIOR

Clients with mania experience psychomotor agitation and seem to be in perpetual motion; sitting still is difficult. This continual movement has many ramifications: clients can become exhausted or injure themselves.

In the manic phase, the client may wear clothes that reflect the elevated mood: brightly colored, flamboyant, attention-getting, and perhaps sexually suggestive. For example, a woman in the manic phase may wear a lot of jewelry and hair ornaments, or her makeup may be garish and heavy, whereas a male client may wear a tight and revealing muscle shirt or go bare-chested.

Clients experiencing a manic episode think, move, and talk fast. Pressured speech, one of the hallmark symptoms, is evidenced by unrelentingly rapid and often loud speech without pauses. Those with pressured speech interrupt and cannot listen to others. They ignore verbal and nonverbal cues indicating that others wish to speak, and they continue with constant intelligible or unintelligible speech, turning from one listener to another or speaking to no one at all. If interrupted, clients with mania often start over from the beginning.

MOOD AND AFFECT

Mania is reflected in periods of euphoria, exuberant activity, grandiosity, and false sense of well-being. Projection of an all-knowing and all-powerful image may be an unconscious defense against underlying low self-esteem. Some clients manifest mania with an angry, verbally aggressive tone and are sarcastic and irritable, especially when others set limits on their behavior. Clients' mood is quite labile, and they may alternate between periods of loud laughter and episodes of tears.

THOUGHT PROCESS AND CONTENT

Cognitive ability or thinking is confused and jumbled with thoughts racing one after another, which is often referred to as flight of ideas. Clients cannot connect concepts, and they jump from one subject to another. Circumstantiality and tangentiality also characterize thinking. At times, clients may be unable to communicate thoughts or needs in ways that others understand.

These clients start many projects at one time but cannot carry any to completion. There is little true planning, but clients talk nonstop about plans and projects to anyone and everyone, insisting on the importance of accomplishing these activities. Sometimes they try to enlist help from others in one or more activities. They do not consider risks or personal experience, abilities, or resources. Clients start these activities as they occur in their thought processes. Examples of these multiple activities are going on shopping sprees, using credit cards excessively while unemployed and broke, starting several business ventures at once, having promiscuous sex, gambling, taking impulsive trips, embarking on illegal endeavors, making risky investments, talking with multiple people, and speeding (APA, 2000).

Some clients experience psychotic features during mania; they express grandiose delusions involving importance, fame, privilege, and wealth. Some may claim to be the president, a famous movie star, or even God or a prophet.

SENSORIUM AND INTELLECTUAL PROCESSES

Clients may be oriented to person and place but rarely to time. Intellectual functioning, such as fund of knowledge, is difficult to assess during the manic phase. Clients may claim to have many abilities they do not possess. The ability to concentrate or to pay attention is grossly impaired. Again, if a client is psychotic, he or she may experience hallucinations.

JUDGMENT AND INSIGHT

People in the manic phase are easily angered and irritated and strike back at what they perceive as censorship by others because they impose no restrictions on themselves. They are impulsive and rarely think before acting or speaking, which makes their judgment poor. Insight is limited because they believe they are "fine" and have no problems. They blame any difficulties on others.

SELF-CONCEPT

Clients with mania often have exaggerated self-esteem; they believe they can accomplish anything. They rarely discuss their self-concept realistically. Nevertheless, a false sense of well-being masks difficulties with chronic low self-esteem.

ROLES AND RELATIONSHIPS

Clients in the manic phase rarely can fulfill role responsibilities. They have trouble at work or school (if they are even attending) and are too distracted and hyperactive to pay attention to children or activities of daily living. Although they may begin many tasks or projects, they complete few.

These clients have a great need to socialize but little understanding of their excessive, overpowering, and confrontational social interactions. Their need for socialization often leads to promiscuity. Clients invade the intimate space and personal business of others. Arguments result when others feel threatened by such boundary invasions. Although the usual mood of manic people is elation, emotions are unstable and can fluctuate (**labile emotions**) readily between euphoria and hostility. Clients with mania can become hostile to others whom they perceive as standing in way of desired goals. They cannot postpone or delay gratification. For example, a manic client tells his wife, "You are the most wonderful woman in the world. Give me $50 so I can buy you a ticket to the opera." When she refuses, he snarls and accuses her of being cheap and selfish and may even strike her.

PHYSIOLOGIC AND SELF-CARE CONSIDERATIONS

Clients with mania can go days without sleep or food and not even realize they are hungry or tired. They may be on the brink of physical exhaustion but are unwilling or unable to stop, rest, or sleep. They often ignore personal hygiene as "boring" when they have "more important things" to do. Clients may throw away possessions or destroy valued items. They may even physically injure themselves and tend to ignore or be unaware of health needs that can worsen.

Data Analysis

The nurse analyzes assessment data to determine priorities and to establish a plan of care. Nursing diagnoses commonly established for clients in the manic phase are as follows:

- Risk for Other-Directed Violence
- Risk for Injury
- Imbalanced Nutrition: Less Than Body Requirements
- Ineffective Coping
- Noncompliance
- Ineffective Role Performance
- Self-Care Deficit
- Chronic Low Self-Esteem
- Disturbed Sleep Pattern

Outcome Identification

Examples of outcomes appropriate to mania are as follows:
- The client will not injure self or others.
- The client will establish a balance of rest, sleep, and activity.
- The client will establish adequate nutrition, hydration, and elimination.
- The client will participate in self-care activities.
- The client will evaluate personal qualities realistically.
- The client will engage in socially appropriate, reality-based interaction.
- The client will verbalize knowledge of his or her illness and treatment.

Intervention

PROVIDING FOR SAFETY

Because of the safety risks that clients in the manic phase take, safety plays a primary role in care, followed by issues related to self-esteem and socialization. A primary nursing responsibility is to provide a safe environment for clients and others. The nurse assesses clients directly for suicidal ideation and plans or thoughts of hurting others. In addition, clients in the manic phase have little insight into their anger and agitation and how their behaviors affect others. They often intrude into others' space, take others' belongings without permission, or appear aggressive in approaching others. This behavior can threaten or anger people who then retaliate. It is important to monitor the clients' whereabouts and behaviors frequently.

The nurse also should tell clients that staff members will help them control their behavior if clients cannot do so alone. For clients who feel out of control, the nurse must establish external controls empathetically and nonjudgmentally. These external controls provide long-term comfort to clients, although their initial response may be aggression. People in the manic phase have labile emotions; it is not unusual for them to strike staff members who have set limits in a way clients dislike.

These clients physically and psychologically invade boundaries. It is necessary to set limits when they cannot set limits on themselves. For example, the nurse might say,

"John, you are too close to my face. Please stand back 2 feet."

or

"It is unacceptable to hug other clients. You may talk to others, but do not touch them."

When setting limits, it is important to clearly identify the unacceptable behavior and the expected, appropriate behavior. All staff must consistently set and enforce limits for those limits to be effective.

MEETING PHYSIOLOGIC NEEDS

Clients with mania may get very little rest or sleep, even if they are on the brink of physical exhaustion. Medication may be helpful, though clients may resist taking it. Decreasing environmental stimulation may assist clients to relax. The nurse provides a quiet environment without noise, television, or other distractions. Establishing a bedtime routine, such as a tepid bath, may help clients to calm down enough to rest.

Nutrition is another area of concern. Manic clients may be too "busy" to sit down and eat, or they may have such poor concentration that they fail to stay interested in food for very long. "Finger foods" or things clients can eat while moving around are the best options to improve nutrition. Such foods also should be as high in calories and protein as possible. For example, celery and carrots are finger foods, but they supply little nutrition. Sandwiches, protein bars, and fortified shakes are better choices. Clients with mania also benefit from food that is easy to eat without much preparation. Meat that must be cut into bite sizes or plates of spaghetti are not likely to be successful options. Having snacks available between meals, so clients can eat whenever possible, is also useful.

The nurse needs to monitor food and fluid intake and hours of sleep until clients routinely meet these needs without difficulty. Observing and supervising clients at meal times are also important to prevent clients from taking food from others.

NURSING INTERVENTIONS FOR MANIA

Provide for client's physical safety and safety of those around client.

- Set limits on client's behavior when needed.
- Remind the client to respect distances between self and others.
- Use short, simple sentences to communicate.
- Clarify the meaning of client's communication.
- Frequently provide finger foods that are high in calories and protein.
- Promote rest and sleep.
- Protect the client's dignity when inappropriate behavior occurs.
- Channel client's need for movement into socially acceptable motor activities.

PROVIDING THERAPEUTIC COMMUNICATION

Clients with mania have short attention spans, so the nurse uses clear, simple sentences when communicating. They may not be able to handle a lot of information at once, so the nurse breaks information into many small segments. It helps to ask clients to repeat brief messages to ensure they have heard and incorporated them.

Clients may need to undergo baseline and follow-up laboratory tests. A brief explanation of the purpose of each test allays anxiety. The nurse gives printed information to reinforce verbal messages, especially those related to rules, schedules, civil rights, treatment, staff names, and client education.

The speech of manic clients may be pressured: rapid, circumstantial, rhyming, noisy, or intrusive with flights of ideas. Such disordered speech indicates thought processes that are flooded with thoughts, ideas, and impulses. The nurse must keep channels of communication open with clients, regardless of speech patterns. The nurse can say,

"Please speak more slowly. I'm having trouble following you."

This puts the responsibility for the communication difficulty on the nurse rather than on the client. This nurse patiently and frequently repeats this request during conversation because clients will return to rapid speech.

Clients in the manic phase often use pronouns when referring to people, making it difficult for listeners to understand who is being discussed and when the conversation has moved to a new subject. While clients are agitatedly talking, they usually are thinking and moving just as quickly, so it is a challenge for the nurse to follow a coherent story. The nurse can ask clients to identify each person, place, or thing being discussed.

When speech includes flight of ideas, the nurse can ask clients to explain the relationship between topics—for example,

"What happened then?"

or

"Was that before of after you got married?"

The nurse also assesses and documents the coherence of messages.

Clients with pressured speech rarely let others speak. Instead, they talk nonstop until they run out of steam or just stand there looking at the other person before moving away. Those with pressured speech do not respond to others' verbal or nonverbal signals that indicate a desire to speak. The nurse avoids becoming involved in power struggles over who will dominate the conversation. Instead, the nurse may talk to clients away from others so there is no "competition" for the nurse's attention. The nurse also sets limits regarding taking turns speaking and listening as well as giving attention to others when they need it. Clients with mania cannot have all requests granted immediately even though that may be their desire.

PROMOTING APPROPRIATE BEHAVIORS

These clients need to be protected from their pursuit of socially unacceptable and risky behaviors. The nurse can direct their need for movement into socially acceptable, large motor activities such as arranging chairs for a community meeting or walking. In acute mania, clients lose the ability to control their behavior and engage in risky activities. Because acutely manic clients feel extraordinarily powerful, they place few restrictions on themselves. They act out impulsive thoughts, have inflated and grandiose perceptions of their abilities, are demanding, and need immediate gratification. This can affect their physical, social, occupational, or financial safety as well as that of others. Clients may make purchases that exceed their ability to pay. They may give away money or jewelry or other possessions. The nurse may need to monitor a client's access to such items until his or her behavior is less impulsive.

In an acute manic episode, clients also may lose sexual inhibitions, resulting in provocative and risky behaviors. Clothing may be flashy or revealing, or clients may undress in public areas. They may engage in unprotected sex with virtual strangers. Clients may ask staff members or other clients (of the same or opposite sex) for sex, graphically describe sexual acts, or display their genitals. The nurse handles such behavior in a matter-of-fact, nonjudgmental manner. For example,

"Mary, let's go to your room and find a sweater."

It is important to treat clients with dignity and respect despite their inappropriate behavior. It is not helpful to "scold" or chastise them; they are not children engaging in willful misbehavior.

In the manic phase, clients cannot understand personal boundaries, so it is the staff's role to keep clients in view for intervention as necessary. For example, a staff member who sees a client invading the intimate space of others can say,

"Jeffrey, I'd appreciate your help in setting up a circle of chairs in the group therapy room."

This large motor activity distracts Jeffrey from his inappropriate behavior, appeals to his need for heightened physical activity, is noncompetitive, and is socially acceptable. The staff's vigilant redirection to a more socially appropriate activity protects clients from the hazards of unprotected sex and reduces embarrassment over such behaviors when they return to normal behavior.

MANAGING MEDICATIONS

Lithium is not metabolized; rather, it is reabsorbed by the proximal tubule and excreted in the urine. Periodic serum lithium levels are used to monitor the client's safety and to ensure that the dose given has increased the serum lithium level to a treatment level or reduced it to a maintenance level. There is a narrow range of safety among maintenance levels (0.5 to 1 mEq/L), treatment levels (0.8 to 1.5 mEq/L), and toxic levels (1.5 mEq/L and above). It is important to assess for signs of toxicity and to ensure that clients and their families have this information before discharge (Table 15.8). Older adults can have symptoms of toxicity at lower serum levels. Lithium is potentially fatal in overdose.

Clients should drink adequate water (approximately 2 liters per day) and continue with the usual amount of dietary table salt. Having too much salt in the diet because of unusually salty foods or the ingestion of salt-containing antacids can reduce receptor availability for lithium and increase lithium excretion, so the lithium level will be too low. If there is too much water, lithium is diluted and the lithium level will be too low to be therapeutic. Drinking too little water or losing fluid through excessive sweating, vomiting, or diarrhea increases the lithium level, which may result in toxicity. Monitoring daily weights and the balance between intake and output and checking for dependent edema can be helpful in monitoring fluid balance. The physician should be contacted if the client has diarrhea, fever, flu, or any condition that leads to dehydration.

Thyroid function tests usually are ordered as a baseline and every 6 months during treatment with lithium. In 6 to 18 months, one third of clients taking lithium have an increased level of thyroid-stimulating hormone, which can cause anxiety, labile emotions, and sleeping difficulties. Decreased levels are implicated in fatigue and depression.

Because most lithium is excreted in the urine, baseline and periodic assessments of renal status are necessary to assess renal function. The reduced renal function in older adults necessitates lower doses. Lithium is contraindicated in people with compromised renal function or urinary retention and those taking low-salt diets or diuretics. Lithium

Table 15.8	SYMPTOMS AND INTERVENTIONS OF LITHIUM TOXICITY	
Serum Lithium Level	**Symptoms of Lithium Toxicity**	**Interventions**
1.5–2 mEq/L	Nausea and vomiting, diarrhea, reduced coordination, drowsiness, slurred speech, muscle weakness	Withhold next dose; call physician. Serum lithium levels are ordered and doses of lithium are usually suspended for a few days or the dose is reduced.
2–3 mEq/L	Ataxia, agitation, blurred vision, tinnitus, giddiness, choreoathetoid movements, confusion, muscle fasciculation, hyperreflexia, hypertonic muscles, myoclonic twitches, pruritus, maculopapular rash, movement of limbs, slurred speech, large output of dilute urine, incontinence of bladder or bowel, vertigo	Withhold future doses, call physician, stat serum lithium level. Gastric lavage may be used to remove oral lithium; IV containing saline and electrolytes used to ensure fluid and electrolyte function and maintain renal function.
3.0 and above	Cardiac arrhythmia, hypotension, peripheral vascular collapse, focal or generalized seizures, reduced levels of consciousness from stupor to coma, myoclonic jerks of muscle groups, and spasticity of muscles	All preceding interventions plus lithium ion excretion is augmented with use of aminophylline, mannitol, or urea. Hemodialysis may also be used to remove lithium from the body. Respiratory, circulatory, thyroid, and immune systems are monitored and assisted as needed.

also is contraindicated in people with brain or cardiovascular damage.

PROVIDING CLIENT AND FAMILY TEACHING

Educating clients about the dangers of risky behavior is necessary; however, clients with acute mania largely fail to heed such teaching because they have little patience or capacity to listen, understand, and see the relevance of this information. Clients with euphoria may not see why the behavior is a problem because they believe they can do anything without impunity. As they begin to cycle toward normalcy, however, risky behavior lessens, and clients become ready and able for teaching.

Manic clients start many tasks, create many goals, and try to carry them out all at once. The result is that they cannot complete any. They move readily between these goals while sometimes obsessing about the importance of one over another, but the goals can quickly change. Clients may invest in a business in which they have no knowledge or experience, go on spending sprees, impulsively travel, speed, make new "best friends," and take the center of attention in any group. They are egocentric and have little concern for others except as listeners, sexual partners, or the means to achieve one of their poorly conceived goals.

Education about the cause of bipolar disorder, medication management, ways to deal with behaviors, and potential problems that manic people can encounter is important for family members. Education reduces the guilt, blame, and shame that accompany mental illness; increases client safety; enlarges the support system for clients and the family members; and promotes compliance. Education takes the

"mystery" out of treatment for mental illness by providing a proactive view: this is what we know, this is what can be done, and this is what you can do to help.

Family members often say they know clients have stopped taking their medication when, for example, clients become more argumentative, talk about buying expensive items that they cannot afford, hotly deny anything is wrong, or demonstrate any other signs of escalating mania. People sometimes need permission to act on their observations, so a family education session is an appropriate place to give this permission and to set up interventions for various behaviors.

Clients should learn to adhere to the established dosage of lithium and not to omit doses or change dosage intervals; unprescribed dosage alterations interfere with maintenance of serum lithium levels. Clients should know about the many drugs that interact with lithium and should tell each physician they consult that they are taking lithium. When a client taking lithium seems to have increased manic behavior, lithium levels should be checked to determine whether there is lithium toxicity. Periodic monitoring of serum lithium levels is necessary to ensure the safety and adequacy of the treatment regimen. Persistent thirst and diluted urine can indicate the need to call a physician and have the serum lithium level checked to see if the dosage needs to be reduced.

Clients and family members should know the symptoms of lithium toxicity and interventions to take, including backup plans if the physician is not immediately available. The nurse should give these in writing and explain them to clients and family.

Evaluation

Evaluation of the treatment of bipolar disorder includes but is not limited to the following:

- Safety issues
- Comparison of mood and affect between start of treatment and present
- Adherence to treatment regimen of medication and psychotherapy
- Changes in client's perception of quality of life
- Achievement of specific goals of treatment including new coping methods

SUICIDE

Suicide is the intentional act of killing oneself. Suicidal thoughts are common in people with mood disorders, especially depression. Each year, more than 30,000 suicides are reported in the United States; suicide attempts are estimated to be 8 to 10 times higher. In the United States, men commit approximately 72% of suicides, which is roughly three times the rate of women, although women are four times more likely than men to attempt suicide. The higher suicide rates for men are partly the result of the method chosen (e.g., shooting, hanging, jumping from a high place). Women are more likely to overdose on medication. Men, young women, whites, and separated and divorced people are at increased risk for suicide. Adults older than age 65 years compose 10% of the population but account for 25% of suicides. Suicide is the second leading cause of death (after accidents) among people 15 to 24 years of age, and the rate of suicide is increasing most rapidly in this age group (Andreasen & Black, 2006).

Clients with psychiatric disorders, especially depression, bipolar disorder, schizophrenia, substance abuse, posttraumatic stress disorder, and borderline personality disorder, are at increased risk for suicide (Rihmer, 2007). Chronic medical illnesses associated with increased risk for suicide include cancer, HIV or AIDS, diabetes, cerebrovascular accidents, and head and spinal cord injury. Environmental factors that increase suicide risk include isolation, recent loss, lack of social support, unemployment, critical life events, and family history of depression or suicide. Behavioral factors that increase risk include impulsivity, erratic or unexplained changes from usual behavior, and unstable lifestyle (Swann et al., 2005; Valente & Saunders, 2005).

Suicidal ideation means thinking about killing oneself. Active suicidal ideation is when a person thinks about and seeks ways to commit suicide. Passive suicidal ideation is when a person thinks about wanting to die or wishes he or she were dead but has no plans to cause his or her death. People with active suicidal ideation are considered more potentially lethal.

Attempted suicide is a suicidal act that either failed or was incomplete. In an incomplete suicide attempt, the person did not finish the act because (1) someone recognized the suicide attempt as a cry for help and responded or (2) the person was discovered and rescued (Sudak, 2005).

Suicide involves ambivalence. Many fatal accidents may be impulsive suicides. It is impossible to know, for example, whether the person who drove into a telephone pole did this intentionally. Hence, keeping accurate statistics on suicide is difficult. There are also many myths and misconceptions about suicide of which the nurse should be aware. The nurse must know the facts and warning signs for those at risk for suicide as described in Box 15.2.

Assessment

A history of previous suicide attempts increases risk for suicide. The first 2 years after an attempt represent the highest risk period, especially the first 3 months. Those with a relative who committed suicide are at increased risk for suicide: the closer the relationship, the greater the risk. One possible explanation is that the relative's suicide offers a sense of "permission" or acceptance of suicide as a method of escaping a difficult situation. This familiarity and acceptance also is believed to contribute to "copycat suicides" by teenagers, who are greatly influenced by their peers' actions (Sudak, 2005).

Many people with depression who have suicidal ideation lack the energy to implement suicide plans. The natural energy that accompanies increased sunlight in spring is believed to explain why most suicides occur in April. Most suicides happen on Monday mornings, when most people return to work (another energy spurt). Research has shown that antidepressant treatment actually can give clients with depression the energy to act on suicidal ideation (Sudak, 2005).

CLIENT/FAMILY EDUCATION FOR MANIA

- Teach about bipolar illness and ways to manage the disorder.
- Teach about medication management, including the need for periodic blood work and management of side effects.
- For clients taking lithium, teach about the need for adequate salt and fluid intake.
- Teach the client and family about signs of toxicity and the need to seek medical attention immediately.
- Educate the client and family about risk-taking behavior and how to avoid it.
- Teach about behavioral signs of relapse and how to seek treatment in early stages.

Box 15.2   MYTHS AND FACTS ABOUT SUICIDE

Myths	Facts
People who talk about suicide never commit suicide.	Suicidal people often send out subtle or not-so-subtle messages that convey their inner thoughts of hopelessness and self-destruction. Both subtle and direct messages of suicide should be taken seriously with appropriate assessments and interventions.
Suicidal people only want to hurt themselves, not others.	Although the self-violence of suicide demonstrates anger turned inward, the anger can be directed toward others in a planned or impulsive action. *Physical harm:* Psychotic people may be responding to inner voices that command the individual to kill others before killing the self. A depressed person who has decided to commit suicide with a gun may impulsively shoot the person who tries to grab the gun in an effort to thwart the suicide. *Emotional harm:* Often, family members, friends, health care professionals, and even police involved in trying to avert a suicide or those who did not realize the person's depression and plans to commit suicide feel intense guilt and shame because of their failure to help and are "stuck" in a never-ending cycle of despair and grief. Some people, depressed after the suicide of a loved one, will rationalize that suicide was a "good way out of the pain" and plan their own suicide to escape pain. Some suicides are planned to engender guilt and pain in survivors; for example, as someone who wants to punish another for rejecting or not returning love.
There is no way to help someone who wants to kill himself or herself.	Suicidal people have mixed feelings (ambivalence) about their wish to die, wish to kill others, or to be killed. This ambivalence often prompts the cries for help evident in overt or covert cues. Intervention can help the suicidal individual get help from situational supports, choose to live, learn new ways to cope, and move forward in life.
Do not mention the word *suicide* to a person you suspect to be suicidal, because this could give him or her the idea to commit suicide.	Suicidal people have already thought of the idea of suicide and may have begun plans. Asking about suicide does not cause a nonsuicidal person to become suicidal.
Ignoring verbal threats of suicide or challenging a person to carry out his or her suicide plans will reduce the individual's use of these behaviors.	Suicidal gestures are a potentially lethal way to act out. Threats should not be ignored or dismissed, nor should a person be challenged to carry out suicidal threats. All plans, threats, gestures, or cues should be taken seriously and immediate help given that focuses on the problem about which the person is suicidal. When asked about suicide, it is often a relief for the client to know that his or her cries for help have been heard and that help is on the way.
Once a suicide risk, always a suicide risk.	Although it is true that most people who successfully commit suicide have made attempts at least once before, most people with suicidal ideation can have positive resolution to the suicidal crisis. With proper support, finding new ways to resolve the problem helps these individuals become emotionally secure and have no further need for suicide as a way to resolve a problem.

WARNINGS OF SUICIDAL INTENT

Most people with suicidal ideation send either direct or indirect signals to others about their intent to harm themselves. The nurse *never* ignores any hint of suicidal ideation regardless of how trivial or subtle it seems and the client's intent or emotional status. Often, people contemplating suicide have ambivalent and conflicting feelings about their desire to die; they frequently reach out to others for help. For example, a client might say,

"I keep thinking about taking my entire supply of medications to end it all" (direct) or "I just can't take it anymore" (indirect).

Box 15.3 provides more examples of client statements about suicide and effective responses from the nurse.

Asking clients directly about thoughts of suicide is important. Psychiatric admission assessment interview forms routinely include such questions. It is also standard practice to inquire about suicide or self-harm thoughts in any setting where people seek treatment for emotional problems.

RISKY BEHAVIORS

A few people who commit suicide give no warning signs. Some artfully hide their distress and suicide plans. Others act impulsively by taking advantage of a situation to carry out the desire to die. Some suicidal people in treatment describe placing themselves in risky or dangerous situations such as speeding in a blinding rainstorm or when intoxicated. This "Russian roulette" approach carries a high risk for harm to clients and innocent bystanders alike. It allows

---

Box 15.3   SUICIDAL IDEATION: CLIENT STATEMENTS AND NURSE RESPONSES

Client Statement	Nurse Responses
"I just want to go to sleep and not think anymore."	"Specifically just how are you planning to sleep and not think anymore?" "By 'sleep,' do you mean 'die'?" "What is it you do not want to think of anymore?"
"I want it to be all over."	"I wonder if you are thinking of suicide." "What is it you specifically want to be over?"
"It will just be the end of the story."	"Are you planning to end your life?" "How do you plan to end your story?"
"You have been a good friend." "Remember me."	"You sound as if you are saying good-bye. Are you?" "Are you planning to commit suicide?" "What is it you really want me to remember about you?"
"Here is my chess set that you have always admired."	"What is going on that you are giving away things to remember you by?"
"If there is ever any need for anyone to know this, my will and insurance papers are in the top drawer of my dresser."	"I appreciate your trust. However, I think there is an important message you are giving me. Are you thinking of ending your life?"
"I can't stand the pain anymore."	"How do you plan to end the pain?" "Tell me about the pain." "Sounds like you are planning to harm yourself."
"Everyone will feel bad soon." "I just can't bear it anymore."	"Who is the person you want to feel bad by killing yourself?" "What is it you cannot bear?" "How do you see an end to this?"
"Everyone would be better off without me."	"Who is one person you believe would be better off without you?" "How do you plan to eliminate yourself, if you think everyone would be better off without you?" "What is one way you perceive others would be better off without you?"
Nonverbal change in behavior from agitated to calm, anxious to relaxed, depressed to smiling, hostile to benign, from being without direction to appearing to be goal-directed	"You seem different today. What is this about?" "I sense you have reached a decision. Share it with me."

Drug Alert!

Antidepressants and Suicide Risk

Depressed clients who begin taking an antidepressant may have a continued or increased risk for suicide in the first few weeks of therapy. They may experience an increase in energy from the antidepressant but remain depressed. This increase in energy may make clients more likely to act on suicidal ideas and able to carry them out. Also, because antidepressants take several weeks to reach their peak effect, clients may become discouraged and act on suicidal ideas because they believe the medication is not helping them. For these reasons, it is extremely important to monitor the suicidal ideation of depressed clients until the risk has subsided.

clients to feel brave by repeatedly confronting death and surviving.

LETHALITY ASSESSMENT

When a client admits to having a "death wish" or suicidal thoughts, the next step is to determine potential lethality. This assessment involves asking the following questions:

- Does the client have a plan? If so, what is it? Is the plan specific?
- Are the means available to carry out this plan? (For example, if the person plans to shoot himself, does he have access to a gun and ammunition?)
- If the client carries out the plan, is it likely to be lethal? (For example, a plan to take 10 aspirin is not lethal; a plan to take a 2-week supply of a tricyclic antidepressant is.)
- Has the client made preparations for death, such as giving away prized possessions, writing a suicide note, or talking to friends one last time?
- Where and when does the client intend to carry out the plan?
- Is the intended time a special date or anniversary that has meaning for the client?

Specific and positive answers to these questions all increase the client's likelihood of committing suicide. It is important to consider whether or not the client believes her or his method is lethal even if it is not. Believing a method to be lethal poses a significant risk.

Outcome Identification

Suicide prevention usually involves treating the underlying disorder, such as mood disorder or psychosis, with psychoactive agents. The overall goals are first to keep the client safe and later to help him or her to develop new coping skills that do not involve self-harm. Other outcomes may relate to activities of daily living, sleep and nourishment needs, and problems specific to the crisis such as stabilization of psychiatric illness/symptoms.

Examples of outcomes for a suicidal person include the following:

- The client will be safe from harming self or others.
- The client will engage in a therapeutic relationship.
- The client will establish a no-suicide contract.
- The client will create a list of positive attributes.
- The client will generate, test, and evaluate realistic plans to address underlying issues.

Intervention

USING AN AUTHORITATIVE ROLE

Intervention for suicide or suicidal ideation becomes the first priority of nursing care. The nurse assumes an authoritative role to help clients stay safe. In this crisis situation, clients see few or no alternatives to resolve their problems. The nurse lets clients know their safety is the primary concern and takes precedence over other needs or wishes. For example, a client may want to be alone in her room to think privately. This is not allowed while she is at increased risk for suicide.

PROVIDING A SAFE ENVIRONMENT

Inpatient hospital units have policies for general environmental safety. Some policies are more liberal than others, but all usually deny clients access to materials on cleaning carts, their own medications, sharp scissors, and penknives. For suicidal clients, staff members remove any item they can use to commit suicide, such as sharp objects, shoelaces, belts, lighters, matches, pencils, pens, and even clothing with drawstrings.

Again, institutional policies for suicide precautions vary, but usually staff members observe clients every 10 minutes if lethality is low. For clients with high potential lethality, one-to-one supervision by a staff person is initiated. This means that clients are in direct sight of and no more than 2 to 3 feet away from a staff member for all activities, including going to the bathroom. Clients are under constant staff observation with no exceptions. This may be frustrating or upsetting to clients, so staff members usually need to explain the purpose of such supervision more than once.

INITIATING A NO-SUICIDE CONTRACT

The nurse can implement a no-suicide contract at home as well as in the inpatient treatment setting. In such contracts, clients agree to keep themselves safe and to notify staff at the first impulse to harm themselves (at home, clients agree to notify their caregivers; the contract must identify backup people in case caregivers are unavailable). The urge to commit suicide may return suddenly, so someone must always be available for support. A list of support people who agree to be readily available should be generated.

Most suicidal people adhere to no-suicide contracts because they appeal to the will to live. These contracts, however, are not a guarantee of safety. Farrow and O'Brien (2003) questioned whether a suicidal person is able to give informed consent to enter into such a contract. Potter and associates (2005) reported that contracts do not prevent self-harm behaviors, but they may assist the nurse in client assessment, and promote interaction about safety issues. At no time should a nurse assume that a client is safe just because a contract is in place.

CREATING A SUPPORT SYSTEM LIST

Suicidal clients often lack social support systems such as relatives and friends or religious, occupational, and community support groups. This lack may result from social withdrawal, behavior associated with a psychiatric or medical disorder, or movement of the person to a new area because of school, work, or change in family structure or financial status. The nurse assesses support systems and the type of help each person or group can give a client. Mental health clinics, hotlines, psychiatric emergency evaluation services, student health services, church groups, and self-help groups are part of the community support system.

The nurse makes a list of specific names and agencies that clients can call for support; he or she obtains client consent to avoid breach of confidentiality. Many suicidal people do not have to be admitted to a hospital and can be treated successfully in the community with the help of these support people and agencies.

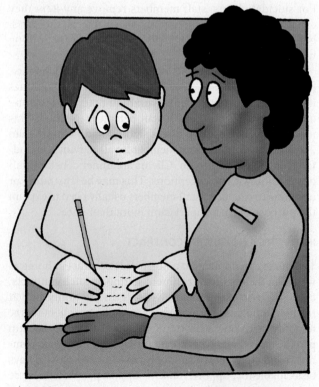

No-suicide contract

Family Response

Suicide is the ultimate rejection of family and friends. Implicit in the act of suicide is the message to others that their help was incompetent, irrelevant, or unwelcome. Some suicides are done to place blame on a certain person—even to the point of planning how that person will be the one to discover the body. Most suicides are efforts to escape untenable situations. Even if a person believes love for family members prompted his or her suicide—as in the case of someone who commits suicide to avoid lengthy legal battles or to save the family the financial and emotional cost of a lingering death—relatives still grieve and may feel guilt, shame, and anger.

Significant others may feel guilty for not knowing how desperate the suicidal person was, angry because the person did not seek their help or trust them, ashamed that their loved one ended his or her life with a socially unacceptable act, and sad about being rejected. Suicide is newsworthy, and there may be whispered gossip and even news coverage. Life insurance companies may not pay survivors' benefits to families of those who kill themselves. Also, the one death may spark "copycat suicides" among family members or others, who may believe they have been given permission to do the same. Families can disintegrate after a suicide.

Nurse's Response

When dealing with a client who has suicidal ideation or attempts, the nurse's attitude must indicate unconditional positive regard not for the act but for the person and his or her desperation. The ideas or attempts are serious signals of a desperate emotional state. The nurse must convey the belief that the person can be helped and can grow and change.

Trying to make clients feel guilty for thinking of or attempting suicide is not helpful; they already feel incompetent, hopeless, and helpless. The nurse does not blame clients or act judgmentally when asking about the details of a planned suicide. Rather, the nurse uses a nonjudgmental tone of voice and monitors his or her body language and facial expressions to make sure not to convey disgust or blame.

Nurses believe that one person can make a difference in another's life. They must convey this belief when caring for suicidal people. Nevertheless, nurses also must realize that no matter how competent and caring interventions are, a few clients will still commit suicide. A client's suicide can be devastating to the staff members who treated him or her, especially if they have gotten to know the person and his or her family well over time. Even with therapy, staff members may end up leaving the health care facility or the profession as a result.

Legal and Ethical Considerations

Assisted suicide is a topic of national legal and ethical debate, with much attention focusing on the court decisions related to the actions of Dr. Jack Kevorkian, a physician who has participated in numerous assisted suicides. Oregon was the first state to adopt assisted suicide into law and has set up safeguards to prevent indiscriminate assisted suicide. Many people believe it should be legal in any state for health care professionals or family to assist those who are terminally ill and want to die. Others view suicide as against the laws of humanity and religion and believe that health care professionals should be prosecuted if they assist those trying to die. Groups such as the Hemlock Society and people such as Dr. Kevorkian are lobbying for changes in laws that would allow health care professionals and family members to assist with suicide attempts for the terminally ill. Controversy and emotion continue to surround the issue.

Often, nurses must care for terminally or chronically ill people with a poor quality of life, such as those with the intractable pain of terminal cancer or severe disability or those kept alive by life-support systems. It is not the nurse's role to decide how long these clients must suffer. It is the nurse's role to provide supportive care for clients and family as they work through the difficult emotional decisions about if and when these clients should be allowed to die; people who have been declared legally dead can be disconnected from life support. Each state has defined legal death and the ways to determine it.

ELDER CONSIDERATIONS

Alexopoulos (2004) reported that depression is common among the elderly and is markedly increased when elders are medically ill. Elders tend to have psychotic features, particularly delusions, more frequently than younger people with depression. Suicide among persons older than age 65 is doubled compared with suicide rates of persons younger than 65. Late-onset bipolar disorder is rare.

Elders are treated for depression with ECT more frequently than younger persons. Elder persons have increased intolerance of side effects of antidepressant medications and may not be able to tolerate doses high enough to effectively treat the depression. Also, ECT produces a more rapid response than medications, which may be desirable if the depression is compromising the medical health of the elder person. Because suicide among the elderly is increased, the most rapid response to treatment becomes even more important (Kellner et al., 2004).

COMMUNITY-BASED CARE

Nurses in any area of practice in the community frequently are the first health care professionals to recognize behaviors consistent with mood disorders. In some cases, a family member may mention distress about a client's withdrawal from activities; difficulty thinking, eating, and sleeping; complaints of being tired all the time; sadness; and agitation (all symptoms of depression). They might also mention cycles of euphoria, spending binges, loss of inhibitions, changes in sleep and eating patterns, and loud clothing styles and colors (all symptoms of the manic phase of bipolar disorder). Documenting and reporting such behaviors can help these people to receive treatment. Estimates are that nearly 40% of people who have been diagnosed with a mood disorder do not receive treatment (Akiskal, 2005). Contributing factors may include the stigma still associated with mental disorders, the lack of understanding about the disruption to life that mood disorders can cause, confusion about treatment choices, or a more compelling medical diagnosis; these combine with the reality of limited time that health care professionals devote to any one client.

People with depression can be treated successfully in the community by psychiatrists, psychiatric advanced practice nurses, and primary care physicians. People with bipolar disorder, however, should be referred to a psychiatrist or psychiatric advanced practice nurse for treatment. The physician or nurse who treats a person with bipolar disorder must understand the drug treatment, dosages, desired effects, therapeutic levels, and potential side effects so that he or she can answer questions and promote compliance with treatment.

MENTAL HEALTH PROMOTION

Many studies have been conducted to determine how to prevent mood disorders and suicide, but prediction of suicide risk in clinical practice remains difficult (Carter et al., 2005). Programs that use an educational approach designed to address the unique stressors that contribute to the increased incidence of depressive illness in women have had some success. These programs focus on increasing self-esteem and reducing loneliness and hopelessness, which in turn decrease the likelihood of depression.

Efforts to improve primary care treatment of depression have built upon a chronic illness care model that includes patient self-management, or helping people be better prepared to deal with life issues and changes. This includes having a partnership with their provider, having a crisis or relapse prevention plan, creating a social support network, and making needed behavioral changes to promote health (Bachman et al., 2006).

Because suicide is a leading cause of death among adolescents, prevention, early detection, and treatment are very important. Strengthening protective factors (those factors associated with a reduction in suicide risk) would improve the mental health of adolescents. Protective factors include close parent–child relationships, academic achievement, family-life stability, and connectedness with peers and others outside the family. School-based programs can be universal (general information for all students) or indicated (targeting young people at risk). Indicated or selective programs have been more successful than universal programs (Horowitz & Garber, 2006; Rapee et al., 2006). Likewise, screening for early detection of risk factors such as family strife, parental alcoholism or mental illness, history of fighting, and access to weapons in the home can lead to referral and early intervention.

SELF-AWARENESS ISSUES

Nurses working with clients who are depressed often empathize with them and also begin to feel sad or agitated. They may unconsciously start to avoid contact with these clients to escape such feelings. The nurse must monitor his or her feelings and reactions closely when dealing with clients with depression to be sure he or she fulfills the responsibility to establish a therapeutic nurse–client relationship.

People with depression are usually negative, pessimistic, and unable to generate new ideas easily. They feel hopeless and incompetent. The nurse easily can become consumed with suggesting ways to fix the problems. Most clients find some reason why the nurse's solutions will not work: "I have tried that," "It would never work," "I don't have the time to do that," or "You just don't understand." Rejection of suggestions can make the nurse feel incompetent and question his or her professional skill. Unless a client is suicidal or is experiencing a crisis, the nurse does not try to solve the client's problems. Instead, the nurse uses therapeutic techniques to encourage clients to generate their own solutions. Studies have shown that clients tend to act on plans or solutions they generate rather than those that others offer (Schultz & Videbeck, 2005). Finding and acting on their own solutions gives clients renewed competence and self-worth.

Working with clients who are manic can be exhausting. They are so hyperactive that the nurse may feel spent or tired after caring for them. The nurse may feel frustrated because these clients engage in the same behaviors repeatedly, such as being intrusive with others, undressing, singing, rhyming, and dancing. It takes hard work to remain patient and calm with the manic client, but it is essential for the nurse to provide limits and redirection in a calm manner until the client can control his or her own behavior independently.

Some health care professionals consider suicidal people to be failures, immoral, or unworthy of care. These negative attitudes may result from several factors. They may reflect society's negative view of suicide: many states still have laws against suicide, although they rarely enforce these laws. Health care professionals may feel inadequate and anxious dealing with suicidal clients, or they may be uncomfortable about their own mortality. Many people have had thoughts about "ending it all," even if for a fleeting moment when life is not going well. The scariness of remembering such flirtations with suicide causes anxiety. If this anxiety is not resolved, the staff person can demonstrate avoidance, demeaning behavior, and superiority to suicidal clients. Therefore, to be effective, the nurse must be aware of his or her own feelings and beliefs about suicide.

Points to Consider When Working With Clients With Mood Disorders

- Remember that clients with mania may seem happy, but they are suffering inside.
- For clients with mania, delay client teaching until the acute manic phase is resolving.
- Schedule specific, short periods with depressed or agitated clients to eliminate unconscious avoidance of them.
- Do not try to fix a client's problems. Use therapeutic techniques to help him or her find solutions.
- Use a journal to deal with frustration, anger, or personal needs.
- If a particular client's care is troubling, talk with another professional about the plan of care, how it is being carried out, and how it is working.

Critical Thinking Questions

1. Is it possible for someone to make a "rational" decision to commit suicide? Under what circumstances?
2. Are laws ethical that permit physician-assisted suicide? Why or why not?
3. A person with bipolar disorder frequently discontinues taking medication when out of the hospital, becomes manic, and engages in risky behavior such as speeding, drinking and driving, and incurring large debts. How do you reconcile the client's right to refuse medication with public or personal safety? Who should make such a decision? How could it be enforced?

KEY POINTS

- Studies have found a genetic component to mood disorders. The incidence of depression is up to three times greater in first-degree relatives of people with diagnosed depression. People with bipolar disorder usually have a blood relative with bipolar disorder.
- Only 9% of people with mood disorders exhibit psychosis.
- Major depression is a mood disorder that robs the person of joy, self-esteem, and energy. It interferes with relationships and occupational productivity.
- Symptoms of depression include sadness, disinterest in previously pleasurable activities, crying, lack of motivation, asocial behavior, and psychomotor retardation (slowed thinking, talking, and movement). Sleep disturbances, somatic complaints, loss of energy, change in weight, and a sense of worthlessness are other common features.
- Several antidepressants are used to treat depression. SSRIs, the newest type, have the fewest side effects. Tricyclic antidepressants are older and have a longer

INTERNET RESOURCES

RESOURCE	INTERNET ADDRESS
• American Association of Suicidology	http://www.suicidology.org
• Centre for Suicide Prevention	http://www.siec.ca
• Depression Information and Support	http://www.depression.about.com
• Depression Issues	http://www.bipolardepressioninfo.com
• National Institute of Mental Health Suicide Research Consortium	http://www.depressionissues.com
• Postpartum Depression Screening Quiz	http://www.nih.gov/research/suicide.htm
• SAD Association	http://babyparenting.about.com/b/a/132722.htm

lag period before reaching adequate serum levels; they are the least expensive type. MAOIs are used least: Clients are at risk for hypertensive crisis if they ingest tyramine-rich foods and fluids while taking these drugs. MAOIs also have a lag period before reaching adequate serum levels.

• People with bipolar disorder cycle between mania, normalcy, and depression. They also may cycle only between mania and normalcy or between depression and normalcy.

• Clients with mania have a labile mood, are grandiose and manipulative, have high self-esteem, and believe they are capable of anything. They sleep little, are always in frantic motion, invade others' boundaries, cannot sit still, and start many tasks. Speech is rapid and pressured, reflects rapid thinking, and may be circumstantial and tangential with features of rhyming, punning, and flight of ideas. Clients show poor judgment with little sense of safety needs and take physical, financial, occupational, or interpersonal risks.

• Lithium is used to treat bipolar disorder. It is helpful for bipolar mania and can partially or completely eradicate cycling toward bipolar depression. Lithium is effective in 75% of clients but has a narrow range of safety; thus, ongoing monitoring of serum lithium levels is necessary to establish efficacy while preventing toxicity. Clients taking lithium must ingest adequate salt and water to avoid overdosing or underdosing because lithium salt uses the same postsynaptic receptor sites as sodium chloride does. Other antimanic drugs include sodium valproate, carbamazepine, other anticonvulsants, and clonazepam, which is also a benzodiazepine.

• For clients with mania, the nurse must monitor food and fluid intake, rest and sleep, and behavior, with a focus on safety, until medications reduce the acute stage and clients resume responsibility for themselves.

• Suicidal ideation means thinking of suicide.

• People with increased rates of suicide include single adults, divorced men, adolescents, older adults, the very poor or very wealthy, urban dwellers, migrants, students, whites, people with mood disorders, substance abusers, people with medical or personality disorders, and people with psychosis.

• The nurse must be alert to clues to a client's suicidal intent—both direct (making threats of suicide) and indirect (giving away prized possessions, putting his or her life in order, making vague good-byes).

• Conducting a suicide lethality assessment involves determining the degree to which the person has planned his or her death, including time, method, tools, place, person to find the body, reason, and funeral plans.

• Nursing interventions for a client at risk for suicide involve keeping the person safe by instituting a no-suicide contract, ensuring close supervision, and removing objects that the person could use to commit suicide.

REFERENCES

Akiskal, H. S. (2005). Mood disorders: Historical introduction and conceptual overview. In B. J. Sadock & V. A. Sadock (Eds.), *Comprehensive textbook of psychiatry* (Vol. 1, 8th ed., 1559–1575). Philadelphia: Lippincott Williams & Wilkins.

Alexopoulos, G. S. (2004). Late-life mood disorders. In J. Sadavoy, L. F. Jarvik, G. T. Grossberg, et al. (Eds.), *Comprehensive textbook of geriatric psychiatry* (3rd ed., pp. 609–653). New York: W. W. Norton and Company.

American Psychiatric Association. (2000). *Diagnostic and statistical manual of mental disorders* (4th ed., text revision). Washington, DC: American Psychiatric Association.

Andreasen, N. C., & Black, D. W. (2006) *Introductory textbook of psychiatry* (4th ed.). Washington DC: American Psychiatric Publishing.

Andrews, M. M., & Boyle, J. S. (2003). *Transcultural concepts in nursing care* (4th ed.). Philadelphia: Lippincott Williams & Wilkins.

Bachman, J, Swensen, S, Reardon, M. E., & Miller, D. (2006). Patient self-management in the primary care treatment of depression. *Administration and Policy in Mental Health, 33*(1), 76–85.

Bowden, C. L. (2006). Valproate. In A. F Schatzberg & Nemeroff, C. B (Eds.), *Essentials of clinical pharmacology* (2nd ed., pp 355–366). Washington DC: American Psychiatric Publishing.

Carter, G., Reith, D. M., Whyte, I. M., & McPherson, M. (2005). Repeated self-poisoning: Increasing severity of self-harm as a predictor of subsequent suicide. *British Journal of Psychiatry, 186*, 253–257.

Eitan, R., & Lerer, B. (2006). Nonpharmacological, somatic treatments of depression: Electroconvulsive therapy and novel brain stimulation modalities. *Dialogues in Clinical Neuroscience, 8*(2), 241–258.

Facts and Comparisons. (2007). *Drug facts and comparisons* (61st ed.). St. Louis: Facts and Comparisons: A Wolters Kluwer Company.

Fallow, T. L., & O'Brien, A. J. (2003). No-suicide contracting in psychiatric inpatient settings. *Archives of Psychiatric Nursing, 15*(3), 99–106.

Fenton, L., Fasula, M., Ostroff, R., & Sanacora, G. (2006). Can cognitive behavioral therapy reduce relapse rates of depression after ECT? A preliminary study. *Journal of ECT, 22*(3), 196–198.

Frederikse, M., Petrides, G., & Kellner, C. (2006). Continuation and maintenance electroconvulsive therapy for the treatment of depressive illness: A response to the National Institute for Clinical Excellence report. (2006). *Journal of ECT, 22*(1), 13–17.

Freeman, M. P., Wiegand, C., & Gelenberg, A. J. (2006). Lithium. In A. F. Schatzberg & Nemeroff, C. B. (Eds.), *Essentials of clinical pharmacology* (2nd ed., pp. 335–354). Washington DC: American Psychiatric Publishing.

Horowitz, J. L., & Garber, J. (2006). The prevention of depressive symptoms in children and adolescents: A meta-analytic review. *Journal of Consulting and Clinical Psychology, 74*(3), 401–415.

Kellner, C. H., Coffey, C. E., & Greenberg, R. M. (2004). Electroconvulsive therapy. In J. Sadavoy, L. F. Jarvik, G. T. Grossberg, et al. (Eds.), *Comprehensive textbook of geriatric psychiatry* (3rd ed., pp. 845–901). New York: W. W. Norton and Company.

Kellner, C. H., Knapp, R. G., Petrides, G., et al. (2006). Continuation electroconvulsive therapy vs pharmacotherapy for relapse prevention in major depression: A multisite study from the consortium for research in electroconvulsive therapy (CORE). *Archives of General Psychiatry, 63*(12), 1337–1344.

Kelsoe, J. R. (2005). Mood disorders: Genetics. In B. J. Sadock & V. A. Sadock (Eds.), *Comprehensive textbook of psychiatry* (Vol. 1, 8th ed., pp. 1582–1594). Philadelphia: Lippincott Williams & Wilkins.

Ketter, T. A., Wang, P. W., & Post, R. M. (2006). Carbamazepine and oxcarbazepine. In A. F. Schatzberg & Nemeroff, C. B. (Eds.). *Essentials of clinical pharmacology* (2nd ed., pp 367–393). Washington DC: American Psychiatric Publishing.

Lurie, S. J., Gawinski, B., Pierce, D., & Rousseau, S. J. Seasonal affective disorder. *American Family Physician, 74*(9), 1521–1524.

Markowitz, J. C., & Milrod, B. (2005). Mood disorders: Intrapsychic and interpersonal aspects. In B. J. Sadock & V. A. Sadock (Eds.), *Comprehensive textbook of psychiatry* (Vol. 1, 8th ed., pp. 1603–1611). Philadelphia: Lippincott Williams & Wilkins.

Potter, M. L., Vitale-Nolen, R., & Dawson, A. M. (2005). Implementation of safety agreements in an acute psychiatric facility. *Journal of the American Psychiatric Nurses Association, 11*(3), 144–155.

Rapee, R. M., Wignall, A., Sheffield, J., et al. (2006). Adolescents' reactions to universal and indicated prevention programs for depression: Perceived stigma and consumer satisfaction. *Prevention Science, 7*(2), 167–177.

Rihmer, Z. (2007). Suicide risk in mood disorders. *Current Opinion in Psychiatry, 20*(1), 17–22.

Rihmer, Z., & Angst, J. (2005). Mood disorders: Epidemiology. In B. J. Sadock & V. A. Sadock (Eds.), *Comprehensive textbook of psychiatry* (Vol. 1, 8th ed., pp. 1575–1582). Philadelphia: Lippincott Williams & Wilkins.

Ross, C. A. (2006). The sham ECT literature: Implications for consent to ECT. *Ethical Human Psychology and Psychiatry, 8*(1), 17–28.

Rush, A. J. (2005). Mood disorders: Treatment of depression. In B. J. Sadock & V. A. Sadock (Eds.), *Comprehensive textbook of psychiatry* (Vol. 1, 8th ed., pp. 1652–1661). Philadelphia: Lippincott Williams & Wilkins.

Schultz, J. M., & Videbeck, S. (2005). *Lippincott's manual of psychiatric nursing care plans* (7th ed.). Philadelphia: Lippincott Williams & Wilkins.

Sit, D., Rothschild, A. J., & Wisner, K. L. (2006). A review of postpartum psychosis. *Journal of Women's Health, 15*(4), 352–368.

Sudak, H. S. (2005). Suicide. In B. J. Sadock & V. A. Sadock (Eds.), *Comprehensive textbook of psychiatry* (Vol. 2, 8th ed., pp. 2442–2453). Philadelphia: Lippincott Williams & Wilkins.

Swann, A. C., Dougherty, D. M., Pazzaglia, P. J., et al. (2005). Increased impulsivity associated with severity of suicide attempt history in patients with bipolar disorder. *American Journal of Psychiatry, 162*(9), 1680–1687.

Tecott, L. H., & Smart, S. L. (2005). Monoamine neurotransmitters. In B. J. Sadock & V. A. Sadock (Eds.), *Comprehensive textbook of psychiatry* (Vol. 1, 8th ed., pp. 49–60). Philadelphia: Lippincott Williams & Wilkins.

Thase, M. E. (2005). Mood disorders: Neurobiology. In B. J. Sadock & V. A. Sadock (Eds.), *Comprehensive textbook of psychiatry* (Vol. 1, 8th ed., pp. 1594–1603). Philadelphia: Lippincott Williams & Wilkins.

Valente, S. M., & Saunders, J. (2005). Screening for depression and suicide: Self-report instruments that work. *Journal of Psychosocial Nursing, 43*(11), 22–31.

ADDITIONAL READINGS

Crocker, L., Clare, L., & Evans, K. (2006). Giving up or finding a solution? The experience of attempted suicide in later life. *Aging & Mental Health, 10*(6), 638–647.

D'Augelli, A. R., Grossman, A. H., Saiter, N. P., et al. (2005). Predicting the suicide attempts of lesbian, gay, and bisexual youth. *Suicide & Life-threatening Behavior, 35*(6), 646–660.

Gorlyn, M. (2005). Impulsivity in the prediction of suicidal behavior in adolescent populations, *International Journal of Adolescent Medicine and Health, 17*(3), 205–209.

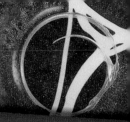

Chapter Study Guide

MULTIPLE-CHOICE QUESTIONS

Select the best answer for each of the following questions.

1. The nurse observes that a client with bipolar disorder is pacing in the hall, talking loudly and rapidly, and using elaborate hand gestures. The nurse concludes that the client is demonstrating which of the following?
   A. Aggression
   B. Anger
   C. Anxiety
   D. Psychomotor agitation

2. A client with bipolar disorder begins taking lithium carbonate (lithium), 300 mg four times a day. After 3 days of therapy, the client says, "My hands are shaking." The best response by the nurse is
   A. "Fine motor tremors are an early effect of lithium therapy that usually subsides in a few weeks."
   B. "It is nothing to worry about unless it continues for the next month."
   C. "Tremors can be an early sign of toxicity, but we'll keep monitoring your lithium level to make sure you're okay."
   D. "You can expect tremors with lithium. You seem very concerned about such a small tremor."

3. What are the most common types of side effects from SSRIs?
   A. Dizziness, drowsiness, dry mouth
   B. Convulsions, respiratory difficulties
   C. Diarrhea, weight gain
   D. Jaundice, agranulocytosis

4. The nurse observes that a client with depression sat at a table with two other clients during lunch. The best feedback the nurse could give the client is
   A. "Do you feel better after talking with others during lunch?"
   B. "I'm so happy to see you interacting with other clients."
   C. "I see you were sitting with others at lunch today."
   D. "You must feel much better than you were a few days ago."

5. Which of the following typifies the speech of a person in the acute phase of mania?
   A. Flight of ideas
   B. Psychomotor retardation
   C. Hesitant
   D. Mutism

6. What is the rationale for a person taking lithium to have enough water and salt in his or her diet?
   A. Salt and water are necessary to dilute lithium to avoid toxicity.
   B. Water and salt convert lithium into a usable solute.
   C. Lithium is metabolized in the liver, necessitating increased water and salt.
   D. Lithium is a salt that has greater affinity for receptor sites than sodium chloride.

7. Identify the serum lithium level for maintenance and safety.
   A. 0.1 to 1.0 mEq/L
   B. 0.5 to 1.5 mEq/L
   C. 10 to 50 mEq/L
   D. 50 to 100 mEq/L

8. A client says to the nurse, "You are the best nurse I've ever met. I want you to remember me." What is an appropriate response by the nurse?
   A. "Thank you. I think you are special too."
   B. "I suspect you want something from me. What is it?"
   C. "You probably say that to all your nurses."
   D. "Are you thinking of suicide?"

9. A client with mania begins dancing around the day room. When she twirled her skirt in front of the male clients, it was obvious she had no underpants on. The nurse distracts her and takes her to her room to put on underpants. The nurse acted as she did to
   A. Minimize the client's embarrassment about her present behavior.
   B. Keep her from dancing with other clients.
   C. Avoid embarrassing the male clients who are watching.
   D. Teach her about proper attire and hygiene.

SHORT-ANSWER QUESTIONS

1. Identify four areas that must be included in a patient teaching plan for a client starting lithium treatment.

2. Identify four client statements that might indicate a subtle message about suicidal ideation.

CLINICAL EXAMPLE

June, 46 years old, is divorced with three children: 10, 13, and 16 years of age. She works in the county clerk's office and has called in sick four times in the past 2 weeks. June has lost 17 pounds in the past 2 months, is spending a lot of time in bed, but still feels exhausted "all the time." During the admission interview, June looks overwhelmingly sad, is tearful, has her head down, and makes little eye contact. She answers the nurse's questions with one or two words. The nurse considers postponing the remainder of the interview because June seems unable to provide much information.

1. What assessment data are crucial for the nurse to obtain before ending the interview?

2. Identify three nursing diagnoses based on the available data.

3. Identify a short-term outcome for each of the nursing diagnoses.

4. Discuss nursing interventions that would be helpful for June.

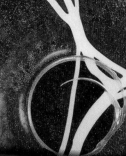

Chapter 16

Personality Disorders

Key Terms

- antisocial personality disorder
- avoidant personality disorder
- borderline personality disorder
- character
- cognitive restructuring
- confrontation
- decatastrophizing
- dependent personality disorder
- depressive personality disorder
- dysphoric
- histrionic personality disorder
- limit setting
- narcissistic personality disorder
- no-self-harm contract
- obsessive-compulsive personality disorder
- paranoid personality disorder
- passive-aggressive personality disorder
- personality
- personality disorders
- positive self-talk
- schizoid personality disorder
- schizotypal personality disorder
- temperament
- thought stopping
- time-out

Learning Objectives

After reading this chapter, you should be able to

1. Describe personality disorders in terms of the client's difficulty in perceiving, relating to, and thinking about self, others, and the environment.

2. Discuss factors thought to influence the development of personality disorders.

3. Apply the nursing process to the care of clients with personality disorders.

4. Provide education to clients, families, and community members to increase their knowledge and understanding of personality disorders.

5. Evaluate personal feelings, attitudes, and responses to clients with personality disorders.

Visit the Point http://thePoint.lww.com for NCLEX-style questions, journal articles, and more!

Personality can be defined as an ingrained enduring pattern of behaving and relating to self, others, and the environment; personality includes perceptions, attitudes, and emotions. These behaviors and characteristics are consistent across a broad range of situations and do not change easily. A person usually is not consciously aware of her or his personality. Many factors influence personality: some stem from biologic and genetic makeup, whereas some are acquired as a person develops and interacts with the environment and other people.

Personality disorders are diagnosed when personality traits become inflexible and maladaptive and significantly interfere with how a person functions in society or cause the person emotional distress. They usually are not diagnosed until adulthood, when personality is more completely formed. Nevertheless, maladaptive behavioral patterns often can be traced to early childhood or adolescence. Although there can be great variance among clients with personality disorders, many experience significant impairment in fulfilling family, academic, employment, and other functional roles.

Diagnosis is made when the person exhibits enduring behavioral patterns that deviate from cultural expectations in two or more of the following areas:

- Ways of perceiving and interpreting self, other people, and events (cognition)
- Range, intensity, lability, and appropriateness of emotional response (affect)
- Interpersonal functioning
- Ability to control impulses or express behavior at the appropriate time and place (impulse control)

Personality disorders are longstanding because personality characteristics do not change easily. Thus, clients with personality disorders continue to behave in their same familiar ways even when these behaviors cause them difficulties or distress. No specific medication alters personality, and therapy designed to help clients make changes is often long-term with very slow progress. Some people with personality disorders believe their problems stem from others or the world in general; they do not recognize their own behavior as the source of difficulty. For these reasons, people with personality disorders are difficult to treat, which may be frustrating for the nurse and other caregivers as well as family and friends. There are also difficulties in diagnosing and treating clients with personality disorders because of similarities and subtle differences between categories or types. Types often overlap, and many people with personality disorders also have coexisting mental illnesses.

CATEGORIES OF PERSONALITY DISORDERS

The *Diagnostic and Statistical Manual of Mental Disorders, 4th edition, Text Revision* (DSM-IV-TR; American Psychiatric Association [APA], 2000) lists personality disorders as a separate and distinct category from other major mental illnesses. They are on axis II of the multiaxial classification system (see Chapter 1). The *DSM-IV-TR* classifies personality disorders into "clusters," or categories, based on the predominant or identifying features (Box 16.1):

- Cluster A includes people whose behavior appears odd or eccentric and includes paranoid, schizoid, and schizotypal personality disorders.
- Cluster B includes people who appear dramatic, emotional, or erratic and includes antisocial, borderline, histrionic, and narcissistic personality disorders.
- Cluster C includes people who appear anxious or fearful and includes avoidant, dependent, and obsessive-compulsive personality disorders.

In psychiatric settings, nurses most often encounter clients with antisocial and borderline personality disorders. Thus, these two disorders are the primary focus of this chapter. Clients with antisocial personality disorder may enter a psychiatric setting as part of a court-ordered evaluation or as an alternative to jail. Clients with borderline personality disorder often are hospitalized because their emotional instability may lead to self-inflicted injuries.

This chapter discusses the other personality disorders briefly. Most clients with these disorders are not treated in acute care settings for these personality disorders. Nurses may encounter these clients in any health care setting or in the psychiatric setting when a client is already hospitalized for another major mental illness.

Two disorders currently being studied for inclusion as personality disorders are depressive and passive-aggressive

Box 16.1 DSM-IV-TR PERSONALITY DISORDER CATEGORIES

Cluster A: Individuals whose behavior appears odd or eccentric (paranoid, schizoid, and schizotypal personality disorders)
Cluster B: Individuals who appear dramatic, emotional, or erratic (antisocial, borderline, histrionic, and narcissistic personality disorders)
Cluster C: Individuals who appear anxious or fearful (avoidant, dependent, and obsessive-compulsive personality disorders)
Proposed personality disorder categories: depressive and passive-aggressive personality disorders

Adapted from American Psychiatric Association. (2000). DSM-IV-TR: Diagnostic and statistical manual of mental disorders (4th ed., text revision). Washington, DC: APA.

personality disorders, both of which are included in the *DSM-IV-TR*. This chapter discusses them briefly as well.

ONSET AND CLINICAL COURSE

Personality disorders are relatively common, occurring in 10% to 13% of the general population. Incidence is even higher for people in lower socioeconomic groups and unstable or disadvantaged populations. Fifteen percent of all psychiatric inpatients have a primary diagnosis of a personality disorder. Forty percent to 45% of those with a primary diagnosis of major mental illness also have a coexisting personality disorder that significantly complicates treatment. In mental health outpatient settings, the incidence of personality disorder is 30% to 50% (Svrakic & Cloninger, 2005). Clients with personality disorders have a higher death rate, especially as a result of suicide; they also have higher rates of suicide attempts, accidents, and emergency department visits and increased rates of separation, divorce, and involvement in legal proceedings regarding child custody (Svrakic & Cloninger, 2005). Personality disorders have been correlated highly with criminal behavior (70% to 85% of criminals have personality disorders), alcoholism (60% to 70% of alcoholics have personality disorders), and drug abuse (70% to 90% of those who abuse drugs have personality disorders; Svrakic & Cloninger, 2005).

People with personality disorders often are described as "treatment resistant." This is not surprising, considering that personality characteristics and behavioral patterns are deeply ingrained. It is difficult to change one's personality; if such changes occur, they evolve slowly. The slow course of treatment can be very frustrating for family, friends, and health care providers.

Another barrier to treatment is that many clients with personality disorders do not perceive their dysfunctional or maladaptive behaviors as a problem; indeed, sometimes these behaviors are a source of pride. For example, a belligerent or aggressive person may perceive himself or herself as having a strong personality and being someone who can't be taken advantage of or pushed around. Clients with personality disorders frequently fail to understand the need to change their behavior and may view changes as a threat.

The difficulties associated with personality disorders persist throughout young and middle adulthood but tend to diminish in the 40s and 50s. Those with antisocial personality disorder are less likely to engage in criminal behavior, although problems with substance abuse and disregard for the feelings of others persist. Clients with **borderline personality disorder** tend to demonstrate decreased impulsive behavior, increased adaptive behavior, and more stable relationships by 50 years of age. This increased stability and improved behavior can occur even without treatment. Some personality disorders, such as schizoid, schizotypal, paranoid, avoidant, and obsessive-compulsive, tend to remain consistent throughout life (Seivewright, Tyrer, & Johnson, 2002).

ETIOLOGY

Biologic Theories

Personality develops through the interaction of hereditary dispositions and environmental influences. **Temperament** refers to the biologic processes of sensation, association, and motivation that underlie the integration of skills and habits based on emotion. Genetic differences account for about 50% of the variances in temperament traits.

The four temperament traits are harm avoidance, novelty seeking, reward dependence, and persistence. Each of these four genetically influenced traits affects a person's automatic responses to certain situations. These response patterns are ingrained by 2 to 3 years of age (Svrakic & Cloninger, 2005).

People with high harm avoidance exhibit fear of uncertainty, social inhibition, shyness with strangers, rapid fatigability, and pessimistic worry in anticipation of problems. Those with low harm avoidance are carefree, energetic, outgoing, and optimistic. High harm-avoidance behaviors may result in maladaptive inhibition and excessive anxiety. Low harm-avoidance behaviors may result in unwarranted optimism and unresponsiveness to potential harm or danger.

A high novelty-seeking temperament results in someone who is quick-tempered, curious, easily bored, impulsive, extravagant, and disorderly. He or she may be easily bored and distracted with daily life, prone to angry outbursts, and fickle in relationships. The person low in novelty seeking is slow-tempered, stoic, reflective, frugal, reserved, orderly, and tolerant of monotony; he or she may adhere to a routine of activities.

Reward dependence defines how a person responds to social cues. People high in reward dependence are tenderhearted, sensitive, sociable, and socially dependent. They may become overly dependent on approval from others and readily assume the ideas or wishes of others without regard for their own beliefs or desires. People with low reward dependence are practical, tough-minded, cold, socially insensitive, irresolute, and indifferent to being alone. Social withdrawal, detachment, aloofness, and disinterest in others can result.

Highly persistent people are hardworking and ambitious overachievers who respond to fatigue or frustration as a personal challenge. They may persevere even when a situation dictates they should change or stop. People with low persistence are inactive, indolent, unstable, and erratic. They tend to give up easily when frustrated and rarely strive for higher accomplishments.

These four genetically independent temperament traits occur in all possible combinations. Some of the previous descriptions of high and low levels of traits correspond closely with the descriptions of the various personality disorders. For example, people with antisocial personality disorder are low in harm-avoidance traits and high in novelty-seeking traits, whereas people with dependent personality disorder are high in reward-dependence traits and harm-avoidance traits.

Psychodynamic Theories

Although temperament is largely inherited, social learning, culture, and random life events unique to each person influence character. **Character** consists of concepts about the self and the external world. It develops over time as a person comes into contact with people and situations and confronts challenges. Three major character traits have been distinguished: self-directedness, cooperativeness, and self-transcendence. When fully developed, these character traits define a mature personality (Svrakic & Cloninger, 2005).

Self-directedness is the extent to which a person is responsible, reliable, resourceful, goal oriented, and self-confident. Self-directed people are realistic and effective and can adapt their behavior to achieve goals. People low in self-directedness are blaming, helpless, irresponsible, and unreliable. They cannot set and pursue meaningful goals.

Cooperativeness refers to the extent to which a person sees himself or herself as an integral part of human society. Highly cooperative people are described as empathic, tolerant, compassionate, supportive, and principled. People with low cooperativeness are self-absorbed, intolerant, critical, unhelpful, revengeful, and opportunistic; that is, they look out for themselves without regard for the rights and feelings of others.

Self-transcendence describes the extent to which a person considers himself or herself to be an integral part of the universe. Self-transcendent people are spiritual, unpretentious, humble, and fulfilled. These traits are helpful when dealing with suffering, illness, or death. People low in self-transcendence are practical, self-conscious, materialistic, and controlling. They may have difficulty accepting suffering, loss of control, personal and material losses, and death.

Character matures in stepwise stages from infancy through late adulthood. Chapter 3 discusses psychological development according to Freud, Erikson, and others. Each stage has an associated developmental task that the person must perform for mature personality development. Failure to complete a developmental task jeopardizes the person's ability to achieve future developmental tasks. For example, if the task of basic trust is not achieved in infancy, mistrust results and subsequently interferes with achievement of all future tasks.

Experiences with family, peers, and others can significantly influence psychosocial development. Social education in the family creates an environment that can support or oppress specific character development. For example, a family environment that does not value and demonstrate cooperation with others (compassion, tolerance) fails to support the development of that trait in its children. Likewise, the person with nonsupportive or difficult peer relationships growing up may have lifelong difficulty relating to others and forming satisfactory relationships.

In summary, personality develops in response to inherited dispositions (temperament) and environmental influences (character), which are experiences unique to each person. Personality disorders result when the combination of temperament and character development produces maladaptive, inflexible ways of viewing self, coping with the world, and relating to others.

CULTURAL CONSIDERATIONS

Judgments about personality functioning must involve a consideration of the person's ethnic, cultural, and social background (APA, 2000). Members of minority groups, immigrants, political refugees, and people from different ethnic backgrounds may display guarded or defensive behavior as a result of language barriers or previous negative experiences; this should not be confused with paranoid personality disorder. People with religious or spiritual beliefs, such as clairvoyance, speaking in tongues, or evil spirits as a cause of disease, could be misinterpreted as having schizotypal personality disorder.

There is also a difference in how some cultural groups view avoidance or dependent behavior, particularly for women. An emphasis on deference, passivity, and politeness should not be confused with a dependent personality disorder. Cultures that value work and productivity may produce citizens with a strong emphasis in these areas; this should not be confused with obsessive-compulsive personality disorder.

Certain personality disorders—for example, antisocial and schizoid personality disorders—are diagnosed more often in men. Borderline and histrionic personality disorders are diagnosed more often in women. Social stereotypes about typical gender roles and behaviors can influence diagnostic decisions if clinicians are unaware of such biases.

TREATMENT

Several treatment strategies are used with clients with personality disorders; these strategies are based on the disorder's type and severity or the amount of distress or functional impairment the client experiences. Combinations of medication and group and individual therapies are more likely to be effective than is any single treatment (Svrakic & Cloninger, 2005). Not all people with personality disorders seek treatment, however, even when significant others urge them to do so. Typically, people with paranoid, schizoid, schizotypal, narcissistic, and passive-aggressive personality disorders are least likely to engage or remain in any treatment. They see other people, rather than their own behavior, as the cause of their problems.

Psychopharmacology

Pharmacologic treatment of clients with personality disorders focuses on the client's symptoms rather than the particular subtype. The four symptom categories that underlie personality disorders are cognitive-perceptual distortions, including psychotic symptoms; affective symptoms and mood dysregulation; aggression and behavioral dysfunction; and anxiety. These four symptom categories relate to the underlying temperaments that distinguish the *DSM-IV-TR* clusters of personality disorders:

- Low reward dependence and cluster A disorders correspond to the categories of affective dysregulation, detachment, and cognitive disturbances.
- High novelty-seeking and cluster B disorders correspond to the target symptoms of impulsiveness and aggression.
- High harm-avoidance and cluster C disorders correspond to the categories of anxiety and depression symptoms.

Cognitive-perceptual disturbances include magical thinking, odd beliefs, illusions, suspiciousness, ideas of reference, and low-grade psychotic symptoms. These chronic symptoms usually respond to low-dose antipsychotic medications (Simeon & Hollander, 2006).

Several types of aggression have been described in people with personality disorders. Aggression may occur in impulsive people (some with a normal electroencephalogram, some with an abnormal one); people who exhibit predatory or cruel behavior; or people with organic-like impulsivity, poor social judgment, and emotional lability. Lithium, anticonvulsant mood stabilizers, and benzodiazepines are used most often to treat aggression. Low-dose neuroleptics may be useful in modifying predatory aggression (Simeon & Hollander, 2006).

Mood dysregulation symptoms include emotional instability, emotional detachment, depression, and dysphoria. Emotional instability and mood swings respond favorably to lithium, carbamazepine (Tegretol), valproate (Depakote), or low-dose neuroleptics such as haloperidol (Haldol). Emotional detachment, cold and aloof emotions, and disinterest in social relations often respond to selective serotonin reuptake inhibitors or atypical antipsychotics such as risperidone (Risperdal), olanzapine (Zyprexa), and quetiapine (Seroquel). Atypical depression is often treated with selective serotonin reuptake inhibitors, monoamine oxidase inhibitor antidepressants, or low-dose antipsychotic medications (Simeon & Hollander, 2006).

Anxiety seen with personality disorders may be chronic cognitive anxiety, chronic somatic anxiety, or severe acute anxiety. Chronic cognitive anxiety responds to selective serotonin reuptake inhibitors and monoamine oxidase inhibitors, as does chronic somatic anxiety or anxiety manifested as multiple physical complaints. Episodes of severe acute anxiety are best treated with monoamine oxidase inhibitors or low-dose antipsychotic medications.

Table 16.1 summarizes drug choices for various target symptoms of personality disorders. These drugs, including

Table 16.1	DRUG CHOICES FOR SYMPTOMS OF PERSONALITY DISORDERS
Target Symptom	**Drug of Choice**
Aggression/impulsivity	
Affective aggression (normal)	Lithium
	Anticonvulsants
	Low-dose antipsychotics
Predatory (hostility/cruelty)	Antipsychotics
	Lithium
Organic-like aggression	Cholinergic agonists (donepezil)
	Imipramine (Tofranil)
Ictal aggression (abnormal)	Carbamazepine (Tegretol)
	Diphenylhydantoin (Dilantin)
	Benzodiazepines
Mood dysregulation	
Emotional lability	Lithium
	Carbamazepine (Tegretol)
	Antipsychotics
Atypical depression/ dysphoria	MAOIs
	SSRIs
	Antipsychotics
Emotional detachment	SSRIs
	Atypical antipsychotics
Anxiety	
Chronic cognitive	SSRIs
	MAOIs
	Benzodiazepines
Chronic somatic	MAOIs
	SSRIs
Severe anxiety	MAOIs
	Low-dose antipsychotics
Psychotic symptoms	
Acute and psychosis	Antipsychotics
Chronic and low-level psychotic-like symptoms	Low-dose antipsychotics

MAOIs, monoamine oxidase inhibitors; SSRIs, selective serotonin reuptake inhibitors.

Adapted from Svrakic, D. M., & Cloninger, C. R. (2005). Personality disorders. In B. J. Sadock & V. A. Sadock (Eds.), *Comprehensive textbook of psychiatry, Vol. 2* (8th ed., pp. 2063–2104). Philadelphia: Lippincott Williams & Wilkins.

side effects and nursing considerations, are discussed in detail in Chapter 2.

Individual and Group Psychotherapy

Therapy helpful to clients with personality disorders varies according to the type and severity of symptoms and the particular disorder. Inpatient hospitalization usually is indicated when safety is a concern, for example, when a person with borderline personality disorder has suicidal ideas or engages in self-injury. Otherwise, hospitalization is not useful and may even result in dependence on the hospital and staff.

Individual and group psychotherapy goals for clients with personality disorders focus on building trust, teaching basic living skills, providing support, decreasing distressing symptoms such as anxiety, and improving interpersonal relationships. Relaxation or meditation techniques can help manage anxiety for clients with cluster C personality disorders. Improvement in basic living skills through the relationship with a case manager or therapist can improve the functional skills of people with schizotypal and schizoid personality disorders. Assertiveness training groups can assist people with dependent and passive-aggressive personality disorders to have more satisfying relationships with others and to build self-esteem.

Cognitive-behavioral therapy has been particularly helpful for clients with personality disorders (Harvard Medical School Health, 2002). Several cognitive restructuring techniques are used to change the way the client thinks about self and others: thought stopping, in which the client stops negative thought patterns; positive self-talk, designed to change negative self-messages; and decatastrophizing, which teaches the client to view life events more realistically and not as catastrophes. Examples of these techniques are presented later in this chapter.

Dialectical behavior therapy was designed for clients with borderline personality disorder (Linehan, 1993). It focuses on distorted thinking and behavior based on the assumption that poorly regulated emotions are the underlying problem (Harvard Medical School Health, 2002). Table 16.2 summa-

Table 16.2	SUMMARY OF SYMPTOMS AND NURSING INTERVENTIONS FOR PERSONALITY DISORDERS	
Personality Disorder	**Symptoms/Characteristics**	**Nursing Interventions**
Paranoid	Mistrust and suspicions of others; guarded, restricted affect	Serious, straightforward approach; teach client to validate ideas before taking action; involve client in treatment planning
Schizoid	Detached from social relationships; restricted affect; involved with things more than people	Improve client's functioning in the community; assist client to find case manager
Schizotypal	Acute discomfort in relationships; cognitive or perceptual distortions; eccentric behavior	Develop self-care skills; improve community functioning; social skills training
Antisocial	Disregard for rights of others, rules, and laws	Limit setting; confrontation; teach client to solve problems effectively and manage emotions of anger or frustration
Borderline	Unstable relationships, self-image, and affect; impulsivity; self-mutilation	Promote safety; help client to cope and control emotions; cognitive restructuring techniques; structure time; teach social skills
Histrionic	Excessive emotionality and attention seeking	Teach social skills; provide factual feedback about behavior
Narcissistic	Grandiose; lack of empathy; need for admiration	Matter-of-fact approach; gain cooperation with needed treatment; teach client any needed self-care skills
Avoidant	Social inhibitions; feelings of inadequacy; hypersensitive to negative evaluation	Support and reassurance; cognitive restructuring techniques; promote self-esteem
Dependent	Submissive and clinging behavior; excessive need to be taken care of	Foster client's self-reliance and autonomy; teach problem-solving and decision-making skills; cognitive restructuring techniques
Obsessive-compulsive	Preoccupation with orderliness, perfectionism, and control	Encourage negotiation with others; assist client to make timely decisions and complete work; cognitive restructuring techniques
Depressive	Pattern of depressive cognitions and behaviors in a variety of contexts	Assess self-harm risk; provide factual feedback; promote self-esteem; increase involvement in activities
Passive-aggressive	Pattern of negative attitudes and passive resistance to demands for adequate performance in social and occupational situations	Help client to identify feelings and express them directly; assist client to examine own feelings and behavior realistically

rizes the symptoms of and nursing interventions for personality disorders.

Cluster A: Personality Disorders

PARANOID PERSONALITY DISORDER

Clinical Picture

Paranoid personality disorder is characterized by pervasive mistrust and suspiciousness of others. Clients with this disorder interpret others' actions as potentially harmful. During periods of stress, they may develop transient psychotic symptoms. Incidence is estimated to be 0.5% to 2.5% of the general population; the disorder is more common in men than in women. Data about prognosis and long-term outcomes are limited because most people with paranoid personality disorder do not readily seek or remain in treatment (APA, 2000).

Clients appear aloof and withdrawn and may remain a considerable physical distance from the nurse; they view this as necessary for their protection. Clients also may appear guarded or hypervigilant; they may survey the room and its contents, look behind furniture or doors, and generally appear alert to any impending danger. They may choose to sit near the door to have ready access to an exit or with their backs against the wall to prevent anyone from sneaking up behind them. They may have a restricted affect and may be unable to demonstrate warm or empathic emotional responses such as "You look nice today" or "I'm sorry you're having a bad day." Mood may be labile, quickly changing from quietly suspicious to angry or hostile. Responses may become sarcastic for no apparent reason. The constant mistrust and suspicion that clients feel toward others and the environment distorts thoughts, thought processing, and content. Clients frequently see malevolence in the actions of others when none exists. They may spend disproportionate time examining and analyzing the behavior and motives of others to discover hidden and threatening meanings. Clients often feel attacked by others and may devise elaborate plans or fantasies for protection.

These clients use the defense mechanism of *projection,* which is blaming other people, institutions, or events for their own difficulties. It is common for such clients to blame the government for personal problems. For example, a client who gets a parking ticket may say it is part of a plot by the police to drive him out of the neighborhood. He may engage in fantasies of retribution or devise elaborate and sometimes violent plans to get even. Although most clients do not carry out such plans, there is a potential danger.

Conflict with authority figures on the job is common; clients may even resent being given directions from a supervisor. Paranoia may extend to feelings of being singled out for menial tasks, treated as stupid, or more closely monitored than other employees.

Nursing Interventions

Forming an effective working relationship with paranoid or suspicious clients is difficult. The nurse must remember that these clients take everything seriously and are particularly sensitive to the reactions and motivations of others. Therefore, the nurse must approach these clients in a formal, business-like manner and refrain from social chitchat or jokes. Being on time, keeping commitments, and being particularly straightforward are essential to the success of the nurse–client relationship.

Because these clients need to feel in control, it is important to involve them in formulating their plans of care. The nurse asks what the client would like to accomplish in concrete terms, such as minimizing problems at work or getting along with others. Clients are more likely to engage in the therapeutic process if they believe they have something to gain. One of the most effective interventions is helping clients to learn to validate ideas before taking action; however, this requires the ability to trust and to listen to one person. The rationale for this intervention is that clients can avoid problems if they can refrain from taking action until they have validated their ideas with another person. This helps prevent clients from acting on paranoid ideas or beliefs. It also assists them to start basing decisions and actions on reality.

SCHIZOID PERSONALITY DISORDER

Clinical Picture

Schizoid personality disorder is characterized by a pervasive pattern of detachment from social relationships and a restricted range of emotional expression in interpersonal settings. It occurs in approximately 0.5% to 7% of the general population and is more common in men than in women. People with schizoid personality disorder avoid treatment as much as they avoid other relationships, unless their life circumstances change significantly (APA, 2000).

Clients with schizoid personality disorder display a constricted affect and little, if any, emotion. They are aloof and indifferent, appearing emotionally cold, uncaring, or unfeeling. They report no leisure or pleasurable activities because they rarely experience enjoyment. Even under stress or adverse circumstances, their response appears passive and disinterested. There is marked difficulty experiencing and expressing emotions, particularly anger or aggression. Oddly, clients do not report feeling distressed about this lack of emotion; it is more distressing to family members. Clients usually have a rich and extensive fantasy life, although they may be reluctant to reveal that information to the nurse or anyone else. The ideal relationships that occur in the client's fantasies are rewarding and gratifying; these fantasies, though, are in stark contrast to real-life experiences. The fantasy relationship often includes someone the client has met only briefly. Nevertheless, these clients can distinguish fantasies from reality, and no disordered or delusional thought processes are evident.

Clients generally are accomplished intellectually and often involved with computers or electronics in hobbies or work. They may spend long hours solving puzzles or mathematical problems, although they see these pursuits as useful or productive rather than fun.

Clients may be indecisive and lack future goals or direction. They see no need for planning and really have no aspirations. They have little opportunity to exercise judgment or decision making because they rarely engage in these activities. Insight might be described as impaired, at least by the social standards of others: these clients do not see their situation as a problem and fail to understand why their lack of emotion or social involvement troubles others. They are self-absorbed and loners in almost all aspects of daily life. Given an opportunity to engage with other people, these clients decline. They also are indifferent to praise or criticism and are relatively unaffected by the emotions or opinions of others. They also experience dissociation from or no bodily or sensory pleasures. For example, the client has little reaction to beautiful scenery, a sunset, or a walk on the beach.

Clients have a pervasive lack of desire for involvement with others in all aspects of life. They do not have or desire friends, rarely date or marry, and have little or no sexual contact. They may have some connection with a first-degree relative, often a parent. Clients may remain in the parental home well into adulthood if they can maintain adequate separation and distance from other family members. They have few social skills, are oblivious to the social cues or overtures of others, and do not engage in social conversation. They may succeed in vocational areas, provided they value their jobs and have little contact with others in work, which typically involves computers or electronics.

Nursing Interventions

Nursing interventions focus on improved functioning in the community. If a client needs housing or a change in living circumstances, the nurse can make referrals to social services or appropriate local agencies for assistance. The nurse can help agency personnel find suitable housing that accommodates the client's desire and need for solitude. For example, the client with a schizoid personality disorder would function best in a board and care facility, which provides meals and laundry service but requires little social interaction. Facilities designed to promote socialization through group activities would be less desirable.

If the client has an identified family member as his or her primary relationship, the nurse must ascertain whether that person can continue in that role. If that person cannot, the client may need to establish at least a working relationship with a case manager in the community. The case manager then can help the client to obtain services and health

care, manage finances, and so on. The client has a greater chance of success if he or she can relate his or her needs to one person (as opposed to neglecting important areas of daily life).

SCHIZOTYPAL PERSONALITY DISORDER
Clinical Picture

Schizotypal personality disorder is characterized by a pervasive pattern of social and interpersonal deficits marked by acute discomfort with and reduced capacity for close relationships as well as by cognitive or perceptual distortions and behavioral eccentricities. Incidence is about 3% to 5% of the population; the disorder is slightly more common in men than in women. Clients may experience transient psychotic episodes in response to extreme stress. An estimated 10% to 20% of people with schizotypal personality disorder eventually develop schizophrenia (APA, 2000).

Clients often have an odd appearance that causes others to notice them. Clients may be unkempt and disheveled, and their clothes are often ill-fitting, do not match, and may be stained or dirty. They may wander aimlessly and, at times, become preoccupied with some environmental detail. Speech is coherent but may be loose, digressive, or vague. Clients often provide unsatisfactory answers to questions and may be unable to specify or to describe information clearly. They frequently use words incorrectly, which makes their speech sound bizarre. For example, in response to a question about sleeping habits, the client might respond, "Sleep is slow, the REMs don't flow." These clients have a restricted range of emotions; that is, they lack the ability to experience and to express a full range of emotions such as anger, happiness, and pleasure. Affect is often flat and sometimes is silly or inappropriate.

Cognitive distortions include ideas of reference, magical thinking, odd or unfounded beliefs, and a preoccupation with parapsychology, including extrasensory perception and clairvoyance. Ideas of reference usually involve the client's belief that events have special meaning for him or her; however, these ideas are not firmly fixed and delusional, as may be seen in clients with schizophrenia. In magical thinking, which is normal in small children, a client believes he or she has special powers—that by thinking about something, he or she can make it happen. In addition, clients may express ideas that indicate paranoid thinking and suspiciousness, usually about the motives of other people.

Clients experience great anxiety around other people, especially those who are unfamiliar. This does not improve with time or repeated exposures; rather, the anxiety may intensify. This results from the belief that strangers cannot be trusted. Clients do not view their anxiety as a problem that arises from a threatened sense of self. Interpersonal relationships are troublesome; therefore, clients may have only one significant relationship, usually with a first-degree relative. They may remain in their parents' home well into the adult years. They have a limited capacity for close relationships, even though they may be unhappy being alone.

Clients cannot respond to normal social cues and hence cannot engage in superficial conversation. They may have skills that could be useful in a vocational setting, but they are not often successful in employment without support or assistance. Mistrust of others, bizarre thinking and ideas, and unkempt appearance can make it difficult for these clients to get and to keep jobs.

Nursing Interventions

The focus of nursing care for clients with schizotypal personality disorder is development of self-care and social skills and improved functioning in the community. The nurse encourages clients to establish a daily routine for hygiene and grooming. Such a routine is important because it does not depend on the client to decide when hygiene and grooming tasks are necessary. It is useful for clients to have an appearance that is not bizarre or disheveled because stares or comments from others can increase discomfort. Because these clients are uncomfortable around others and this is not likely to change, the nurse must help them function in the community with minimal discomfort. It may help to ask clients to prepare a list of people in the community with whom they must have contact, such as a landlord, store clerk, or pharmacist. The nurse can then role-play interactions that clients would have with each of these people; this allows clients to practice clear and logical requests to obtain services or to conduct personal business. Because face-to-face contact is more uncomfortable, clients may be able to make written requests or to use the telephone for business. Social skills training may help clients to talk clearly with others and to reduce bizarre conversations. It helps to identify one person with whom clients can discuss unusual or bizarre beliefs, such as a social worker or family member. Given an acceptable outlet for these topics, clients may be able to refrain from these conversations with people who might react negatively.

Cluster B: Personality Disorders

ANTISOCIAL PERSONALITY DISORDER

Antisocial personality disorder is characterized by a pervasive pattern of disregard for and violation of the rights of others—and with the central characteristics of deceit and manipulation. This pattern also has been referred to as psychopathy, sociopathy, or dyssocial personality disorder. It occurs in about 3% of the general population and is three to four times more common in men than in women. In prison populations, about 50% are diagnosed with antisocial personality disorder. Antisocial behaviors tend to peak in the 20s and diminish significantly after 45 years of age (APA, 2000).

APPLICATION OF THE NURSING PROCESS: ANTISOCIAL PERSONALITY DISORDER

Assessment

Clients are skillful at deceiving others, so during assessment, it helps to check and to validate information from other sources.

HISTORY

Onset is in childhood or adolescence, although formal diagnosis is not made until the client is 18 years of age. Childhood histories of enuresis, sleepwalking, and syntonic acts of cruelty are characteristic predictors. In adolescence, clients may have engaged in lying, truancy, sexual promiscuity, cigarette smoking, substance use, and illegal activities that brought them into contact with police (McGue & Iacono, 2005). Families have high rates of depression, substance abuse, antisocial personality disorder, poverty, and divorce. Erratic, neglectful, harsh, or even abusive parenting frequently marks the childhoods of these clients.

GENERAL APPEARANCE AND MOTOR BEHAVIOR

Appearance usually is normal; these clients may be quite engaging and even charming. Depending on the circumstances of the interview, they may exhibit signs of mild or

---

CLINICAL VIGNETTE: ANTISOCIAL PERSONALITY DISORDER

Steve found himself in the local jail again after being arrested for burglary. Steve had told the police it wasn't breaking and entering; he had his friend's permission to use his parents' home, but they'd just forgotten to leave the key. Steve has a long juvenile record of truancy, fighting, and marijuana use, which he blames on "having the wrong friends." This is his third arrest, and Steve claims the police are picking on him ever since an elderly lady in the community gave him $5,000

when he was out of work. He intends to pay her back when his ship comes in. Steve's wife of 3 years left him recently, claiming he couldn't hold a decent job and was running up bills they couldn't pay. Steve was tired of her nagging and was ready for a new relationship anyway. He wishes he could win the lottery and find a beautiful girl to love him. He's tired of people demanding that he grow up, get a job, and settle down. They just don't understand that he's got more exciting things to do.

- Violation of the rights of others
- Lack of remorse for behavior
- Shallow emotions
- Lying
- Rationalization of own behavior
- Poor judgment
- Impulsivity
- Irritability and aggressiveness
- Lack of insight
- Thrill-seeking behaviors
- Exploitation of people in relationships
- Poor work history
- Consistent irresponsibility

Adapted from DSM-IV-TR, 2000.

moderate anxiety, especially if another person or agency arranged the assessment.

MOOD AND AFFECT

Clients often display false emotions chosen to suit the occasion or to work to their advantage. For example, a client who is forced to seek treatment instead of going to jail may appear engaging or try to evoke sympathy by sadly relating a story of his or her "terrible childhood." The client's actual emotions are quite shallow.

These clients cannot empathize with the feelings of others, which enables them to exploit others without guilt. Usually, they feel remorse only if they are caught breaking the law or exploiting someone.

THOUGHT PROCESS AND CONTENT

Clients do not experience disordered thoughts, but their view of the world is narrow and distorted. Because coercion and personal profit motivate them, they tend to believe that others are similarly governed. They view the world as cold and hostile and therefore rationalize their behavior. Clichés such as "It's a dog-eat-dog world" represent their viewpoint. Clients believe they are only taking care of themselves because no one else will.

SENSORIUM AND INTELLECTUAL PROCESSES

Clients are oriented, have no sensory-perceptual alterations, and have average or above-average IQs.

JUDGMENT AND INSIGHT

These clients generally exercise poor judgment for various reasons. They pay no attention to the legality of their actions

and do not consider morals or ethics when making decisions. Their behavior is determined primarily by what they want, and they perceive their needs as immediate. In addition to seeking immediate gratification, these clients also are impulsive. Such impulsivity ranges from simple failure to use normal caution (waiting for a green light to cross a busy street) to extreme thrill-seeking behaviors such as driving recklessly.

Clients lack insight and almost never see their actions as the cause of their problems. It is always someone else's fault: some external source is responsible for their situation or behavior.

SELF-CONCEPT

Superficially, clients appear confident, self-assured, and accomplished, perhaps even flip or arrogant. They feel fearless, disregard their own vulnerability, and usually believe they cannot be caught in lies, deceit, or illegal actions. They may be described as egocentric (believing the world revolves around them), but actually the self is quite shallow and empty; these clients are devoid of personal emotions. They realistically appraise their own strengths and weaknesses.

ROLES AND RELATIONSHIPS

Clients manipulate and exploit those around them. They view relationships as serving their needs and pursue others only for personal gain. They never think about the repercussions of their actions to others. For example, a client is caught scamming an older person out of her entire life savings. The client's only comment when caught is "Can you believe that's all the money I got? I was cheated! There should have been more."

These clients often are involved in many relationships, sometimes simultaneously. They may marry and have children, but they cannot sustain long-term commitments. They usually are unsuccessful as spouses and parents and leave others abandoned and disappointed. They may obtain employment readily with their adept use of superficial social skills, but over time their work history is poor. Problems may result from absenteeism, theft, or embezzlement, or they may simply quit out of boredom.

Data Analysis

People with antisocial personality disorder generally do not seek treatment voluntarily unless they perceive some personal gain from doing so. For example, a client may choose a treatment setting as an alternative to jail or to gain sympathy from an employer; they may cite stress as a reason for absenteeism or poor performance. Inpatient treatment settings are not necessarily effective for these clients and may, in fact, bring out their worst qualities.

Nursing diagnoses commonly used when working with these clients include the following:

- Ineffective Coping
- Ineffective Role Performance
- Risk for Other-Directed Violence

Outcome Identification

The treatment focus often is behavioral change. Although treatment is unlikely to affect the client's insight or view of the world and others, it is possible to make changes in behavior. Treatment outcomes may include the following:

- The client will demonstrate nondestructive ways to express feelings and frustration.
- The client will identify ways to meet his or her own needs that do not infringe on the rights of others.
- The client will achieve or maintain satisfactory role performance (e.g., at work, as a parent).

Intervention

FORMING A THERAPEUTIC RELATIONSHIP AND PROMOTING RESPONSIBLE BEHAVIOR

The nurse must provide structure in the therapeutic relationship, identify acceptable and expected behaviors, and be consistent in those expectations. The nurse must minimize attempts by these clients to manipulate and to control the relationship.

Limit setting is an effective technique that involves three steps:

1. Stating the behavioral limit (describing the unacceptable behavior)
2. Identifying the consequences if the limit is exceeded
3. Identifying the expected or desired behavior

Consistent limit setting in a matter-of-fact nonjudgmental manner is crucial to success. For example, a client may approach the nurse flirtatiously and attempt to gain personal information. The nurse would use limit setting by saying,

> *"It is not acceptable for you to ask personal questions. If you continue, I will terminate our interaction. We need to use this time to work on solving your job-related problems."*

The nurse should not become angry or respond to the client harshly or punitively.

Confrontation is another technique designed to manage manipulative or deceptive behavior. The nurse points out a client's problematic behavior while remaining neutral and matter-of-fact; he or she avoids accusing the client. The nurse also can use confrontation to keep clients focused on the topic and in the present. The nurse can focus on the behavior itself rather than on attempts by clients to justify it. For example:

> *Nurse:* "You've said you're interested in learning to manage angry outbursts, but you've missed the last three group meetings."
> *Client:* "Well, I can tell no one in the group likes me. Why should I bother?"
> *Nurse:* "The group meetings are designed to help you and the others, but you can't work on issues if you're not there."

HELPING CLIENTS SOLVE PROBLEMS AND CONTROL EMOTIONS

Clients with antisocial personality disorder have an established pattern of reacting impulsively when confronted with problems. The nurse can teach problem-solving skills and help clients to practice them. Problem-solving skills include identifying the problem, exploring alternative solutions and related consequences, choosing and implementing an alternative, and evaluating the results. Although these clients have the cognitive ability to solve problems, they need to learn a step-by-step approach to deal with them. For example, a client's car isn't running, so he stops going to work. The problem is transportation to work; alternative solutions might be taking the bus, asking a coworker for a ride, and getting the car fixed. The nurse can help the client to discuss the various options and choose one so that he can go back to work.

Managing emotions, especially anger and frustration, can be a major problem. When clients are calm and not upset, the nurse can encourage them to identify sources of frustration, how they respond to it, and the consequences. In this way, the nurse assists clients to anticipate stressful situations and to learn ways to avoid negative future consequences. Taking a **time-out** or leaving the area and going to a neutral place to regain internal control is often a helpful strategy. Time-outs help clients to avoid impulsive reactions and angry outbursts in emotionally charged situations, regain control of emotions, and engage in constructive problem solving.

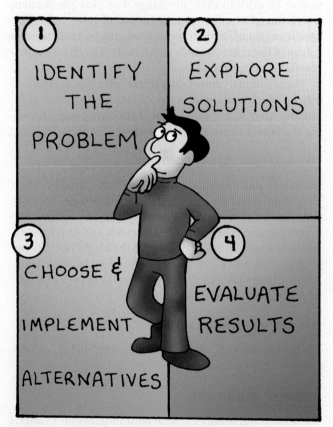

Problem-solving skills

ENHANCING ROLE PERFORMANCE

The nurse helps clients to identify specific problems at work or home that are barriers to success in fulfilling roles. Assessing use of alcohol and other drugs is essential when examining role performance because many clients use or abuse these substances. These clients tend to blame others for their failures and difficulties, and the nurse must redirect them to examine the source of their problems realistically. Referrals to vocational or job programs may be indicated.

Evaluation

The nurse evaluates the effectiveness of treatment based on attainment of or progress toward outcomes. If a client can maintain a job with acceptable performance, meet basic family responsibilities, and avoid committing illegal or immoral acts, then treatment has been successful.

BORDERLINE PERSONALITY DISORDER

Borderline personality disorder is characterized by a pervasive pattern of unstable interpersonal relationships, self-image, and affect as well as marked impulsivity. About 2% to 3% of the general population has borderline personality disorder; it is five times more common in those with a first-degree relative with the diagnosis. Borderline personality disorder is the most common personality disorder found in clinical settings. It is three times more common in women

---

Nursing Care Plan *Antisocial Personality Disorder*

Nursing Diagnosis

Ineffective Coping: *Inability to form a valid appraisal of the stressors, inadequate choices of practiced responses, and/or inability to use available resources*

ASSESSMENT DATA

- Low frustration tolerance
- Impulsive behavior
- Inability to delay gratification
- Poor judgment
- Conflict with authority
- Difficulty following rules and obeying laws
- Lack of feelings of remorse
- Socially unacceptable behavior
- Dishonesty
- Ineffective interpersonal relationships
- Manipulative behavior
- Failure to learn or change behavior based on past experience or punishment
- Failure to accept or handle responsibility

EXPECTED OUTCOMES

Immediate
The client will
- Not harm self or others
- Identify behaviors leading to hospitalization
- Function within limits of therapeutic milieu

Stabilization
The client will
- Demonstrate nondestructive ways to deal with stress and frustration
- Identify ways to meet own needs that do not infringe on the rights of others

Community
The client will
- Achieve or maintain satisfactory work performance
- Meet own needs without exploiting or infringing on the rights of others

IMPLEMENTATION

Nursing Interventions *denotes collaborative interventions

Encourage the client to identify the actions that precipitated hospitalization (e.g., debts, marital problems, law violation).

Rationale

These clients frequently deny responsibility for consequences of their own actions.

continued ···▸

Nursing Care Plan: Antisocial Personality Disorder, cont.

IMPLEMENTATION

Nursing Interventions *denotes collaborative interventions	Rationale
Give positive feedback for honesty. The client may try to avoid responsibility by acting as though he or she is "sick" or helpless.	Honest identification of the consequences of the client's behavior is necessary for future behavior change.
Identify unacceptable behaviors, either general (stealing others' possessions) or specific (embarrassing Ms. X by telling lewd jokes).	You must supply clear, concrete limits when the client is unable or unwilling to do so.
Develop specific consequences for unacceptable behaviors (e.g., the client may not watch television).	Unpleasant consequences may help decrease or eliminate unacceptable behaviors. The consequences must be related to something the client enjoys to be effective.
Avoid any discussion about why requirements exist. State the requirement in a matter-of-fact manner. Avoid arguing with the client.	The client may attempt to bend the rules "just this once" with numerous excuses and justifications. Your refusal to be manipulated or charmed will help decrease manipulative behavior.
Inform the client of unacceptable behaviors and the resulting consequences in advance of their occurrence.	The client must be aware of expectations and consequences.
*Communicate and document in the client's care plan all behaviors and consequences in specific terms.	The client may attempt to gain favor with individual staff members or play one staff member against another. ("Last night the nurse told me I could do that.") If all team members follow the written plan, the client will not be able to manipulate changes.
Avoid discussing another staff member's actions or statements unless the other staff member is present.	The client may try to manipulate staff members or focus attention on others to decrease attention to himself or herself.
*Be consistent and firm with the care plan. Do not make independent changes in rules or consequences. Any change should be made by the staff as a group and conveyed to all staff members working with this client. (You may designate a primary staff person to be responsible for minor decisions and refer all questions to this person.)	Consistency is essential. If the client can find just one person to make independent changes, any plan will become ineffective.
Avoid trying to coax or convince the client to do the "right thing."	The client must decide to accept responsibility for his or her behavior and its consequences.
When the client exceeds a limit, provide consequences immediately after the behavior in a matter-of-fact manner.	Consequences are most effective when they closely follow the unacceptable behavior. Do not react to the client in an angry or punitive manner. If you show anger toward the client, the client may take advantage of it. It is better to get out of the situation if possible and let someone else handle it
Point out the client's responsibility for his or her behavior in a nonjudgmental manner.	The client needs to learn the connection between behavior and the consequences, but blame and judgment are not appropriate.
Provide immediate positive feedback or reward for acceptable behavior.	Immediate positive feedback will help to increase acceptable behavior. The client must receive attention for positive behaviors, not just unacceptable ones.

continued ⋯⟩

Nursing Care Plan: Antisocial Personality Disorder, cont.

IMPLEMENTATION

Nursing Interventions *denotes collaborative interventions	**Rationale**
Gradually, require longer periods of acceptable behavior and greater rewards, and inform the client of changes as decisions are made. For example, at first the client must demonstrate acceptable behavior for 2 hours to earn 1 hour of television time. Gradually, the client could progress to 5 days of acceptable behavior and earn a 2-day weekend pass.	This gradual progression will help to develop the client's ability to delay gratification. This is necessary if the client is to function effectively in society.
Encourage the client to identify sources of frustration, how he or she dealt with it previously, and any unpleasant consequences that resulted.	This may facilitate the client's ability to accept responsibility for his or her own behavior.
Explore alternative, socially and legally acceptable methods of dealing with identified frustrations.	The client has the opportunity to learn to make alternative choices.
Help the client to try alternatives as situations arise. Give positive feedback when the client uses alternatives successfully.	The client can role-play alternatives in a nonthreatening environment.
*Discuss job seeking, work attendance, court appearances, and so forth when working with the client in anticipation of discharge.	Dealing with consequences and working are responsible behaviors. The client may have had little or no successful experience in these areas and may benefit from assistance.

Adapted from Schultz, J. M., & Videbeck, S. L. (2005). Lippincott's manual of psychiatric nursing care plans (7th ed.). Philadelphia: Lippincott Williams & Wilkins.

NURSING INTERVENTIONS FOR ANTISOCIAL PERSONALITY DISORDER

- Promoting responsible behavior
  Limit setting
    State the limit.
    Identify consequences of exceeding the limit.
    Identify expected or acceptable behavior.
  Consistent adherence to rules and treatment plan
  Confrontation
    Point out problem behavior.
    Keep client focused on self.
- Helping clients solve problems and control emotions
  Effective problem-solving skills
  Decreased impulsivity
  Expressing negative emotions such as anger or frustration
  Taking a time-out from stressful situations
- Enhancing role performance
  Identifying barriers to role fulfillment
  Decreasing or eliminating use of drugs and alcohol

than in men. Under stress, transient psychotic symptoms are common. Eight percent to 10% of people with this diagnosis commit suicide, and many more suffer permanent damage from self-mutilation injuries such as cutting or burning (APA, 2000). Typically, recurrent self-mutilation is a cry for help, an expression of intense anger or helplessness, or a form of self-punishment. The resulting physical pain is also a means to block emotional pain. Clients who engage in self-mutilation do so to reinforce that they are still alive; they seek to experience physical pain in the face of emotional numbing (Paris, 2005).

CLIENT/FAMILY EDUCATION FOR ANTISOCIAL PERSONALITY DISORDER

- Avoiding use of alcohol and other drugs
- Appropriate social skills
- Effective problem-solving skills
- Managing emotions such as anger and frustration
- Taking a time-out to avoid stressful situations

Working with clients who have borderline personality disorder can be frustrating. They may cling and ask for help one minute and then become angry, act out, and reject all offers of help in the next minute. They may attempt to manipulate staff to gain immediate gratification of needs and at times sabotage their own treatment plans by purposely failing to do what they have agreed. Their labile mood, unpredictability, and diverse behaviors can make it seem as if the staff is always "back to square one" with them.

APPLICATION OF THE NURSING PROCESS: BORDERLINE PERSONALITY DISORDER

Assessment

HISTORY

Many of these clients report disturbed early relationships with their parents that often begin at 18 to 30 months of age. Commonly, early attempts by these clients to achieve developmental independence were met with punitive responses from parents or threats of withdrawal of parental support and approval. Fifty percent of these clients have experienced childhood sexual abuse; others have experienced physical and verbal abuse and parental alcoholism (Meissner, 2005). Clients tend to use transitional objects (e.g., teddy bears, pillows, blankets, dolls) extensively; this may continue into adulthood. Transitional objects are often similar to favorite items from childhood that the client used for comfort or security.

DSM-IV-TR DIAGNOSTIC CRITERIA:
SYMPTOMS OF BORDERLINE
PERSONALITY DISORDER

- Fear of abandonment, real or perceived
- Unstable and intense relationships
- Unstable self-image
- Impulsivity or recklessness
- Recurrent self-mutilating behavior or suicidal threats or gestures
- Chronic feelings of emptiness and boredom
- Labile mood
- Irritability
- Polarized thinking about self and others ("splitting")
- Impaired judgment
- Lack of insight
- Transient psychotic symptoms such as hallucinations demanding self-harm

Adapted from DSM-IV-TR, 2000.

GENERAL APPEARANCE AND MOTOR BEHAVIOR

Clients experience a wide range of dysfunction—from severe to mild. Initial behavior and presentation may vary widely depending on a client's present status. When dysfunction is severe, clients may appear disheveled and may be unable to sit still, or they may display very labile emotions. In other cases, initial appearance and motor behavior may seem normal. The client seen in the emergency room threatening suicide or self-harm may seem out of control, whereas a client seen in an outpatient clinic may appear fairly calm and rational.

MOOD AND AFFECT

The pervasive mood is **dysphoric**, involving unhappiness, restlessness, and malaise. Clients often report intense loneliness, boredom, frustration, and feeling "empty." They rarely experience periods of satisfaction or well-being. Although there is a pervasive depressed affect, it is unstable and erratic. Clients may become irritable, even hostile or sarcastic, and complain of episodes of panic anxiety. They experience intense emotions such as anger and rage but rarely express them productively or usefully. They usually are hypersensitive to others' emotions, which can easily trigger reactions. Minor changes may precipitate a severe emotional crisis, for example, when an appointment must be changed from one day to the next. Commonly, these clients experience major emotional trauma when their therapists take vacations.

THOUGHT PROCESS AND CONTENT

Thinking about self and others is often polarized and extreme, which is sometime referred to as *splitting*. Clients tend to adore and idealize other people even after a brief acquaintance but then quickly devalue them if these others do not meet their expectations in some way. Clients have excessive and chronic fears of abandonment even in normal situations; this reflects their intolerance of being alone. They also may engage in obsessive rumination about almost anything, regardless of the issue's relative importance.

Clients may experience dissociative episodes (periods of wakefulness when they are unaware of their actions). Self-harm behaviors often occur during these dissociative episodes, although other times clients may be fully aware of injuring themselves. As stated earlier, under extreme stress, clients may develop transient psychotic symptoms such as delusions or hallucinations.

SENSORIUM AND INTELLECTUAL PROCESSES

Intellectual capacities are intact, and clients are fully oriented to reality. The exception is transient psychotic symptoms; during such episodes, reports of auditory hallucinations encouraging or demanding self-harm are most common. These symptoms usually abate when the stress is relieved. Many clients also report flashbacks of previous abuse or trauma. These experiences are consistent with posttraumatic

CLINICAL VIGNETTE: BORDERLINE PERSONALITY DISORDER

Sally had been calling her therapist all day, ever since their session this morning. But the therapist hadn't called her back, even though all her messages said this was an emergency. She was sure her therapist was angry at her and was probably going to drop her as a client. Then she'd have no one; she'd be abandoned by the only person in the world she could talk to. Sally was upset and crying as she began to run the razor blade across her arm. As the blood trickled out, she began to calm down. Then her therapist called and asked what the problem was. Sally was sobbing as she told her therapist that she was cutting her arm because the therapist didn't care anymore, that she was abandoning Sally just like everyone else in her life—her parents, her best friend, every man she had a relationship with. No one was ever there for her when she needed them.

stress disorder, which is common in clients with borderline personality disorder (see Chapter 11).

JUDGMENT AND INSIGHT

Clients frequently report behaviors consistent with impaired judgment and lack of care and concern for safety, such as gambling, shoplifting, and reckless driving. They make decisions impulsively based on emotions rather than facts.

Clients have difficulty accepting responsibility for meeting needs outside a relationship. They see life's problems and failures as a result of others' shortcomings. Because others are always to blame, insight is limited. A typical reaction to a problem is "I wouldn't have gotten into this mess if so-and-so had been there."

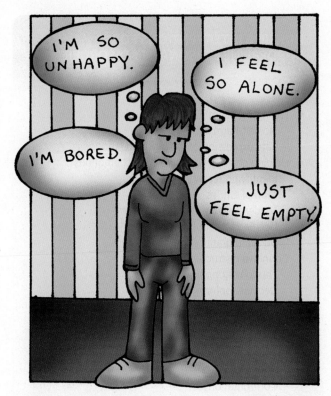

Unstable, unhappy affect of borderline personality disorder

SELF-CONCEPT

Clients have an unstable view of themselves that shifts dramatically and suddenly. They may appear needy and dependent one moment and angry, hostile, and rejecting the next. Sudden changes in opinions and plans about career, sexual identity, values, and types of friends are common. Clients view themselves as inherently bad or evil and often report feeling as if they don't really exist at all.

Suicidal threats, gestures, and attempts are common. Self-harm and mutilation, such as cutting, punching, or burning, are common. These behaviors must be taken very seriously because these clients are at increased risk for completed suicide, even if numerous previous attempts have not been life threatening. These self-inflicted injuries cause much pain and often require extensive treatment; some result in massive scarring or permanent disability such as paralysis or loss of mobility from injury to nerves, tendons, and other essential structures.

ROLES AND RELATIONSHIPS

Clients hate being alone, but their erratic, labile, and sometimes dangerous behaviors often isolate them. Relationships are unstable, stormy, and intense; the cycle repeats itself continually. These clients have extreme fears of abandonment and difficulty believing a relationship still exists once the person is away from them. They engage in many desperate behaviors, even suicide attempts, to gain or to maintain relationships. Feelings for others are often distorted, erratic, and inappropriate. For example, they may view someone they have only met once or twice as their best and only friend or the "love of my life." If another person does not immediately reciprocate their feelings, they may feel rejected, become hostile, and declare him or her to be their enemy. These erratic emotional changes can occur in the space of 1 hour. Often, these situations precipitate self-mutilating behavior; occasionally, clients may attempt to harm others physically.

Clients usually have a history of poor school and work performance because of constantly changing career goals and shifts in identity or aspirations, preoccupation with maintaining relationships, and fear of real or perceived abandonment. Clients lack the concentration and self-discipline to follow through on sometimes mundane tasks associated with work or school.

PHYSIOLOGIC AND SELF-CARE CONSIDERATIONS

In addition to suicidal and self-harm behavior, clients also may engage in binging (excessive overeating) and purging (self-induced vomiting), substance abuse, unprotected sex, or reckless behavior such as driving while intoxicated. They usually have difficulty sleeping.

Data Analysis

Nursing diagnoses for clients with borderline personality disorder may include the following:
• Risk for Suicide
• Risk for Self-Mutilation
• Risk for Other-Directed Violence
• Ineffective Coping
• Social Isolation

Outcome Identification

Treatment outcomes may include the following:
• The client will be safe and free of significant injury.
• The client will not harm others or destroy property.
• The client will demonstrate increased control of impulsive behavior.
• The client will take appropriate steps to meet his or her own needs.
• The client will demonstrate problem-solving skills.
• The client will verbalize greater satisfaction with relationships.

Interventions

Clients with borderline personality disorder often are involved in long-term psychotherapy to address issues of family dysfunction and abuse. The nurse is most likely to have contact with these clients during crises, when they are exhibiting self-harm behaviors or transient psychotic symptoms. Brief hospitalizations often are used to manage these difficulties and to stabilize the client's condition.

PROMOTING CLIENTS' SAFETY

Clients' physical safety is always a priority. The nurse must always seriously consider suicidal ideation with the presence of a plan, access to means for enacting the plan, and self-harm behaviors and institute appropriate interventions (see Chapter 15). Clients often experience chronic suicidality or ongoing intermittent ideas of suicide over months or years. The challenge for the nurse, in concert with clients, is to determine when suicidal ideas are likely to be translated into action.

Clients may enact self-harm urges by cutting, burning, or punching themselves, which sometimes causes permanent physical damage. Self-injury can occur when a client is enraged or experiencing dissociative episodes or psychotic symptoms, or it may occur for no readily apparent reason. Helping clients to avoid self-injury can be difficult when antecedent conditions vary greatly. Sometimes, clients may discuss self-harm urges with the nurse if they feel comfortable doing so. The nurse must remain nonjudgmental when discussing this topic. The nurse can encourage clients to enter a **no-self-harm contract**, in which a client promises to not engage in self-harm and to report to the nurse when he or she is losing control. The nurse emphasizes that the no-self-harm contract is not a promise to the nurse but is the client's promise to himself or herself to be safe. This distinction is critical to avoid blurring the boundaries between nurse and client.

When clients are relatively calm and thinking clearly, it is helpful for the nurse to explore self-harm behavior. The nurse avoids sensational aspects of the injury; the focus is on identifying mood and affect, level of agitation and distress, and circumstances surrounding the incident. In this way, clients can begin to identify trigger situations, moods, or emotions that precede self-harm and to use more effective coping skills to deal with the trigger issues.

If clients do injure themselves, the nurse assesses the injury and need for treatment in a calm, matter-of-fact manner. Lecturing or chastising clients is punitive and has no positive effect on self-harm behaviors. Deflecting attention from the actual physical act is usually desirable.

NURSING INTERVENTIONS FOR BORDERLINE PERSONALITY DISORDER

• Promoting client's safety
  No-self-harm contract
  Safe expression of feelings and emotions
• Helping client to cope and control emotions
  Identifying feelings
  Journal entries
  Moderating emotional responses
  Decreasing impulsivity
  Delaying gratification
• Cognitive restructuring techniques
  Thought stopping
  Decatastrophizing
• Structuring time
• Teaching social skills
• Teaching effective communication skills
• Therapeutic relationship
  Limit setting
  Confrontation

PROMOTING THE THERAPEUTIC RELATIONSHIP

Regardless of the clinical setting, the nurse must provide structure and limit setting in the therapeutic relationship. In a clinic setting, this may mean seeing the client for scheduled appointments of a predetermined length rather than whenever the client appears and demands the nurse's immediate attention. In the hospital setting, the nurse would plan to spend a specific amount of time with the client working on issues or coping strategies rather than giving the client exclusive access when he or she has had an outburst. Limit-setting and confrontation techniques, which are described earlier, are also helpful.

ESTABLISHING BOUNDARIES IN RELATIONSHIPS

Clients have difficulty maintaining satisfying interpersonal relationships. Personal boundaries are unclear, and clients often have unrealistic expectations. Erratic patterns of thinking and behaving often alienate them from others. This may be true for both professional and personal relationships. Clients easily can misinterpret the nurse's genuine interest and caring as a personal friendship, and the nurse may feel flattered by a client's compliments. The nurse must be quite clear about establishing the boundaries of the therapeutic relationship to ensure that neither the client's nor the nurse's boundaries are violated. For example:

> **Client:** *"You're better than my family and the doctors. You understand me more than anyone else."*
> **Nurse:** *"I'm interested in helping you get better, just as the other staff members are."* (establishing boundaries)

TEACHING EFFECTIVE COMMUNICATION SKILLS

It is important to teach basic communication skills such as eye contact, active listening, taking turns talking, validating the meaning of another's communication, and using "I" statements ("I think . . . ," "I feel . . . ," "I need . . ."). The nurse can model these techniques and engage in role-playing with clients. The nurse asks how clients feel when interacting and gives feedback about nonverbal behavior, such as "I noticed you were looking at the floor when discussing your feelings."

HELPING CLIENTS TO COPE AND TO CONTROL EMOTIONS

Clients often react to situations with extreme emotional responses without actually recognizing their feelings. The nurse can help clients to identify their feelings and learn to tolerate them without exaggerated responses such as destruction of property or self-harm. Keeping a journal often helps clients gain awareness of feelings. The nurse can review journal entries as a basis for discussion.

Another aspect of emotional regulation is decreasing impulsivity and learning to delay gratification. When clients have an immediate desire or request, they must learn that it is unreasonable to expect it to be granted without delay. Clients can use distraction such as taking a walk or listening to music to deal with the delay, or they can think about ways to meet needs themselves. Clients can write in their journals about their feelings when gratification is delayed.

RESHAPING THINKING PATTERNS

These clients view everything, people and situations, in extremes—totally good or totally bad. **Cognitive restructuring** is a technique useful in changing patterns of thinking by helping clients to recognize negative thoughts and feelings and to replace them with positive patterns of thinking. **Thought stopping** is a technique to alter the process of negative or self-critical thought patterns such as "I'm dumb, I'm stupid, I can't do anything right." When the thoughts begin, the client may actually say "Stop!" in a loud voice to stop the negative thoughts. Later, more subtle means such as forming a visual image of a stop sign will be a cue to interrupt the negative thoughts. The client then learns to replace recurrent negative thoughts of worthlessness with more positive thinking. In **positive self-talk**, the client reframes negative thoughts into positive ones: "I made a mistake, but it's not the end of the world. Next time, I'll know what to do" (Andreasen & Black, 2006).

Decatastrophizing is a technique that involves learning to assess situations realistically rather than always assuming a catastrophe will happen. The nurse asks, "So what is the worst thing that could happen?" or "How likely do you think that is?" or "How do you suppose other people might deal with that?" or "Can you think of any exceptions to that?" In this way, the client must consider other points of view and actually think about the situation; in time, his or her thinking may become less rigid and inflexible (Andreasen & Black, 2006).

STRUCTURING THE CLIENTS' DAILY ACTIVITIES

Feelings of chronic boredom and emptiness, fear of abandonment, and intolerance of being alone are common problems.

CLIENT/FAMILY EDUCATION FOR BORDERLINE PERSONALITY DISORDER

- Teaching social skills
  - Maintaining personal boundaries
  - Realistic expectations of relationships
- Teaching time structuring
  - Making a written schedule of activities
  - Making a list of solitary activities to combat boredom
- Teaching self-management through cognitive restructuring
  - Decatastrophizing situation
  - Thought stopping
  - Positive self-talk
- Using assertiveness techniques such as "I" statements
- Use of distraction such as walking or listening to music

Clients often are at a loss about how to manage unstructured time, become unhappy and ruminative, and may engage in frantic and desperate behaviors (e.g., self-harm) to change the situation. Minimizing unstructured time by planning activities can help clients to manage time alone. Clients can make a written schedule that includes appointments, shopping, reading the paper, and going for a walk. They are more likely to follow the plan if it is in written form. This also can help clients to plan ahead to spend time with others instead of frantically calling others when in distress. The written schedule also allows the nurse to help clients to engage in more healthful behaviors such as exercising, planning meals, and cooking nutritious food.

Evaluation

As with any personality disorder, changes may be small and slow. The degree of functional impairment of clients with borderline personality disorder may vary widely. Clients with severe impairment may be evaluated in terms of their ability to be safe and to refrain from self-injury. Other clients may be employed and have fairly stable interpersonal relationships. Generally, when clients experience fewer crises less frequently over time, treatment has been effective.

HISTRIONIC PERSONALITY DISORDER

Clinical Picture

Histrionic personality disorder is characterized by a pervasive pattern of excessive emotionality and attention seeking. It occurs in 2% to 3% of the general population and in 10% to 15% of the clinical population. It is seen more often in women than in men. Clients usually seek treatment for depression, unexplained physical problems, and difficulties in relationships (APA, 2000).

The tendency of these clients to exaggerate the closeness of relationships or to dramatize relatively minor occurrences can result in unreliable data. Speech is usually colorful and theatrical, full of superlative adjectives. It becomes apparent, however, that although colorful and entertaining, descriptions are vague and lack detail. Overall appearance is normal, although clients may overdress (e.g., wear an evening dress and high heels for a clinical interview). Clients are overly concerned with impressing others with their appearance and spend inordinate time, energy, and money to this end. Dress and flirtatious behavior are not limited to social situations or relationships but also occur in occupational and professional settings. The nurse may feel these clients are charming or even seducing him or her.

Clients are emotionally expressive, gregarious, and effusive. They often exaggerate emotions inappropriately. For example, a client says "He is the most wonderful doctor! He is so fantastic! He has changed my life!" to describe a physician she has seen once or twice. In such a case, the client cannot specify why she views the doctor so highly.

Expressed emotions, although colorful, are insincere and shallow; this is readily apparent to others but not to clients. They experience rapid shifts in moods and emotions and may be laughing uproariously one moment and sobbing the next. Thus, their displays of emotion may seem phony or forced to observers. Clients are self-absorbed and focus most of their thinking on themselves with little or no thought about the needs of others. They are highly suggestible and will agree with almost anyone to gain attention. They express strong opinions very firmly, but because they base them on little evidence or facts, the opinions often shift under the influence of someone they are trying to impress.

Clients are uncomfortable when they are not the center of attention and go to great lengths to gain that status. They use their physical appearance and dress to gain attention. At times, they may fish for compliments in unsubtle ways, fabricate unbelievable stories, or create public scenes to attract attention. They may even faint, become ill, or fall to the floor. They brighten considerably when given attention after some of these behaviors; this leaves others feeling that they have been used. Any comment or statement that could be interpreted as uncomplimentary or unflattering may produce a strong response such as a temper tantrum or crying outburst.

Clients tend to exaggerate the intimacy of relationships. They refer to almost all acquaintances as "dear, dear friends." They may embarrass family members or friends by flamboyant and inappropriate public behavior such as hugging and kissing someone who has just been introduced or sobbing uncontrollably over a minor incident. Clients may ignore old friends if someone new and interesting has been introduced. People with whom these clients have relationships often describe being used, manipulated, or exploited shamelessly.

Clients may have a wide variety of vague physical complaints or relate exaggerated versions of physical illness. These episodes usually involve the attention clients received (or failed to receive) rather than any particular physiologic concern.

Nursing Interventions

The nurse gives clients feedback about their social interactions with others, including manner of dress and nonverbal behavior. Feedback should focus on appropriate alternatives, not merely criticism. For example, the nurse might say,

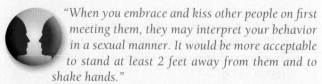

"When you embrace and kiss other people on first meeting them, they may interpret your behavior in a sexual manner. It would be more acceptable to stand at least 2 feet away from them and to shake hands."

It also may help to discuss social situations to explore clients' perceptions of others' reactions and behavior. Teaching social skills and role-playing those skills in a safe, nonthreatening environment can help clients to gain confidence in their ability to interact socially. The nurse must be specific in describing and modeling social skills, including establishing eye contact, engaging in active listening, and respecting personal space. It also helps to outline topics of discussion appropriate for casual acquaintances, closer friends or family, and the nurse only.

Clients may be quite sensitive to discussing self-esteem and may respond with exaggerated emotions. It is important to explore personal strengths and assets and to give specific feedback about positive characteristics. Encouraging clients to use assertive communication, such as "I" statements, may promote self-esteem and help them to get their needs met more appropriately. The nurse must convey genuine confidence in the client's abilities.

NARCISSISTIC PERSONALITY DISORDER

Clinical Picture

Narcissistic personality disorder is characterized by a pervasive pattern of grandiosity (in fantasy or behavior), need for admiration, and lack of empathy. It occurs in 1% to 2% of the general population and in 2% to 16% of the clinical population. Fifty percent to 75% of people with this diagnosis are men. Narcissistic traits are common in adolescence and do not necessarily indicate that a personality disorder will develop in adulthood. Individual psychotherapy is the most effective treatment, and hospitalization is rare unless comorbid conditions exist for which the client requires inpatient treatment (APA, 2000).

Clients may display an arrogant or haughty attitude. They lack the ability to recognize or to empathize with the feelings of others. They may express envy and begrudge others any recognition or material success because they believe it rightfully should be theirs. Clients tend to disparage, belittle, or discount the feelings of others. They may express their grandiosity overtly, or they quietly may expect to be recognized for their perceived greatness. They often are preoccupied with fantasies of unlimited success, power, brilliance, beauty, or ideal love. These fantasies reinforce their sense of superiority. Clients may ruminate about long-overdue admiration and privilege and compare themselves favorably with famous or privileged people.

Thought-processing is intact, but insight is limited or poor. Clients believe themselves to be superior and special and are unlikely to consider that their behavior has any relation to their problems: they view their problems as the fault of others.

Underlying self-esteem is almost always fragile and vulnerable. These clients are hypersensitive to criticism and need constant attention and admiration. They often display a sense of entitlement (unrealistic expectation of special treatment or automatic compliance with wishes). They may believe that only special or privileged people can appreciate their unique qualities or are worthy of their friendship. They expect special treatment from others and often are puzzled or even angry when they do not receive it. They often form and exploit relationships to elevate their own status. Clients assume total concern from others about their welfare. They discuss their own concerns in lengthy detail with no regard for the needs and feelings of others and often become impatient or contemptuous of those who discuss their own needs and concerns.

At work, these clients may experience some success because they are ambitious and confident. Difficulties are common, however, because they have trouble working with others (whom they consider to be inferior) and have limited ability to accept criticism or feedback. They also are likely to believe they are underpaid and underappreciated or should have a higher position of authority even though they are not qualified.

Nursing Interventions

Clients with narcissistic personality disorder can present one of the greatest challenges to the nurse. The nurse must use self-awareness skills to avoid the anger and frustration that these clients' behavior and attitude can engender. Clients may be rude and arrogant, unwilling to wait, and harsh and critical of the nurse. The nurse must not internalize such criticism or take it personally. The goal is to gain cooperation of these clients with other treatment as indicated. The nurse teaches about comorbid medical or psychiatric conditions, medication regimen, and any needed self-care skills in a matter-of-fact manner. He or she sets limits on rude or verbally abusive behavior and explains his or her expectations of the client.

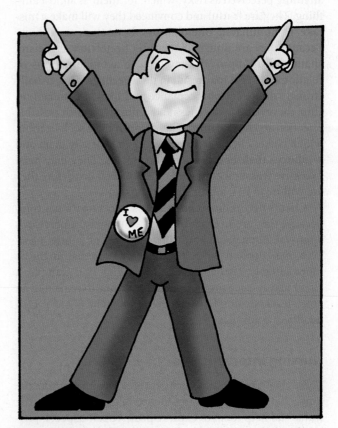

Narcissistic personality

Cluster C: Personality Disorders

AVOIDANT PERSONALITY DISORDER

Clinical Picture

Avoidant personality disorder is characterized by a pervasive pattern of social discomfort and reticence, low self-esteem, and hypersensitivity to negative evaluation. It occurs in 0.5% to 1% of the general population and in 10% of the clinical population. It is equally common in men and women. Clients are good candidates for individual psychotherapy (APA, 2000).

These clients are likely to report being overly inhibited as children and that they often avoid unfamiliar situations and people with an intensity beyond that expected for their developmental stage. This inhibition, which may have continued throughout upbringing, contributes to low self-esteem and social alienation. Clients are apt to be anxious and may fidget in chairs and make poor eye contact with the nurse. They may be reluctant to ask questions or to make requests. They may appear sad as well as anxious. They describe being shy, fearful, socially awkward, and easily devastated by real or perceived criticism. Their usual response to these feelings is to become more reticent and withdrawn.

Clients have very low self-esteem. They are hypersensitive to negative evaluation from others and readily believe themselves to be inferior. Clients are reluctant to do anything perceived as risky, which, for them, is almost anything. They are fearful and convinced they will make a mistake, be humiliated, or embarrass themselves and others. Because they are unusually fearful of rejection, criticism, shame, or disapproval, they tend to avoid situations or relationships that may result in these feelings. They usually strongly desire social acceptance and human companionship: they wish for closeness and intimacy but fear possible rejection and humiliation. These fears hinder socialization, which makes clients seem awkward and socially inept and reinforces their beliefs about themselves. They may need excessive reassurance of guaranteed acceptance before they are willing to risk forming a relationship.

Clients may report some success in occupational roles because they are so eager to please or to win a supervisor's approval. Shyness, awkwardness, or fear of failure, however, may prevent them from seeking jobs that might be more suitable, challenging, or rewarding. For example, a client may reject a promotion and continue to remain in an entry-level position for years even though he or she is well qualified to advance.

Nursing Interventions

These clients require much support and reassurance from the nurse. In the nonthreatening context of the relationship, the nurse can help them to explore positive self-aspects, positive responses from others, and possible reasons for self-criticism. Helping clients to practice self-affirmations and positive self-talk may be useful in promoting self-esteem. Other cognitive restructuring techniques such as reframing and decatastrophizing (described previously) can enhance self-worth. The nurse can teach social skills and help clients to practice them in the safety of the nurse–client relationship. Although these clients have many social fears, those are often counterbalanced by their desire for meaningful social contact and relationships. The nurse must be careful and patient with clients and not expect them to implement social skills too rapidly.

DEPENDENT PERSONALITY DISORDER

Clinical Picture

Dependent personality disorder is characterized by a pervasive and excessive need to be taken care of, which leads to submissive and clinging behavior and fears of separation. These behaviors are designed to elicit caretaking from others. The disorder occurs in as much as 15% of the population and is seen three times more often in women than in men. It runs in families and is most common in the youngest child. People with dependent personality disorder often seek treatment for anxious, depressed, or somatic symptoms (APA, 2000).

Clients are frequently anxious and may be mildly uncomfortable. They are often pessimistic and self-critical; other people hurt their feelings easily. They commonly report feeling unhappy or depressed; this is associated most likely with the actual or threatened loss of support from another. They are preoccupied excessively with unrealistic fears of being left alone to care for themselves. They believe they would fail on their own, so keeping or finding a relationship occupies much of their time. They have tremendous difficulty making decisions, no matter how minor. They seek advice and repeated reassurances about all types of decisions, from what to wear to what type of job to pursue. Although they can make judgments and decisions, they lack the confidence to do so.

Clients perceive themselves as unable to function outside a relationship with someone who can tell them what to do. They are very uncomfortable and feel helpless when alone, even if the current relationship is intact. They have difficulty initiating projects or completing simple daily tasks independently. They believe they need someone else to assume responsibility for them, a belief that far exceeds what is age or situation appropriate. They may even fear gaining competence because doing so would mean an eventual loss of support from the person on whom they depend. They may do almost anything to sustain a relationship, even one of poor quality. This includes doing unpleasant tasks, going places they dislike, or, in extreme cases, tolerating abuse. Clients are reluctant to express disagreement for fear of losing the other person's support or approval; they may even consent to activities that are wrong or illegal to avoid that loss.

When these clients do experience the end of a relationship, they urgently and desperately seek another. The unspoken motto seems to be "Any relationship is better than none at all."

Nursing Interventions

The nurse must help clients to express feelings of grief and loss over the end of a relationship while fostering autonomy and self-reliance. Helping clients to identify their strengths and needs is more helpful than encouraging the overwhelming belief that "I can't do anything alone!" Cognitive restructuring techniques such as reframing and decatastrophizing may be beneficial.

Clients may need assistance in daily functioning if they have little or no past success in this area. Included are such things as planning menus, doing the weekly shopping, budgeting money, balancing a checkbook, and paying bills. Careful assessment to determine areas of need is essential. Depending on the client's abilities and limitations, referral to agencies for services or assistance may be indicated.

The nurse also may need to teach problem solving and decision making and help clients apply them to daily life. He or she must refrain from giving advice about problems or making decisions for clients even though clients may ask the nurse to do so. The nurse can help the client to explore problems, serve as a sounding board for discussion of alternatives, and provide support and positive feedback for the client's efforts in these areas.

OBSESSIVE-COMPULSIVE PERSONALITY DISORDER

Clinical Picture

Obsessive-compulsive personality disorder is characterized by a pervasive pattern of preoccupation with perfectionism, mental and interpersonal control, and orderliness at the expense of flexibility, openness, and efficiency. It occurs in about 1% to 2% of the population, affecting twice as many men as women. This increases to 3% to 10% in clients in mental health settings. Incidence is increased in oldest children and people in professions involving facts, figures, or methodical focus on detail. These people often seek treatment because they recognize that their life is pleasureless or they are experiencing problems with work or relationships. Clients frequently benefit from individual therapy (APA, 2000).

The demeanor of these clients is formal and serious, and they answer questions with precision and much detail. They often report feeling the need to be perfect beginning in childhood. They were expected to be good and to do the right thing to win parental approval. Expressing emotions or asserting independence was probably met with harsh disapproval and emotional consequences. Emotional range is usually quite constricted. They have difficulty expressing emotions, and any emotions they do express are rigid, stiff, and formal, lacking spontaneity. Clients can be very stubborn and reluctant to relinquish control, which makes it difficult for them to be vulnerable to others by expressing feelings. Affect is also restricted: they usually appear anxious and fretful or stiff and reluctant to reveal underlying emotions.

Clients are preoccupied with orderliness and try to maintain it in all areas of life. They strive for perfection as though it were attainable and are preoccupied with details, rules, lists, and schedules to the point of often missing "the big picture." They become absorbed in their own perspective, believe they are right, and do not listen carefully to others because they have already dismissed what is being said. Clients check and recheck the details of any project or activity; often, they never complete the project because of "trying to get it right." They have problems with judgment and decision making—specifically actually reaching a decision. They consider and reconsider alternatives, and the desire for perfection prevents reaching a decision. Clients interpret rules or guidelines literally and cannot be flexible or modify decisions based on circumstances. They prefer written rules for each and every activity at work. Insight is limited, and they are often oblivious that their behavior annoys or frustrates others. If confronted with this annoyance, these clients are stunned, unable to believe others "don't want me to do a good job."

These clients have low self-esteem and are always harsh, critical, and judgmental of themselves; they believe that they "could have done better" regardless of how well the job has been done. Praise and reassurance do not change this belief. Clients are burdened by extremely high and unattainable standards and expectations. Although no one could live up to these expectations, they feel guilty and worthless for being unable to achieve them. They tend to evaluate self and others solely on deeds or actions without regard for personal qualities.

These clients have much difficulty in relationships, few friends, and little social life. They do not express warm or tender feelings to others; attempts to do so are very stiff and formal and may sound insincere. For example, if a significant other expresses love and affection, a client's response might be "The feeling is mutual."

Marital and parental–child relationships are often difficult because these clients can be harsh and unrelenting. For example, most clients are frugal, do not give gifts or want to discard old items, and insist that those around them do the same. Shopping for something new to wear may seem frivolous and wasteful. Clients cannot tolerate lack of control and hence may organize family outings to the point that no one enjoys them. These behaviors can cause daily strife and discord in family life.

At work, clients may experience some success, particularly in fields when precision and attention to detail are desirable. They may miss deadlines, however, while trying to achieve perfection or may fail to make needed decisions while searching for more data. They fail to make timely decisions because of continually striving for perfection.

They have difficulty working collaboratively, preferring to "do it myself" so it is done correctly. If clients do accept help from others, they may give such detailed instructions and watch the other person so closely that coworkers are insulted, annoyed, and refuse to work with them. Given this excessive need for routine and control, new situations and compromise are also difficult.

Nursing Interventions

Nurses may be able to help clients to view decision making and completion of projects from a different perspective. Rather than striving for the goal of perfection, clients can set a goal of completing the project or making the decision by a specified deadline. Helping clients to accept or to tolerate less-than-perfect work or decisions made on time may alleviate some difficulties at work or home. Clients may benefit from cognitive restructuring techniques. The nurse can ask, "What is the worst that could happen?" or "How might your boss (or your wife) see this situation?" These questions may challenge some rigid and inflexible thinking.

Encouraging clients to take risks, such as letting someone else plan a family activity, may improve relationships. Practicing negotiation with family or friends also may help clients to relinquish some of their need for control.

Other Related Disorders

Researchers are studying the following two disorders, depressive personality disorder and passive-aggressive disorder, for inclusion as personality disorders. The *DSM-IV-TR* currently lists and describes these conditions.

DEPRESSIVE PERSONALITY DISORDER

Clinical Picture

Depressive personality disorder is characterized by a pervasive pattern of depressive cognitions and behaviors in various contexts. It occurs equally in men and women and more often in people with relatives who have major depressive disorders. People with depressive personality disorders often seek treatment for their distress and generally have a favorable response to antidepressant medications (APA, 2000).

Although clients with depressive personality disorder may seem to have similar behavior characteristics as clients with major depression (e.g., moodiness, brooding, joylessness, pessimism), the personality disorder is much less severe. Clients with depressive personality disorder usually do not experience the severity and long duration of major depression or the hallmark symptoms of sleep disturbances, loss of appetite, recurrent thoughts of death, and total disinterest in all activities. Major depressive episode is discussed in Chapter 15.

These clients have a sad, gloomy, or dejected affect. They express persistent unhappiness, cheerlessness, and hopelessness, regardless of the situation. They often report the inability to experience joy or pleasure in any activity; they cannot relax and do not display a sense of humor. Clients may repress or not express anger. They brood and worry over all aspects of daily life. Thinking is negative and pessimistic; these clients rarely see any hope for future improvement. They view this pessimism as "being realistic." Regardless of positive outcomes in a given situation, negative thinking continues. Judgment or decision-making skills are usually intact but dominated by pessimistic thinking; clients often blame themselves or others unjustly for situations beyond anyone's control.

Self-esteem is quite low, with feelings of worthlessness and inadequacy even when clients have been successful. Self-criticism often leads to punitive behavior and feelings of guilt or remorse. Clients may appear overtly quiet and passive; they prefer to follow others rather than be leaders in any work or social situation. Although clients feel dependent on approval from others, they tend to be overly critical and quick to reject others first. These clients, who need and want the approval and attention of others, actually drive others away; this reinforces feelings of being unworthy of anyone's attention.

Nursing Interventions

When working with clients who report depressed feelings, it is always important to assess whether there is risk for self-harm. If a client expresses suicidal ideation or has urges for self-injury, the nurse must provide interventions and plan care as indicated (see Chapter 15).

The nurse explains that the client must take action, rather than wait, to feel better. Encouraging the client to become involved in activities or engaged with others provides opportunities to interrupt the cyclical, negative thought patterns.

Giving factual feedback, rather than general praise, reinforces attempts to interact with others and gives specific positive information about improved behaviors. An example of general praise is

"Oh, you're doing so well today."

This statement does not identify specific positive behaviors. Allowing the client to identify specific positive behaviors often helps to promote self-esteem. An example of specific praise is

"You talked to Mrs. Jones for 10 minutes, even though it was difficult. I know that took a lot of effort."

This statement gives the client a clear message about what specific behavior was effective and positive—the client's ability to talk to someone else.

Chapter 16 • PERSONALITY DISORDERS **361**

Cognitive restructuring techniques such as thought stopping or positive self-talk (discussed previously) also can enhance self-esteem. Clients learn to recognize negative thoughts and feelings and learn new positive patterns of thinking about themselves.

It may be necessary to teach the client effective social skills such as eye contact, attentive listening, and topics appropriate for initial social conversation (e.g., the weather, current events, local news). Even if the client knows these social skills, practicing them is important—first with the nurse and then with others. Practicing with the nurse is initially less threatening. Another simple but effective technique is to help the client practice giving others compliments. This requires the client to identify something positive rather than negative in others. Giving compliments also promotes receiving compliments, which further enhances positive feelings.

PASSIVE-AGGRESSIVE PERSONALITY DISORDER

Clinical Picture

Passive-aggressive personality disorder is characterized by a negative attitude and a pervasive pattern of passive resistance to demands for adequate social and occupational performance. It occurs in 1% to 3% of the general population and in 2% to 8% of the clinical population. It is thought to be slightly more prevalent in women than in men (APA, 2000).

These clients may appear cooperative, even ingratiating, or sullen and withdrawn, depending on the circumstances. Their mood may fluctuate rapidly and erratically, and they may be easily upset or offended. They may alternate between hostile self-assertion such as stubbornness or fault finding and excessive dependence, expressing contrition and guilt. There is a pervasive attitude that is negative, sullen, and defeatist. Affect may be sad or angry. The negative attitude influences thought content: Clients perceive and anticipate difficulties and disappointments where none exist. They view the future negatively, believing that nothing good ever lasts. Their ability to make judgments or decisions is often impaired. Clients are frequently ambivalent and indecisive, preferring to allow others to make decisions that these clients then criticize. Insight is also limited: Clients tend to blame others for their own feelings and misfortune. Rather than accepting reasonable responsibility for the situation, these clients may alternate blaming behavior with exaggerated remorse and contrition.

Clients experience intense conflict between dependence on others and a desire for assertion. Self-confidence is low despite the bravado shown. Clients may complain they are misunderstood and unappreciated by others and may report feeling cheated, victimized, and exploited. They habitually resent, oppose, and resist demands to function at a level expected by others. This opposition occurs most frequently in work situations but also can be evident in social functioning. They express such resistance through procrastination,

forgetfulness, stubbornness, and intentional inefficiency, especially in response to tasks assigned by authority figures. They also may obstruct the efforts of coworkers by failing to do their share. In social or family relationships, these clients may play the role of the martyr who "sacrifices everything for others" or who may be aggrieved and misunderstood. These behaviors sometimes are effective in manipulating others to do as clients wish, without clients needing to make a direct request.

These clients often have various vague or generalized somatic complaints and may even adopt a sick role. They then can be angry or bitter, complaining, "No one can figure out what's wrong with me. I just have to suffer. It's my bad luck!"

Nursing Interventions

The nurse may encounter much resistance from the client in identifying feelings and expressing them directly. Often, clients do not recognize that they feel angry and may express it indirectly. The nurse can help them examine the relationship between feelings and subsequent actions. For example, a client may intend to complete a project at work but then procrastinates, forgets, or becomes "ill" and misses the deadline. Or the client may intend to participate in a family outing but becomes ill, forgets, or has "an emergency" when it is time. By focusing on the behavior, the nurse can help the client to see what is so annoying or troubling to others. The nurse also can help the client to learn appropriate ways to express feelings directly, especially negative feelings such as anger. Methods such as having the client write about the feelings or role-play are effective. If the client is unwilling to engage in this process, however, the nurse cannot force him or her to do so.

ELDER CONSIDERATIONS

Personality disorders are not first diagnosed in elder persons but may persist from young adulthood into older age. Abrams and Sadavoy (2004) wrote that personality disorders from clusters A and C are more prevalent in older age and are closely correlated with depression. Some persons with personality disorders tend to stabilize and experience fewer difficulties in later life. Others are described as "aging badly," that is, they are unable or unwilling to acknowledge limitations that come with aging, they refuse to accept help when needed, and they do not make reasonable decisions about their health care, finances, or living situation. These individuals seems chronically angry, unhappy, or dissatisfied, resulting in strained relationships and even alienation from family, friends, caregivers, and health care providers.

COMMUNITY-BASED CARE

Caring for clients with personality disorders occurs primarily in community-based settings. Acute psychiatric settings such as hospitals are useful for safety concerns for short periods. The nurse uses skills to deal with clients who have personality disorders in clinics, outpatient settings, doctors' offices, and many medical settings. Often, the personality disorder is not the focus of attention; rather, the client may be seeking treatment for a physical condition.

Most people with personality disorders are treated in group or individual therapy settings, community support programs, or self-help groups. Others will not seek treatment for their personality disorder but may be treated for a major mental illness. Wherever the nurse encounters clients with personality disorders, including in his or her own life, the interventions discussed in this chapter can prove useful.

MENTAL HEALTH PROMOTION

The treatment of individuals with a personality disorder often focuses on mood stabilization, decreasing impulsivity, and developing social and relationship skills. Hayward, Slade, and Moran (2006) studied clients with personality disorders in terms of clients' perceptions of their unmet needs. They found that clients perceived unmet needs in five areas: self-care (keeping clean and tidy); sexual expression (dissatisfaction with sex life); budgeting (managing daily finances); psychotic symptoms; and psychological distress. Although psychotic symptoms and psychological distress are usually addressed by health care providers, the other three areas are not. This suggests that dealing with those areas in the treatment of a client might result in a greater sense of well-being and improved health.

Children who have a greater number of "protective factors" are less likely to develop antisocial behavior as adults. These protective factors include school commitment or importance of school, parent or peer disapproval of antisocial behavior, and being involved in a religious community. Interestingly, the study found that children at risk for abuse and children who were not at risk were less likely to have antisocial behavior as adults if these protective factors were present in their environment. Children lacking these protective factors are much more likely to develop antisocial behavior as adults (Herrenkohl et al., 2005).

SELF-AWARENESS ISSUES

Because clients with personality disorders take a long time to change their behaviors, attitudes, or coping skills, nurses working with them easily can become frustrated or angry. These clients continually test the limits, or boundaries, of the nurse–client relationship with attempts at manipulation. Nurses must discuss feelings of anger or frustration with colleagues to help them recognize and cope with their own feelings.

The overall appearance of clients with personality disorders can be misleading. Unlike clients who are psychotic or severely depressed, clients with personality disorders look as though they are capable of functioning more effec-

tively. The nurse can easily but mistakenly believe the client simply lacks motivation or the willingness to make changes and may feel frustrated or angry. It is easy for the nurse to think, "Why does the client continue to do that? Can't he see it only gets him into difficulties?" This reaction is similar to reactions the client has probably received from others.

Clients with personality disorders also challenge the ability of therapeutic staff to work as a team. For example, clients with antisocial or borderline personalities often manipulate staff members by splitting them—that is, causing staff members to disagree or to contradict one another in terms of the limits of the treatment plan. This can be quite disruptive. In addition, team members may have differing opinions about individual clients. One staff member may believe that a client needs assistance, whereas another may believe the client is overly dependent. Ongoing communication is necessary to remain firm and consistent about expectations for clients.

Points to Consider When Working With Clients With Personality Disorders

- Talking to colleagues about feelings of frustration will help you to deal with your emotional responses so you can be more effective with clients.
- Clear, frequent communication with other health care providers can help to diminish the client's manipulation.
- Do not take undue flattery or harsh criticism personally; it is a result of the client's personality disorder.
- Set realistic goals and remember that behavior changes in clients with personality disorders take a long time. Progress can be very slow.

Critical Thinking Questions

1. Where do you see yourself in relation to the four types of temperament (harm avoidance, novelty seeking, reward dependence, and persistence)?
2. What has been the most significant influence on your development as a person?
3. There is a significant correlation between the diagnosis of antisocial personality disorder and criminal behavior. The *DSM-IV-TR* includes "violation of the rights of others" in the definition of this disorder. Is this personality disorder more a social than a mental health problem? Why?

KEY POINTS

- People with personality disorders have traits that are inflexible and maladaptive and cause either significant functional impairment or subjective distress.

- Personality disorders are relatively common and diagnosed in early adulthood, although some behaviors are evident in childhood or adolescence.
- Rapid or substantial changes in personality are unlikely. This can be a primary source of frustration for family members, friends, and health care professionals.
- Schizotypal personality disorder is characterized by social and interpersonal deficits, cognitive and perceptual distortions, and eccentric behavior.
- People with paranoid personality disorders are suspicious, mistrustful, and threatened by others.
- People with depressive personality disorder are sad, gloomy, and negative; experience no pleasure; and tend to brood or ruminate about their lives.
- Schizoid personality disorder includes marked detachment from others, restricted emotions, indifference, and fantasy.
- People with antisocial personality disorder often appear glib and charming, but they are suspicious, insensitive, and uncaring and often exploit others for their own gain.
- People with borderline personality disorder have markedly unstable mood, affect, self-image, interpersonal relationships, and impulsivity; they often engage in self-harm behavior.
- People with obsessive-compulsive personality disorder are preoccupied with orderliness, perfection, and interpersonal control at the expense of flexibility, openness, and efficiency.
- Histrionic personality disorder is characterized by excessive emotionality and dramatic, attention-seeking, and seductive or provocative behavior.
- Narcissistic personality disorder is characterized by grandiosity, need for admiration, lack of empathy for others, and a sense of entitlement.
- Avoidant personality disorder is characterized by social discomfort and reticence in all situations, low self-esteem, and hypersensitivity to negative evaluation.
- Dependent personality disorder is characterized by a pervasive and excessive need to be taken care of, which leads to submissive and clinging behaviors and fears of separation and abandonment.
- People with passive-aggressive personality disorder demonstrate passive resistance to demands for adequate social and occupational performance and negativity; they often play the role of a martyr.
- The therapeutic relationship is crucial in caring for clients with personality disorders. Nurses can help clients to identify their feelings and dysfunctional behaviors and to develop appropriate coping skills and positive behaviors. Therapeutic communication and role modeling help to promote appropriate social interactions, which help to improve interpersonal relationships.
- Several therapeutic strategies are effective when working with clients with personality disorders. Cognitive restructuring techniques such as thought stopping, positive self-talk, and decatastrophizing are useful; self-help skills aid the client to function better in the community.
- Psychotropic medications are prescribed for clients with personality disorders based on the type and severity of symptoms the client experiences in aggression and impulsivity, mood dysregulation, anxiety, and psychotic symptoms.
- Clients with borderline personality disorder often have self-harm urges that they enact by cutting, burning, or punching themselves; this behavior sometimes causes permanent physical damage. The nurse can encourage the client to enter into a no-self-harm contract in which the client promises to try to keep from harming himself or herself and to report to the nurse when he or she is having self-harm urges.
- Nurses must use self-awareness skills to minimize client manipulation and deal with feelings of frustration.

INTERNET RESOURCES

RESOURCE	INTERNET ADDRESS
Avoidant Personality Disorder	http://www.mentalhealth.com
Borderline Personality Disorder	http://www.borderlinepersonalitytoday.com/main
Cognitive Behavioral Therapy	http://www.bpdcentral.com
Dependent Personality Disorder	http://www.nacbt.org/whatiscbt.htm
Dialectical Behavior Therapy	http://www.mentalhealth.com
Histrionic Personality Disorder	http://www.brainencyclopedia.com/encyclopedia/c/co/ cognitive_therapy.htm
Narcissistic Personality Disorder	http://www.mentalhealth.com
Paranoid Personality Disorder	http://www.mentalhealth.com
Personality Disorders	http://www.mentalhealth.com
Schizoid Personality Disorder	http://www.mentalhelp.net/poc/center_index.php?id-8
Schizotypal Personality Disorder	http://www.nmha.org/infactr/factsheet/91.cfm

REFERENCES

Abrams, R. C., & Sadavoy, J. (2004). Personality disorders. In J. Sadavoy, L. F. Jarvik, G. T. Grossberg, et al. (Eds.), *Comprehensive textbook of geriatric psychiatry* (3rd ed., pp. 701–721). New York: W. W. Norton and Company.

American Psychiatric Association. (2000). *Diagnostic and statistical manual of mental disorders* (4th ed., text revision). Washington, DC: American Psychiatric Association.

Andreasen, N. C., & Black, D. W. (2006). *Introductory textbook of psychiatry* (4th ed.). Washington DC: American Psychiatric Publishing.

Harvard Medical School Health. (2002). Borderline personality disorder: New recommendations. *Harvard Medical Health Letter, 18*(9), 4–6.

Hayward, M., Slade, M., & Moran, P. A. (2006). Personality disorders and unmet needs among psychiatric inpatients. *Psychiatric Services, 57*(4), 538–543.

Herrenkohl, T. I., Tajima, E. A., Whitney, S. D., & Huang, B. (2005). Protection against antisocial behavior in children exposed to physically abusive discipline. *Journal of Adolescent Health, 36*(6), 457–465.

Linehan, M. M. (1993). *Cognitive-behavioral treatment of borderline personality disorder*. New York: Guilford Press.

McGue, M., & Iacono, W. G. (2005). The association of early adolescent problem behavior with adult psychopathology. *American Journal of Psychiatry, 162*(6), 1118–1124.

Meissner, W. W. (2005). Classic Psychoanalysis. In B. J. Sadock & V. A. Sadock (Eds.). *Comprehensive textbook of psychiatry* (Vol. 1, 8th ed, pp. 701–746). Philadelphia: Lippincott Williams & Wilkins.

Paris, J. (2005). Understanding self-mutilation in borderline personality disorder. *Harvard Review of Psychiatry, 13*(3), 179–185.

Schultz, J. M., & Videbeck, S. L. (2005). *Lippincott's manual of psychiatric nursing care plans* (7th ed.). Philadelphia: Lippincott Williams & Wilkins.

Seivewright, H., Tyrer, P., & Johnson, T. (2002). Change in personality status in neurotic disorders. *Lancet, 359*(9325), 2253–2254.

Simeon, D., & Hollander, E. (2006). Treatment of personality disorders. In A. F. Schatzberg & C. B. Nereroff (Eds.), *Essentials of clinical psychopharmacology* (2nd ed., pp. 689–705). Washington DC: American Psychiatric Publishing.

Svrakic, D. M., & Cloninger, C. R. (2005). Personality disorders. In B. J. Sadock & V. A. Sadock (Eds.), *Comprehensive textbook of psychiatry* (Vol. 2, 8th ed., pp. 2063–2104). Philadelphia: Lippincott Williams & Wilkins.

ADDITIONAL READINGS

McQuillan, A., Nicastro, R., Guenot, F., Girard, M., Lissner, C., & Ferrero, F. (2005). Intensive dialectic behavior therapy for outpatients with borderline personality disorder who are in crisis. *Psychiatric Services, 56*(2), 193–197.

Oldham, J. M. (2006). Borderline personality disorder and suicidality. *American Journal of Psychiatry, 163*(1), 20–26.

Paris, J. (2005). The development of impulsivity in borderline personality disorder. *Development and Psychopathology, 17*(4), 1091–1104.

Swenson, C. R., Torrey, W. C., & Koerner, K. (2002). Implementing dialectical behavior therapy. *Psychiatric Services, 53*(2), 171–178.

Chapter Study Guide

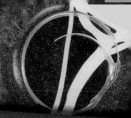

MULTIPLE-CHOICE QUESTIONS

Select the best answer for each of the following questions.

1. When working with a client with a paranoid personality disorder, the nurse would use which of the following approaches?
   A. Cheerful
   B. Friendly
   C. Serious
   D. Supportive

2. Which of the following underlying emotions is commonly seen in a passive-aggressive personality disorder?
   A. Anger
   B. Depression
   C. Fear
   D. Guilt

3. Cognitive restructuring techniques include all the following except
   A. Decatastrophizing
   B. Positive self-talk
   C. Reframing
   D. Relaxation

4. Transient psychotic symptoms that occur with borderline personality disorder are most likely treated with which of the following?
   A. Anticonvulsant mood stabilizers
   B. Antipsychotics
   C. Benzodiazepines
   D. Lithium

5. Clients with a histrionic personality disorder are most likely to benefit from which of the following nursing interventions?
   A. Cognitive restructuring techniques
   B. Improving community functioning
   C. Providing emotional support
   D. Teaching social skills

6. When interviewing any client with a personality disorder, the nurse would assess for which of the following?
   A. Ability to charm and manipulate people
   B. Desire for interpersonal relationships
   C. Disruption in some aspects of his or her life
   D. Increased need for approval from others

7. The nurse would assess for which of the following characteristics in a client with narcissistic personality disorder?
   A. Entitlement
   B. Fear of abandonment
   C. Hypersensitivity
   D. Suspiciousness

8. The most important short-term goal for the client who tries to manipulate others would be to
   A. Acknowledge own behavior
   B. Express feelings verbally
   C. Stop initiating arguments
   D. Sustain lasting relationships

FILL-IN-THE-BLANK QUESTIONS

Identify the personality disorder that is described in each of the following.

_____ Unstable relationships, affect, and self-image

_____ Disregard for the rights of others

_____ Detachment from social relationships, restricted affect

_____ Social inhibitions, feelings of inadequacy

SHORT-ANSWER QUESTIONS

Describe the behavior associated with each of the following temperament traits.

Harm avoidance: High

Harm avoidance: Low

Novelty seeking: High

Novelty seeking: Low

Reward dependence: High

Reward dependence: Low

Persistence: High

Persistence: Low

CLINICAL EXAMPLE

Susan Marks, 25 years old, is diagnosed with borderline personality disorder. She has been attending college sporadically but has only 15 completed credits and no real career goal. She is angry because her parents have told her she must get a job to support herself. Last week, she met a man in the park and fell in love with him on the first date. She has been calling him repeatedly, but he will not return her calls. Declaring that her parents have deserted her and her boyfriend doesn't love her anymore, she slashes her forearms with a sharp knife. She then calls 911, stating, "I'm about to die! Please help me!" She is taken by ambulance to the emergency room and is admitted to the inpatient psychiatry unit.

1. Identify two priority nursing diagnoses that would be appropriate for Susan on her admission to the unit.

2. Write an expected outcome for each of the identified nursing diagnoses.

3. List three nursing interventions for each of the identified nursing diagnoses.

4. What community resources or referrals would be beneficial for Susan?

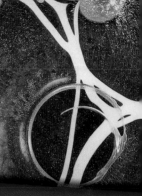

Key Terms

- 12-step program
- blackout
- codependence
- controlled substance
- denial
- detoxification
- dual diagnosis
- flushing
- hallucinogen
- inhalant
- intoxication
- opioid
- polysubstance abuse
- spontaneous remission
- stimulants
- substance abuse
- substance dependence
- tapering
- tolerance
- tolerance break
- withdrawal syndrome

Learning Objectives

After reading this chapter, you should be able to

1. Explain the trends in substance abuse and discuss the need for related prevention programs.

2. Discuss the characteristics, risk factors, and family dynamics prevalent with substance abuse.

3. Describe the principles of a 12-step treatment approach for substance abuse.

4. Apply the nursing process to the care of clients with substance abuse issues.

5. Provide education to clients, families, and community members to increase knowledge and understanding of substance use and abuse.

6. Discuss the nurse's role in dealing with the chemically impaired professional.

7. Evaluate your feelings, attitudes, and responses to clients and families with substance use and abuse.

Substance use/abuse and related disorders are a national health problem. More than 15 million Americans are dependent on alcohol, and 500,000 are between the ages of 9 and 12 years. Almost 7 million persons are binge drinkers between the ages of 12 and 20 years—under the legal age limit for drinking in most states (Narconon, 2005). The actual prevalence of substance abuse is difficult to determine precisely because many people meeting the criteria for diagnosis do not seek treatment and surveys conducted to estimate prevalence are based on self-reported data that may be inaccurate.

Drug and alcohol abuse costs business and industry an estimated $100 billion annually. Alcoholism alone accounts for 500 million lost days of work. Up to 40% of industrial fatalities and 47% of workplace injuries are linked to alcoholism and alcohol consumption. Estimates of motor vehicle fatalities related to alcohol are 50% (Substance Abuse and Mental Health Services Administration, 2005). In the United States, one person is killed every 30 minutes in an alcohol-related traffic accident.

The number of infants suffering the physiologic and emotional consequences of prenatal exposure to alcohol or drugs (e.g., fetal alcohol syndrome, "crack babies") is increasing at alarming rates. Chemical abuse also results in increased violence, including domestic abuse, homicide, and child abuse and neglect. These rising statistics regarding substance abuse do not bode well for future generations.

Forty-three percent of all Americans have been exposed to alcoholism in their families. Children of alcoholics are four times more likely than the general population to develop problems with alcohol (National Institute on Alcohol Abuse and Alcoholism, 2007). Many people in treatment programs as adults report having had their first drink of alcohol as a young child, when they were younger than age 10. This first drink was often a taste of the drink of a parent or family member. With the increasing rates of use being reported among young people today, this problem could spiral out of control unless great strides can be made through programs for prevention, early detection, and effective treatment.

TYPES OF SUBSTANCE ABUSE

Many substances can be used and abused; some can be obtained legally, whereas others are illegal. This discussion includes alcohol and prescription medications as substances that can be abused. Abuse of more than one substance is termed **polysubstance abuse.**

The *Diagnostic and Statistical Manual of Mental Disorders, 4th edition, Text Revision (DSM-IV-TR)*, lists 11 diagnostic classes of substance abuse:

- Alcohol
- Amphetamines or similarly acting sympathomimetics
- Caffeine
- Cannabis
- Cocaine
- Hallucinogens
- Inhalants
- Nicotine
- Opioids
- Phencyclidine (PCP) or similarly acting drugs
- Sedatives, hypnotics, or anxiolytics

It also categorizes substance-related disorders into two groups: those that include disorders of abuse and dependence and substance-induced disorders such as intoxication, withdrawal, delirium, dementia, psychosis, mood disorder, anxiety, sexual dysfunction, and sleep disorder.

This chapter describes the specific symptoms of intoxication, overdose, withdrawal, and detoxification for each substance with the exception of caffeine and nicotine. Although caffeine and nicotine abuse can cause significant physiologic health problems and result in substance-induced disorders such as sleep disorders, anxiety, and withdrawal, treatment of these two substances usually is not viewed as falling into the mental health arena.

Intoxication is use of a substance that results in maladaptive behavior. **Withdrawal syndrome** refers to the negative psychological and physical reactions that occur when use of a substance ceases or dramatically decreases. **Detoxification** is the process of safely withdrawing from a substance. The treatment of other substance-induced disorders such as psychosis and mood disorders is discussed in depth in separate chapters.

Substance abuse can be defined as using a drug in a way that is inconsistent with medical or social norms and despite negative consequences. The *DSM-IV-TR* distinguishes substance abuse from dependence for purposes of medical diagnosis. Substance abuse denotes problems in social, vocational, or legal areas of the person's life, whereas **substance dependence** also includes problems associated with addiction such as tolerance, withdrawal, and unsuccessful attempts to stop using the substance. This distinction between abuse and dependence frequently is viewed as unclear and unnecessary (Jaffe & Anthony, 2005) because the distinction does not affect clinical decisions once withdrawal or detoxification has been completed. Hence, the terms *substance abuse* and *substance dependence* or *chemical dependence* can be used interchangeably. In this chapter, the term *substance use* is used to include both abuse and dependence; it is not meant to refer to the occasional or one-time user.

ONSET AND CLINICAL COURSE

Much research on substance use has focused on alcohol because it is legal and more widely used; thus, more is known about alcohol's effects. The prognosis for alcohol use in general is unclear because usually only people seeking treatment for problems with alcohol are studied.

The early course of alcoholism typically begins with the first episode of intoxication between 15 and 17 years of age (Schuckit, 2005); the first evidence of minor alcohol-related problems is seen in the late teens. These events do not differ significantly from the experiences of people who do not go on to develop alcoholism. A pattern of more severe difficulties for people with alcoholism begins to emerge in the middle 20s to the middle 30s; these difficulties can be the alcohol-related breakup of a significant relationship, an arrest for public intoxication or driving while intoxicated, evidence of alcohol withdrawal, early alcohol-related health problems, or significant interference with functioning at work or school. During this time, the person experiences his or her first **blackout**, which is an episode during which the person continues to function but has no conscious awareness of his or her behavior at the time or any later memory of the behavior.

As the person continues to drink, he or she often develops a **tolerance** for alcohol; that is, he or she needs more alcohol to produce the same effect. After continued heavy drinking, the person experiences a **tolerance break**, which means that very small amounts of alcohol intoxicate the person.

The later course of alcoholism, when the person's functioning definitely is affected, is often characterized by periods of abstinence or temporarily controlled drinking. Abstinence may occur after some legal, social, or interpersonal crisis, and the person may then set up rules about drinking such as drinking only at certain times or drinking only beer. This period of temporarily controlled drinking soon leads to an escalation of alcohol intake, more problems, and a subsequent crisis. The cycle repeats continuously (Schuckit, 2005).

For many people, substance use is a chronic illness characterized by remissions and relapses to former levels of use (Jaffe & Anthony, 2005). The highest rates for successful recovery are for people who abstain from substances, are highly motivated to quit, and have a past history of life success (i.e., satisfactory experiences in coping, work, relationships, and so forth). Although an estimated 60% to 70% of people in alcoholism treatment remain sober after 1 year (Schuckit, 2005), this estimate may be optimistic—and misleading—because most relapses occur during the second year after treatment.

Evidence shows that some people with alcohol-related problems can modify or quit drinking on their own without a treatment program; this is called **spontaneous remission** or natural recovery (Bischof et al., 2005). The abstinence was often in response to a crisis or a promise to a loved one and was accomplished by engaging in alternative activities; relying on relationships with family and friends; and avoiding alcohol, alcohol users, and social cues associated with drinking. Spontaneous remission can occur in as many as 20% of alcoholics, although it is highly unlikely that people in the late stage of alcoholism can recover without treatment (Schuckit, 2005).

Poor outcomes have been associated with an earlier age at onset, longer periods of substance use, and the coexistence of a major psychiatric illness. With extended use, the risk for mental and physical deterioration and infectious disease such as HIV and AIDS, hepatitis, and tuber-culosis increases, especially for those with a history of intravenous drug use. In addition, people addicted to alcohol and drugs have a rate of suicide that is 20% higher than that of the general population.

RELATED DISORDERS

Substance-induced disorders such as anxiety, mood disorders, and dementia are discussed in other chapters. For instance, Chapter 21 discusses delirium, which may be seen in severe alcohol withdrawal. A clinical care plan for a client receiving treatment for substance abuse is featured near the end of this chapter. The effects on adults who grew up in a home with an alcoholic parent are discussed later, as are the special needs of clients with a dual diagnosis of substance use and a major psychiatric disorder.

ETIOLOGY

The exact causes of drug use, dependence, and addiction are not known, but various factors are thought to contribute to the development of substance-related disorders (Jaffe & Anthony, 2005). Much of the research on biologic and genetic factors has been done on alcohol abuse, but psychological, social, and environmental studies have examined other drugs as well.

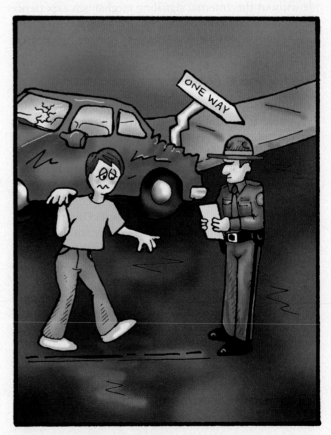

Drugs and alcohol can lead to legal problems

Biologic Factors

Children of alcoholic parents are at higher risk for developing alcoholism and drug dependence than are children of nonalcoholic parents. This increased risk is partly the result of environmental factors, but evidence points to the importance of genetic factors as well. Several studies of twins have shown a higher rate of concordance (when one twin has it, the other twin gets it) among identical than among fraternal twins. Adoption studies have shown higher rates of alcoholism in sons of biologic fathers with alcoholism than in those of nonalcoholic biologic fathers. These studies led theorists to describe the genetic component of alcoholism as a genetic vulnerability that is then influenced by various social and environmental factors (Jaffe & Anthony, 2005). Dick and Beirut (2006) found that 50% to 60% of the variation in causes of alcoholism was the result of genetics, with the remainder caused by environmental influences.

Neurochemical influences on substance use patterns have been studied primarily in animal research (Jaffe & Anthony, 2005). The ingestion of mood-altering substances stimulates dopamine pathways in the limbic system, which produces pleasant feelings or a "high" that is a reinforcing, or positive, experience. Distribution of the substance throughout the brain alters the balance of neurotransmitters that modulate pleasure, pain, and reward responses. Researchers have proposed that some people have an internal alarm that limits the amount of alcohol consumed to one or two drinks, so that they feel a pleasant sensation but go no further. People without this internal signaling mechanism experience the high initially but continue to drink until central nervous system depression is marked and they are intoxicated.

Psychological Factors

In addition to the genetic links to alcoholism, family dynamics are thought to play a part. Children of alcoholics are four times as likely to develop alcoholism (Schuckit, 2005) compared with the general population. Some theorists believe that inconsistency in the parent's behavior, poor role modeling, and lack of nurturing pave the way for the child to adopt a similar style of maladaptive coping, stormy relationships, and substance abuse. Others hypothesize that even children who abhorred their family lives are likely to abuse substances as adults because they lack adaptive coping skills and cannot form successful relationships (NIMH, 2007).

Some people use alcohol as a coping mechanism or to relieve stress and tension, increase feelings of power, and decrease psychological pain. High doses of alcohol, however, actually increase muscle tension and nervousness (Schuckit, 2005).

Social and Environmental Factors

Cultural factors, social attitudes, peer behaviors, laws, cost, and availability all influence initial and continued use of substances (Jaffe & Anthony, 2005). In general, younger experimenters use substances that carry less social disapproval such as alcohol and cannabis, whereas older people use drugs such as cocaine and opioids that are more costly and rate higher disapproval. Alcohol consumption increases in areas where availability increases and decreases in areas where costs of alcohol are higher because of increased taxation. Many people view the social use of cannabis, although illegal, as not very harmful; some even advocate legalizing the use of marijuana for social purposes. Urban areas where cocaine and opioids are readily available also have high crime rates, high unemployment, and substandard school systems that contribute to high rates of cocaine and opioid use and low rates of recovery. Thus, environment and social customs can influence a person's use of substances.

CULTURAL CONSIDERATIONS

Attitudes toward substance use, patterns of use, and physiologic differences to substances vary in different cultures. Muslims do not drink alcohol, but wine is an integral part of Jewish religious rites. Some Native American tribes use peyote, a hallucinogen, in religious ceremonies. It is important to be aware of such beliefs when assessing for a substance abuse problem.

Certain ethnic groups have genetic traits that either predispose them to or protect them from developing alcoholism. For instance, **flushing**, a reddening of the face and neck as a result of increased blood flow, has been linked to variants of genes for enzymes involved in alcohol metabolism. Even small amounts of alcohol can produce flushing, which may be accompanied by headaches and nausea. The flushing reaction is highest among people of Asian ancestry (Wakabayashi & Masuda, 2006).

Another genetic difference between ethnic groups is found in other enzymes involved in metabolizing alcohol in the liver. Variations have been found in the structure and activity levels of the enzymes among Asians, African Americans, and whites. One enzyme found in people of Japanese descent has been associated with faster elimination of alcohol from the body. Other enzyme variations are being studied to determine their effects on the metabolism of alcohol among various ethnic groups (National Institute on Alcohol Abuse and Alcoholism, 2005a).

Statistics for individual tribes vary, but alcohol abuse overall plays a part in the five leading causes of death for Native Americans and Alaska Natives (motor vehicle crashes, alcoholism, cirrhosis, suicide, and homicide). Among tribes with high rates of alcoholism, an estimated 75% of all accidents are alcohol-related (National Institute on Alcohol Abuse and Alcoholism, 2005a). Alaska Natives are 7 times more likely than the general population to die of alcohol-related problems (Malcolm et al., 2006).

In Japan, alcohol consumption has quadrupled since 1960. The Japanese do not regard alcohol as a drug, and there are no religious prohibitions against drinking. Milne (2002) described a traditionally indulgent attitude toward those who drink too much, stating "In a tightly knit society where concealing emotions and frustrations is a highly developed and necessary part of maintaining consensus, getting drunk is a socially sanctioned safety valve" (p. 388).

In Russia, high rates of alcohol abuse, suicide, cigarette smoking, accidents, violence, and cardiovascular disease are found in the male population. Life expectancy for Russian males is 60.5 years, whereas it is 74 years for females. This is a trend mirrored across the entire former Soviet Union (Grogan, 2006).

TYPES OF SUBSTANCES AND TREATMENT

The classes of mood-altering substances have some similarities and differences in terms of intended effect, intoxication effects, and withdrawal symptoms. Treatment approaches after detoxification, however, are quite similar. This section presents a brief overview of seven classes of substances and the effects of intoxication, overdose, withdrawal, and detoxification, and it highlights important elements of which the nurse should be aware.

Alcohol

INTOXICATION AND OVERDOSE

Alcohol is a central nervous system depressant that is absorbed rapidly into the bloodstream. Initially, the effects are relaxation and loss of inhibitions. With intoxication, there is slurred speech, unsteady gait, lack of coordination, and impaired attention, concentration, memory, and judgment. Some people become aggressive or display inappropriate sexual behavior when intoxicated. The person who is intoxicated may experience a blackout.

An overdose, or excessive alcohol intake in a short period, can result in vomiting, unconsciousness, and respiratory depression. This combination can cause aspiration pneumonia or pulmonary obstruction. Alcohol-induced hypotension can lead to cardiovascular shock and death. Treatment of an alcohol overdose is similar to that for any central nervous system depressant: gastric lavage or dialysis to remove the drug and support of respiratory and cardiovascular functioning in an intensive care unit. The administration of central nervous system stimulants is contraindicated (Lehne, 2006). The physiologic effects of repeated intoxication and long-term use are listed in Box 17.1.

WITHDRAWAL AND DETOXIFICATION

Symptoms of withdrawal usually begin 4 to 12 hours after cessation or marked reduction of alcohol intake. Symptoms include coarse hand tremors, sweating, elevated pulse and blood pressure, insomnia, anxiety, and nausea or vomiting. Severe or untreated withdrawal may progress to transient hallucinations, seizures, or delirium—called

Box 17.1	PHYSIOLOGIC EFFECTS OF LONG-TERM ALCOHOL USE

- Cardiac myopathy
- Wernicke's encephalopathy
- Korsakoff's psychosis
- Pancreatitis
- Esophagitis
- Hepatitis
- Cirrhosis
- Leukopenia
- Thrombocytopenia
- Ascites

delirium tremens, or DTs. Alcohol withdrawal usually peaks on the second day and is over in about 5 days (American Psychiatric Association [APA], 2000). This can vary, however, and withdrawal may take 1 to 2 weeks.

Because alcohol withdrawal can be life-threatening, detoxification needs to be accomplished under medical supervision. If the client's withdrawal symptoms are mild and he or she can abstain from alcohol, he or she can be treated safely at home. For more severe withdrawal or for clients who cannot abstain during detoxification, a short admission of 3 to 5 days is the most common setting. Some psychiatric units also admit clients for detoxification, but this is less common.

Safe withdrawal usually is accomplished with the administration of benzodiazepines such as lorazepam (Ativan), chlordiazepoxide (Librium), or diazepam (Valium) to suppress the withdrawal symptoms. Withdrawal can be accomplished by fixed-schedule dosing known as tapering or symptom-triggered dosing in which the presence and severity of withdrawal symptoms determine the amount of medication needed and the frequency of administration. Often, the protocol used is based on an assessment tool such as the Clinical Institute Withdrawal Assessment of Alcohol Scale, Revised, shown in Box 17.2. Total scores less than 8 indicate mild withdrawal; scores from 8 to 15 indicate moderate withdrawal (marked arousal); and scores greater than 15 indicate severe withdrawal. Clients on symptom-triggered dosing receive medication based on scores of this scale alone, whereas clients on fixed-dose tapers also can receive additional doses depending on the level of scores from this scale. Both methods of medicating clients are safe and effective (Bayard et al., 2004).

Sedatives, Hypnotics, and Anxiolytics

INTOXICATION AND OVERDOSE

This class of drugs includes all central nervous system depressants: barbiturates, nonbarbiturate hypnotics, and

Box 17.2   ADDICTION RESEARCH FOUNDATION CLINICAL INSTITUTE
WITHDRAWAL ASSESSMENT FOR ALCOHOL, REVISED (CIWA-AR)

NAUSEA AND VOMITING—Ask "Do you feel sick to your stomach? Have you vomited?" Observation.
0 no nausea and no vomiting
1 mild nausea with no vomiting
2
3
4 intermittent nausea with dry heaves
5
6
7 constant nausea, frequent dry heaves and vomiting

TREMOR—Arms extended and fingers spread apart. Observation.
0 no tremor
1 not visible, but can be felt fingertip to fingertip
2
3
4 moderate, with patient's arms extended
5
6
7 severe, flapping tremors

PAROXYSMAL SWEATS—Observation.
0 no sweat visible
1 barely perceptible sweating, palms moist
2
3
4 beads of sweat obvious on forehead
5
6
7 drenching sweats

ANXIETY—Ask, "Do you feel nervous?" Observation.
0 no anxiety, at ease
1 mildly anxious
2
3
4 moderately anxious, or guarded, so anxiety is inferred
5
6
7 equivalent to acute panic states as seen in severe delirium or acute psychotic reactions

AGITATION—Observation.
0 normal activity
1 somewhat more than normal activity
2
3
4 moderately fidgety and restless
5

6
7 paces back and forth during most of the interview, or constantly thrashes about

TACTILE DISTURBANCES—Ask, "Have you any itching, pins and needles sensations, any burning, any numbness or do you feel bugs crawling on or under your skin?" Observation.
0 none
1 very mild itching, pins and needles, burning or numbness
2 mild itching, pins and needles, burning or numbness
3 moderate itching, pins and needles, burning or numbness
4 moderately severe hallucinations
5 severe hallucinations
6 extremely severe hallucinations
7 continuous hallucinations

AUDITORY DISTURBANCES—Ask, "Are you more aware of sounds around you? Are they harsh? Do they frighten you? Are you hearing anything that is disturbing to you? Are you hearing things you know are not there?" Observation.
0 not present
1 very mild harshness or ability to frighten
2 mild harshness or ability to frighten
3 moderate harshness or ability to frighten
4 moderately severe hallucinations
5 severe hallucinations
6 extremely severe hallucinations
7 continuous hallucinations

VISUAL DISTURBANCES—Ask, "Does the light appear too bright? Is its color different? Does it hurt your eyes? Are you seeing anything that is disturbing to you? Are you seeing things you know are not there?" Observation.
0 not present
1 very mild sensitivity
2 mild sensitivity
3 moderate sensitivity
4 moderately severe hallucinations
5 severe hallucinations
6 extremely severe hallucinations
7 continuous hallucinations

HEADACHE, FULLNESS IN HEAD—Ask, "Does your head feel different? Does it feel like there is a band around your head?" Do not rate for dizziness or lightheadedness. Otherwise, rate severity. Observation.
0 not present
1 very mild
2 mild
3 moderate

continued ⋯⟩

Box 17.2: Addiction Research Foundation Clinical Institute Withdrawal Assessment for Alcohol, Revised (CIWA-AR), cont.

4 moderately severe

5 severe

6 very severe

7 extremely severe

ORIENTATION AND CLOUDING OF SENSORIUM—Ask, "What day is this? Where are you? Who am I?" Observation.

0 oriented and can do serial additions

1 cannot do serial additions or is uncertain about date

2 disoriented for date by no more than 2 calendar days

3 disoriented for date by more than 2 calendar days

4 disoriented for place and/or person

Maximum Possible Score 67

A score of less than 10 usually indicates no need for additional withdrawal medication.

---

anxiolytics, particularly benzodiazepines. Benzodiazepines and barbiturates are the most frequently abused drugs in this category (Ciraulo & Sarid-Segal, 2005). The intensity of the effect depends on the particular drug. The effects of the drugs, symptoms of intoxication, and withdrawal symptoms are similar to those of alcohol. In the usual prescribed doses, these drugs cause drowsiness and reduce anxiety, which is the intended purpose. Intoxication symptoms include slurred speech, lack of coordination, unsteady gait, labile mood, impaired attention or memory, and even stupor and coma.

Benzodiazepines alone, when taken orally in overdose, are rarely fatal, but the person is lethargic and confused. Treatment includes gastric lavage followed by ingestion of activated charcoal and a saline cathartic; dialysis can be used if symptoms are severe (Lehne, 2006). The client's confusion and lethargy improve as the drug is excreted.

Barbiturates, in contrast, can be lethal when taken in overdose. They can cause coma, respiratory arrest, cardiac failure, and death. Treatment in an intensive care unit is required using lavage or dialysis to remove the drug from the system and to support respiratory and cardiovascular function.

WITHDRAWAL AND DETOXIFICATION

The onset of withdrawal symptoms depends on the half-life of the drug (see Chapter 2). Medications such as lorazepam, whose actions typically last about 10 hours, produce withdrawal symptoms in 6 to 8 hours; longer-acting medications such as diazepam may not produce withdrawal symptoms for 1 week (APA, 2000). The withdrawal syndrome is characterized by symptoms that are the opposite of the acute effects of the drug: that is, autonomic hyperactivity (increased pulse, blood pressure, respirations, and temperature), hand tremor, insomnia, anxiety, nausea, and psychomotor agitation. Seizures and hallucinations occur only rarely in severe benzodiazepine withdrawal (Ciraulo & Sarid-Segal, 2005).

Detoxification from sedatives, hypnotics, and anxiolytics is often managed medically by tapering the amount of the drug the client receives over a period of days or weeks, depending on the drug and the amount the client had been using. **Tapering**, or administering decreasing doses of a medication, is essential with barbiturates to prevent coma and death that occur if the drug is stopped abruptly. For example, when tapering the dosage of a benzodiazepine, the client may be given Valium, 10 mg four times a day; the

---

CLINICAL VIGNETTE: DETOXIFICATION

　　John, 62 years old, was admitted 5 AM this morning for an elective knee replacement surgery. The surgical procedure, including the anesthetic, went smoothly. John was stabilized in the recovery room in about 3 hours. His blood pressure was 124/82, temperature 98.8°F, pulse 76, respirations 16. John was alert, oriented, and verbally responsive, so he was transferred to a room on the orthopedic unit.

　　By 10 PM, John is agitated, sweating, and saying, "I have to get out of here!" His blood pressure is 164/98, pulse 98, and

respirations 28. His surgical dressing is dry and intact, and he has no complaints of pain. The nurse talks with John's wife and asks about his usual habits of alcohol consumption. John's wife says he consumes three or four drinks each evening after work and has beer or wine with dinner. John did not report his alcohol consumption to his doctor before surgery. John's wife says, "No one ever asked me about how much he drank, so I didn't think it was important."

dose is decreased every 3 days, and the number of times a day the dose is given also is decreased until the client is safely withdrawn from the drug.

[handwritten margin notes: "C" COKE, DUST, GIRL, TOOT, LINE, NOSE CANDY, SNOW, BLOW, SNEEZE, POWDER, CRACK, ROCK, FLAKE, CAIN, "WHITE LADY", THE LADY, NEUROCAIN]

[handwritten above heading: SPEED, BENNIES, GLASS, CRYSTAL, CRANK, PEP PILLS]

Stimulants (Amphetamines, Cocaine)

Stimulants are drugs that stimulate or excite the central nervous system. Although the *DSM-IV-TR* categorizes amphetamines, cocaine, and central nervous system stimulants separately, the effects, intoxication, and withdrawal symptoms of these drugs are virtually identical. They are grouped together here for this reason.

Stimulants have limited clinical use (with the exception of stimulants used to treat attention deficit hyperactivity disorder; see Chapter 20) and a high potential for abuse. Amphetamines ("uppers") were popular in the past; they were used by people who wanted to lose weight or to stay awake. Cocaine, an illegal drug with virtually no clinical use in medicine, is highly addictive and a popular recreational drug because of the intense and immediate feeling of euphoria it produces.

Methamphetamine is particularly dangerous. It is highly addictive and causes psychotic behavior. Brain damage related to its use is frequent, primarily as a result of the substances used to make it—that is, liquid agricultural fertilizer. The percentage of people admitted to inpatient settings for methamphetamine abuse has increased in 49 of the 50 states in the United States (Substance Abuse and Mental Health Services Administration, 2005).

INTOXICATION AND OVERDOSE

Intoxication from stimulants develops rapidly; effects include the high or euphoric feeling, hyperactivity, hypervigilance, talkativeness, anxiety, grandiosity, hallucinations, stereotypic or repetitive behavior, anger, fighting, and impaired judgment. Physiologic effects include tachycardia, elevated blood pressure, dilated pupils, perspiration or chills, nausea, chest pain, confusion, and cardiac dysrhythmias. Overdoses of stimulants can result in seizures and coma; deaths are rare (Jaffe et al., 2005). Treatment with chlorpromazine (Thorazine), an antipsychotic, controls hallucinations, lowers blood pressure, and relieves nausea (Lehne, 2006).

WITHDRAWAL AND DETOXIFICATION

Withdrawal from stimulants occurs within a few hours to several days after cessation of the drug and is not life-threatening. Marked dysphoria is the primary symptom and is accompanied by fatigue, vivid and unpleasant dreams, insomnia or hypersomnia, increased appetite, and psychomotor retardation or agitation. Marked withdrawal symptoms are referred to as "crashing"; the person may experience depressive symptoms, including suicidal ideation, for several days. Stimulant withdrawal is not treated pharmacologically.

Cannabis (Marijuana)

[handwritten margin notes: POT, WEED, GANJA GRASS, HASHISH, BHANG, REEFER, BOOM, BLUNTS, GANGSTER, SKUN, DANK, HERB]

Cannabis sativa is the hemp plant that is widely cultivated for its fiber used to make rope and cloth and for oil from its seeds. It has become widely known for its psychoactive resin (Hall & Degenhardt, 2005). This resin contains more than 60 substances, called cannabinoids, of which delta-9-tetrahydrocannabinol is thought to be responsible for most of the psychoactive effects. Marijuana refers to the upper leaves, flowering tops, and stems of the plant; hashish is the dried resinous exudate from the leaves of the female plant. Cannabis is most often smoked in cigarettes ("joints"), but it can be eaten.

Cannabis is the most widely used illicit substance in the United States. Research has shown that cannabis has short-term effects of lowering intraocular pressure, but it is not approved for the treatment of glaucoma. It also has been studied for its effectiveness in relieving the nausea and vomiting associated with cancer chemotherapy and the anorexia and weight loss of AIDS. Currently, two cannabinoids, dronabinol (Marinol) and nabilone (Cesamet), have been approved for treating nausea and vomiting from cancer chemotherapy.

INTOXICATION AND OVERDOSE

Cannabis begins to act less than 1 minute after inhalation. Peak effects usually occur in 20 to 30 minutes and last at least 2 to 3 hours. Users report a high feeling similar to that with alcohol, lowered inhibitions, relaxation, euphoria, and increased appetite. Symptoms of intoxication include impaired motor coordination, inappropriate laughter, impaired judgment and short-term memory, and distortions of time and perception. Anxiety, dysphoria, and social withdrawal may occur in some users. Physiologic effects, in addition to increased appetite, include conjunctival injection (bloodshot eyes), dry mouth, hypotension, and tachycardia. Excessive use of cannabis may produce delirium or, rarely, cannabis-induced psychotic disorder, both of which are treated symptomatically. Overdoses of cannabis do not occur (Hall & Degenhardt, 2005).

WITHDRAWAL AND DETOXIFICATION

Although some people have reported withdrawal symptoms of muscle aches, sweating, anxiety, and tremors, no clinically significant withdrawal syndrome is identified (Lehne, 2006).

Opioids

Opioids are popular drugs of abuse because they desensitize the user to both physiologic and psychological pain and induce a sense of euphoria and well-being. Opioid compounds include both potent prescription analgesics such as morphine, meperidine (Demerol), codeine, hydromorphone, oxycodone, methadone, oxymorphone, hydrocodone, and propoxyphene as well as illegal substances such as heroin

[handwritten margin note: HEROIN = SKAG, BLACK TAR, "H", HORSE, SMACK, DOPE, BOY, CHIVA, SKUNK, JUNK, BROWN SUGAR]

and normethadone. People who abuse opioids spend a great deal of their time obtaining the drugs; they often engage in illegal activity to get them. Health care professionals who abuse opioids often write prescriptions for themselves or divert prescribed pain medication for clients to themselves (APA, 2000).

INTOXICATION AND OVERDOSE

Opioid intoxication develops soon after the initial euphoric feeling; symptoms include apathy, lethargy, listlessness, impaired judgment, psychomotor retardation or agitation, constricted pupils, drowsiness, slurred speech, and impaired attention and memory. Severe intoxication or opioid overdose can lead to coma, respiratory depression, pupillary constriction, unconsciousness, and death. Administration of naloxone (Narcan), an opioid antagonist, is the treatment of choice because it reverses all signs of opioid toxicity. Naloxone is given every few hours until the opioid level drops to nontoxic; this process may take days (Lehne, 2006).

WITHDRAWAL AND DETOXIFICATION

Opioid withdrawal develops when drug intake ceases or decreases markedly, or it can be precipitated by the administration of an opioid antagonist. Initial symptoms are anxiety, restlessness, aching back and legs, and cravings for more opioids (Jaffe & Strain, 2005). Symptoms that develop as withdrawal progresses include nausea, vomiting, dysphoria, lacrimation, rhinorrhea, sweating, diarrhea, yawning, fever, and insomnia. Symptoms of opioid withdrawal cause significant distress but do not require pharmacologic intervention to support life or bodily functions. Short-acting drugs such as heroin produce withdrawal symptoms in 6 to 24 hours; the symptoms peak in 2 to 3 days and gradually subside in 5 to 7 days. Longer-acting substances such as methadone may not produce significant withdrawal symptoms for 2 to 4 days, and the symptoms may take 2 weeks to subside. Methadone can be used as a replacement for the opioid, and the dosage is then decreased over 2 weeks. Substitution of methadone during detoxification reduces symptoms to no worse than a mild case of flu (Lehne, 2006). Withdrawal symptoms such as anxiety, insomnia, dysphoria, anhedonia, and drug craving may persist for weeks or months.

Hallucinogens

Hallucinogens are substances that distort the user's perception of reality and produce symptoms similar to psychosis, including hallucinations (usually visual) and depersonalization. Hallucinogens also cause increased pulse, blood pressure, and temperature; dilated pupils; and hyperreflexia. Examples of hallucinogens are mescaline, psilocybin, lysergic acid diethylamide, and "designer drugs" such as Ecstasy. PCP, developed as an anesthetic, is included in this section because it acts similarly to hallucinogens.

[handwritten margin note: ECSTASY = X, XTC, ROLLS, LOVE DRUG, HUG DRUG, CLUB DRUG, DISCO BISCUITS, WHITE DOVES, NEW YORKERS, LOVERS SPEED, MBDB, MDEA, FCB, MDE, MDA]

INTOXICATION AND OVERDOSE

[handwritten margin note: PCP = ANGEL DUST, HOG, OZONE, ROCKET FUEL, CRYSTAL, EMBALMING FLUID, WACK]

Hallucinogen intoxication is marked by several maladaptive behavioral or psychological changes: anxiety, depression, paranoid ideation, ideas of reference, fear of losing one's mind, and potentially dangerous behavior such as jumping out a window in the belief that one can fly (Jones, 2005). Physiologic symptoms include sweating, tachycardia, palpitations, blurred vision, tremors, and lack of coordination. PCP intoxication often involves belligerence, aggression, impulsivity, and unpredictable behavior.

Toxic reactions to hallucinogens (except PCP) are primarily psychological; overdoses as such do not occur. These drugs are not a direct cause of death, although fatalities have occurred from related accidents, aggression, and suicide. Treatment of toxic reactions is supportive. Psychotic reactions are managed best by isolation from external stimuli; physical restraints may be necessary for the safety of the client and others. PCP toxicity can include seizures, hypertension, hyperthermia, and respiratory depression. Medications are used to control seizures and blood pressure. Cooling devices such as hyperthermia blankets are used, and mechanical ventilation is used to support respirations (Lehne, 2006).

WITHDRAWAL AND DETOXIFICATION

No withdrawal syndrome has been identified for hallucinogens, although some people have reported a craving for the drug. Hallucinogens can produce flashbacks, which are transient recurrences of perceptual disturbances like those experienced with hallucinogen use. These episodes occur even after all traces of the hallucinogen are gone and may persist for a few months up to 5 years.

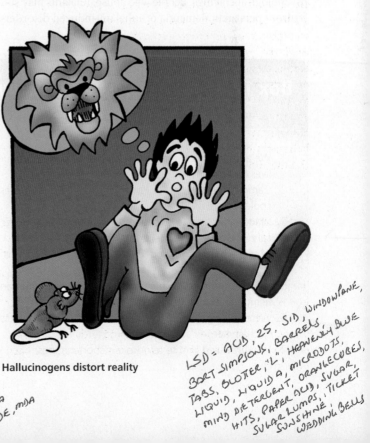

Hallucinogens distort reality

[handwritten margin note: LSD = ACID, 25, SID, WINDOWPANE, BART SIMPSONS, BARRELS, HEAVENLY BLUE, TABS, BLOTTER, "L", MICRODOTS, LIQUID, LIQUID A, MIND DETERGENT, ORANGE CUBES, HITS, PAPER ACID, SUGAR, SUGAR LUMPS, TICKET, SUNSHINE, WEDDING BELLS]

Inhalants = GATEWAY DRUGS   huffing

Inhalants are a diverse group of drugs that includes anesthetics, nitrates, and organic solvents that are inhaled for their effects. The most common substances in this category are aliphatic and aromatic hydrocarbons found in gasoline, glue, paint thinner, and spray paint. Less frequently used halogenated hydrocarbons include cleaners, correction fluid, spray can propellants, and other compounds containing esters, ketones, and glycols (APA, 2000). Most of the vapors are inhaled from a rag soaked with the compound, from a paper or plastic bag, or directly from the container. Inhalants can cause significant brain damage, peripheral nervous system damage, and liver disease.

INTOXICATION AND OVERDOSE

Inhalant intoxication involves dizziness, nystagmus, lack of coordination, slurred speech, unsteady gait, tremor, muscle weakness, and blurred vision. Stupor and coma can occur. Significant behavioral symptoms are belligerence, aggression, apathy, impaired judgment, and inability to function. Acute toxicity causes anoxia, respiratory depression, vagal stimulation, and dysrhythmias. Death may occur from bronchospasm, cardiac arrest, suffocation, or aspiration of the compound or vomitus (Crowley & Sakai, 2005). Treatment consists of supporting respiratory and cardiac functioning until the substance is removed from the body. There are no antidotes or specific medications to treat inhalant toxicity.

WITHDRAWAL AND DETOXIFICATION

There are no withdrawal symptoms or detoxification procedures for inhalants as such, although frequent users report psychological cravings. People who abuse inhalants may suffer from persistent dementia or inhalant-induced disorders such as psychosis, anxiety, or mood disorders even if the inhalant abuse ceases. These disorders are all treated symptomatically (Crowley & Sakai, 2005).

TREATMENT AND PROGNOSIS

Current treatment modalities are based on the concept of alcoholism (and other addictions) as a medical illness that is progressive, chronic, and characterized by remissions and relapses (Jaffe & Anthony, 2005). Until the 1970s, organized treatment programs and clinics for substance abuse were scarce. Before the illness of addiction was fully understood, most of society and even the medical community viewed chemical dependency as a personal problem; the user was advised to "pull yourself together" and "get control of your problem." Founded in 1949, the Hazelden Clinic in Minnesota is the noted exception; because of its success, many programs are based on the Hazelden model of treatment.

Today, treatment for substance use is available in a variety of community settings, not all of which involve health professionals. Alcoholics Anonymous (AA) was founded in the 1930s by alcoholics. This self-help group developed the **12-step program** model for recovery (Box 17.3), which is based on the philosophy that total abstinence is essential and that alcoholics need the help and support of others to maintain sobriety. Key slogans reflect the ideas in the 12 steps, such as "one day at a time" (approach sobriety one day at a time), "easy does it" (don't get frenzied about daily life and problems), and "let go and let God" (turn your life over to a higher power). People who are early in recovery are encouraged to have a sponsor to help them progress through the 12 steps of AA. Once sober, a member can be a sponsor for another person.

Box 17.3 TWELVE STEPS OF ALCOHOLICS ANONYMOUS

1. We admitted we were powerless over alcohol, that our lives had become unmanageable.
2. Came to believe that a Power greater than ourselves could restore us to sanity.
3. Made a decision to turn our wills and lives over to the care of God as we understood Him.
4. Made a searching and fearless moral inventory of ourselves.
5. Admitted to God, to ourselves, and to another human being the exact nature of our wrongs.
6. Were entirely ready to have God remove all these defects of character.
7. Humbly asked Him to remove our shortcomings.
8. Made a list of all persons we had harmed, and became willing to make amends to them all.
9. Made direct amends to such people whenever possible, except when to do so would injure them or others.
10. Continued to take personal inventory and when we were wrong promptly admitted it.
11. Sought through prayer and meditation to improve our conscious contact with God as we understood Him, praying only for knowledge of His will for us and the power to carry that out.
12. Having had a spiritual awakening as a result of these steps, we tried to carry this message to alcoholics and to practice these principles in all our affairs.

Regular attendance at meetings is emphasized. Meetings are available daily in large cities and at least weekly in smaller towns or rural areas. AA meetings may be "closed" (only those who are pursuing recovery can attend) or "open" (anyone can attend). Meetings may be educational with a featured speaker; other meetings focus on a reading, daily meditation, or a theme, and then offer the opportunity for members to relate their battles with alcohol and to ask the others for help staying sober.

Many treatment programs, regardless of setting, use the 12-step approach and emphasize participation in AA. They also include individual counseling and a wide variety of groups. Group experiences involve education about substances and their use, problem-solving techniques, and cognitive techniques to identify and to modify faulty ways of thinking. An overall theme is coping with life, stress, and other people without the use of substances.

Although traditional treatment programs and AA have been successful for many people, they are not effective for everyone. Some object to the emphasis on God and spirituality; others do not respond well to the confrontational approach sometimes used in treatment or to identifying himself or herself as an alcoholic or an addict. Women and minorities have reported feeling overlooked or ignored by an essentially "white, male, middle-class" organization. Treatment programs have developed to meet these needs, such as Women for Sobriety (exclusively for women) and Rainbow Recovery (for gay and lesbian individuals). AA groups may also be designated for women or gay and lesbian people.

The 12-step concept of recovery has been used for other drugs as well. Such groups include Narcotics Anonymous; Al-Anon, a support group for spouses, partners, and friends of alcoholics; and AlaTeen, a group for children of parents with substance problems. This same model has been used in self-help groups for people with gambling problems and eating disorders. National addresses for these groups are listed in Box 17.4.

Treatment Settings and Programs

Clients being treated for intoxication and withdrawal or detoxification are encountered in a wide variety of medical settings from emergency departments to outpatient clinics. Clients needing medically supervised detoxification often are treated on medical units in the hospital setting and then referred to an appropriate outpatient treatment setting when they are medically stable.

Health professionals provide extended or outpatient treatment in various settings, including clinics or centers offering day and evening programs, halfway houses, residential settings, or special chemical dependency units in hospitals. Generally, the type of treatment setting selected is based on the client's needs as well as on his or her insurance coverage. For example, for someone who has limited insurance coverage, is working, and has a supportive family, the outpatient setting may be chosen first because it is less expensive, the client can continue to work, and the family can provide support. If the client cannot remain sober during outpatient treatment, then inpatient treatment may be required. Clients with repeated treatment experiences may need the structure of a halfway house with a gradual transition into the community.

Pharmacologic Treatment

Pharmacologic treatment in substance abuse has two main purposes: to permit safe withdrawal from alcohol, sedative-hypnotics, and benzodiazepines and to prevent relapse. Table 17.1 summarizes drugs used in substance abuse treatment. For clients whose primary substance is alcohol, vitamin B_1 (thiamine) often is prescribed to prevent or to treat Wernicke-Korsakoff syndrome, which are neurologic conditions that can result from heavy alcohol use. Cyanocobalamin (vitamin B_{12}) and folic acid often are prescribed for clients with nutritional deficiencies.

Alcohol withdrawal usually is managed with a benzodiazepine anxiolytic agent, which is used to suppress the

---

Box 17.4   NATIONAL ADDRESSES FOR SELF-HELP GROUPS AND TREATMENT PROGRAMS

Alcoholics Anonymous
PO Box 459, Grand Central Station
New York, NY 10163
1-212-870-3400

Al-Anon Family Group Headquarters, Inc.
1600 Corporate Landing Parkway
Virginia Beach, VA 23454-5617
1-757-563-1600

Women for Sobriety
PO Box 618
Quakertown, PA 18951
1-215-536-8026

Rainbow Recovery Inc.
10833 US Highway 41 South
Gibsonton, FL 33534
1-800-281-5919

Table 17.1   DRUGS USED FOR SUBSTANCE ABUSE TREATMENT

Drug	Use	Dosage	Nursing Considerations
Lorazepam (Ativan)	Alcohol withdrawal	2–4 mg every 2–4 hours PRN	Monitor vital signs and global assessments for effectiveness; may cause dizziness or drowsiness
Chlordiazepoxide (Librium)	Alcohol withdrawal	50–100 mg, repeat in 2–4 hours if necessary; not to exceed 300 mg/day	Monitor vital signs and global assessments for effectiveness; may cause dizziness or drowsiness
Disulfiram (Antabuse)	Maintain abstinence from alcohol	500 mg/day for 1–2 weeks, then 250 mg/day	Teach client to read labels to avoid products with alcohol
Methadone (Dolophine)	Maintain abstinence from heroin	Up to 120 mg/day for maintenance	May cause nausea and vomiting
Levomethadyl (ORLAAM)	Maintain abstinence from opiates	60–90 mg 3 times a week for maintenance	Do not take drug on consecutive days; take-home doses are not permitted
Naltrexone (ReVia, Trexan)	Blocks the effects of opiates; reduces alcohol cravings	350 mg/week, divided into 3 doses for opiate-blocking effect; 50 mg/day for up to 12 weeks for alcohol cravings	Client may not respond to narcotics used to treat cough, diarrhea, or pain; take with food or milk; may cause headache, restlessness, or irritability
Clonidine (Catapres)	Suppresses opiate withdrawal symptoms	0.1 mg every 6 hours PRN	Take blood pressure before each dose; withhold if client is hypotensive
Thiamine (vitamin B_1)	Prevent or treat Wernicke-Korsakoff syndrome in alcoholism	100 mg/day	Teach client about proper nutrition
Folic acid (folate)	Treat nutritional deficiencies	1–2 mg/day	Teach client about proper nutrition; urine may be dark yellow
Cyanocobalamin (vitamin B_{12})	Treat nutritional deficiencies	25–250 mcg/day	Teach client about proper nutrition

symptoms of abstinence. The most commonly used benzo-diazepines are lorazepam, chlordiazepoxide, and diazepam. These medications can be administered on a fixed schedule around the clock during withdrawal. Giving these medications on an as-needed basis according to symptom parameters, however, is just as effective and results in a speedier withdrawal (Lehne, 2006).

Disulfiram (Antabuse) may be prescribed to help deter clients from drinking. If a client taking disulfiram drinks alcohol, a severe adverse reaction occurs with flushing, a throbbing headache, sweating, nausea, and vomiting. In severe cases, severe hypotension, confusion, coma, and even death may result (see Chapter 2). The client also must avoid a wide variety of products that contain alcohol such as cough syrup, lotions, mouthwash, perfume, aftershave, vinegar, and vanilla and other extracts. The client must read product labels carefully because any product containing alcohol can produce symptoms. Ingestion of alcohol may cause unpleasant symptoms for 1 to 2 weeks after the last dose of disulfiram.

Acamprosate (Campral) may be prescribed for clients recovering from alcohol abuse or dependence to help reduce cravings for alcohol and decrease the physical and emotional discomfort that occurs especially in the first few months of recovery. These include sweating, anxiety, and sleep disturbances. The dosage is two tablets (333 mg each) or 666 mg, three times a day. Persons with renal impairment cannot take this drug. Side effects are reported as mild and include diarrhea, nausea, flatulence, and pruritus.

Methadone, a potent synthetic opiate, is used as a substitute for heroin in some maintenance programs. The client takes one daily dose of methadone, which meets the physical need for opiates but does not produce cravings for more. Methadone does not produce the high associated with heroin. The client has essentially substituted his or her addiction to heroin for an addiction to methadone; however, methadone is safer because it is legal, controlled by a physician, and available in tablet form. The client avoids the risks of intravenous drug use, the high cost of heroin (which often leads to criminal acts), and the questionable content of street drugs.

Levomethadyl is a narcotic analgesic whose only purpose is the treatment of opiate dependence. It is used in the same manner as methadone.

Naltrexone (ReVia) is an opioid antagonist often used to treat overdose. It blocks the effects of any opioids that might be ingested, thereby negating the effects of using more opioids. It also has been found to reduce the cravings for alcohol in abstinent clients (O'Brien, 2005).

There are four medications that are sometimes prescribed for the off-label use of decreasing craving for cocaine. They are disulfiram (discussed earlier); modafinil (Provigil), an antinarcoleptic; propranolol (Inderal), a beta-blocker; and topiramate (Topamax), an anticonvulsant also used to stabilize moods and treat migraines.

Clonidine (Catapres) is an alpha-2-adrenergic (α_2-adrenergic) agonist used to treat hypertension. It is given to clients with opiate dependence to suppress some effects of withdrawal or abstinence. It is most effective against nausea, vomiting, and diarrhea but produces modest relief from muscle aches, anxiety, and restlessness (Lehne, 2006).

Ondansetron (Zofran), a 5-HT$_3$ antagonist that blocks the vagal stimulation effects of serotonin in the small intestine, is used as an antiemetic. It has been used in young males at high risk for alcohol dependence or with early-onset alcohol dependence. It is being studied for treatment of methamphetamine addiction.

Dual Diagnosis

The client with both substance abuse and another psychiatric illness is said to have a **dual diagnosis**. Dual diagnosis clients who have schizophrenia, schizoaffective disorder, or bipolar disorder present the greatest challenge to health care professionals. It is estimated that 50% of people with a substance abuse disorder also have a mental health diagnosis (Jaffe & Anthony, 2005). Traditional methods of treatment for major psychiatric illness or primary substance abuse often have little success in these clients for the following reasons:

- Clients with a major psychiatric illness may have impaired abilities to process abstract concepts; this is a major barrier in substance abuse programs.
- Substance use treatment emphasizes avoidance of all psychoactive drugs. This may not be possible for the client who needs psychotropic drugs to treat his or her mental illness.
- The concept of "limited recovery" is more acceptable in the treatment of psychiatric illnesses, but substance abuse has no limited recovery concept.
- The notion of lifelong abstinence, which is central to substance use treatment, may seem overwhelming and impossible to the client who lives "day to day" with a chronic mental illness.

- The use of alcohol and other drugs can precipitate psychotic behavior; this makes it difficult for professionals to identify whether symptoms are the result of active mental illness or substance abuse.

Clients with a dual diagnosis (substance use and mental illness) present challenges that traditional settings cannot meet. Studies of successful treatment and relapse prevention strategies for this population found several key elements that need to be addressed. These include healthy, nurturing, supportive living environments; assistance with fundamental life changes, such as finding a job, abstinent friends; connections with other recovering people; and treatment of their comorbid conditions (Drake et al., 2005). Clients identified the need for stable housing, positive social support, using prayer or relying on a higher power, participation in meaningful activity, eating regularly, getting sufficient sleep, and looking presentable as important components of relapse prevention (Davis & O'Neill, 2005).

APPLICATION OF THE NURSING PROCESS

Identifying people with substance use problems can be difficult. Substance use typically includes the use of defense mechanisms, especially **denial**. Clients may deny directly having any problems or may minimize the extent of problems or actual substance use. In addition, the nurse may encounter clients with substance problems in various settings unrelated to mental health. A client may come to a clinic for treatment of medical problems related to alcohol use, or a client may develop withdrawal symptoms while in the hospital for surgery or an unrelated condition. The nurse must be alert to the possibility of substance use in these situations and be prepared to recognize their existence and to make appropriate referrals.

The Alcohol Use Disorders Identification Test (AUDIT) is a useful screening device to detect hazardous drinking patterns that may be precursors to full-blown substance use disorders (Bohn et al., 1995). This tool (Box 17.5) promotes recognition of problem drinking in the early stage, when resolution without formal treatment is more likely. Early detection and treatment are associated with more positive outcomes.

Detoxification is the initial priority. A nursing care plan for the client in alcohol withdrawal is included at the end of this chapter. Priorities for individual clients are based on their physical needs and may include safety, nutrition, fluids, elimination, and sleep. The remainder of this section focuses on care of the client being treated for substance abuse after detoxification.

Assessment

HISTORY

Clients with a parent or other family members with substance abuse problems may report a chaotic family life, although this is not always the case. They generally describe

Box 17.5 ALCOHOL USE DISORDER IDENTIFICATION TEST (AUDIT)

The following questionnaire will give you an indication of the level of risk associated with your current drinking pattern. To accurately assess your situation, you will need to be honest in your answers. This questionnaire was developed by the World Health Organization and is used in many countries to assist people to better understand their current level of risk in relation to alcohol consumption.

1. How often do you have a drink containing alcohol? (0) Never, (1) Monthly or less, (2) 2 to 4 times a month, (3) 2 to 3 times a week, (4) 4 or more times a week.
2. How many standard drinks do you have on a typical day when you are drinking? (0) 1 or 2, (1) 3 or 4, (2) 5 or 6, (3) 7 to 9, (4) 10 or more.
3. How often do you have six or more drinks on one occasion? (0) Never, (1) Less than monthly, (2) Monthly, (3) Weekly, (4) Daily or almost daily.
4. How often during the last year have you found that you were not able to stop drinking once you had started? (0) Never, (1) Less than monthly, (2) Monthly, (3) Weekly, (4) Daily or almost daily.
5. How often during the past year have you failed to do what was normally expected of you because of drinking? (0) Never, (1) Less than monthly, (2) Monthly, (3) Weekly, (4) Daily or almost daily.
6. How often during the last year have you needed a drink in the morning to get yourself going after a heavy drinking session? (0) Never, (1) Less than monthly, (2) Monthly, (3) Weekly, (4) Daily or almost daily.
7. How often during the last year have you had a feeling of guilt or remorse after drinking? (0) Never, (1) Less than monthly, (2) Monthly, (3) Weekly, (4) Daily or almost daily.
8. How often during the last year have you been unable to remember what happened the night before because you had been drinking? (0) Never, (1) Less than monthly, (2) Monthly, (3) Weekly, (4) Daily or almost daily.
9. Have you or someone else been injured as a result of your drinking? (0) Never, (1) Less than monthly, (2) Monthly, (3) Weekly, (4) Daily or almost daily.
10. Has a relative, a doctor, or other health worker been concerned about your drinking or suggested that you cut down? (0) No, (2) Yes, but not in the last year, (4) Yes, during the last year.

Adapted from Babor, T., de la Fuente, J. R., Saunders, J., et al. (1992). Alcohol Use Disorders Identification Test (AUDIT): Guidelines for use in primary health care. World Health Organization, Geneva. Used with permission. Bohn, Babor, & Kranzler (1995).

CLINICAL VIGNETTE: ALCOHOLISM

Sam, age 38, is married with two children. Sam's father was an alcoholic, and his childhood was chaotic. His father was seldom around for Sam's school activities or family events, and when he was present, his drunken behavior spoiled the occasion. When Sam graduated from high school and left home, he vowed he would never be like his father.

Initially, Sam had many hopes and dreams about becoming an architect and raising a family with love and affection, and he pictured himself as a devoted and loving spouse. But he'd had some bad luck. He got into trouble for underage drinking in college, and his grades slipped because he missed classes after celebrating with his friends. Sam believes life has treated him unfairly—after all, he only has a few beers with friends to relax. Sometimes he overdoes it and he drinks more than he intended—but doesn't everybody? Sam's big plans for the future are on hold.

Today, Sam's boss told him he would be fired if he was late or absent from work in the next 30 days. Sam tells himself that the boss is being unreasonable; after all, Sam is an excellent worker, when he's there. The last straw was when Sam's wife told him she was tired of his drinking and irresponsible behavior. She threatened to leave if Sam did not stop drinking. Her parting words were, "You're just like your father!"

DSM-IV-TR DIAGNOSTIC CRITERIA: SYMPTOMS OF SUBSTANCE ABUSE

- Denial of problems
- Minimizes use of substance
- Rationalization
- Blaming others for problems
- Anxiety
- Irritability
- Impulsivity
- Feelings of guilt and sadness or anger and resentment
- Poor judgment
- Limited insight
- Low self-esteem
- Ineffective coping strategies
- Difficulty expressing genuine feelings
- Impaired role performance
- Strained interpersonal relationships
- Physical problems such as sleep disturbances and inadequate nutrition

Adapted from DSM-IV-TR, 2000.

some crisis that precipitated entry into treatment, such as physical problems or development of withdrawal symptoms while being treated for another condition. Usually, other people such as an employer threatening loss of a job or a spouse or partner threatening loss of a relationship are involved in a client's decision to seek treatment. Rarely do clients decide to seek treatment independently with no outside influence.

GENERAL APPEARANCE AND MOTOR BEHAVIOR

Assessment of general appearance and behavior usually reveals appearance and speech to be normal. Clients may appear anxious, tired, and disheveled if they have just completed a difficult course of detoxification. Depending on their overall health status and any health problems resulting from substance use, clients may appear physically ill. Most clients are somewhat apprehensive about treatment, resent being in treatment, or feel pressured by others to be there. This may be the first time in a long time that clients have had to deal with any difficulty without the help of a psychoactive substance.

MOOD AND AFFECT

Wide ranges of mood and affect are possible. Some clients are sad and tearful, expressing guilt and remorse for their behavior and circumstances. Others may be angry and sarcastic or quiet and sullen, unwilling to talk to the nurse. Irritability is common because clients are newly free of substances. Clients may be pleasant and seemingly happy,

appearing unaffected by the situation, especially if they are still in denial about the substance use.

THOUGHT PROCESS AND CONTENT

During assessment of thought process and content, clients are likely to minimize their substance use, blame others for their problems, and rationalize their behavior. They may believe they cannot survive without the substance or may express no desire to do so. They may focus their attention on finances, legal issues, or employment problems as the main source of difficulty rather than their substance use. They may believe that they could quit "on their own" if they wanted to, and they continue to deny or minimize the extent of the problem.

SENSORIUM AND INTELLECTUAL PROCESSES

Clients generally are oriented and alert unless they are experiencing lingering effects of withdrawal. Intellectual abilities are intact unless clients have experienced neurologic deficits from long-term alcohol use or inhalant use.

JUDGMENT AND INSIGHT

Clients are likely to have exercised poor judgment, especially while under the influence of the substance. Judgment may still be affected: clients may behave impulsively such as leaving treatment to obtain the substance of choice. Insight usually is limited regarding substance use. Clients may have difficulty acknowledging their behavior while using or may not see loss of jobs or relationships as connected to the substance use. They may still believe they can control the substance use.

SELF-CONCEPT

Clients generally have low self-esteem, which they may express directly or cover with grandiose behavior. They do not feel adequate to cope with life and stress without the substance and often are uncomfortable around others when not using. They often have difficulty identifying and expressing true feelings; in the past, they have preferred to escape feelings and to avoid any personal pain or difficulty with the help of the substance.

ROLES AND RELATIONSHIPS

Clients usually have experienced many difficulties with social, family, and occupational roles. Absenteeism and poor work performance are common. Often, family members have told these clients that the substance use was a concern, and it may have been the subject of family arguments. Relationships in the family often are strained. Clients may be angry with family members who were instrumental in bringing them to treatment or who threatened loss of a significant relationship.

PHYSIOLOGIC CONSIDERATIONS

Many clients have a history of poor nutrition (using rather than eating) and sleep disturbances that persist beyond detoxification. They may have liver damage from drinking alcohol, hepatitis or HIV infection from intravenous drug use, or lung or neurologic damage from using inhalants.

Data Analysis

Each client has nursing diagnoses specific to his or her physical health status. These may include the following:

- Imbalanced Nutrition: Less Than Body Requirements
- Risk for Infection
- Risk for Injury
- Diarrhea
- Excess Fluid Volume
- Activity Intolerance
- Self-Care Deficits

Nursing diagnoses commonly used when working with clients with substance use include the following:

- Ineffective Denial
- Ineffective Role Performance
- Dysfunctional Family Processes: Alcoholism
- Ineffective Coping

Outcome Identification

Treatment outcomes for clients with substance use may include the following:

- The client will abstain from alcohol and drug use.
- The client will express feelings openly and directly.
- The client will verbalize acceptance of responsibility for his or her own behavior.
- The client will practice nonchemical alternatives to deal with stress or difficult situations.
- The client will establish an effective after-care plan.

Intervention

PROVIDING HEALTH TEACHING FOR CLIENT AND FAMILY

Clients and family members need facts about the substance, its effects, and recovery. The nurse must dispel the following myths and misconceptions:

- "It's a matter of will power."
- "I can't be an alcoholic if I only drink beer or if I only drink on weekends."
- "I can learn to use drugs socially."
- "I'm okay now; I could handle using once in a while."

Education about relapse is important. Family members and friends should be aware that clients who begin to revert to old behaviors, return to substance-using acquaintances, or believe they can "handle myself now" are at high risk for relapse, and loved ones need to take action. Whether a client plans to attend a self-help group or has other resources, a specific plan for continued support and involvement after treatment increases the client's chances for recovery.

ADDRESSING FAMILY ISSUES

Alcoholism (and other substance abuse) often is called a family illness. All those who have a close relationship with a person who abuses substances suffer emotional, social, and sometimes physical anguish.

Codependence is a maladaptive coping pattern on the part of family members or others that results from a prolonged relationship with the person who uses substances. Characteristics of codependence are poor relationship skills, excessive anxiety and worry, compulsive behaviors, and resistance to change. Family members learn these dysfunctional behavior patterns as they try to adjust to the behavior of the substance user. One type of codependent behavior is called enabling, which is a behavior that seems helpful on the surface but actually perpetuates the substance use. For example, a wife who continually calls in to report that her husband is sick when he is really drunk or hung-over prevents the husband from having to face the true implications and repercussions of his behavior. What appears to be a helpful action really just assists the husband to avoid the consequences of his behavior and to continue abusing the substance.

Roles may shift dramatically, such as when a child actually looks out for or takes care of a parent. Codependent behaviors also have been identified in health care professionals when they make excuses for a client's behavior or do things for clients that clients can do for themselves.

An adult child of an alcoholic is someone who was raised in a family in which one or both parents were addicted to alcohol and who has been subjected to the many dysfunctional aspects associated with parental alcoholism. In addition to being at high risk for alcoholism and eating disorders, children of alcoholics often develop an inability to trust, an extreme need to control, an excessive sense of responsibility, and denial of feelings; these characteristics persist into adulthood. Many people growing up in homes with parental alcoholism believe their problems will be solved when they are old enough to leave and escape the situation. They may begin to have problems in relationships, low self-esteem, and excessive fears of abandonment or insecurity as adults (Kelley et al., 2005). Never having experienced normal family life, they may find that they do not know what "normal" is.

Without support and help to understand and cope, many family members may develop substance abuse problems of their own, thus perpetuating the dysfunctional cycle. Treatment and support groups are available to address the issues of family members. Clients and family also need information about support groups, their purpose, and their locations in the community.

PROMOTING COPING SKILLS

Nurses can encourage clients to identify problem areas in their lives and to explore the ways that substance use may have intensified those problems. Clients should not believe that all life's problems will disappear with sobriety; rather, sobriety will assist them to think about the problems clearly. The nurse may need to redirect a client's attention to his or her behavior and how it influenced his or her problems. The nurse should not allow clients to focus on external events or other people without discussing their role in the problem.

tion, successful treatment should result in more stable role performance, improved interpersonal relationships, and increased satisfaction with quality of life.

ELDER CONSIDERATIONS

Onset of initial drinking problems after the age of 50 years is not uncommon (Atkinson, 2004). Some elders with alcohol use problems are those who had a drinking problem early in life, had a significant period of abstinence, and then resumed drinking again in later life. Others may have been heavy or reactive consumers of alcohol early in life. However, estimates are that 30% to 60% of elders in treatment programs began drinking abusively after age 60.

Risk factors for late-onset substance abuse in elders include chronic illness that causes pain, long-term use of prescription medication (sedative-hypnotics, anxiolytics), life stress, loss, social isolation, grief, depression, and an abundance of discretionary time and money (Atkinson, 2004). Elders may experience physical problems associated with substance abuse rather quickly, especially if their overall medical health is compromised by other illnesses.

COMMUNITY-BASED CARE

Many people receiving treatment for substance abuse do so in community-based settings such as outpatient treatment, freestanding substance abuse treatment facilities, and recovery programs such as AA and Rational Recovery. Follow-up or after-care for clients in the community is based on the client's preferences or the programs available. Some clients remain active in self-help groups. Others attend after-care program sessions sponsored by the agency where they completed treatment. Still others seek individual or family counseling. In addition to formal after-care, the nurse also may encounter recovering clients in clinics or physicians' offices.

CLIENT/FAMILY EDUCATION FOR SUBSTANCE ABUSE

- Substance abuse is an illness.
- Dispel myths about substance abuse.
- Abstinence from substances is not a matter of willpower.
- Any alcohol, whether beer, wine, or liquor, can be an abused substance.
- Prescribed medication can be an abused substance.
- Feedback from family about relapse signs, e.g., a return to previous maladaptive coping mechanisms, is vital.
- Continued participation in an after-care program is important.

Nurse: *"Can you describe some problems you've been having?"*
Client: *"My wife is always nagging—nothing is ever good enough—so we don't get along very well."*
Nurse: *"How do you communicate with your wife?"*
Client: *"I can't talk to her about anything; she won't listen."*
Nurse: *"Are you saying that you don't talk to her very much?"*

It may be helpful to role-play situations that clients have found difficult. This is also an opportunity to help clients learn to solve problems or to discuss situations with others calmly and more effectively. In the group setting in treatment, it is helpful to encourage clients to give and to receive feedback about how others perceive their interaction or ability to listen.

The nurse also can help clients to find ways to relieve stress or anxiety that do not involve substance use. Relaxing, exercising, listening to music, or engaging in activities may be effective. Clients also may need to develop new social activities or leisure pursuits if most of their friends or habits of socializing involved the use of substances.

The nurse can help clients to focus on the present, not the past. It is not helpful for clients to dwell on past problems and regrets. Rather, they must focus on what they can do now regarding their behavior or relationships. Clients may need support from the nurse to view life and sobriety in feasible terms—taking it one day at a time. The nurse can encourage clients to set attainable goals such as, "What can I do today to stay sober?" instead of feeling overwhelmed by thinking "How can I avoid substances for the rest of my life?" Clients need to believe that they can succeed.

Evaluation

The effectiveness of substance abuse treatment is based heavily on the client's abstinence from substances. In addi-

---

NURSING INTERVENTIONS FOR SUBSTANCE ABUSE

- Health teaching for the client and family
- Dispel myths surrounding substance abuse
- Decrease codependent behaviors among family members
- Make appropriate referrals for family members
- Promote coping skills
- Role-play potentially difficult situations
- Focus on the here-and-now with clients
- Set realistic goals such as staying sober today

MENTAL HEALTH PROMOTION

A person only has to watch television or read a magazine to see many advertisements targeted at the promotion of responsible drinking or encouraging parents to be an "antidrug" for their children. Increasing public awareness and educational advertising have not made any significant change in the rates of substance abuse in the United States (National Institute for Mental Health, 2005b). Two populations currently identified for prevention programs are older adults and college-aged adults.

Menninger (2002) described drinking problems among older adults as falling into two distinct patterns: early-onset alcoholism (two thirds), which includes those clients who have been drinking all their lives; and late-onset alcoholism (one third), which includes those clients who develop alcoholism late in life. Late-onset alcoholism is usually milder and more amenable to treatment, yet health care professionals overlook it more frequently. Menninger suggested use of a screening tool such as AUDIT in all primary care settings to promote early identification of older adults with alcoholism. He believed that brief intervention at an early stage will arrest or prevent the development of late-onset alcoholism in this population.

The College Drinking Prevention Program, which is government sponsored, is a response to some of the following statistics about college students between 18 and 24 years of age (National Institute on Alcohol Abuse and Alcoholism, 2005b):

- 1700 students die annually from alcohol-related unintentional injuries.
- 599,000 students are unintentionally injured while under the influence of alcohol.
- 606,000 students are assaulted by another student under the influence of alcohol.
- 97,000 students are victims of alcohol-related assault or date rape.
- One third of first-year students fail to enroll for their second year.

This prevention program was designed to help college students avoid the "predictable" or expected binge drinking common at U.S. colleges and universities. Some campuses offer alcohol and drug-free dormitories for students, and some college-wide activities no longer allow alcohol to be served. Educational programs (about the previous statistics) are designed to raise student awareness about excessive drinking. Students who wish to abstain from alcohol are encouraged to socialize together and to provide support to one another for this lifestyle choice.

SUBSTANCE ABUSE IN HEALTH PROFESSIONALS

Physicians, dentists, and nurses have far higher rates of dependence on **controlled substances** such as opioids, stimulants, and sedatives than other professionals of comparable educational achievement such as lawyers. One reason is thought to be the ease of obtaining controlled substances (Jaffe & Anthony, 2005). Health care professionals also have higher rates of alcoholism than the general population.

The issue of reporting colleagues with suspected substance abuse is an important and extremely sensitive one. It is difficult for colleagues and supervisors to report their peers for suspected abuse. Nurses may hesitate to report suspected behaviors for several reasons: They have difficulty believing that a trained health care professional would engage in abuse; they may feel guilty or fear falsely accusing someone; or they may simply want to avoid conflict. Substance abuse by health professionals is very serious, however, because it can endanger clients. Nurses have an ethical responsibility to report suspicious behavior to a supervisor and, in some states, a legal obligation as defined in the state's nurse practice act. Nurses should not try to handle such situations alone by warning the coworker; this often just allows the coworker to continue to abuse the substance without suffering any repercussions.

General warning signs of abuse include poor work performance, frequent absenteeism, unusual behavior, slurred speech, and isolation from peers. More specific behaviors and signs that might indicate substance abuse include the following:

- Incorrect drug counts
- Excessive controlled substances listed as wasted or contaminated
- Reports by clients of ineffective pain relief from medications, especially if relief had been adequate previously
- Damaged or torn packaging on controlled substances
- Increased reports of "pharmacy error"
- Consistent offers to obtain controlled substances from pharmacy
- Unexplained absences from the unit
- Trips to the bathroom after contact with controlled substances
- Consistent early arrivals at or late departures from work for no apparent reason

Nurses can become involved in substance abuse just as any other person might. Nurses with abuse problems deserve the opportunity for treatment and recovery as well. Reporting suspected substance abuse could be the crucial first step toward a nurse getting the help he or she needs.

SELF-AWARENESS ISSUES

The nurse must examine his or her beliefs and attitudes about substance abuse. A history of substance use in the nurse's family can influence strongly his or her interaction with clients. The nurse may be overly harsh and critical, telling the client that he or she should "realize how you're hurting your family." Conversely, the nurse may unknowingly act out old family roles and engage in enabling behavior such as sympathizing with the client's reasons for using substances. Examining one's own substance use or the use by close friends and family may be difficult and unpleasant but is necessary if the nurse is to have therapeutic relationships with clients.

The nurse also might have different attitudes about various substances of abuse. For example, a nurse may have empathy for clients who are addicted to prescription medication but disgusted by clients who use heroin or other illegal substances. It is important to remember that the treatment process and underlying issues of substance abuse, remission, and relapse are quite similar regardless of the substance.

Many clients experience periodic relapses. For some, being sober is a lifelong struggle. The nurse may become cynical or pessimistic when clients return for multiple attempts at substance use treatment. Such thoughts as "he deserves health problems if he keeps drinking" or "she should expect to get hepatitis or HIV infection if she keeps doing intravenous drugs" are signs that the nurse has some self-awareness problems that prevent him or her from working effectively with clients and their families.

Points to Consider When Working With Clients and Families With Substance Abuse Problems

- Remember that substance abuse is a chronic, recurring disease for many people, just like diabetes or heart disease. Even though clients look like they should be able to control their substance abuse easily, they cannot without assistance and understanding.
- Examine substance abuse problems in your own family and friends even though it may be painful. Recognizing your own background, beliefs, and attitudes is the first step toward managing those feelings effectively so that they do not interfere with the care of clients and families.
- Approach each treatment experience with an open and objective attitude. The client may be successful in maintaining abstinence after his or her second or third (or more) treatment experience.

Nursing Care Plan *Dual Diagnosis*

Nursing Diagnosis

Ineffective Coping: *Inability to form a valid appraisal of the stressors, inadequate choices of practiced responses, and/or inability to use available resources.*

ASSESSMENT DATA

- Poor impulse control
- Low self-esteem
- Lack of social skills
- Dissatisfaction with life circumstances
- Lack of purposeful daily activity

EXPECTED OUTCOMES

Immediate
The client will
- Take only prescribed medication
- Interact appropriately with staff and other clients
- Express feelings openly
- Develop plans to manage unstructured time

Stabilization
The client will
- Demonstrate appropriate or adequate social skills
- Identify social activities in drug- and alcohol-free environments
- Assess own strengths and weaknesses realistically

Community
The client will
- Maintain contact or relationship with a professional in the community
- Verbalize plans to join a community support group that meets the needs of clients with a dual diagnosis, if available
- Participate in drug- and alcohol-free programs and activities

continued ⋯⟶

Nursing Care Plan: Dual Diagnosis, cont.

IMPLEMENTATION

Nursing Interventions *denotes collaborative interventions	**Rationale**
Encourage open expression of feelings.	Verbalizing feelings is an initial step toward dealing constructively with those feelings.
Validate the client's frustration or anger in dealing with dual problems (e.g., "I know this must be very difficult.").	Expressing feelings outwardly, especially negative ones, may relieve some of the client's stress and anxiety.
Consider alcohol or substance use as a factor that influences the client's ability to live in the community, similar to such factors as taking medications, keeping appointments, and so forth.	Substance use is not necessarily the major problem the client with a dual diagnosis experiences, only one of several problems. Overemphasis on any single factor does not guarantee success.
Maintain frequent contact with the client, even if it is only brief telephone calls.	Frequent contact decreases the length of time the client feels "stranded" or left alone to deal with problems.
Give positive feedback for abstinence on a day-by-day basis.	Positive feedback reinforces abstinent behavior.
If drinking or substance use occurs, discuss the events that led to the incident with the client in a nonjudgmental manner.	The client may be able to see the relatedness of the events or a pattern of behavior while discussing the situation.
Discuss ways to avoid similar circumstances in the future.	Anticipatory planning may prepare the client to avoid similar circumstances in the future.
Assess the amount of unstructured time with which the client must cope.	The client is more likely to experience frustration or dissatisfaction, which can lead to substance use, when he or she has excessive amounts of unstructured time.
Assist the client to plan daily or weekly schedules of purposeful activities: errands, appointments, taking walks, and so forth.	Scheduled events provide the client with something to anticipate or look forward to doing.
Writing the schedule on a calendar may be beneficial.	Visualization of the schedule provides a concrete reference for the client.
Encourage the client to record activities, feelings, and thoughts in a journal.	A journal can provide a focus for the client and yield information that is useful in future planning but may otherwise be forgotten or overlooked.
Teach the client social skills. Describe and demonstrate specific skills, such as eye contact, attentive listening, nodding, and so forth. Discuss the kind of topics that are appropriate for social conversation, such as the weather, news, local events, and so forth.	The client may have little or no knowledge of social interaction skills. Modeling the skills provides a concrete example of the desired skills.
Give positive support to the client for appropriate use of social skills.	Positive feedback will encourage the client to continue socialization attempts and enhance self-esteem.
*Refer the client to volunteer or vocational services if indicated.	Purposeful activity makes better use of the client's unstructured time and can enhance the client's feelings of worth and self-esteem.
*Refer the client to community support services that address mental health and substance dependence-related needs.	Clients with dual diagnosis have complicated and long-term problems that require ongoing, extended assistance.

Adapted from Schultz, J. M., & Videbeck, S. L. (2005). Lippincott's manual of psychiatric nursing care plans (7th ed). Philadelphia: Lippincott Williams & Wilkins.

INTERNET RESOURCES

RESOURCE	INTERNET ADDRESS
• Al-Anon/Alateen	http://www.al-anon.org
• Alcoholics Anonymous	http://www.alcoholics-anonymous.org
• Alcoholics Anonymous Meetings Database	http://www.meetingfinder.org
• Center for Substance Abuse Treatment	http://www.samhsa.gov/csat/csat.html
• Narcotics Anonymous	http://www.na.org
• National Council on Alcoholism and Drug Dependence	http://www.ncadd.org
• National Institute of Mental Health	http://nimh.nih.gov
• National Institute on Alcohol Abuse and Alcoholism	http://www.niaaa.nih.gov
• Online AA Recovery Resources	http://www.recovery.org/aa
• Women for Sobriety	http://www.womenforsobriety.org

Critical Thinking Questions

1. You discover that another nurse on your hospital unit has taken Valium from a client's medication supply. You confront the nurse, and she replies, "I'm under a lot of stress at home. I've never done anything like this before, and I promise it will never happen again." What should you do, and why?

2. In England, medical clinics provide daily doses of drugs such as heroin at no charge to persons who are addicted in efforts to decrease illegal drug traffic and lower crime rates. Is this an effective method? Would you advocate trying this in the United States? Why or why not?

KEY POINTS

- Substance use and substance-related disorders can involve alcohol, stimulants, cannabis, opioids, hallucinogens, inhalants, sedatives, hypnotics, anxiolytics, caffeine, and nicotine.
- Substance use and dependence include major impairment in the user's social and occupational functioning and behavioral and psychological changes.
- Alcohol is the substance abused most often in the United States; cannabis is second.
- Intoxication is the use of a substance that results in maladaptive behavior.
- *Withdrawal syndrome* is defined as negative psychological and physical reactions when use of a substance ceases or dramatically decreases.
- Detoxification is the process of safely withdrawing from a substance. Detoxification from alcohol and barbiturates can be life-threatening and requires medical supervision.

- The most significant risk factors for alcoholism are having an alcoholic parent, genetic vulnerability, and growing up in an alcoholic home.
- Routine screening with tools such as the AUDIT in a wide variety of settings (clinics, physicians' offices, through emergency services) can be used to detect substance use problems.
- After detoxification, treatment of substance use continues in various outpatient and inpatient settings. Approaches often are based on the 12-step philosophy of abstinence, altered lifestyles, and peer support.
- Substance abuse is a family illness, meaning that it affects all members in some way. Family members and close friends need education and support to cope with their feelings toward the abuser. Many support groups are available to family members and close friends.
- Clients who are dually diagnosed with substance use problems and major psychiatric illness do poorly in traditional treatment settings and need specialized attention.
- Nursing interventions for clients being treated for substance abuse include teaching clients and families about substance abuse, dealing with family issues, and helping clients to learn more effective coping skills.
- Health care professionals have increased rates of substance use problems, particularly involving opioids, stimulants, and sedatives. Reporting suspected substance abuse in colleagues is an ethical (and sometimes legal) responsibility of all health care professionals.

REFERENCES

American Psychiatric Association. (2000). *Diagnostic and statistical manual of mental disorders* (4th ed., text revision). Washington, DC: American Psychiatric Association.

Atkinson, R. M. (2004). Substance abuse. In J. Sadavoy, L. F. Jarvik, G. T. Greenberg, et al. (Eds.), *Comprehensive textbook of geriatric psychiatry* (3rd ed., pp. 723–761). New York: W. W. Norton and Company.

Bayard, M., McIntyre, J., Hill, K. R., & Woodside, J., Jr. (2004). Alcohol withdrawal syndrome. *American Family Physician, 69*(6), 1443–1450.

Bischof, G., Rumpf, H. J., Meyer, C., et al. (2005). Influence of psychiatric comorbidity in alcohol-dependent subjects in a representative population survey on treatment utilization and natural recovery. *Addiction, 100*(3), 405–413.

Bohn, M. J., Babor, T. F., & Kranzler, H. R. (1995). The alcohol use disorder identification test (AUDIT): Validation of a screening instrument for use in medical settings. *Journal of Studies on Alcohol, 56*(4), 423–432.

Ciraulo, D. A., & Sarid-Segal, O. (2005). Sedative-, hypnotic- or anxiolytic-related abuse. In B. J. Sadock & V. A. Sadock (Eds.), *Comprehensive textbook of psychiatry* (Vol. 1, 8th ed., pp. 1300–1318). Philadelphia: Lippincott Williams & Wilkins.

Crowley, T. J., & Sakai, J. (2005). Inhalant-related disorders. In B. J. Sadock & V. A. Sadock (Eds.), *Comprehensive textbook of psychiatry* (Vol. 1, 8th ed., pp. 1247–1257). Philadelphia: Lippincott Williams & Wilkins.

Davis, K. E., & O'Neill, S. J. (2005). A focus group analysis of relapse prevention strategies for persons with substance use and mental disorders. *Psychiatric Services, 56*(10), 1288–1291.

Dick, D. M., & Bierut, L. J. (2006). The genetics of alcohol dependence. *Current Psychiatry Reports, 8*(2), 151–157.

Drake, R. E., Wallach, M. A., & McGovern, M. P. (2005). Future directions in preventing relapse to substance abuse among clients with severe mental illness. *Psychiatric Services, 56*(10), 1297–1302.

Grogan, L. (2006). Alcoholism, tobacco and drug use in the countries of central and eastern Europe and the former Soviet Union. *Substance Use & Misuse, 41*(4), 567–571.

Hall, W., & Degenhardt, L. (2005). Cannabis-related disorders. In B. J. Sadock & V. A. Sadock (Eds.), *Comprehensive textbook of psychiatry* (Vol. 1, 8th ed., pp. 1211–1220). Philadelphia: Lippincott Williams & Wilkins.

Jaffe, J. H., & Anthony, J. C. (2005). Substance-related disorders: Introduction and overview. In B. J. Sadock & V. A. Sadock (Eds.), *Comprehensive textbook of psychiatry* (Vol. 1, 8th ed., pp. 1137–1168). Philadelphia: Lippincott Williams & Wilkins.

Jaffe, J. H., Ling, W., & Rawson, R. A. (2005). Amphetamine (or amphetamine-like) related disorders. In B. J. Sadock & V. A. Sadock (Eds.), *Comprehensive textbook of psychiatry* (Vol. 1, 8th ed., pp. 1188–1201). Philadelphia: Lippincott Williams & Wilkins.

Jaffe, J. H., & Strain, E. C. (2005). Opioid-related disorders. In B. J. Sadock & V. A. Sadock (Eds.), *Comprehensive textbook of psychiatry* (Vol. 1, 8th ed., pp. 1265–1291). Philadelphia: Lippincott Williams & Wilkins.

Jones, R. T. (2005). Hallucinogen-related disorders. In B. J. Sadock & V. A. Sadock (Eds.), *Comprehensive textbook of psychiatry* (Vol. 1, 8th ed., pp. 1238–1247). Philadelphia: Lippincott Williams & Wilkins.

Kelley, M. L., Nair, V., Rawlings, T., et al. (2005). Retrospective reports of parenting received in their families of origin: Relationships to adult attachment in adult children of alcoholics. *Addictive Behaviors, 30*(8), 1479–1495.

Lehne, R. A. (2006). *Pharmacology for nursing care* (6th ed.). Philadelphia: W. B. Saunders.

Malcolm, B. P., Hesselbrock, M. N., Segal, B. (2006). Multiple substance dependence and course of alcoholism among Alaska native men and women. *Substance Use & Misuse, 41*(5), 729–741.

Menninger, J. A. (2002). Assessment and treatment of alcoholism and substance-related disorders in the elderly. *Bulletin of the Menninger Clinic, 66*(2), 166–183.

Milne, D. (2002). Alcohol consumption in Japan. *Canadian Medical Association Journal, 167*(4), 388.

Narconon. (2005). Alcohol statistics. Available: http://www.usnodrugs.com/alcohol-statistics.htm.

National Institute on Alcohol Abuse and Alcoholism. (2007). A family history of alcoholism. Available: http://www.pubs.niaaa.nih.gov/publications/FamilyHistory/famhist.htm.

National Institute on Alcohol Abuse and Alcoholism. (2005a). *Alcohol and minorities.* Available: http://www.niaaa.nih.gov/.

National Institute on Alcohol Abuse and Alcoholism. (2005b). A snapshot of high-risk college drinking consequences. Available: http://www.collegedrinkingprevention.gov.

O'Brien, C. P. (2005). Anticraving medications for relapse prevention: A possible new class of psychoactive medications. *American Journal of Psychiatry, 162*(8), 1423–1431.

Schuckit, M. A. (2005). Alcohol-related disorders. In B. J. Sadock & V. A. Sadock (Eds.), *Comprehensive textbook of psychiatry* (Vol. 1, 8th ed., pp. 1168–1188). Philadelphia: Lippincott Williams & Wilkins.

Substance Abuse and Mental Health Services Administration. (2005). Statistics for alcoholism and drug dependency. United States Department of Health and Human Services. Available: http://www.oas.samhsa.gov.

Wakabayashi, I., & Masuda, H. (2006). Influence of drinking alcohol on atherosclerotic risk in alcohol flushers and non-flushers of Oriental patients with type 2 diabetes mellitus. *Alcohol and Alcoholism, 41*(6), 672–677.

ADDITIONAL READINGS

Javitt, D., & Zukin, S. R. (2005). Phencyclidine (or phencyclidine-like) related disorders. In B. J. Sadock & V. A. Sadock (Eds.), *Comprehensive textbook of psychiatry* (Vol. 1, 8th ed., pp. 1291–1300). Philadelphia: Lippincott Williams & Wilkins.

Jersild, D. (2002). Alcohol in the vulnerable lives of college women. *Chronicle of Higher Education, 48*(38), B10–B11.

Rajemdram R., Lewison, G., & Preedy, V. R. (2006). Worldwide alcohol-related research and the disease burden. *Alcohol and Alcoholism, 41*(1), 99–106.

Stolberg, V. B. (2006). A review of perspectives on alcohol and alcoholism in the history of American health and medicine. *Journal of Ethnicity in Substance Abuse, 5*(4), 39–106.

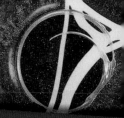

Chapter Study Guide

MULTIPLE-CHOICE QUESTIONS

Select the best answer for each of the following questions.

1. Which of the following statements would indicate that teaching about naltrexone (ReVia) has been effective?
   A. "I'll get sick if I use heroin while taking this medication."
   B. "This medication will block the effects of any opioid substance I take."
   C. "If I use opioids while taking naltrexone, I'll become extremely ill."
   D. "Using naltrexone may make me dizzy."

2. Clonidine (Catapres) is prescribed for symptoms of opioid withdrawal. Which of the following nursing assessments is essential before giving a dose of this medication?
   A. Assess the client's blood pressure.
   B. Determine when the client last used an opiate.
   C. Monitor the client for tremors.
   D. Complete a thorough physical assessment.

3. Which of the following would the nurse recognize as signs of alcohol withdrawal?
   A. Coma, disorientation, and hypervigilance
   B. Tremulousness, sweating, and elevated blood pressure
   C. Increased temperature, lethargy, and hypothermia
   D. Talkativeness, hyperactivity, and blackouts

4. Which of the following behaviors would indicate stimulant intoxication?
   A. Slurred speech, unsteady gait, impaired concentration
   B. Hyperactivity, talkativeness, euphoria
   C. Relaxed inhibitions, increased appetite, distorted perceptions
   D. Depersonalization, dilated pupils, visual hallucinations

5. The 12 Steps of AA teach that
   A. Acceptance of being an alcoholic will prevent urges to drink.
   B. A Higher Power will protect individuals if they feel like drinking.
   C. Once a person has learned to be sober, he or she can graduate and leave AA.
   D. Once a person is sober, he or she remains at risk to drink.

6. The nurse has provided an in-service program on impaired professionals. She knows that teaching has been effective when staff identify the following as the greatest risk for substance abuse among professionals:
   A. Most nurses are codependent in their personal and professional relationships.
   B. Most nurses come from dysfunctional families and are at risk for developing addiction.
   C. Most nurses are exposed to various substances and believe they are not at risk to develop the disease.
   D. Most nurses have preconceived ideas about what kind of people become addicted.

7. A client comes to day treatment intoxicated, but says he is not. The nurse identifies that the client is exhibiting symptoms of
   A. Denial
   B. Reaction formation
   C. Projection
   D. Transference

8. The client tells the nurse that she takes a drink every morning to calm her nerves and stop her tremors. The nurse realizes the client is at risk for
   A. An anxiety disorder
   B. A neurologic disorder
   C. Physical dependence
   D. Psychological addiction

FILL-IN-THE-BLANK QUESTIONS

Give two examples of drugs for each of the following categories.

_____ Stimulants

_____ Opioids

_____ Hallucinogens

_____ Inhalants

SHORT-ANSWER QUESTIONS

1. List four behaviors that might lead the nurse to suspect another health care professional of substance abuse.

2. Explain the concept of tapering medications during detoxification.

CLINICAL EXAMPLE

Sharon, 43 years of age, is attending an outpatient treatment program for alcohol abuse. She is divorced, and her two children live with their father. Sharon broke up with her boyfriend of 3 years just last week. She recently was arrested for the second time for driving while intoxicated, which is why she is in this treatment program. Sharon tells anyone who will listen that she is "not an alcoholic" but is in this program only to avoid serving time in jail.

1. Identify two nursing diagnoses for Sharon.

2. Write an expected outcome for each identified diagnosis.

3. List three interventions for each of the diagnoses.

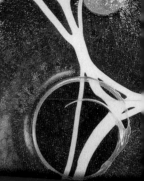

Key Terms

- alexithymia
- anorexia nervosa
- binge eating
- body image
- body image disturbance
- bulimia nervosa
- enmeshment
- purging
- satiety
- self-monitoring

Learning Objectives

After reading this chapter, you should be able to

1. Compare and contrast the symptoms of anorexia nervosa and bulimia nervosa.

2. Discuss various etiologic theories of eating disorders.

3. Identify effective treatment for clients with eating disorders.

4. Apply the nursing process to the care of clients with eating disorders.

5. Provide teaching to clients, families, and community members to increase knowledge and understanding of eating disorders.

6. Evaluate your feelings, beliefs, and attitudes about clients with eating disorders.

Eating is part of everyday life. It is necessary for survival, but it is also a social activity and part of many happy occasions. People go out for dinner, invite friends and family for meals in their homes, and celebrate special events such as marriages, holidays, and birthdays with food. Yet for some people, eating is a source of worry and anxiety. Are they eating too much? Do they look fat? Is some new weight loss promotion going to be the answer?

Obesity has been identified as a major health problem in the United States; some call it an epidemic. The number of obesity-related illnesses among children has increased dramatically. At the same time, millions of women are either starving themselves or engaging in chaotic eating patterns that can lead to death.

This chapter focuses on anorexia nervosa and bulimia nervosa, the two most common eating disorders found in the mental health setting. It discusses strategies for early identification and prevention of these disorders.

OVERVIEW OF EATING DISORDERS

Although many believe that eating disorders are relatively new, documentation from the Middle Ages indicates willful dieting leading to self-starvation in female saints who fasted to achieve purity. In the late 1800s, doctors in England and France described young women who apparently used self-starvation to avoid obesity. It was not until the 1960s, however, that anorexia nervosa was established as a mental disorder. Bulimia nervosa was first described as a distinct syndrome in 1979 (Anderson & Yager, 2005).

Eating disorders can be viewed on a continuum, with clients with anorexia eating too little or starving themselves, clients with bulimia eating chaotically, and clients with obesity eating too much. There is much overlap among the eating disorders: 30% to 35% of normal-weight people with bulimia have a history of anorexia nervosa and low body weight, and about 50% of people with anorexia nervosa exhibit bulimic behavior. The distinguishing features of anorexia include an earlier age at onset and below-normal body weight; the person fails to recognize the eating behavior as a problem. Clients with bulimia have a later age at onset and near-normal body weight. They usually are ashamed and embarrassed by the eating behavior.

More than 90% of cases of anorexia nervosa and bulimia occur in females (American Psychiatric Association [APA], 2000). Although fewer men than women suffer from eating disorders, the number of men with anorexia or bulimia may be much higher than previously believed (Woodside et al., 2002). Men, however, are less likely to seek treatment. The prevalence of both eating disorders is estimated to be 1% to 3% of the general population in the United States (Anderson & Yager, 2005).

Anorexia Nervosa

Anorexia nervosa is a life-threatening eating disorder characterized by the client's refusal or inability to maintain a minimally normal body weight, intense fear of gaining weight or becoming fat, significantly disturbed perception of the shape or size of the body, and steadfast inability or refusal to acknowledge the seriousness of the problem or even that one exists (APA, 2000). Clients with anorexia have a body weight that is 85% or less of that expected for their age and height, have experienced amenorrhea for at least three consecutive cycles, and have a preoccupation with food and food-related activities.

For *Diagnostic and Statistical Manual of Mental Disorders, 4th edition, Text Revision* (*DSM-IV-TR*; APA, 2000) diagnostic criteria for anorexia nervosa, please refer to the box below.

DSM-IV-TR DIAGNOSTIC CRITERIA: SYMPTOMS OF ANOREXIA NERVOSA

Fear of gaining weight or becoming fat even when severely underweight
Body image disturbance
Amenorrhea
Depressive symptoms such as depressed mood, social withdrawal, irritability, and insomnia
Preoccupation with thoughts of food
Feelings of ineffectiveness
Inflexible thinking
Strong need to control environment
Limited spontaneity and overly restrained emotional expression

Complaints of constipation and abdominal pain
Cold intolerance
Lethargy
Emaciation
Hypotension, hypothermia, and bradycardia
Hypertrophy of salivary glands
Elevated BUN (blood urea nitrogen)
Electrolyte imbalances
Leukopenia and mild anemia
Elevated liver function studies

Adapted from *DSM-IV-TR*, 2000.

Clients with anorexia nervosa can be classified into two subgroups depending on how they control their weight. Clients with the restricting subtype lose weight primarily through dieting, fasting, or excessive exercising. Those with the binge eating and purging subtype engage regularly in binge eating followed by purging. **Binge eating** means consuming a large amount of food (far greater than most people eat at one time) in a discrete period of usually 2 hours or less. **Purging** means the compensatory behaviors designed to eliminate food by means of self-induced vomiting or misuse of laxatives, enemas, and diuretics. Some clients with anorexia do not binge but still engage in purging behaviors after ingesting small amounts of food.

Clients with anorexia become totally absorbed in their quest for weight loss and thinness. The term *anorexia* is actually a misnomer: These clients do not lose their appetites. They still experience hunger but ignore it and signs of physical weakness and fatigue; they often believe that if they eat anything, they will not be able to stop eating and will become fat. Clients with anorexia often are preoccupied with food-related activities such as grocery shopping, collecting recipes or cookbooks, counting calories, creating fat-free meals, and cooking family meals. They also may engage in unusual or ritualistic food behaviors such as refusing to eat around others, cutting food into minute pieces, or not allowing the food they eat to touch their lips. These behaviors increase their sense of control. Excessive exercise is common; it may occupy several hours a day.

Anorexia nervosa typically begins between 14 and 18 years of age. In the early stages, clients often deny they have a negative body image or anxiety regarding their appearance. They are very pleased with their ability to control their weight and may express this. When they initially come for treatment, they may be unable to identify or to explain their emotions about life events such as school or relationships with family or friends. A profound sense of emptiness is common.

As the illness progresses, depression and lability in mood become more apparent. As dieting and compulsive behaviors increase, clients isolate themselves. This social isolation can lead to a basic mistrust of others and even paranoia. Clients may believe their peers are jealous of their weight loss and may believe that family and health care professionals are trying to make them "fat and ugly."

In long-term studies of clients with anorexia nervosa, Anderson and Yager (2005) reported that 30% were well, 30% were partially improved, 30% were chronically ill, and 10% had died of anorexia-related causes. Clients with the lowest body weights and longest durations of illness tended to relapse most often and have the poorest outcomes. Clients who abuse laxatives are at a greater risk for medical complications. Table 18.1 lists common medical complications of eating disorders.

Table 18.1 MEDICAL COMPLICATIONS OF EATING DISORDERS

Body System	Symptoms
Related to weight loss	
Musculoskeletal	Loss of muscle mass, loss of fat, osteoporosis, and pathologic fractures
Metabolic	Hypothyroidism (symptoms include lack of energy, weakness, intolerance to cold, and bradycardia), hypoglycemia, and decreased insulin sensitivity
Cardiac	Bradycardia, hypotension, loss of cardiac muscle, small heart, cardiac arrhythmias (including atrial and ventricular premature contractions, prolonged QT interval, ventricular tachycardia), and sudden death
Gastrointestinal	Delayed gastric emptying, bloating, constipation, abdominal pain, gas, and diarrhea
Reproductive	Amenorrhea and low levels of luteinizing and follicle-stimulating hormones
Dermatologic	Dry, cracking skin due to dehydration, lanugo (i.e., fine, baby-like hair over body), edema, and acrocyanosis (i.e., blue hands and feet)
Hematologic	Leukopenia, anemia, thrombocytopenia, hypercholesterolemia, and hypercarotenemia
Neuropsychiatric	Abnormal taste sensation, apathetic depression, mild organic mental symptoms, and sleep disturbances
Related to purging (vomiting and laxative abuse)	
Metabolic	Electrolyte abnormalities, particularly hypokalemia, hypochloremic alkalosis, hypomagnesemia, and elevated blood urea nitrogen (BUN)
Gastrointestinal	Salivary gland and pancreas inflammation and enlargement with an increase in serum amylase, esophageal and gastric erosion or rupture, dysfunctional bowel, and superior mesenteric artery syndrome
Dental	Erosion of dental enamel (perimyolysis), particularly front teeth
Neuropsychiatric	Seizures (related to large fluid shifts and electrolyte disturbances), mild neuropathies, fatigue, weakness, and mild organic mental symptoms

Adapted from Anderson, A. E., & Yager, J. (2005). Eating disorders. In B. J. Sadock & V. A. Sadock (Eds.), *Comprehensive textbook of psychiatry,* (Vol. 2, 8th ed., pp. 2002–2021). Philadelphia: Lippincott Williams & Wilkins.

CLINICAL VIGNETTE: ANOREXIA NERVOSA

Maggie, 15 years old, is 5 feet, 7 inches tall and weighs 92 pounds. Though it is August, she is wearing sweatpants and three layers of shirts. Her hair is dry, brittle, and uncombed, and she wears no makeup. Maggie's family physician has referred her to the eating disorders unit because she has lost 20 pounds in the last 4 months and her menstrual periods have ceased. She also is lethargic and weak yet has trouble sleeping. Maggie is an avid ballet student and believes she still needs to lose more weight to achieve the figure she wants. Her ballet instructor has expressed concern to Maggie's parents about her appearance and fatigue.

Maggie's family reports that she has gone from being an A and B student to barely passing in school. She spends much of her time isolated in her room and is often exercising for long hours, even in the middle of the night. Maggie seldom goes out with friends, and they have stopped calling her. The nurse interviews Maggie but gains little information, as Maggie is reluctant to discuss her eating. Maggie does say she is too fat and has no interest in gaining weight. She does not understand why her parents are forcing her to come to "this place where all they want to do is fatten you up and keep you ugly."

Bulimia Nervosa

Bulimia nervosa, often simply called bulimia, is an eating disorder characterized by recurrent episodes (at least twice a week for 3 months) of binge eating followed by inappropriate compensatory behaviors to avoid weight gain such as purging (self-induced vomiting or use of laxatives, diuretics, enemas, or emetics), fasting, or excessively exercising (APA, 2000). The amount of food consumed during a binge episode is much larger than a person would normally eat. The client often engages in binge eating secretly. Between binges, the client may eat low-calorie foods or fast. Binging or purging episodes are often precipitated by strong emotions and followed by guilt, remorse, shame, or self-contempt.

The weight of clients with bulimia usually is in the normal range, although some clients are overweight or underweight. Recurrent vomiting destroys tooth enamel, and incidence of dental caries and ragged or chipped teeth increases in these clients. Dentists are often the first health care professionals to identify clients with bulimia.

Bulimia nervosa usually begins in late adolescence or early adulthood; 18 or 19 years is the typical age at onset. Binge eating frequently begins during or after dieting. Between binging and purging episodes, clients may eat restrictively, choosing salads and other low-calorie foods. This restrictive eating effectively sets them up for the next episode of binging and purging, and the cycle continues.

Clients with bulimia are aware that their eating behavior is pathologic and go to great lengths to hide it from others. They may store food in their cars, desks, or secret locations around the house. They may drive from one fast-food restaurant to another, ordering a normal amount of food at each but stopping at six places in 1 or 2 hours. Such patterns may exist for years until family or friends discover the client's behavior or medical complications develop for which the client seeks treatment.

Follow-up studies with clients with bulimia show that 10 years after treatment, 30% continued to engage in recurrent binge-eating and purging behaviors, whereas 38% to 47% were fully recovered (Anderson & Yager, 2005). One third of fully recovered clients relapse. Clients with a comorbid personality disorder tend to have poorer outcomes than those without. The death rate from bulimia is estimated at 3% or less.

For *DSM-IV-TR* diagnostic criteria for bulimia nervosa, please refer to the box below.

Related Disorders

Eating disorders usually first diagnosed in infancy and childhood include *rumination disorder, pica,* and *feeding disorder* (see Chapter 20). Common elements in clients with these disorders are family dysfunction and parent–child conflicts.

Binge eating disorder is listed as a research category in the *DSM-IV-TR* (APA, 2000); it is being investigated to determine its classification as a mental disorder. The essential features are recurrent episodes of binge eating; no regular use of inappropriate compensatory behaviors such as purging or excessive exercise or abuse of laxatives; guilt, shame, and disgust about eating behaviors; and marked psychological distress. Binge eating disorder frequently affects people over age 35, and it occurs often in men (Pope et al., 2006). Individuals are more likely to be overweight or obese, overweight as children, and teased about their weight at an early age. Thirty-five percent reported that binge eating preceded dieting; 65% reported dieting before binge eating.

Night eating syndrome is characterized by morning anorexia, evening hyperphagia (consuming 50% of daily calories after the last evening meal), and nighttime awakenings (at least once a night) to consume snacks. It is associated with life stress, low self-esteem, anxiety, depression, and adverse reactions to weight loss. Most people with night eating syndrome are obese. (O'Reardon et al., 2005). Treatment with SSRI antidepressants has shown positive effects.

Comorbid psychiatric disorders are common in clients with anorexia nervosa and bulimia nervosa. Mood disorders, anxiety disorders, and substance abuse/dependence are frequently seen in clients with eating disorders. Of those, depression and obsessive-compulsive disorder are most common (Anderson & Yager, 2005). Anorexia and bulimia are both characterized by perfectionism, obsessive-compulsiveness, neuroticism, negative emotionality, harm avoidance, low self-directedness, low cooperativeness, and traits associated with avoidant personality disorder. In addition, clients with bulimia may also exhibit high impulsivity, sensation seeking, novelty seeking, and traits associated with borderline personality disorder (Cassin & von Ranson, 2005).

Eating disorders often are linked to a history of sexual abuse, especially if the abuse occurred before puberty (Preti et al., 2006). Such a history may be a factor contributing to problems with intimacy, sexual attractiveness, and low interest in sexual activity. Clients with eating disorders and a history of sexual abuse also have higher levels of depression and anxiety, lower self-esteem, more interpersonal problems, and more severe obsessive-compulsive symptoms (Carter et al., 2006). Whether or not sexual abuse has a cause-and-effect relationship with the development of eating disorders, however, remains unclear.

ETIOLOGY

A specific cause for eating disorders is unknown. Initially, dieting may be the stimulus that leads to their development. Biologic vulnerability, developmental problems, and family and social influences can turn dieting into an eating disorder (Table 18.2). Psychological and physiologic reinforcement of maladaptive eating behavior sustains the cycle (Andersen & Yager, 2005).

Biologic Factors

Studies of anorexia nervosa and bulimia nervosa have shown that these disorders tend to run in families. Genetic vulnerability also might result from a particular personality type or a general susceptibility to psychiatric disorders. Or it may directly involve a dysfunction of the hypothalamus. A family history of mood or anxiety disorders (e.g., obsessive-compulsive disorder) places a person at risk for an eating disorder (Andersen & Yager, 2005).

Disruptions of the nuclei of the hypothalamus may produce many of the symptoms of eating disorders. Two sets of nuclei are particularly important in many aspects of hunger

CLINICAL VIGNETTE: BULIMIA NERVOSA

Susan is driving home from the grocery store and eating from the grocery bags as she drives. In the 15-minute trip, she has already consumed a package of cookies, a large bag of potato chips, and a pound of ham from the deli. She thinks "I have to hurry, I'll be home soon. No one can see me like this!" She knew when she bought these food items that she would never get home with them.

Susan hurriedly drops the groceries on the kitchen counter and races for the bathroom. Tears are streaming down her face as she vomits to get rid of what she has just eaten. She feels guilty and ashamed and does not understand why she cannot stop her behavior. If only she did not eat those things. She thinks, "I'm 30 years old, married with two beautiful daughters, and a successful interior design consultant. What would my clients say if they could see me now? If my husband and daughters saw me, they would be disgusted." As Susan leaves the bathroom to put away the remainder of the groceries, she promises herself to stay away from all those bad foods. If she just does not eat them, this won't happen. This is a promise she has made many times before.

| Table 18.2 | | RISK FACTORS FOR EATING DISORDERS | | |

Disorder	Biologic Risk Factors	Developmental Risk Factors	Family Risk Factors	Sociocultural Risk Factors
Anorexia nervosa	Obesity; dieting at an early age	Issues of developing autonomy and having control over self and environment; developing a unique identity; dissatisfaction with body image	Family lacks emotional support; parental maltreatment; cannot deal with conflict	Cultural ideal of being thin; media focus on beauty, thinness, fitness; preoccupation with achieving the ideal body
Bulimia nervosa	Obesity; early dieting; possible serotonin and norepinephrine disturbances; chromosome 1 susceptibility	Self-perceptions of being overweight, fat, unattractive, and undesirable; dissatisfaction with body image	Chaotic family with loose boundaries; parental maltreatment including possible physical or sexual abuse	Same as above; weight-related teasing

and **satiety** (satisfaction of appetite): the lateral hypothalamus and the ventromedial hypothalamus. Deficits in the lateral hypothalamus result in decreased eating and decreased responses to sensory stimuli that are important to eating. Disruption of the ventromedial hypothalamus leads to excessive eating, weight gain, and decreased responsiveness to the satiety effects of glucose, which are behaviors seen in bulimia.

Many neurochemical changes accompany eating disorders, but it is difficult to tell whether they cause or result from eating disorders and the characteristic symptoms of starvation, binging, and purging. For example, norepinephrine levels rise normally in response to eating, allowing the body to metabolize and to use nutrients. Norepinephrine levels do not rise during starvation, however, because few nutrients are available to metabolize. Therefore, low norepinephrine levels are seen in clients during periods of restricted food intake. Also, low epinephrine levels are related to the decreased heart rate and blood pressure seen in clients with anorexia.

Increased levels of the neurotransmitter serotonin and its precursor tryptophan have been linked with increased satiety. Low levels of serotonin as well as low platelet levels of monoamine oxidase have been found in clients with bulimia and the binge and purge subtype of anorexia nervosa (Andersen & Yager, 2005); this may explain binging behavior. The positive response of some clients with bulimia to treatment with selective serotonin reuptake inhibitor antidepressants supports the idea that serotonin levels at the synapse may be low in these clients.

Developmental Factors

ANOREXIA NERVOSA

Onset of anorexia nervosa usually occurs during adolescence or young adulthood. Some researchers believe its causes are related to developmental issues.

Two essential tasks of adolescence are the struggle to develop autonomy and the establishment of a unique identity. Autonomy, or exerting control over oneself and the environment, may be difficult in families that are overprotective or in which **enmeshment** (lack of clear role boundaries) exists. Such families do not support members' efforts to gain independence, and teenagers may feel as though they have little or no control over their lives. They begin to control their eating through severe dieting and thus gain control over their weight. Losing weight becomes reinforcing: by continuing to lose, these clients exert control over one aspect of their lives.

It is important to identify potential risk factors for developing eating disorders so that prevention programs can target those at greatest risk. Johnson and Wardle (2005) found that adolescent girls who expressed body dissatisfaction were most likely to experience adverse outcomes such as emotional eating, binge eating, abnormal attitudes about eating and weight, low self-esteem, stress, and depression. In a study of almost 3,000 dieters, 104 developed an eating disorder within 2 years of screening. Characteristics of those who developed an eating disorder included disturbed eating habits; disturbed attitudes toward food; eating in secret; preoccupation with food, eating, shape, or weight; fear of losing control over eating; and wanting to have a completely empty stomach (Fairburn et al., 2005).

The need to develop a unique identity, or a sense of whom one is as a person, is another essential task of adolescence. It coincides with the onset of puberty, which initiates many emotional and physiologic changes. Self-doubt and confusion can result if the adolescent does not measure up to the person she or he wants to be.

Advertisements, magazines, and movies that feature thin models reinforce the cultural belief that slimness is attractive. Excessive dieting and weight loss may be the way an adolescent chooses to achieve this ideal. **Body image** is how a person perceives his or her body, that is, a mental self-image. For most people, body image is consistent with how others view them. For people with anorexia nervosa, however, their body image differs greatly from the perception of others. They perceive themselves as fat, unattractive, and undesirable even when they are severely underweight and malnourished. **Body image disturbance** occurs when there is an extreme discrepancy between one's body image and the perceptions of others and extreme dissatisfaction with one's body image.

BULIMIA NERVOSA

Self-perceptions of the body can influence the development of identity in adolescence greatly, and often persist into adulthood. Self-perceptions that include being overweight lead to the belief that dieting is necessary before one can be happy or satisfied. Clients with bulimia nervosa report dissatisfaction with their bodies as well as the belief that they are fat, unattractive, and undesirable. The binging and purging cycle of bulimia can begin at any time—after dieting has been unsuccessful, before the severe dieting begins, or at the same time as part of a "weight loss plan."

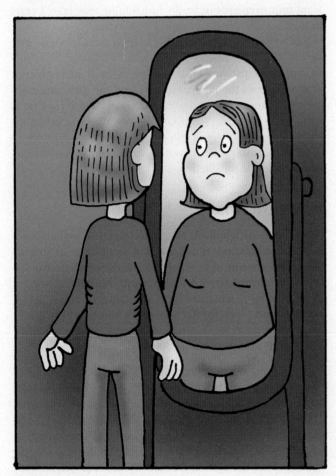

Body image disturbance

Family Influences

Girls growing up amid family problems and abuse are at higher risk for both anorexia and bulimia. Disordered eating is a common response to family discord. Girls growing up in families without emotional support often try to escape their negative emotions. They place an intense focus outward on something concrete: physical appearance. Disordered eating becomes a distraction from emotions.

Childhood adversity has been identified as a significant risk factor in the development of problems with eating or weight in adolescence or early adulthood. Adversity is defined as physical neglect, sexual abuse, or parental maltreatment that included little care, affection, and empathy as well as excessive paternal control, unfriendliness, or overprotectiveness.

Sociocultural Factors

In the United States and other Western countries, the media fuels the image of the "ideal woman" as thin. The culture equates beauty, desirability, and, ultimately, happiness with being very thin, perfectly toned, and physically fit. Adolescents often idealize actresses and models as having the perfect "look" or body even though many of these celebrities are underweight or use special effects to appear thinner than they are. Books, magazines, dietary supplements, exercise equipment, plastic surgery advertisements, and weight loss programs abound; the dieting industry is a billion-dollar business. The culture considers being overweight a sign of laziness, lack of self-control, or indifference; it equates pursuit of the "perfect" body with beauty, desirability, success, and will power. Thus, many women speak of being "good" when they stick to their diet and "bad" when they eat desserts or snacks.

Pressure from others also may contribute to eating disorders. Pressure from coaches, parents, and peers and the emphasis placed on body form in sports such as gymnastics, ballet, and wrestling can promote eating disorders in athletes (Waldrop, 2005). Parental concern over a girl's weight and teasing from parents or peers reinforces a girl's body dissatisfaction and her need to diet or control eating in some way.

CULTURAL CONSIDERATIONS

Both anorexia nervosa and bulimia nervosa are far more prevalent in industrialized societies, where food is abundant and beauty is linked with thinness. In the United States, anorexia nervosa is less frequent among African Americans (Andreasen & Black, 2006). For example, before 1995, there was little television on the island of Fiji. Eating disorders were almost nonexistent, and being "plump" was considered the ideal shape for girls and women. In the 5 years following the widespread introduction of television, the number of eating disorders in Fiji skyrocketed.

Eating disorders are most common in the United States, Canada, Europe, Australia, Japan, New Zealand, and South Africa. Immigrants from cultures in which eating disorders are rare may develop eating disorders as they assimilate the thin-body ideal (APA, 2000).

Eating disorders appear to be equally common among Hispanic and white women and less common among African American and Asian women (Anderson-Yager, 2005). Minority women who are younger, better educated, and more closely identified with white, middle-class values are at increased risk for developing an eating disorder.

During the past several years, eating disorders have shown an increase among all U.S. social classes and ethnic groups (Anderson & Yager, 2005). With today's technology, the entire world is exposed to the Western ideal, which equates thinness with beauty and desirability. As this ideal becomes widespread to non-Western cultures, anorexia and bulimia will likely increase there as well.

TREATMENT

Anorexia Nervosa

Clients with anorexia nervosa can be very difficult to treat because they are often resistant, appear uninterested, and deny their problems. Treatment settings include inpatient specialty eating disorder units, partial hospitalization or day treatment programs, and outpatient therapy. The choice of setting depends on the severity of the illness, such as weight loss, physical symptoms, duration of binging and purging, drive for thinness, body dissatisfaction, and comorbid psychiatric conditions. Major life-threatening complications that indicate the need for hospital admission include severe fluid, electrolyte, and metabolic imbalances; cardiovascular complications; severe weight loss and its consequences (Andreasen & Black, 2006); and risk for suicide. Short hospital stays are most effective for clients who are amenable to weight gain, and gain weight rapidly while hospitalized. Longer inpatient stays are required for those who gain weight more slowly and are more resistant to gaining additional weight (Willer et al., 2005). Outpatient therapy has the best success with clients who have been ill for less than 6 months, are not binging and purging, and have parents likely to participate effectively in family therapy. Cognitive behavior therapy can also be effective in preventing relapse and improving overall outcomes.

MEDICAL MANAGEMENT

Medical management focuses on weight restoration, nutritional rehabilitation, rehydration, and correction of electrolyte imbalances. Clients receive nutritionally balanced meals and snacks that gradually increase caloric intake to a normal level for size, age, and activity. Severely malnourished clients may require total parenteral nutrition, tube feedings, or hyperalimentation to receive adequate nutritional intake. Generally, access to a bathroom is supervised

to prevent purging as clients begin to eat more food. Weight gain and adequate food intake are most often the criteria for determining the effectiveness of treatment.

PSYCHOPHARMACOLOGY

Several classes of drugs have been studied, but few have shown clinical success. Amitriptyline (Elavil) and the antihistamine cyproheptadine (Periactin) in high doses (up to 28 mg/day) can promote weight gain in inpatients with anorexia nervosa. Olanzapine (Zyprexa) has been used with success because of both its antipsychotic effect (on bizarre body image distortions) and associated weight gain. Fluoxetine (Prozac) has shown some effectiveness in preventing relapse in clients whose weight has been partially or completely restored (Andreasen & Black, 2005); however, close monitoring is needed because weight loss can be a side effect.

PSYCHOTHERAPY

Family therapy may be beneficial for families of clients younger than 18 years. Families who demonstrate enmeshment, unclear boundaries among members, and difficulty handling emotions and conflict can begin to resolve these issues and improve communication. Family therapy also is useful to help members to be effective participants in the client's treatment. However, in a dysfunctional family, significant improvements in family functioning may take 2 years or more.

Individual therapy for clients with anorexia nervosa may be indicated in some circumstances such as if the family cannot participate in family therapy, if the client is older or separated from the nuclear family, or if the client has individual issues requiring psychotherapy. Therapy that is focused on the client's particular issues and circumstances, such a coping skills, self-esteem, self-acceptance, interpersonal relationships, assertiveness, can improve overall functioning and life satisfaction.

Bulimia Nervosa

Most clients with bulimia are treated on an outpatient basis. Hospital admission is indicated if binging and purging behaviors are out of control and the client's medical status is compromised. Most clients with bulimia have near-normal weight, which reduces the concern about severe malnutrition—a factor in clients with anorexia nervosa.

COGNITIVE-BEHAVIORAL THERAPY

Cognitive-behavioral therapy (CBT) has been found to be the most effective treatment for bulimia. This outpatient approach often requires a detailed manual to guide treatment. Strategies designed to change the client's thinking (cognition) and actions (behavior) about food focus on interrupting the cycle of dieting, binging, and purging and altering dysfunctional thoughts and beliefs about food, weight, body image, and overall self-concept. CBT enhanced with assertiveness training and self-esteem enhancement has produced positive results (Shiina et al., 2005).

PSYCHOPHARMACOLOGY

Since the 1980s, several controlled studies have been conducted to evaluate the effectiveness of antidepressants to treat bulimia. Drugs such as desipramine (Norpramin), imipramine (Tofranil), amitriptyline (Elavil), nortriptyline (Pamelor), phenelzine (Nardil), and fluoxetine (Prozac) were prescribed in the same dosages used to treat depression (see Chapter 2). In all the studies, the antidepressants were more effective than were the placebos in reducing binge eating. They also improved mood and reduced preoccupation with shape and weight. Most of the positive results, however, were short term, with about one third relapsing within a 2-year period (Agras, 2006).

APPLICATION OF THE NURSING PROCESS

Although anorexia and bulimia have several differences, many similarities are found in assessing, planning, implementing, and evaluating nursing care for clients with these disorders. Thus, this section addresses both eating disorders and highlights differences where they exist.

Assessment

Several specialized tests have been developed for eating disorders. An assessment tool such as the Eating Attitudes Test often is used in studies of anorexia and bulimia. This test also can be used at the end of treatment to evaluate outcomes because it is sensitive to clinical changes.

HISTORY

Family members often describe clients with anorexia nervosa as perfectionists with above-average intelligence, achievement oriented, dependable, eager to please, and seeking approval before their condition began. Parents describe clients as being "good, causing us no trouble" until the onset of anorexia. Likewise, clients with bulimia often are focused on pleasing others and avoiding conflict. Clients with bulimia, however, often have a history of impulsive behavior such as substance abuse and shoplifting as well as anxiety, depression, and personality disorders (Schultz & Videbeck, 2005).

GENERAL APPEARANCE AND MOTOR BEHAVIOR

Clients with anorexia appear slow, lethargic, and fatigued; they may be emaciated, depending on the amount of weight loss. They may be slow to respond to questions and have difficulty deciding what to say. They are often reluctant to answer questions fully because they do not want to acknowledge any problem. They often wear loose-fitting clothes in layers, regardless of the weather, both to hide weight loss and to keep warm (clients with anorexia are generally

cold). Eye contact may be limited. Clients may turn away from the nurse, indicating their unwillingness to discuss problems or to enter treatment.

Clients with bulimia may be underweight or overweight but are generally close to expected body weight for age and size. General appearance is not unusual, and they appear open and willing to talk.

MOOD AND AFFECT

Clients with eating disorders have labile moods that usually correspond to their eating or dieting behaviors. Avoiding "bad" or fattening foods gives them a sense of power and control over their bodies, whereas eating, binging, or purging leads to anxiety, depression, and feeling out of control. Clients with eating disorders often seem sad, anxious, and worried. Those with anorexia seldom smile, laugh, or enjoy any attempts at humor; they are somber and serious most of the time. In contrast, clients with bulimia are initially pleasant and cheerful as though nothing is wrong. The pleasant façade usually disappears when they begin describing binge eating and purging; they may express intense guilt, shame, and embarrassment.

It is important to ask clients with eating disorders about thoughts of self-harm or suicide. It is not uncommon for these clients to engage in self-mutilating behaviors such as cutting. Concern about self-harm and suicidal behavior should increase when clients have a history of sexual abuse (see Chapters 11 and 15).

THOUGHT PROCESSES AND CONTENT

Clients with eating disorders spend most of the time thinking about dieting, food, and food-related behavior. They are preoccupied with their attempts to avoid eating or eating "bad" or "wrong" foods. Clients cannot think about themselves without thinking about weight and food. The body image disturbance can be almost delusional; even if clients are severely underweight, they can point to areas on their buttocks or thighs that are "still fat," thereby fueling their need to continue dieting. Clients with anorexia who are severely underweight may have paranoid ideas about their family and health care professionals, believing they are their "enemies" who are trying to make them fat by forcing them to eat.

SENSORIUM AND INTELLECTUAL PROCESSES

Generally, clients with eating disorders are alert and oriented; their intellectual functions are intact. The exception is clients with anorexia who are severely malnourished and showing signs of starvation such as mild confusion, slowed mental processes, and difficulty with concentration and attention.

JUDGMENT AND INSIGHT

Clients with anorexia have very limited insight and poor judgment about their health status. They do not believe they have a problem; rather, they believe others are trying to interfere with their ability to lose weight and to achieve the desired body image. Facts about failing health status are not enough to convince these clients of their true problems. Clients with anorexia continue to restrict food intake or to engage in purging despite the negative effect on health.

In contrast, clients with bulimia are ashamed of the binge eating and purging. They recognize these behaviors as abnormal and go to great lengths to hide them. They feel out of control and unable to change even though they recognize their behaviors as pathologic. Box 18.1 shows an Eating Attitudes Test.

SELF-CONCEPT

Low self-esteem is prominent in clients with eating disorders. They see themselves only in terms of their ability to control their food intake and weight. They tend to judge themselves harshly and see themselves as "bad" if they eat certain foods or fail to lose weight. They overlook or ignore other personal characteristics or achievements as less important than thinness. Clients often perceive themselves as helpless, powerless, and ineffective. This feeling of lack of control over themselves and their environment only strengthens their desire to control their weight.

ROLES AND RELATIONSHIPS

Eating disorders interfere with the ability to fulfill roles and to have satisfying relationships. Clients with anorexia may begin to fail at school, which is in sharp contrast to previously successful academic performance. They withdraw from peers and pay little attention to friendships. They believe that others will not understand or fear they will begin out-of-control eating with others.

Clients with bulimia feel great shame about their binge eating and purging behaviors. As a result, they tend to lead secret lives that include sneaking behind the backs of friends and family to binge and purge in privacy. The time spent buying and eating food and then purging can interfere with role performance both at home and at work.

PHYSIOLOGIC AND SELF-CARE CONSIDERATIONS

The health status of clients with eating disorders relates directly to the severity of self-starvation, purging behaviors, or both (see Table 18.1). In addition, clients may exercise excessively, almost to the point of exhaustion, in an effort to control weight. Many clients have sleep disturbances such as insomnia, reduced sleep time, and early-morning wakening. Those who frequently vomit have many dental problems such as loss of tooth enamel, chipped and ragged teeth, and dental caries. Frequent vomiting also may result in sores in the mouth. Complete medical and dental examinations are essential.

Data Analysis

Nursing diagnoses for clients with eating disorders include the following:

- Imbalanced Nutrition: Less Than/More Than Body Requirements
- Ineffective Coping
- Disturbed Body Image

Other nursing diagnoses may be pertinent, such as Deficient Fluid Volume, Constipation, Fatigue, and Activity Intolerance.

Outcome Identification

For severely malnourished clients, their medical condition must be stabilized before psychiatric treatment can begin. Medical stabilization may include parenteral fluids, total parenteral nutrition, and cardiac monitoring.

Examples of expected outcomes for clients with eating disorders include the following:

- The client will establish adequate nutritional eating patterns.
- The client will eliminate use of compensatory behaviors such as excessive exercise and use of laxatives and diuretics.
- The client will demonstrate coping mechanisms not related to food.
- The client will verbalize feelings of guilt, anger, anxiety, or an excessive need for control.
- The client will verbalize acceptance of body image with stable body weight.

Interventions

ESTABLISHING NUTRITIONAL EATING PATTERNS

Typically, inpatient treatment is for clients with anorexia nervosa who are severely malnourished and clients with bulimia whose binge eating and purging behaviors are out of control. Primary nursing roles are to implement and to supervise the regimen for nutritional rehabilitation. Total parenteral nutrition or enteral feedings may be prescribed initially when a client's health status is severely compromised.

When clients can eat, a diet of 1,200 to 1,500 calories per day is ordered, with gradual increases in calories until clients are ingesting adequate amounts for height, activity level, and growth needs. Typically, allotted calories are divided into three meals and three snacks. A liquid protein supplement is given to replace any food not eaten to ensure consumption of the total number of prescribed calories. The nurse is responsible for monitoring meals and snacks and often initially will sit with a client during eating at a table away from other clients. Depending on the treatment program, diet beverages and food substitutions may be prohibited, and a specified time may be set for consuming each meal or snack. Clients also may be discouraged from performing food rituals such as cutting food into tiny pieces or mixing food in unusual combinations. The nurse must be alert for any attempts by clients to hide or to discard food.

Box 18.1 EATING ATTITUDES TEST

Please place an (X) under the column that applies best to each of the numbered statements. All the results will be strictly confidential. Most of the questions relate to food or eating, although other types of questions have been included. Please answer each question carefully. Thank you.

	Always	Very Often	Often	Sometimes	Rarely	Never
1. Like eating with other people.						X
2. Prepare foods for others but do not eat what I cook.	X					
3. Become anxious prior to eating.	X					
4. Am terrified about being overweight.	X					
5. Avoid eating when I am hungry.	X					
6. Find myself preoccupied with food.	X					
7. Have gone on eating binges where I feel that I may not be able to stop.	X					
8. Cut food into small pieces.	X					
9. Aware of the calorie content of foods that I eat.	X					
10. Particularly avoid foods with a high carbohydrate content (e.g., bread, potatoes, rice, etc.).	X					
11. Feel bloated after meals.	X					
12. Feel that others would prefer I ate more.	X					
13. Vomit after I have eaten.	X					
14. Feel extremely guilty after eating.	X					
15. Am preoccupied with a desire to be thinner.	X					
16. Exercise strenuously to burn off calories.	X					
17. Weigh myself several times a day.	X					
18. Like my clothes to fit tightly.						X
19. Enjoy eating meat.						X
20. Wake up early in the morning.	X					
21. Eat the same foods day after day.	X					
22. Think about burning up calories when I exercise.	X					
23. Have regular menstrual periods.						X
24. Other people think I am too thin.	X					
25. Am preoccupied with the thought of having fat on my body.	X					
26. Take longer than others to eat.	X					
27. Enjoy eating at restaurants.						X
28. Take laxatives.	X					
29. Avoid foods with sugar in them.	X					
30. Eat diet foods.	X					
31. Feel that food controls my life.	X					
32. Display self-control around food.	X					
33. Feel that others pressure me to eat.	X					
34. Give too much time and thought to food.	X					
35. Suffer from constipation.		X				
36. Feel uncomfortable after eating sweets.	X					
37. Engage in dieting behavior.	X					
38. Like my stomach to be empty.	X					
39. Enjoy trying new rich foods.						X
40. Have impulse to vomit after meals.	X					

Scoring: The patient is given the questionnaire without the X's, just blank. Three points are assigned to endorsements that coincide with the X's; the adjacent alternatives are weighted as 2 points and 1 point, respectively. A total score of over 30 indicates significant concerns with eating behavior.

After each meal or snack, clients may be required to remain in view of staff for 1 to 2 hours to ensure they do not empty the stomach by vomiting. Some treatment programs limit client access to bathrooms without supervision, particularly after meals, to discourage vomiting. As clients begin to gain weight and to become more independent in eating behavior, these restrictions are lessened gradually.

In most treatment programs, clients are weighed only once daily, usually on awakening and after they have emptied the bladder. Clients should wear minimal clothing, such as a hospital gown, each time they are weighed. They may attempt to place objects in their clothing to give the appearance of weight gain.

Clients with bulimia often are treated on an outpatient basis. The nurse must work closely with clients to establish normal eating patterns and to interrupt the binge and purge cycle. He or she encourages clients to eat meals with their families or, if they live alone, with friends. Clients always should sit at a table in a designated eating area such as a kitchen or dining room. It is easier for clients to follow a nutritious eating plan if it is written in advance and groceries are purchased for the planned menus. Clients must avoid buying foods frequently consumed during binges, such as cookies, candy bars, and potato chips. They should discard or move to the kitchen food that was kept at work, in the car, or in the bedroom.

IDENTIFYING EMOTIONS AND DEVELOPING COPING STRATEGIES

Because clients with anorexia have problems with self-awareness, they often have difficulty identifying and expressing feelings (**alexithymia**). Therefore, they often express these feelings in terms of somatic complaints such as feeling fat or bloated. The nurse can help clients begin to recognize emotions such as anxiety or guilt by asking them to describe how they are feeling and allowing adequate time for response. The nurse should not ask, "Are you sad?" or "Are you anxious?" because a client may quickly agree rather than struggle for an answer. The nurse encourages the client to describe her or his feelings. This approach can eventually help clients to recognize their emotions and to connect them to their eating behaviors.

Self-monitoring is a cognitive-behavioral technique designed to help clients with bulimia. It may help clients to identify behavior patterns and then implement techniques to avoid or to replace them (Carter et al., 2003). Self-monitoring techniques raise client awareness about behavior and help them to regain a sense of control. The nurse encourages clients to keep a diary of all food eaten throughout the day, including binges, and to record moods, emotions, thoughts, circumstances, and interactions surrounding eating and binging or purging episodes. In this way, clients begin to see connections between emotions and situations and eating behaviors. The nurse can then help clients

NURSING INTERVENTIONS FOR EATING DISORDERS

- **Establishing nutritional eating patterns**
  Sit with the client during meals and snacks.
  Offer liquid protein supplement if client is unable to complete meal.
  Adhere to treatment program guidelines regarding restrictions.
  Observe client following meals and snacks for 1 to 2 hours.
  Weigh client daily in uniform clothing.
  Be alert for attempts to hide or discard food or inflate weight.
- **Helping the client identify emotions and develop non–food-related coping strategies**
  Ask the client to identify feelings.
  Self-monitoring using a journal
  Relaxation techniques
  Distraction
  Assist client to change stereotypical beliefs.
- **Helping the client deal with body image issues**
  Recognize benefits of a more near-normal weight.
  Assist to view self in ways not related to body image.
  Identify personal strengths, interests, talents.
- **Providing client and family education** (See Client/Family Education for Eating Disorders)

to develop ways to manage emotions such as anxiety by using relaxation techniques or distraction with music or another activity. This is an important step toward helping clients find ways to cope with people, emotions, or situations that do not involve food.

DEALING WITH BODY IMAGE ISSUES

The nurse can help clients to accept a more normal body image. This may involve clients agreeing to weigh more than they would like, to be healthy, and to stay out of the hospital. When clients experience relief from emotional distress, have increased self-esteem, and are meeting emotional needs in healthy ways, they are more likely to accept their weight and body image.

The nurse also can help clients to view themselves in terms other than weight, size, shape, and satisfaction with body image. Helping clients to identify areas of personal strength that are not food related broadens clients' perceptions of themselves. This includes identifying talents, interests, and positive aspects of character unrelated to body shape or size.

The nurse explains to family and friends that they can be most helpful by providing emotional support, love, and attention. They can express concern about the client's health, but it is rarely helpful to focus on food intake, calories, and weight.

Evaluation

The nurse can use assessment tools such as the Eating Attitudes Test to detect improvement for clients with eating disorders. Both anorexia and bulimia are chronic for many clients. Residual symptoms such as dieting, compulsive exercising, and experiencing discomfort when eating in a social setting are common. Treatment is considered successful if the client maintains a body weight within 5% to 10% of normal with no medical complications from starvation or purging.

COMMUNITY-BASED CARE

Treatment for clients with eating disorders usually occurs in community settings. Hospital admission is indicated only for medical necessity such as for clients with dangerously low weight, electrolyte imbalances, or renal, cardiac, or hepatic complications. Clients who cannot control the cycle of binge eating and purging may be treated briefly in an inpatient setting. Other treatment settings include partial hospitalization or day treatment programs, individual or group outpatient therapy, and self-help groups.

MENTAL HEALTH PROMOTION

Nurses can educate parents, children, and young people about strategies to prevent eating disorders. Important aspects include realizing that the "ideal" figures portrayed in advertisements and magazines are unrealistic, developing realistic ideas about body size and shape, resisting peer pressure to diet, improving self-esteem, and learning coping strategies for dealing with emotions and life issues.

The Atlanta Center for Eating Disorders (2006) offers the following advice:

- Read the research about fad diets: They don't work. No-fat diets are unhealthy, and claims about diets that use special combinations of food are unfounded.
- Send the right message to children about food and body image issues. Parents who are constantly worrying about or talking about weight or are always "on a diet" powerfully influence their children. Give up dieting and eat well-balanced meals.
- Listen to your conversations. Weight, dieting, and appearance are among the most common topics for women. Make a pact with friends to stop talking about your bodies negatively.
- Focus on the positive aspects of yourself and others that have nothing to do with physical appearance.
- Encourage healthy expression of emotions. Learn positive ways to communicate.

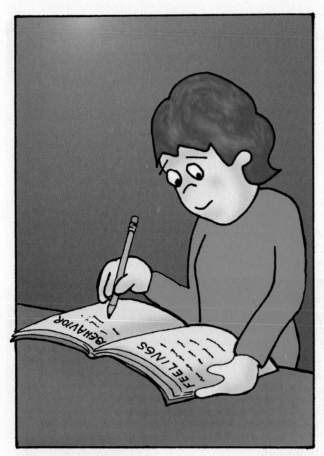

Keeping a feelings diary

PROVIDING CLIENT AND FAMILY EDUCATION

One primary nursing role in caring for clients with eating disorders is providing education to help them take control of nutritional requirements independently. This teaching can be done in the inpatient setting during discharge planning or in the outpatient setting. The nurse provides extensive teaching about basic nutritional needs and the effects of restrictive eating, dieting, and the binge and purge cycle. Clients need encouragement to set realistic goals for eating throughout the day (Muscari, 2002). Eating only salads and vegetables during the day may set up clients for later binges as a result of too little fat and carbohydrates.

For clients who purge, the most important goal is to stop. Teaching should include information about the harmful effects of purging by vomiting and laxative abuse. The nurse explains that purging is an ineffective means of weight control and only disrupts the neuroendocrine system. In addition, purging promotes binge eating by decreasing the anxiety that follows the binge. The nurse explains that if clients can avoid purging, they may be less likely to engage in binge eating. The nurse also teaches the techniques of distraction and delay because they are useful against both binging and purging. The longer clients can delay either binging or purging, the less likely they are to carry out the behavior.

- Give up wanting to be thin before doing anything, and get on with enjoying your life.
- Increase physical activity by focusing on the enjoyment of movement, not on how many calories you'll burn.

School nurses, student health nurses at colleges and universities, and nurses in clinics and doctors' offices may encounter clients in various settings who are at risk for developing or who already have an eating disorder. In these settings, early identification and appropriate referral are primary responsibilities of the nurse. Routine screening of all young women in these settings would help identify those at risk for an eating disorder. Box 18.2 contains a sample of questions that can be used for such screening. Such early identification could result in early intervention and prevention of a full-blown eating disorder.

Box 18.2   SAMPLE SCREENING QUESTIONS

- How often do you feel dissatisfied with your body shape or size?
- Do you think you are fat or need to lose weight, even when others say you are thin?
- Do thoughts about food, weight, dieting, and eating dominate your life?
- Do you eat to make yourself feel better emotionally, and then feel guilty about it?

Nursing Care Plan   *Bulimia*

Nursing Diagnosis

Ineffective Coping: *Inability to form a valid appraisal of the stressors, inadequate choices of practiced responses, and/or inability to use available resources.*

ASSESSMENT DATA

- Inability to meet basic needs
- Inability to ask for help
- Inability to problem solve
- Inability to change behaviors
- Self-destructive behavior
- Suicidal thoughts or behavior
- Inability to delay gratification
- Poor impulse control
- Stealing or shoplifting behavior
- Desire for perfection
- Feelings of worthlessness
- Feelings of inadequacy or guilt
- Unsatisfactory interpersonal relationships
- Self-deprecatory verbalization
- Denial of feelings, illness, or problems
- Anxiety
- Sleep disturbances
- Low self-esteem
- Excessive need to control
- Feelings of being out of control
- Preoccupation with weight, food, or diets
- Distortions of body image
- Overuse of laxatives, diet pills, or diuretics
- Secrecy regarding eating habits or amounts eaten
- Fear of being fat
- Recurrent vomiting
- Binge eating
- Compulsive eating
- Substance use

EXPECTED OUTCOMES

Immediate

The client will

- Be free from self-inflicted harm
- Identify methods not related to food of dealing with stress or crises
- Verbalize feelings of guilt, anxiety, anger, or an excessive need for control

Stabilization

The client will

- Demonstrate more satisfying interpersonal relationships
- Demonstrate alternative methods of dealing with stress or crises
- Eliminate shoplifting or stealing behaviors
- Express feelings in ways not related to food
- Verbalize understanding of disease process and safe use of medications, if any

Community

The client will

- Verbalize more realistic body image
- Follow through with discharge planning, including support groups or therapy as indicated
- Verbalize increased self-esteem and self-confidence

Nursing Care Plan: Bulimia, cont.

IMPLEMENTATION

Nursing Interventions *denotes collaborative interventions	Rationale
Set limits with the client about eating habits, e.g., food will be eaten in a dining room setting, at a table, only at conventional mealtimes.	Limits will discourage binge behavior, such as hiding, sneaking, and gulping food, and help the client return to normal eating patterns. Eating three meals a day will prevent starvation and subsequent overeating in the evening.
Encourage the client to eat with other clients, when tolerated.	Eating with other people will discourage secrecy about eating, though initially the client's anxiety may be too high to join others at mealtime.
Encourage the client to express feelings, such as anxiety and guilt about having eaten.	Expressing feelings can help decrease the client's anxiety and the urge to engage in purging behaviors.
Ask the client directly about thoughts of suicide or self-harm.	The client's safety is a priority. You will not give the client ideas about suicide by addressing the issue directly.
Encourage the client to use a diary to write types and amounts of foods eaten and feelings that occur before, during, and after eating, especially related to urges to engage in binge or purge behavior.	A diary can help the client explore food intake, feelings, and relationships among these feelings and behaviors. Initially, the client may be able to write about these feelings and behaviors more easily than talk about them.
Encourage the client to describe and discuss feelings verbally. Begin to separate dealing with feelings from eating or purging behaviors. Maintain a nonjudgmental approach.	Being nonjudgmental gives the client permission to discuss feelings that may be negative or unacceptable to him or her without fear of rejection or reprisal.
Discuss the types of foods that are soothing to the client and that relieve anxiety.	You may be able to help the client see how he or she has used food to deal with feelings.
Help the client explore ways to relieve anxiety, express feelings, and experience pleasure that are not related to food or eating.	It is important to help the client separate emotional issues from food and eating behaviors.
Give positive feedback for the client's efforts to discuss feelings.	Your sincere praise can promote the client's attempts to deal openly and honestly with anxiety, anger, and other feelings.
*Teach the client and significant others about bulimic behaviors, physical complications, nutrition, and so forth. Refer the client to a dietitian if indicated.	The client and significant others may have little knowledge of the illness, food, and nutrition. Factual information can be useful in dispelling incorrect beliefs and in separating food from emotional issues.
*Teach the client and significant others about the purpose, action, timing, and possible adverse effects of medications, if any.	Antidepressant and other medications may be prescribed for bulimia. Remember, some antidepressant medications may take several weeks to achieve a therapeutic effect.
Teach the client about the use of the problem-solving process.	Successful use of the problem-solving process can help increase the client's self-esteem and confidence.
Explore with the client his or her personal strengths. Making a written list is sometimes helpful.	You can help the client discover his or her strengths; he or she needs to identify them, so it will not be useful for you to make a list for the client.
Discuss with the client the idea of accepting a less than "ideal" body weight.	The client's previous expectations or perception of an ideal weight may have been unrealistic, and even unhealthy.

continued ⋯⇢

Nursing Care Plan: Bulimia, cont.

IMPLEMENTATION

Nursing Interventions *denotes collaborative interventions	Rationale
Encourage the client to incorporate fattening (or "bad") foods into the diet as he or she tolerates.	This will enhance the client's sense of control of overeating.
Encourage the client to express his or her feelings about family members and significant others, their roles and relationships.	Expressing feelings can help the client to identify, accept, and work through feelings in a direct manner.
*Refer the client to assertiveness training books or classes if indicated.	Many bulimic clients are passive in interpersonal relationships. Assertiveness training may foster a sense of increased confidence and healthier relationship dynamics.
*Refer the client to long-term therapy if indicated. Contracting with the client may be helpful to promote follow through with continuing therapy.	Treatment for eating disorders often is a long-term process. The client may be more likely to engage in ongoing therapy if he or she has contracted to do this.
*Ongoing therapy may need to include significant others to sustain the client's non–food-related coping skills.	Dysfunctional relationships with significant others often are a primary issue for clients with eating disorders.
*Refer the client and family and significant others to support groups in the community or via the Internet (e.g., Anorexia Nervosa and Associated Disorders, Overeaters Anonymous).	These groups can offer support, education, and resources to clients and their families or significant others.
*Refer the client to a substance dependence treatment program or substance dependence support group (e.g., Alcoholics Anonymous), if appropriate.	Substance use is common among clients with bulimia.

Adapted from Schultz, J. M., & Videbeck, S. L. (2005). Lippincott's manual of psychiatric nursing care plans (7th ed.). Philadelphia: Lippincott Williams & Wilkins.

CLIENT/FAMILY EDUCATION FOR EATING DISORDERS

Client
- Basic nutritional needs
- Harmful effects of restrictive eating, dieting, purging
- Realistic goals for eating
- Acceptance of healthy body image

Family and Friends
- Provide emotional support.
- Express concern about client's health.
- Encourage client to seek professional help.
- Avoid talking only about weight, food intake, calories.
- Become informed about eating disorders.
- It is not possible for family and friends to force the client to eat. The client needs professional help from a therapist or psychiatrist.

SELF-AWARENESS ISSUES

An emaciated, starving client with anorexia can be a shocking sight, and the nurse may want to "take care of this child" and nurse her back to health. When the client rejects this help and resists the nurse's caring actions, the nurse can become angry and frustrated and feel incompetent to handle the situation.

The client initially may view the nurse, who is responsible for making the client eat, as the enemy. The client may hide or throw away food or become overtly hostile as anxiety about eating increases. The nurse must remember that the client's behavior is a symptom of anxiety and fear about gaining weight and not personally directed toward the nurse. Taking the client's behavior personally may cause the nurse to feel angry and behave in a rejecting manner.

Because eating is such a basic part of everyday life, the nurse may wonder why the client cannot just eat "like everyone else." The nurse also may find it difficult to understand how a 75-pound client sees herself as fat when she looks in the mirror. Likewise, when working with a client who binges and purges, the nurse may wonder why the client cannot exert the willpower to stop. The nurse must remember that the client's eating behavior has gotten out of control. Eating disorders are mental illnesses, just like schizophrenia and bipolar affective disorder.

Points to Consider When Working With Clients With Eating Disorders

- Be empathetic and nonjudgmental, although this is not easy. Remember the client's perspective and fears about weight and eating.
- Avoid sounding parental when teaching about nutrition or why laxative use is harmful. Presenting information factually without chiding the client will obtain more positive results.
- Do not label clients as "good" when they avoid purging or eat an entire meal. Otherwise, clients will believe they are "bad" on days when they purge or fail to eat enough food.

Critical Thinking Questions

1. You notice a friend or family member has been losing weight, has strange eating rituals, and constantly talks about dieting. You suspect an eating disorder. How would you approach this person?
2. A client has the right to refuse treatment. How would the nurse address this right when working with a client with anorexia who doesn't want treatment?

KEY POINTS

- Anorexia nervosa is a life-threatening eating disorder characterized by body weight less than 85% of normal, an intense fear of being fat, a severely distorted body image, and refusal to eat or binge eating and purging.
- Bulimia nervosa is an eating disorder that involves recurrent episodes of binge eating and compensatory behaviors such as purging, using laxatives and diuretics, or exercising excessively.
- Ninety percent of clients with eating disorders are female. Anorexia begins between the ages of 14 and 18, and bulimia begins around age 18 or 19.
- Many neurochemical changes are present in individuals with eating disorders, but it is uncertain whether these changes cause or are a result of the eating disorders.
- Persons with eating disorders feel unattractive and ineffective and may be poorly equipped to deal with the challenges of maturity.
- Societal attitudes regarding thinness, beauty, desirability, and physical fitness may influence the development of eating disorders.
- Severely malnourished clients with anorexia nervosa may require intensive medical treatment to restore homeostasis before psychiatric treatment can begin.
- Family therapy is effective for clients with anorexia; cognitive-behavioral therapy is most effective for clients with bulimia.
- Interventions for clients with eating disorders include establishing nutritional eating patterns, helping the client to identify emotions and to develop coping strategies not related to food, helping the client to deal with body image issues, and providing client and family education.

INTERNET RESOURCES

RESOURCE	INTERNET ADDRESS
About Face (changing attitudes about body image)	http://www.about-face.org
Academy for Eating Disorders	http://www.aedweb.org
Body Positive	http://www.bodypositive.com
Eating Disorder Referral and Information Center	http://www.edreferral.com
Eating Disorders Association	http://www.edauk.com
National Association of Anorexia Nervosa & Associated Eating Disorders	http://www.anad.org
National Eating Disorders Association	http://www.nationaleatingdisorders.org/p.asp?webpage_ID-337

- Focus on healthy eating and pleasurable physical exercise; avoid fad or stringent dieting.
- Parents must become aware of their own behavior and attitudes and the way they influence children.

REFERENCES

Agras, W. S. (2006). Treatment of eating disorders. In A. F. Schatzberg & C. B. Nemeroff (Eds.), *Essentials of clinical psychopharmacology* (2nd ed., pp. 669–687). Washington DC: American Psychiatric Publishing.

American Psychiatric Association. (2000). *Diagnostic and statistical manual of mental disorders* (4th ed., text revision). Washington, DC: American Psychiatric Association.

Anderson, A. E., & Yager, J. (2005). Eating disorders. In B. J. Sadock & V. A. Sadock (Eds.), *Comprehensive textbook of psychiatry* (Vol. 1, 8th ed., pp. 2002–2021). Philadelphia: Lippincott Williams & Wilkins.

Andreasen, N. C., & Black, D. W. (2006). *Introductory textbook of psychiatry* (4th ed.). Washington DC: American Psychiatric Publishing.

Atlanta Center for Eating Disorders. (2006). How can you help prevent eating disorders? Available: http://eatingdisorders.home.mindspring.com/causes2.htm.

Carter, J. C., Bewell, C., Blackmore, E., & Woodside, D. B. (2006). The impact of childhood sexual abuse in anorexia nervosa. *Child Abuse & Neglect, 30*(3), 257–269.

Carter, J. C., Olmsed, M. P., Kaplan, A. S., et al. (2003). Self-help for bulimia nervosa: A randomized controlled trial. *American Journal of Psychiatry, 160*(5), 973–978.

Cassin, S. E., & von Ranson, K. M. (2005). Personality and eating disorders: A decade in review. *Clinical Psychology Review, 25*(7), 895–916.

Fairburn, C. G., Cooper, Z., Doll, H. A., & Davies, B. A. (2005). Identifying dieters who will develop an eating disorder: A prospective, population-based study. *American Journal of Psychiatry, 162*(12), 2249–2255.

Johnson, F., & Wardle, J. (2005). Dietary restraint, body dissatisfaction, and psychological distress: A prospective analysis. *Journal of Abnormal Psychology, 114*(1), 119–125.

Muscari, M. (2002). Effective management of adolescents with anorexia and bulimia. *Journal of Psychosocial Nursing, 40*(2), 23–31.

O'Reardon, J. P., Peshek, A., & Allison K. C. (2005). Night eating syndrome: Diagnosis, epidemiology, and management. *CNS Drugs, 19*(12), 997–1008.

Pope, H. G., Jr., Lalonde, J. K., Pindyck, L. J., et al. (2006). Binge eating disorder: A stable syndrome. *American Journal of Psychiatry, 163*(12), 2181–2183.

Preti, A., Incani, E., Camboni, M. V., et al. (2006). Sexual abuse and eating disorder symptoms: The mediator role of bodily dissatisfaction. *Comprehensive Psychiatry, 47*(6), 475–481.

Schultz, J. M., & Videbeck, S. L. (2005). *Lippincott's manual of psychiatric nursing care plans* (7th ed.). Philadelphia: Lippincott Williams & Wilkins.

Shiina, A., Nakazato, M., Mitsumori, M., et al. (2005). An open trial of outpatient group therapy for bulimic disorders: Combination program of cognitive behavioral therapy with assertive training and self-esteem enhancement. *Psychiatry and Clinical Neurosciences, 59*(6), 690–696.

Waldrop, J. (2005). Early identification and interventions for female athlete triad. *Journal of Pediatric Health Care, 19*(4), 213–220.

Willer, M. G., Thuras, P., & Crow, S. J. (2005). Implications of the changing use of hospitalization to treat anorexia nervosa. *American Journal of Psychiatry, 162*(12), 2374–2376.

Woodside, B. D., Bulik, C. M., Halmi, K. A., et al. (2002). Personality, perfectionism, and attitudes toward eating in parents of individuals with eating disorders. *International Journal of Eating Disorders, 31*(3), 290–299.

ADDITIONAL READINGS

Daee, A., Robinson, P., Lawson, M., et al. (2002). Psychologic and physiologic effects of dieting during adolescence. *Southern Medical Journal, 95*(9), 1031–1032.

Morgan, R. (2002). The men in the mirror. *Higher Chronicle of Education, 49*(5), A53–A54.

Picker, L. (2002). New hope for bulimia. *Shape,* 66–67.

Wiser, S., & Telch, C. F. (1999). Dialectic behavior therapy for binge eating disorder. *Journal of Clinical Psychology, 55*(6), 755–768.

Chapter Study Guide

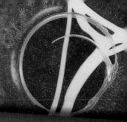

MULTIPLE-CHOICE QUESTIONS

Select the best answer for each of the following questions.

1. Treating clients with anorexia nervosa with a selective serotonin reuptake inhibitor antidepressant such as fluoxetine (Prozac) may present which of the following problems?
   A. Clients object to the side effect of weight gain.
   B. Fluoxetine can cause appetite suppression and weight loss.
   C. Fluoxetine can cause clients to become giddy and silly.
   D. Clients with anorexia get no benefit from fluoxetine.

2. Which of the following is an example of a cognitive-behavioral technique?
   A. Distraction
   B. Relaxation
   C. Self-monitoring
   D. Verbalization of emotions

3. The nurse is working with a client with anorexia nervosa. Even though the client has been eating all her meals and snacks, her weight has remained unchanged for 1 week. Which of the following interventions is indicated?
   A. Supervise the client closely for 2 hours after meals and snacks.
   B. Increase the daily caloric intake from 1,500 to 2,000 calories.
   C. Increase the client's fluid intake.
   D. Request an order from the physician for fluoxetine.

4. Which of the following statements is true?
   A. Anorexia nervosa was not recognized as an illness until the 1960s.
   B. Cultures where beauty is linked to thinness have an increased risk for eating disorders.
   C. Eating disorders are a major health problem only in the United States and Europe.
   D. Persons with anorexia nervosa are popular with their peers as a result of their thinness.

5. All but which of the following are initial goals for treating the severely malnourished client with anorexia nervosa?
   A. Correction of body image disturbance
   B. Correction of electrolyte imbalances
   C. Nutritional rehabilitation
   D. Weight restoration

6. The nurse is evaluating the progress of a client with bulimia. Which of the following behaviors would indicate that the client is making positive progress?
   A. The client can identify calorie content for each meal.
   B. The client identifies healthy ways of coping with anxiety.
   C. The client spends time resting in her room after meals.
   D. The client verbalizes knowledge of former eating patterns as unhealthy.

7. A teenaged girl is being evaluated for an eating disorder. Which of the following would suggest anorexia nervosa?
   A. Guilt and shame about eating patterns
   B. Lack of knowledge about food and nutrition
   C. Refusal to talk about food-related topics
   D. Unrealistic perception of body size

8. A client with bulimia is learning to use the technique of self-monitoring. Which of the following interventions by the nurse would be most beneficial for this client?
   A. Ask the client to write about all feelings and experiences related to food.
   B. Assist the client to make out daily meal plans for 1 week.
   C. Encourage the client to ignore feelings and impulses related to food.
   D. Teach the client about nutrition content and calories of various foods.

FILL-IN-THE-BLANK QUESTIONS

Identify each of the following characteristics as being typical of anorexia nervosa, bulimia nervosa, or both.

_____   Client puts on a pleasant and cheerful face for others.

_____   Client spends the majority of time thinking about food and food-related activities.

_____   Client believes if she starts eating, she will not be able to stop.

_____   Client believes there is no problem with her dieting behavior.

_____   Client is guilty and ashamed about her eating behavior.

SHORT ANSWER QUESTIONS

1. Identify four compensatory behaviors that clients with bulimia use to avoid weight gain.

2. Describe the concept of body image disturbance.

CLINICAL EXAMPLE

Judy is a 17-year-old high school junior who is active in gymnastics. She is 5 feet, 7 inches tall, weighs 85 pounds, and has not had a menstrual period for 5 months. The family physician referred her to the inpatient eating disorders unit with a diagnosis of anorexia nervosa. During the admission interview, Judy is defensive about her weight loss, stating she needs to be thin to be competitive in her sport. Judy points to areas on her buttocks and thighs, saying, "See this? I still have plenty of fat. Why can't everyone just leave me alone?"

1. Identify two nursing diagnoses that would be pertinent for Judy.

2. Write an expected outcome for each identified nursing diagnosis.

3. List three nursing interventions for each nursing diagnosis.

Chapter 19

Somatoform Disorders

Key Terms

- body dysmorphic disorder
- conversion disorder
- disease conviction
- disease phobia
- emotion-focused coping strategies
- factitious disorders
- hypochondriasis
- hysteria
- internalization
- *la belle indifférence*
- malingering
- Munchausen syndrome
- Munchausen syndrome by proxy
- pain disorder
- primary gain
- problem-focused coping strategies
- psychosomatic
- secondary gain
- somatization
- somatization disorder
- somatoform disorders

Learning Objectives

After reading this chapter, you should be able to

1. Explain what is meant by "psychosomatic illness."

2. Describe somatoform disorders and identify their three central features.

3. Discuss the etiologic theories related to somatoform disorders.

4. Discuss the characteristics and dynamics of specific somatoform disorders.

5. Distinguish somatoform disorders from factitious disorders and malingering.

6. Apply the nursing process to the care of clients with somatoform disorders.

7. Provide education to clients, families, and the community to increase knowledge and understanding of somatoform disorders.

8. Evaluate your feelings, beliefs, and attitudes regarding clients with somatoform disorders.

In the early 1800s, the medical field began to consider the various social and psychological factors that influence illness. The term **psychosomatic** began to be used to convey the connection between the mind (*psyche*) and the body (*soma*) in states of health and illness. Essentially, the mind can cause the body to create physical symptoms or to worsen physical illnesses. Real symptoms can begin, continue, or be worsened as a result of emotional factors. Examples include diabetes, hypertension, and colitis, all of which are medical illnesses influenced by stress and emotions. When a person is under a lot of stress or is not coping well with stress, symptoms of these medical illnesses worsen. In addition, stress can cause physical symptoms unrelated to a diagnosed medical illness. After a stressful day at work, many people experience "tension headaches" that can be quite painful. The headaches are a manifestation of stress rather than a symptom of an underlying medical problem.

The term **hysteria** refers to multiple physical complaints with no organic basis; the complaints are usually described dramatically. The concept of hysteria probably originated in Egypt and is about 4,000 years old. In the Middle Ages, hysteria was associated with witchcraft, demons, and sorcerers. People with hysteria, usually women, were considered evil or possessed by evil spirits. Paul Briquet and Jean Martin Charcot, both French physicians, identified hysteria as a disorder of the nervous system.

Sigmund Freud, working with Charcot, observed that people with hysteria improved with hypnosis and experienced relief from their physical symptoms when they recalled memories and expressed emotions. This development led Freud to propose that people can convert unexpressed emotions into physical symptoms (Hollifield, 2005), a process now referred to as *somatization*. This chapter discusses somatoform disorders, which are based on the concept of somatization.

OVERVIEW OF SOMATOFORM DISORDERS

Somatization is defined as the transference of mental experiences and states into bodily symptoms. **Somatoform disorders** can be characterized as the presence of physical symptoms that suggest a medical condition without a demonstrable organic basis to account fully for them. The three central features of somatoform disorders are as follows:

- Physical complaints suggest major medical illness but have no demonstrable organic basis.
- Psychological factors and conflicts seem important in initiating, exacerbating, and maintaining the symptoms.
- Symptoms or magnified health concerns are not under the client's conscious control (Hollifield, 2005).

Clients are convinced they harbor serious physical problems despite negative results during diagnostic testing. They actually experience these physical symptoms as well as the accompanying pain, distress, and functional limitations such symptoms induce. Clients do not willfully control the physical symptoms. Although their illnesses are psychiatric in nature, many clients do not seek help from mental health professionals. Unfortunately, many health care professionals who do not understand the nature of somatoform disorders are not sympathetic to these clients' complaints (Andreasen & Black, 2006). Nurses must remember that these clients really experience the symptoms they describe and cannot voluntarily control them.

The five specific somatoform disorders are as follows (American Psychiatric Association [APA], 2000):

- **Somatization disorder** is characterized by multiple physical symptoms. It begins by 30 years of age, extends over several years, and includes a combination of pain and gastrointestinal, sexual, and pseudoneurologic symptoms.
- **Conversion disorder**, sometimes called conversion reaction, involves unexplained, usually sudden deficits in sensory or motor function (e.g., blindness, paralysis). These deficits suggest a neurologic disorder but are associated with psychological factors. An attitude of *la belle indifférence,* a seeming lack of concern or distress, is a key feature.
- **Pain disorder** has the primary physical symptom of pain, which generally is unrelieved by analgesics and greatly affected by psychological factors in terms of onset, severity, exacerbation, and maintenance.
- **Hypochondriasis** is preoccupation with the fear that one has a serious disease (**disease conviction**) or will get a serious disease (**disease phobia**). It is thought that clients with this disorder misinterpret bodily sensations or functions.
- **Body dysmorphic disorder** is preoccupation with an imagined or exaggerated defect in physical appearance such as thinking one's nose is too large or teeth are crooked and unattractive.

Somatization disorder, conversion disorder, and pain disorder are more common in women than in men; hypochondriasis and body dysmorphic disorder are distributed equally by gender. Somatization disorder occurs in 0.2% to 2% of the general population. Conversion disorder occurs in less than 1% of the population. Pain disorder is commonly seen in medical practice, with 10% to 15% of people in the United States reporting work disability related to back pain alone (APA, 2000). Hypochondriasis is estimated to occur in 4% to 9% of people seen in general medical practice. No statistics of the incidence of body dysmorphic disorder are available.

ONSET AND CLINICAL COURSE

Clients with somatization disorder and body dysmorphic disorder often experience symptoms in adolescence, although these diagnoses may not be made until early adulthood (about 25 years of age). Conversion disorder usually occurs between 10 and 35 years of age. Pain disorder and hypochondriasis can occur at any age (APA, 2000).

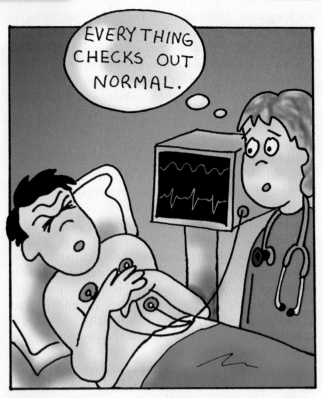

Somatoform disorders

All the somatoform disorders are either chronic or recurrent, lasting for decades for many people. Clients with somatization disorder and conversion disorder most likely seek help from mental health professionals after they have exhausted efforts at finding a diagnosed medical condition. Clients with hypochondriasis, pain disorder, and body dysmorphic disorder are unlikely to receive treatment in mental health settings unless they have a comorbid condition. Clients with somatoform disorders tend to go from one physician or clinic to another, or they may see multiple providers at once in an effort to obtain relief of symptoms. They tend to be pessimistic about the medical establishment and often believe their disease could be diagnosed if providers were more competent.

RELATED DISORDERS

Somatoform disorders need to be distinguished from other body-related mental disorders such as malingering and factitious disorders, in which people feign or intentionally produce symptoms for some purpose or gain. In malingering and factitious disorders, people willfully control the symptoms. In somatoform disorders, clients do not voluntarily control their physical symptoms.

Malingering is the intentional production of false or grossly exaggerated physical or psychological symptoms; it is motivated by external incentives such as avoiding work, evading criminal prosecution, obtaining financial compensation, or obtaining drugs. People who malinger have no real physical symptoms or grossly exaggerate relatively minor symptoms. Their purpose is some external incentive or outcome that they view as important and results directly from the illness. People who malinger can stop the physical symptoms as soon as they have gained what they wanted (Wang et al., 2005).

Factitious disorder occurs when a person intentionally produces or feigns physical or psychological symptoms solely to gain attention. People with factitious disorder may even inflict injury on themselves to receive attention. The common term for factitious disorder is **Munchausen syndrome**. A variation of factitious disorder, **Munchausen syndrome by proxy**, occurs when a person inflicts illness or injury on someone else to gain the attention of emergency medical personnel or to be a "hero" for saving the victim. An example would be a nurse who gives excess intravenous

CLINICAL VIGNETTE: CONVERSION DISORDER

Matthew, 13, has just been transferred from a medical unit to the adolescent psychiatric unit. He had been on the medical unit for 3 days, undergoing extensive tests to determine the cause of a sudden onset of blindness. No organic pathology was discovered, and Matthew was diagnosed with a conversion disorder.

As the nurse interviews Matthew, she notices that he is calm and speaks of his inability to see in a matter-of-fact manner, demonstrating no distress at his blindness. Matthew seems to have the usual interests of a 13-year-old, describing his activities at school and with his friends. However, the nurse finds that Matthew has little to say about his parents, his younger brother, or activities at home.

Later, the nurse has a chance to talk with Matthew's mother when she comes to the unit after work. Soon, Matthew's mother is crying, telling the nurse that her husband has a drinking problem and has been increasingly violent at home. She admitted that two days before Matthew's symptoms developed, Matthew witnessed one of his father's rages, which included breaking furniture and hitting her. When Matthew tried to help his mother, his father called him spineless and worthless and told him to go to the basement and stay there. The nurse understands that the violence Matthew has witnessed and his inability to change the situation may be the triggering event for his conversion disorder.

DSM-IV-TR DIAGNOSTIC CRITERIA:
SYMPTOMS OF SOMATIZATION DISORDER

Pain symptoms: complaints of headache; pain in the abdomen, head, joints, back, chest, rectum; pain during urination, menstruation, or sexual intercourse

Gastrointestinal symptoms: nausea, bloating, vomiting (other than during pregnancy), diarrhea, or intolerance of several foods

Sexual symptoms: sexual indifference, erectile or ejaculatory dysfunction, irregular menses, excessive menstrual bleeding, vomiting throughout pregnancy

Pseudoneurologic symptoms: conversion symptoms such as impaired coordination or balance, paralysis or localized weakness, difficulty swallowing or lump in throat, aphonia, urinary retention, hallucinations, loss of touch or pain sensation, double vision, blindness, deafness, seizures; dissociative symptoms such as amnesia; or loss of consciousness other than fainting

Adapted from American Psychiatric Association. (2000). Diagnostic and statistical manual of mental disorders (4th ed., text revision). Washington, DC: APA.

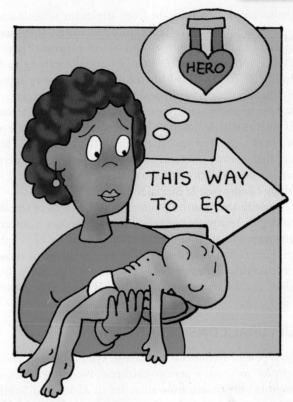

Munchausen syndrome by proxy

potassium to a client and then "saves his life" by performing cardiopulmonary resuscitation. Although factitious disorders are uncommon, they occur most often in people who are in or familiar with medical professions, such as nurses, physicians, medical technicians, or hospital volunteers. People who injure clients or their children through Munchausen syndrome by proxy generally are arrested and prosecuted in the legal system (Ragaisis, 2004).

ETIOLOGY
Psychosocial Theories

Psychosocial theorists believe that people with somatoform disorders keep stress, anxiety, or frustration inside rather than expressing them outwardly. This is called **internalization**. Clients express these internalized feelings and stress through physical symptoms (somatization). Both internalization and somatization are unconscious defense mechanisms. Clients are not consciously aware of the process, and they do not voluntarily control it.

People with somatoform disorders do not readily and directly express their feelings and emotions verbally. They have tremendous difficulty dealing with interpersonal conflict. When placed in situations involving conflict or emotional stress, their physical symptoms appear to worsen. The worsening of physical symptoms helps them to meet psychological needs for security, attention, and affection through primary and secondary gain (Hollifield, 2005). **Primary gains** are the direct external benefits that being sick provides, such as relief of anxiety, conflict, or distress. **Secondary gains** are the internal or personal benefits received from others because one is sick, such as attention from family members and comfort measures (e.g., being brought tea, receiving a back rub). The person soon learns that he or she "needs to be sick" to have their emotional needs met.

Somatization is associated most often with women, as evidenced by the old term *hysteria* (Greek for "wandering uterus"). Ancient theorists believed that unexplained female pains resulted from migration of the uterus throughout the woman's body. Psychosocial theorists posit that increased incidence of somatization in women may be related to various factors:

- Boys in the United States are taught to be stoic and to "take it like a man," causing them to offer fewer physical complaints as adults.
- Women seek medical treatment more often than men, and it is more socially acceptable for them to do so.
- Childhood sexual abuse, which is related to somatization, happens more frequently to girls.
- Women more often receive treatment for psychiatric disorders with strong somatic components such as depression.

Biologic Theories

Research has shown differences in the way that clients with somatoform disorders regulate and interpret stimuli. These clients cannot sort relevant from irrelevant stimuli and respond equally to both types. In other words, they may experience a normal body sensation such as peristalsis and attach a pathologic rather than a normal meaning to it (Hollifield, 2005). Too little inhibition of sensory input amplifies awareness of physical symptoms and exaggerates response to bodily sensations. For example, minor discomfort such as muscle tightness becomes amplified because of the client's concern and attention to the tightness. This amplified sensory awareness causes the person to experience somatic sensations as more intense, noxious, and disturbing (Andreasen & Black, 2006).

Somatization disorder is found in 10% to 20% of female first-degree relatives of people with this disorder. Conversion symptoms are found more often in relatives of people with conversion disorder. First-degree relatives of those with pain disorder are more likely to have depressive disorders, alcohol dependence, and chronic pain (APA, 2000).

CULTURAL CONSIDERATIONS

The type and frequency of somatic symptoms and their meaning may vary across cultures. Pseudoneurologic symptoms of somatization disorder in Africa and South Asia include burning hands and feet and the nondelusional sensation of worms in the head or ants under the skin. Symptoms related to male reproduction are more common in some countries or cultures—for example, men in India often have *dhat*, which is a hypochondriacal concern about loss of semen. Somatization disorder is rare in men in the United States but more common in Greece and Puerto Rico.

Many culture-bound syndromes have corresponding somatic symptoms not explained by a medical condition (Table 19.1). *Koro* occurs in Southeast Asia and may be related to body dysmorphic disorder. It is characterized by the belief that the penis is shrinking and will disappear into the abdomen, causing the man to die. Falling-out episodes, found in the southern United States and the Caribbean islands, are characterized by a sudden collapse during which the person cannot see or move. *Hwa-byung* is a Korean folk syndrome attributed to the suppression of anger and includes insomnia, fatigue, panic, indigestion, and generalized aches and pains. *Sangue dormido* ("sleeping blood") occurs among Portuguese Cape Verde Islanders who report pain, numbness, tremors, paralysis, seizures, blindness, heart attacks, and miscarriages. *Shenjing shuariuo* occurs in China and includes physical and mental fatigue, dizziness, headache, pain, sleep disturbance, memory loss, gastrointestinal problems, and sexual dysfunction (Mojtabai, 2005).

TREATMENT

Treatment focuses on managing symptoms and improving quality of life. The health care provider must show empathy and sensitivity to the client's physical complaints (Karvonen et al., 2004). A trusting relationship helps to ensure that clients stay with and receive care from one provider instead of "doctor shopping."

For many clients, depression may accompany or result from somatoform disorders. Thus, antidepressants help in some cases. Selective serotonin reuptake inhibitors such as fluoxetine (Prozac), sertraline (Zoloft), and paroxetine (Paxil) are used most commonly (Table 19.2).

For clients with pain disorder, referral to a chronic pain clinic may be useful. Clients learn methods of pain management such as visual imaging and relaxation. Services such as physical therapy to maintain and build muscle tone help to improve functional abilities. Providers should avoid prescribing and administering narcotic analgesics to these

Table 19.1   CULTURE-BOUND SYNDROMES

Syndrome	Culture	Characteristics
Dhat	India	Hypochondriacal concern about semen loss
Koro	Southeast Asia	Belief that penis is shrinking and will disappear into abdomen, resulting in death
Falling-out episodes	Southern United States, Caribbean islands	Sudden collapse; person cannot see or move
Hwa-byung	Korea	Suppressed anger causes insomnia, fatigue, panic, indigestion, and generalized aches and pains
Sangue dormido ("sleeping blood")	Portuguese Cape Verde Islands	Pain, numbness, tremors, paralysis, seizures, blindness, heart attack, miscarriage
Shenjing shuariuo	China	Physical and mental fatigue, dizziness, headache, pain, sleep disturbance, memory loss, GI problems, sexual dysfunction

Adapted from Mojtabai, R. (2005). Culture-bound syndromes with psychotic features. In B. J. Sadock & V. A. Sadock (Eds.), *Comprehensive textbook of psychiatry* (Vol. 1, 8th ed., pp. 1538–1542). Philadelphia: Lippincott Williams & Wilkins. © American Psychiatric Association. Reprinted with permission.

Table 19.2	ANTIDEPRESSANTS USED TO TREAT SOMATOFORM DISORDERS	
Drug	**Usual Dose (mg/day)**	**Nursing Considerations**
Fluoxetine (Prozac)	20–60	Monitor for rash, hives, insomnia, headache, anxiety, drowsiness, nausea, loss of appetite; avoid alcohol
Paroxetine (Paxil)	20–60	Monitor for nausea, loss of appetite, dizziness, dry mouth, somnolence or insomnia, sweating, sexual dysfunction; avoid alcohol
Sertraline (Zoloft)	50–200	Monitor for nausea, loss of appetite, diarrhea, headache, insomnia, sexual dysfunction; avoid alcohol

clients because of the risk for dependence or abuse. Clients can use nonsteroidal anti-inflammatory agents to help reduce pain.

Involvement in therapy groups is beneficial for some people with somatoform disorders. Studies of clients with somatization disorder who participated in a structured cognitive-behavioral group showed evidence of improved physical and emotional health 1 year later (Hollifield, 2005). The overall goals of the group were offering peer support, sharing methods of coping, and perceiving and expressing emotions. Abramowitz and Braddock (2006) found that clients with hypochondriasis who were willing to participate in cognitive-behavioral therapy and take medications were able to alter their erroneous perceptions of threat (of illness) and improve. Cognitive-behavioral therapy also produced significant improvement in clients with somatization disorder (Allen et. al., 2006).

In terms of prognosis, somatoform disorders tend to be chronic or recurrent. With treatment, conversion disorder often remits in a few weeks but recurs in 25% of clients. Somatization disorder, hypochondriasis, and pain disorder often last for many years, and clients report being in poor

health. People with body dysmorphic disorder may be preoccupied with the same or a different perceived body flaw throughout their lives (APA, 2000).

APPLICATION OF THE NURSING PROCESS

The underlying mechanism of somatization is consistent for clients with somatoform disorders of all types. This section discusses application of the nursing process for clients with somatization; differences among the disorders are highlighted in the appropriate places.

Assessment

The nurse must investigate physical health status thoroughly to ensure there is no underlying pathology requiring treatment. Box 19.1 contains a useful screening test for symptoms of somatization disorder. When a client has been diagnosed with a somatoform disorder, it is important not to dismiss all future complaints because at any time the client could develop a physical condition that would require medical attention.

Box 19.1	ASSESSMENT QUESTIONS FOR SYMPTOMS IN SCREENING TEST FOR SOMATIZATION DISORDER

1. Have you ever had trouble breathing?
2. Have you ever had trouble with menstrual cramps?
3. Have you ever had burning sensations in your sexual organs, mouth, or rectum?
4. Have you ever had difficulties swallowing or had an uncomfortable lump in your throat that stayed for at least an hour?
5. Have you ever found that you could not remember what you had been doing for hours or days at a time? If yes, did this happen even though you had not been drinking or using drugs?
6. Have you ever had trouble with frequent vomiting?
7. Have you ever had frequent pain in your fingers or toes?

Adapted from Othmer, E., & DeSouza, C. (1983). A screening test for somatization disorder (hysteria). American Journal of Psychiatry, 142(10), 1146–1149.
© American Psychiatric Association. Reprinted with permission.

HISTORY

Clients usually provide a lengthy and detailed account of previous physical problems, numerous diagnostic tests, and perhaps even a number of surgical procedures. It is likely that they have seen multiple health care providers over several years. Clients may express dismay or anger at the medical community with comments such as "They just can't find out what's wrong with me" or "They're all incompetent, and they're trying to tell me I'm crazy!" The exception may be clients with conversion disorder, who show little emotion when describing physical limitations or lack of a medical diagnosis (*la belle indifférence*).

GENERAL APPEARANCE AND MOTOR BEHAVIOR

Overall appearance usually is not remarkable. Often, clients walk slowly or with an unusual gait because of the pain or disability caused by the symptoms. They may exhibit a facial expression of discomfort or physical distress. In many cases, they brighten and look much better as the assessment interview begins because they have the nurse's undivided attention. Clients with somatization disorder usually describe their complaints in colorful, exaggerated terms but often lack specific information.

MOOD AND AFFECT

Mood is often labile, shifting from seeming depressed and sad when describing physical problems to looking bright and excited when talking about how they had to go to the hospital in the middle of the night by ambulance. Emotions are often exaggerated, as are reports of physical symptoms. Clients describing a series of personal crises related to their physical health may appear pleased rather than distressed about these situations. Clients with conversion disorder display an unexpected lack of distress.

THOUGHT PROCESS AND CONTENT

Clients who somatize do not experience disordered thought processes. The content of their thinking is primarily about often exaggerated physical concerns; for example, when they have a simple cold, they may be convinced it is pneumonia. They may even talk about dying and what music they want played at their funeral.

Clients are unlikely to be able to think about or to respond to questions about emotional feelings. They will answer questions about how they feel in terms of physical health or sensations. For example, the nurse may ask, "How did you feel about having to quit your job?" The client might respond, "Well, I thought I'd feel better with the extra rest, but my back pain was just as bad as ever."

Clients with hypochondriasis focus on the fear of serious illness rather than the existence of illness, as seen in clients with other somatoform disorders. However, they are just as preoccupied with physical concerns as other somatizing clients and are likewise very limited in their abilities to iden-

tify emotional feelings or interpersonal issues. Fink and colleagues (2004) found that clients with hypochondriasis were preoccupied with bodily functions, ruminated about illness, were fascinated about medical information, and had unrealistic fears about potential infection and prescription medications.

SENSORIUM AND INTELLECTUAL PROCESSES

Clients are alert and oriented. Intellectual functions are unimpaired.

JUDGMENT AND INSIGHT

Exaggerated responses to their physical health may affect clients' judgment. They have little or no insight into their behavior. They are firmly convinced their problem is entirely physical and often believe that others don't understand.

SELF-CONCEPT

Clients focus only on the physical part of themselves. They are unlikely to think about personal characteristics or strengths and are uncomfortable when asked to do so. Clients who somatize have low self-esteem and seem to deal with it by totally focusing on physical concerns. They lack confidence, have little success in work situations, and have difficulty managing daily life issues, which they relate solely to their physical status.

ROLES AND RELATIONSHIPS

Clients are unlikely to be employed, although they may have a past work history. They often lose jobs because of excessive absenteeism or inability to perform work; clients may have quit working voluntarily because of poor physical health. Consumed with seeking medical care, they have difficulty fulfilling family roles. It is likely that these clients have few friends and spend little time in social activities. They may decline to see friends or to go out socially for fear that they would become desperately ill away from home. Most socialization takes place with members of the health care community.

Clients may report a lack of family support and understanding. Family members may tire of the ceaseless complaints and the client's refusal to accept the absence of a medical diagnosis. The illnesses and physical conditions often interfere with planned family events such going on vacations or attending family gatherings. Home life is often chaotic and unpredictable.

PHYSIOLOGIC AND SELF-CARE CONCERNS

In addition to the multitude of physical complaints, these clients often have legitimate needs in terms of their health practices (Box 19.2). Clients who somatize often have sleep pattern disturbances, lack basic nutrition, and get no exercise. In addition, they may be taking multiple prescriptions for pain or other complaints. If a client has been

Box 19.2   CLINICAL NURSE ALERT

Just because a client has been diagnosed with a somatoform disorder, do not automatically dismiss all future complaints. They should be completely assessed because the client could, at any time, develop a physical condition that would require medical attention.

using anxiolytics or medications for pain, the nurse must consider the possibility of withdrawal (see Chapter 17).

Data Analysis

Nursing diagnoses commonly used when working with clients who somatize include the following:
- Ineffective Coping
- Ineffective Denial
- Impaired Social Interaction
- Anxiety
- Disturbed Sleep Pattern
- Fatigue
- Pain

Clients with conversion disorder may be at risk for disuse syndrome from having pseudoneurologic paralysis symptoms. In other words, if clients do not use a limb for a long time, the muscles may weaken or atrophy from lack of use.

Outcome Identification

Treatment outcomes for clients with a somatoform disorder may include the following:
- The client will identify the relationship between stress and physical symptoms.
- The client will verbally express emotional feelings.
- The client will follow an established daily routine.
- The client will demonstrate alternative ways to deal with stress, anxiety, and other feelings.
- The client will demonstrate healthier behaviors regarding rest, activity, and nutritional intake.

Intervention

PROVIDING HEALTH TEACHING

The nurse must help the client to establish a daily routine that includes improved health behaviors. Adequate nutritional intake, improved sleep patterns, and a realistic balance of activity and rest are all areas with which the client may need assistance. The nurse should expect resistance, including protests from the client that she or he does not feel well enough to do these things. The challenge for the

nurse is to validate the client's feelings while encouraging her or him to participate in activities.

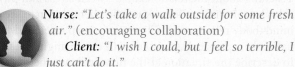

> **Nurse:** *"Let's take a walk outside for some fresh air."* (encouraging collaboration)
> **Client:** *"I wish I could, but I feel so terrible, I just can't do it."*
> **Nurse:** *"I know this is difficult, but some exercise is essential. It will be a short walk."* (validation; encouraging collaboration)

The nurse can use a similar approach to gain client participation in eating more nutritious foods, getting up and dressed at a certain time every morning, and setting a regular bedtime. The nurse also can explain that inactivity and poor eating habits perpetuate discomfort and that often it is necessary to engage in behaviors even when one doesn't feel like it.

> **Client:** *"I just can't eat anything. I have no appetite."*
> **Nurse:** *"I know you don't feel well, but it is important to begin eating."* (validation; encouraging collaboration)
> **Client:** *"I promise I'll eat just as soon as I'm hungry."*
> **Nurse:** *"Actually, if you begin to eat a few bites, you'll begin to feel better, and your appetite may improve."* (encouraging collaboration)

The nurse should not strip clients of their somatizing defenses until he or she has collected adequate assessment data and clients have learned other coping mechanisms. The nurse should not attempt to confront clients about somatic symptoms or attempt to tell them that these symptoms are not "real." They are very real to clients, who actually experience the symptoms and associated distress.

CLIENT/FAMILY EDUCATION FOR SOMATOFORM DISORDERS

- Establish daily health routine, including adequate rest, exercise, and nutrition.
- Teach about relationship of stress and physical symptoms and mind–body relationship.
- Educate about proper nutrition, rest, and exercise.
- Educate client in relaxation techniques: progressive relaxation, deep breathing, guided imagery, and distraction such as music or other activities.
- Educate client by role-playing social situations and interactions.
- Encourage family to provide attention and encouragement when client has fewer complaints.
- Encourage family to decrease special attention when client is in "sick" role.

ASSISTING THE CLIENT TO EXPRESS EMOTIONS

Teaching about the relationship between stress and physical symptoms is a useful way to help clients begin to see the mind–body relationship. Clients may keep a detailed journal of their physical symptoms. The nurse might ask them to describe the situation at the time such as whether they were alone or with others, whether any disagreements were occurring, and so forth. The journal may help clients to see when physical symptoms seemed worse or better and what other factors may have affected that perception.

Limiting the time that clients can focus on physical complaints alone may be necessary. Encouraging them to focus on emotional feelings is important, although this can be difficult for clients. The nurse should provide attention and positive feedback for efforts to identify and discuss feelings.

It may help for the nurse to explain to the family about primary and secondary gains. For example, if the family can provide attention to clients when they are feeling better or fulfilling responsibilities, clients are more likely to continue doing so. If family members have lavished attention on clients when they have physical complaints, the nurse can encourage the relatives to stop reinforcing the sick role.

TEACHING COPING STRATEGIES

Two categories of coping strategies are important for clients to learn and to practice: **emotion-focused coping strategies**, which help clients relax and reduce feelings of stress, and **problem-focused coping strategies**, which help to resolve or change a client's behavior or situation or manage life stressors. Emotion-focused strategies include progressive relaxation, deep breathing, guided imagery, and distractions such as music or other activities. Many approaches to stress

relief are available for clients to try. The nurse should help clients to learn and practice these techniques, emphasizing that their effectiveness usually improves with routine use. Clients must not expect such techniques to eliminate their pain or physical symptoms; rather, the focus is helping them to manage or diminish the intensity of the symptoms.

Problem-focused coping strategies include learning problem-solving methods, applying the process to identified problems, and role-playing interactions with others. For example, a client may complain that no one comes to visit or that she has no friends. The nurse can help the client to plan social contact with others, can role-play what to talk about (other than the client's complaints), and can improve the client's confidence in making relationships. The nurse also can help clients to identify stressful life situations and plan strategies to deal with them. For example, if a client finds it difficult to accomplish daily household tasks, the nurse can help him to plan a schedule with difficult tasks followed by something the client may enjoy.

Evaluation

Somatoform disorders are chronic or recurrent, so changes are likely to occur slowly. If treatment is effective, the client should make fewer visits to physicians as a result of physical complaints, use less medication and more positive coping techniques, and increase functional abilities. Improved family and social relationships are also a positive outcome that may follow improvements in the client's coping abilities.

COMMUNITY-BASED CARE

Health care professionals often encounter clients with somatoform disorders in clinics, physicians' offices, or settings other than those related to mental health. Building a trusting relationship with the client, providing empathy and support, and being sensitive to rather than dismissive of complaints are skills that the nurse can use in any setting where clients are seeking assistance. Making appropriate referrals such as to a pain clinic for clients with pain disorder or providing information about support groups in the community may be helpful. Encouraging clients to find pleasurable activities or hobbies may help to meet their needs for attention and security, thus diminishing the psychological needs for somatic symptoms.

MENTAL HEALTH PROMOTION

A common theme in somatoform disorders is their occurrence in people who do not express conflicts, stress, and emotions verbally. They express themselves through physical symptoms; the resulting attention and focus on their physical ailments somewhat meet their needs. As these clients are better able to express their emotions and needs directly, physical symptoms subside. Thus, assisting them to deal with emotional issues directly is a strategy for mental health promotion.

NURSING INTERVENTIONS FOR SOMATOFORM DISORDERS

- Health teaching
  Establish a daily routine.
  Promote adequate nutrition and sleep.
- Expression of emotional feelings
  Recognize relationship between stress/coping and physical symptoms.
  Keep a journal.
  Limit time spent on physical complaints.
  Limit primary and secondary gains.
- Coping strategies
  Emotion-focused coping strategies such as relaxation techniques, deep breathing, guided imagery, and distraction
  Problem-focused coping strategies such as problem-solving strategies and role-playing

Micale (2000) wrote that "hysteria" and neuroses (now called somatization disorder) have decreased in the United States since 1900. He cited the following reasons for this decline:

- People now have more "psychological self-knowledge."
- The sexual confinement, emotional oppression, and social suffocation of the Victorian era have dissipated.
- The interaction of mind and body now has a scientific foundation.

As people continue to gain knowledge about themselves and to express their emotional needs and desires directly, the incidence of coping through physical symptoms should continue to decline.

SELF-AWARENESS ISSUES

Clients who cope through physical symptoms can be frustrating for the nurse. Initially, they are unwilling to consider that anything other than major physical illness is the root of all their problems. When health professionals tell clients there is no physical illness and refer them to mental health professionals, the response often is anger: Clients may express anger directly or passively at the medical community and be highly critical of the inadequate care they believe they have received. The nurse must not respond with anger to such outbursts or criticism.

The client's progress is slow and painstaking, if any happens at all. Clients coping with somatization have been doing so for years. Changes are not rapid or drastic. The nurse may feel frustrated because, after giving the client his or her best efforts, the client returns time after time with the same focus on physical symptoms. The nurse should be realistic about the small successes that can be achieved in any given period. To enhance the ongoing relationship, the nurse must be able to accept the client and his or her continued complaints and criticisms while remaining nonjudgmental.

Points to Consider When Working With Clients With Somatoform Disorders

- Carefully assess the client's physical complaints. Even when a client has a history of a somatoform disorder, the nurse must not dismiss physical complaints or assume they are psychological. The client actually may have a medical condition.
- Validate the client's feelings while trying to engage him or her in treatment; for example, use a reflective yet engaging comment such as "I know you're not feeling well, but it is important to get some exercise each day."
- Remember that the somatic complaints are not under the client's voluntary control. The client will have fewer somatic complaints when he or she improves coping skills and interpersonal relationships.

(text continues on p. 427)

Nursing Care Plan   *Hypochondriasis*

Nursing Diagnosis

Ineffective Coping: *Inability to form a valid appraisal of the stressors, inadequate choices of practiced responses, and/or inability to use available resources.*

ASSESSMENT DATA

- Denial of emotional problems
- Difficulty identifying and expressing feelings
- Lack of insight
- Self-preoccupation, especially with physical functioning
- Fears of or rumination on disease
- Numerous somatic complaints (may involve many different organs or systems)
- Sensory complaints (pain, loss of taste sensation, olfactory complaints)
- Reluctance or refusal to participate in psychiatric treatment program or activities
- Reliance on medications or physical treatments (such as laxative dependence)

EXPECTED OUTCOMES

Immediate
The client will
- Participate in the treatment program
- Decrease the number and frequency of physical complaints
- Demonstrate compliance with medical therapy and medications
- Demonstrate adequate energy, food, and fluid intake
- Identify life stresses and anxieties
- Identify the relationship between stress and physical symptoms
- Express feelings verbally
- Identify alternative ways to deal with stress, anxiety, or other feelings

continued ⋯⋗

Nursing Care Plan: Hypochondriasis, cont.

ASSESSMENT DATA

- Extensive use of over-the-counter medications, home remedies, enemas, and so forth
- Ritualistic behaviors (such as exaggerated bowel routines)
- Tremors
- Limited gratification from interpersonal relationships
- Lack of emotional support system
- Anxiety
- Secondary gains received for physical problems
- History of repeated visits to physicians or hospital admissions
- History of repeated medical evaluations with no findings of abnormalities

EXPECTED OUTCOMES

Stabilization
The client will
- Decrease ritualistic behaviors
- Decrease physical attention-seeking complaints
- Verbalize increased insight into the dynamics of hypochondriacal behavior, including secondary gains
- Verbalize an understanding of therapeutic regimens and medications, if any

Community
The client will
- Eliminate overuse of medications or physical treatments
- Demonstrate alternative ways to deal with stress, anxiety, or other feelings

IMPLEMENTATION

Nursing Interventions *denotes collaborative interventions	**Rationale**
The initial nursing assessment should include a complete physical assessment, a history of previous complaints and treatment, and a consideration of each current complaint.	The nursing assessment provides a baseline from which to begin planning care.
*The nursing staff should note the medical staff's assessment of each complaint on the client's admission.	Genuine physical problems must be noted and treated.
*Each time the client voices a new complaint, the client should be referred to the medical staff for assessment (and treatment if appropriate).	It is unsafe to assume that all physical complaints are hypochondriacal—the client could really be ill or injured. The client may attempt to establish the legitimacy of complaints by being genuinely injured or ill.
*Minimize the amount of time and attention given to complaints. When the client makes a complaint, refer him or her to the medical staff (if it is a new complaint) or follow the team treatment plan; then tell the client you will discuss something else but not bodily complaints. Tell the client that you are interested in the client as a person, not just in his or her physical complaints. If the complaint is not acute, ask the client to discuss the complaint during a regular appointment with the medical staff.	If physical complaints are unsuccessful in gaining attention, they should decrease in frequency over time.
Withdraw your attention if the client insists on making complaints the sole topic of conversation. Tell the client your reason for withdrawal and that you will return later to discuss other topics.	It is important to make clear to the client that attention is withdrawn from physical complaints, not from the client as a person.

Nursing Care Plan: Hypochondriasis, cont.

IMPLEMENTATION

Nursing Interventions *denotes collaborative interventions	Rationale
Allow the client a specific time limit (like 5 minutes per hour) to discuss physical complaints with one person. The remaining staff will discuss only other issues with the client.	Because physical complaints have been the client's primary coping strategy, it is less threatening to the client if you limit this behavior initially rather than forbid it. If the client is denied this coping mechanism before new skills can be developed, hypochondriacal behavior may increase.
Acknowledge the complaint as the client's perception and then follow the previous approaches; do not argue about the somatic complaints.	Arguing gives the client's complaints attention, albeit negative, and the client is able to avoid discussing feelings.
Use minimal objective reassurance in conjunction with questions to explore the client's feelings. ("Your tests have shown that you have no lesions. Do you still feel that you do? What are your feelings about this?")	This approach helps the client make the transition to discussing feelings.
Encourage the client to discuss his or her feelings about the fears rather than the fears themselves.	The focus is on feelings of fear, not fear of physical problems.
Explore the client's feelings of lack of control over stress and life events.	The client may have helpless feelings but may not recognize this independently.
Initially, carefully assess the client's self-image, social patterns, and ways of dealing with anger, stress, and so forth.	This assessment provides a knowledge base regarding hypochondriacal behaviors.
Talk with the client about sources of satisfaction and dissatisfaction, relationships, employment, and so forth.	Open-ended discussion usually is nonthreatening and helps the client begin self-assessment.
After some discussion of the above and developing a trust relationship, talk more directly with the client and encourage him or her to identify specific stresses, recent and ongoing.	The client's perception of stressors forms the basis of his or her behavior and usually is more significant than others' perception of those stressors.
If the client is using denial as a defense mechanism, point out apparent or possible stresses (in a non-threatening way) and ask the client for feedback.	If the client is in denial, more direct approaches may produce anger or hostility and threaten the trust relationship.
Gradually, help the client identify possible connections between anxiety and the occurrence of physical symptoms, such as: What makes the client more or less comfortable? What is the client doing or what is going on around the client when he or she experiences symptoms?	The client can begin to see the relatedness of stress and physical problems at his or her own pace. Self-realization will be more acceptable to the client than the nurse telling the client the problem.
Encourage the client to keep a diary of situations, stresses, and occurrence of symptoms and use it to identify relationships between stresses and symptoms.	Reflecting on written items may be more accurate and less threatening to the client.
Talk with the client at least once per shift, focusing on the client's identifying and expressing feelings.	Demonstrating consistent interest in the client facilitates the relationship and can desensitize the discussion of emotional issues.
Encourage the client to ventilate feelings by talking or crying, through physical activities, and so forth.	The client may have difficulty expressing feelings directly. Your support may help him or her develop these skills.

continued ⋯⊁

Nursing Care Plan: Hypochondriasis, cont.

IMPLEMENTATION

Nursing Interventions *denotes collaborative interventions	Rationale
*Teach the client and his or her family or significant others about the dynamics of hypochondriacal behavior and the treatment plan, including plans after discharge.	The client and his or her family or significant others may have little or no knowledge of these areas. Knowledge of the treatment plan will promote long-term behavior change.
*Talk with the client and significant others about secondary gains and together develop a plan to reduce those gains. Identify the needs the client is attempting to meet with secondary gains (such as attention or escape from responsibilities).	Maintaining limits to reduce secondary gain requires everyone's participation to be successful. The client's family and significant others must be aware of the client's needs if they want to be effective in helping to meet those needs.
Help the client plan to meet his or her needs in more direct ways. Show the client that he or she can gain attention when he or she does not exhibit symptoms, deals with responsibilities directly, or asserts himself or herself in the face of stress.	Positive feedback and support for healthier behavior tend to make that behavior recur more frequently. The client's family and significant others also must use positive reinforcement.
Reduce the benefits of illness as much as possible. Do not allow the client to avoid responsibilities or allow special privileges, such as staying in bed by voicing somatic discomfort.	If physical problems do not get the client what he or she wants, the client is less likely to cope in that manner.
*Work with the medical staff to limit the number, variety, strength, and frequency of medications, enemas, and so forth that are made available to the client.	A team effort helps to prevent the client's manipulation of staff members to obtain additional medication.
When the client requests a medication or treatment, encourage the client to identify what precipitated his or her complaint and to deal with it in other ways.	If the client can obtain stress relief in a nonchemical, nonmedical way, he or she is less likely to use the medication or treatment.
Observe and record the circumstances related to complaints; talk about your observations with the client.	Alerting the client to situations surrounding the complaint helps him or her see the relatedness of stress and physical symptoms.
Help the client identify and use nonchemical methods of pain relief, such as relaxation techniques.	Using nonchemical pain relief shifts the focus of coping away from medications and increases the client's sense of control.
Teach the client more healthful daily living habits, including diet, stress management techniques, daily exercise, rest, possible connection between caffeine and anxiety symptoms, and so forth.	Optimal physical wellness is especially important with clients using physical symptoms as a coping strategy.
Encourage the client to ventilate feelings by talking or crying, through physical activities, and so forth.	The client may have difficulty expressing feelings. Your support may help the client develop these skills.
Encourage the client to express feelings directly, especially feelings with which the client is uncomfortable (such as anger or resentment).	Direct expression of feelings will minimize the need to use physical symptoms to express them.
Notice the client's interactions with others and give positive feedback for self-assertion and expressing feelings, especially anger, resentment, and other so-called negative emotions.	The client needs to know that appropriate expressions of anger or other negative emotions are acceptable and that he or she can feel better physically as a result of these expressions.

Adapted from Schultz, J. M., & Videbeck, S. L. (2005). Lippincott's manual of psychiatric nursing care plans (7th ed.). Philadelphia: Lippincott Williams & Wilkins.

Critical Thinking Questions

1. When a client has somatoform pain disorder, powerful analgesics such as narcotics are generally contraindicated, even though the client is suffering unremitting pain. How might the nurse feel when working with this client? How does the nurse respond when the client says, "You know I'm in pain! Why won't you do anything? Why do you let me suffer?"

2. Should there be limits on expensive medical tests and procedures for clients with somatoform disorder? Who should decide when health care benefits are limited?

3. A mother is found to have caused a medical crisis by giving her 6-year-old child a medication to which the child has a known severe allergy. The mother is diagnosed as having Munchausen syndrome by proxy. Should she be treated in the mental health setting? Charged with a criminal act? Why?

KEY POINTS

- Somatization means transforming mental experiences and states into bodily symptoms.
- The three central features of somatoform disorders are physical complaints that suggest major medical illness but have no demonstrable organic basis; psychological factors and conflicts that seem important in initiating, exacerbating, and maintaining the symptoms; and symptoms or magnified health concerns that are not under the client's conscious control.
- Somatoform disorders include somatization disorder, conversion disorder, hypochondriasis, pain disorder, and body dysmorphic disorder.
- Malingering means feigning physical symptoms for some external gain such as avoiding work.

- Factitious disorders are characterized by physical symptoms that are feigned or inflicted for the sole purpose of drawing attention to oneself and gaining the emotional benefits of assuming the sick role.
- Internalization and somatization are the chief defense mechanisms seen in somatoform disorders.
- Clients with somatization disorder and conversion reactions eventually may be treated in mental health settings. Clients with other somatoform disorders typically are seen in medical settings.
- Clients who cope with stress through somatizing are reluctant or unable to identify emotional feelings and interpersonal issues and have few coping abilities unrelated to physical symptoms.
- Nursing interventions that may be effective with clients who somatize involve providing health teaching, identifying emotional feelings and stress, and using alternative coping strategies.
- Coping strategies that are helpful to clients with somatoform disorders include relaxation techniques such as guided imagery and deep breathing, distractions such as music, and problem-solving strategies such as identifying stressful situations, learning new methods of managing them, and role-playing social interactions.
- Clients with somatization disorder actually experience symptoms and the associated discomfort and pain. The nurse should never try to confront the client about the origin of these symptoms until the client has learned other coping strategies.
- Somatoform disorders are chronic or recurrent, so progress toward treatment outcomes can be slow and difficult.
- Nurses caring for clients with somatoform disorders must show patience and understanding toward them as they struggle through years of recurrent somatic complaints and attempts to learn new emotion- and problem-focused coping strategies.

INTERNET RESOURCES

RESOURCE	INTERNET ADDRESS
American Psychosomatic Society	http://www.psychosomatic.org
Body Dysmorphic Disorder	http://www.psychcentral.com/disorders/sx42.htm
Conversion Disorder	http://www.emedicine.com/emerg/topic112.htm
Munchausen Syndrome by Proxy Resources	http://www.vachss.com/help_text/msp.html
Psych Central: Hypochondriasis	http://www.psychcentral.com/disorders/sx57.htm

REFERENCES

Abramowitz, J. S., & Braddock, A. E. (2006). Hypochondriasis: Conceptualization, treatment, and relationship to obsessive-compulsive disorder. *Psychiatric Clinics of North America, 29*(2), 503–519.

Allen, L. A., Woolfolk, R. L., Escobar, J. I., Gara, M. A., & Hamer, R. M. (2006). Cognitive-behavioral therapy for somatization disorder: A randomized controlled trial. *Archives of Internal Medicine, 166*(14), 1512–1518.

American Psychiatric Association. (2000). *Diagnostic and statistical manual of mental disorders* (4th ed., text revision). Washington, DC: American Psychiatric Association.

Andreasen, N. C., & Black, D. W. (2006). *Introductory textbook of psychiatry* (2nd ed.). Washington, DC: American Psychiatric Publishing.

Fink, P., Ornbol, E., Toft, T., et al. (2004). A new empirically established hypochondriasis diagnosis. *American Journal of Psychiatry, 161*(9), 1680–1691.

Hollifield, M. A. (2005). Somatoform disorders. In B. J. Sadock & V. A. Sadock (Eds.), *Comprehensive textbook of psychiatry* (Vol. 1., 8th ed., pp. 1800–1828). Philadelphia: Lippincott Williams & Wilkins.

Karvonen, J. T., Veijola, J., Jokelainen, J., et al. (2004). Somatisation disorder in young adult population. *General Hospital Psychiatry, 26*(1), 9–12.

Micale, M. S. (2000). The decline of hysteria. *Harvard Mental Health Letter, 17*(1), 4–6.

Mojtabai, R. (2005). Culture-bound syndromes with psychotic features. In B. J. Sadock & V. A. Sadock (Eds.), *Comprehensive textbook of psychiatry* (Vol. 1, 8th ed., pp. 1538–1541). Philadelphia: Lippincott Williams & Wilkins.

Ragaisis, K. (2004). When the system works: Rescuing a child from Munchausen's syndrome by proxy. *Journal of Child and Adolescent Psychiatric Nursing, 17*(4), 173–176.

Schultz, J. M., & Videbeck, S. L. (2005). *Lippincott's manual of psychiatric nursing care plans* (7th ed.). Philadelphia: Lippincott Williams & Wilkins.

Wang, D., Nadiga, D. N., & Jenson, J. J. (2005). Factitious disorders. In B. J. Sadock & V. A. Sadock (Eds.), *Comprehensive textbook of psychiatry* (Vol. 1, 8th ed., pp. 1829–1843). Philadelphia: Lippincott Williams & Wilkins.

ADDITIONAL READINGS

Bahtia, M. S., & Sapra, S. (2005). Pseudoseizures in children: A profile of 50 cases. *Clinical Pediatrics, 44*(7), 617–621.

Creed, F. (2006). Should general psychiatry ignore somatization and hypochondriasis? *World Psychiatry, 5*(3) 146–150.

Gregory, R. J., & Jindal, S. (2006). Factitious disorder on an inpatient psychiatry ward. *American Journal of Orthopsychiatry, 76*(1), 31–36.

Weardon, A., Perryman, K., & Ward, V. (2006). Adult attachment, reassurance seeking, and hypochondriacal concerns in college students. *Journal of Health Psychology, 11*(6), 877–886.

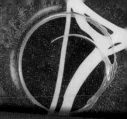

Chapter Study Guide

MULTIPLE-CHOICE QUESTIONS

Select the best answer for each of the following questions.

1. The nurse is caring for a client with a conversion disorder. Which of the following assessments will the nurse expect to see?
   A. Extreme distress over the physical symptom
   B. Indifference about the physical symptom
   C. Labile mood
   D. Multiple physical complaints

2. Which of the following statements would indicate that teaching about somatization disorder has been effective?
   A. "The doctor believes I am faking my symptoms."
   B. "If I try harder to control my symptoms, I will feel better."
   C. "I will feel better when I begin handling stress more effectively."
   D. "Nothing will help me feel better physically."

3. Paroxetine (Paxil) has been prescribed for a client with a somatoform disorder. The nurse instructs the client to watch for which of the following side effects?
   A. Constipation
   B. Increased appetite
   C. Increased flatulence
   D. Nausea

4. Emotion-focused coping strategies are designed to accomplish which of the following outcomes?
   A. Helping the client manage difficult situations more effectively
   B. Helping the client manage the intensity of symptoms
   C. Teaching the client the relationship between stress and physical symptoms
   D. Relieving the client's physical symptoms

5. Which of the following is true about clients with hypochondriasis?
   A. They may interpret normal body sensations as signs of disease.
   B. They often exaggerate or fabricate physical symptoms for attention.
   C. They do not show signs of distress about their physical symptoms.
   D. All the above are true statements.

6. The client's family asks the nurse, "What is hypochondriasis?" The best response by the nurse is, "Hypochondriasis is
   A. A persistent preoccupation with getting a serious disease."
   B. An illness not fully explained by a diagnosed medical condition."
   C. Characterized by a variety of symptoms over a number of years."
   D. The eventual result of excessive worrying about diseases."

7. A client with somatization disorder has been attending group therapy. Which of the following statements indicates that therapy is having a positive outcome for this client?
   A. "I feel better physically just from getting a chance to talk."
   B. "I haven't said much, but I get a lot from listening to others."
   C. "I shouldn't complain too much; my problems aren't as bad as others."
   D. "The other people in this group have emotional problems."

8. A client who developed numbness in the right hand could not play the piano at a scheduled recital. The consequence of the symptom, not having to perform, is best described as
   A. Emotion-focused coping
   B. Phobia
   C. Primary gain
   D. Secondary gain

FILL-IN-THE-BLANK QUESTIONS

Identify the type of somatoform disorder that is described by each of the following statements.

_____ Preoccupation with an imagined or exaggerated body defect

_____ Multiple physical symptoms including pain and gastrointestinal, sexual, and pseudoneurologic symptoms

_____ Sudden, unexplained deficits in sensory or motor function

_____ Pain that is unrelieved by analgesics and greatly affected by psychological factors

_____ Preoccupation with the fear of having or acquiring a serious illness

SHORT-ANSWER QUESTIONS

Define each of the following and provide an example.

Primary gain

Secondary gain

La belle indifférence

CLINICAL EXAMPLE

Mary Jones, 34 years old, was referred to a chronic pain clinic with a diagnosis of pain disorder. She has been unable to work for 7 months because of back pain. Mary has seen several doctors, has had an MRI, and has tried various anti-inflammatory medications. She tells the nurse that she is at the clinic as a last resort because none of her doctors will "do anything" for her. Mary's gait is slow, her posture is stiff, and she grimaces frequently while trying to sit in a chair. She reports being unable to drive a car, play with her children, do housework, or enjoy any of her previous leisure activities.

1. Identify three nursing diagnoses that would be pertinent for Mary's plan of care.

2. Identify two expected outcomes for Mary's plan of care.

3. Describe five interventions that the nurse might implement to achieve the outcomes.

4. What other disciplines might make a contribution to Mary's care at the clinic?

5. Identify any community referrals the nurse might make for Mary.

Chapter 20

Child and Adolescent Disorders

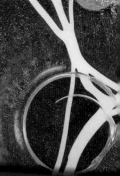

Key Terms

- attention deficit hyperactivity disorder (ADHD)
- autistic disorder
- conduct disorder
- encopresis
- enuresis
- limit setting
- pervasive developmental disorders
- pica
- stereotypic movements
- therapeutic play
- tic
- time-out
- Tourette's disorder

Learning Objectives

After reading this chapter, you should be able to

1. Discuss the characteristics, risk factors, and family dynamics of psychiatric disorders of childhood and adolescence.

2. Apply the nursing process to the care of children and adolescents with psychiatric disorders and their families.

3. Provide education to clients, families, teachers, caregivers, and community members for young clients with psychiatric disorders.

4. Discuss the nurse's role as an advocate for children and adolescents.

5. Evaluate your feelings, beliefs, and attitudes about clients with psychiatric disorders and their parents and caregivers.

Visit thePoint http://thePoint.lww.com for NCLEX-style questions, journal articles, and more!

Psychiatric disorders are not diagnosed as easily in children as they are in adults. Children usually lack the abstract cognitive abilities and verbal skills to describe what is happening. Because they constantly are changing and developing, children have limited sense of a stable, normal self to allow them to discriminate unusual or unwanted symptoms from normal feelings and sensations. Additionally, behaviors that are normal in a child of one age may indicate problems in a child of another age. For example, an infant who cries and wails when separated from her mother is normal. If the same child at 5 years of age cries and shows extreme anxiety when separated only briefly from her or his mother, however, this behavior would warrant investigation.

Children and adolescents experience some of the same mental health problems as adults, such as mood and anxiety disorders, and are diagnosed with these disorders using the same criteria as for adults. Eating disorders, especially anorexia, usually begin in adolescence and continue into adulthood. Discussions of mood, anxiety, and eating disorders are presented in separate chapters of this text.

This chapter focuses on those psychiatric disorders usually first diagnosed in infancy, childhood, or adolescence (Box 20.1); many of these can persist into adulthood. The childhood psychiatric disorders most common in mental health settings and specialized treatment units include pervasive developmental disorders, attention deficit hyperactivity disorder (ADHD), and disruptive behavior disorders. For this reason, the chapter presents an in-depth discussion of ADHD and conduct disorder (the most prevalent disruptive behavior disorder) with appropriate nursing diagnoses and interventions as well as sample nursing care plans. It discusses less common disorders briefly; generally, most of these disorders are not treated in inpatient psychiatric units unless they coexist with other disorders.

Box 20.1 DISORDERS FIRST DIAGNOSED IN INFANCY, CHILDHOOD, AND ADOLESCENCE

MENTAL RETARDATION

- Mild
- Moderate
- Severe
- Profound

LEARNING DISORDERS

- Reading disorder
- Mathematics disorder
- Disorder of written expression

MOTOR SKILLS DISORDER

- Developmental coordination disorder

COMMUNICATION DISORDERS

- Expressive language disorder
- Mixed receptive and expressive language disorder
- Phonologic disorder
- Stuttering

PERVASIVE DEVELOPMENTAL DISORDERS

- Autistic disorder
- Rett's disorder
- Childhood disintegrative disorder
- Asperger's disorder

ATTENTION DEFICIT AND DISRUPTIVE BEHAVIOR DISORDERS

- Attention deficit hyperactivity disorder
- Conduct disorder
- Oppositional defiant disorder

FEEDING AND EATING DISORDERS

- Pica
- Rumination disorder
- Feeding disorder of infancy or early childhood

TIC DISORDERS

- Tourette's disorder
- Chronic motor or tic disorder
- Transient tic disorder

ELIMINATION DISORDERS

- Encopresis
- Enuresis

OTHER DISORDERS OF INFANCY, CHILDHOOD, OR ADOLESCENCE

- Separation anxiety disorder
- Selective mutism
- Reactive attachment disorder
- Stereotypic movement disorder

Each category except feeding and eating disorders has an additional diagnosis "Not Otherwise Specified" (NOS) for similar problems that do not meet the criteria for other diagnoses in the category (DSM-IV-TR, 2000). Adapted from DSM-IV-TR (2000).

Mental Retardation

The essential feature of mental retardation is below-average intellectual functioning (intelligence quotient [IQ] less than 70) accompanied by significant limitations in areas of adaptive functioning such as communication skills, self-care, home living, social or interpersonal skills, use of community resources, self-direction, academic skills, work, leisure, and health and safety (King et al., 2005). The degree of retardation is based on IQ and greatly affects the person's ability to function:

- Mild retardation: IQ 50 to 70
- Moderate retardation: IQ 35 to 50
- Severe retardation: IQ 20 to 35
- Profound retardation: IQ less than 20

Causes of mental retardation include hereditary conditions such as Tay-Sachs disease or fragile X chromosome syndrome; early alterations in embryonic development such as trisomy 21 or maternal alcohol intake that causes fetal alcohol syndrome; pregnancy or perinatal problems such as fetal malnutrition, hypoxia, infections, and trauma; medical conditions of infancy such as infection or lead poisoning; and environmental influences such as deprivation of nurturing or stimulation.

Some people with mental retardation are passive and dependent; others are aggressive and impulsive. Children with mild to moderate mental retardation usually receive treatment in their homes and communities and make periodic visits to physicians. Those with severe or profound mental retardation may require residential placement or day care services.

Learning Disorders

A learning disorder is diagnosed when a child's achievement in reading, mathematics, or written expression is below that expected for age, formal education, and intelligence. Learning problems interfere with academic achievement and life activities requiring reading, math, or writing (American Psychiatric Association [APA], 2000). Reading and written expression disorders usually are identified in the first grade; math disorder may go undetected until the child reaches fifth grade. About 5% of children in U.S. public schools are diagnosed with a learning disorder. The school dropout rate for students with learning disorders is 1.5 times higher than the average rate for all students (APA, 2000).

Low self-esteem and poor social skills are common in children with learning disorders. As adults, some have problems with employment or social adjustment; others have minimal difficulties. Early identification of the learning disorder, effective intervention, and no coexisting problems are associated with better outcomes. Children with learning disorders are assisted with academic achievement through special education classes in public schools.

Motor Skills Disorder

The essential feature of *developmental coordination disorder* is impaired coordination severe enough to interfere with academic achievement or activities of daily living (APA, 2000). This diagnosis is not made if the problem with motor coordination is part of a general medical condition such as cerebral palsy or muscular dystrophy. This disorder becomes evident as a child attempts to crawl or walk or as an older child tries to dress independently or manipulate toys such as building blocks. Developmental coordination disorder often coexists with a communication disorder. Its course is variable; sometimes lack of coordination persists into adulthood (APA, 2000). Schools provide adaptive physical education and sensory integration programs to treat motor skills disorder. Adaptive physical education programs emphasize inclusion of movement games such as kicking a football or soccer ball. Sensory integration programs are specific physical therapies prescribed to target improvement in areas where the child has difficulties. For example, a child with tactile defensiveness (discomfort at being touched by another person) might be involved in touching and rubbing skin surfaces (Pataki & Spence, 2005).

Communication Disorders

A communication disorder is diagnosed when a communication deficit is severe enough to hinder development, academic achievement, or activities of daily living, including socialization. *Expressive language disorder* involves an impaired ability to communicate through verbal and sign language. The child has difficulty learning new words and speaking in complete and correct sentences; his or her speech is limited. *Mixed receptive-expressive language disorder* includes the problems of expressive language disorder along with difficulty understanding (receiving) and determining the meaning of words and sentences. Both disorders can be present at birth (developmental) or may be acquired as a result of neurologic injury or insult to the brain. *Phonologic disorder* involves problems with articulation (forming sounds that are part of speech). *Stuttering* is a disturbance of the normal fluency and time patterning of speech. Phonologic disorder and stuttering run in families and occur more frequently in boys than in girls.

Communication disorders may be mild to severe. Difficulties that persist into adulthood are related most closely to the severity of the disorder. Speech and language therapists work with children who have communication disorders to improve their communication skills and to teach parents to continue speech therapy activities at home (Johnson & Beitchman, 2005).

Pervasive Developmental Disorders

Pervasive developmental disorders are characterized by pervasive and usually severe impairment of reciprocal social interaction skills, communication deviance, and restricted stereotypical behavioral patterns (Volkmar et al., 2005). This category of disorders also is called *autism spectrum disorders* and includes autistic disorder (classic autism), Rett's disorder, childhood disintegrative disorder, and Asperger's disorder. Approximately 75% of children with pervasive developmental disorders have mental retardation (APA, 2000).

AUTISTIC DISORDER

Autistic disorder, the best known of the pervasive developmental disorders, is more prevalent in boys than in girls and is identified usually by 18 months and no later than 3 years of age. Children with autism display little eye contact with and make few facial expressions toward others; they use limited gestures to communicate. They have limited capacity to relate to peers or parents. They lack spontaneous enjoyment, express no moods or emotional affect, and cannot engage in play or make-believe with toys. There is little intelligible speech. These children engage in stereotyped motor behaviors such as hand flapping, body twisting, or head banging.

Eighty percent of cases of autism are early onset, with developmental delays starting in infancy. The other 20% of children with autism have seemingly normal growth and development until 2 or 3 years of age, when developmental regression or loss of abilities begins. They stop talking and relating to parents and peers and begin to demonstrate the behaviors described previously (Volkmar et al., 2005).

Autism was once thought to be rare and was estimated to occur in 4 to 5 children per 10,000 in the 1960s. Current estimates suggest that 1 in 1,000 to 1 in 500 U.S. children from 1 to 15 years of age have autism (National Institute of Child and Human Development, 2006). Figures on the prevalence of autism in adults are unreliable.

Autism does have a genetic link; many children with autism have a relative with autism or autistic traits. Controversy continues about whether measles, mumps, and rubella (MMR) vaccinations contribute to the development of late-onset autism. The National Institute of Child Health and Human Development (2006) states there is no relationship and that the MMR vaccine is safe. Congressional hearings continue to review testimony from those who believe a link exists.

Autism tends to improve, in some cases substantially, as children start to acquire and to use language to communicate with others. If behavior deteriorates in adolescence, it may reflect the effects of hormonal changes or the difficulty meeting increasingly complex social demands. Autistic traits persist into adulthood, and most people with autism remain dependent to some degree on others. Manifestations vary from little speech and poor daily living skills throughout life to adequate social skills that allow relatively independent functioning. Social skills rarely improve enough to permit marriage and child rearing. Adults with autism may

be viewed as merely odd or reclusive, or they may be given a diagnosis of obsessive-compulsive disorder, schizoid personality disorder, or mental retardation.

Until the mid-1970s, children with autism usually were treated in segregated, specialty outpatient, or school programs. Those with more severe behaviors were referred to residential programs. Since then, most residential programs have been closed; children with autism are being "mainstreamed" into local school programs whenever possible. Short-term inpatient treatment is used when behaviors such as head banging or tantrums are out of control. When the crisis is over, community agencies support the child and family.

The goals of treatment of children with autism are to reduce behavioral symptoms (e.g., stereotyped motor behaviors) and to promote learning and development, particularly the acquisition of language skills (Cashin, 2005). Comprehensive and individualized treatment, including special education and language therapy, is associated with more favorable outcomes. Pharmacologic treatment with antipsychotics such as haloperidol (Haldol) or risperidone (Risperdal) may be effective for specific target symptoms such as temper tantrums, aggressiveness, self-injury, hyperactivity, and stereotyped behaviors. Other medications such as naltrexone (ReVia), clomipramine (Anafranil), clonidine (Catapres), and stimulants to diminish self-injury and hyperactive and obsessive behaviors have had varied but unremarkable results (Volkmar et al., 2005).

RETT'S DISORDER

Rett's disorder is a pervasive developmental disorder characterized by the development of multiple deficits after a period of normal functioning. It occurs exclusively in girls, is rare, and persists throughout life. Rett's disorder develops between birth and 5 months of age. The child loses motor skills and begins showing stereotyped movements instead. She loses interest in the social environment, and severe impairment of expressive and receptive language becomes evident as she grows older. Treatment is similar to that of autism.

CHILDHOOD DISINTEGRATIVE DISORDER

Childhood disintegrative disorder is characterized by marked regression in multiple areas of functioning after at least 2 years of apparently normal growth and development (APA, 2000). Typical age at onset is between 3 and 4 years. Children with childhood disintegrative disorder have the same social and communication deficits and behavioral patterns seen with autistic disorder. This rare disorder occurs slightly more often in boys than in girls.

ASPERGER'S DISORDER

Asperger's disorder is a pervasive developmental disorder characterized by the same impairments of social interaction and restricted stereotyped behaviors seen in autistic disorder, but there are no language or cognitive delays. This rare disorder occurs more often in boys than in girls, and the effects are generally lifelong.

Attention Deficit and Disruptive Behavior Disorders

ATTENTION DEFICIT HYPERACTIVITY DISORDER

Attention deficit hyperactivity disorder (ADHD) is characterized by inattentiveness, overactivity, and impulsiveness. ADHD is a common disorder, especially in boys, and probably accounts for more child mental health referrals than any other single disorder (Hechtman, 2005). The essential feature of ADHD is a persistent pattern of inattention and/or hyperactivity and impulsivity more common than generally observed in children of the same age.

ADHD affects an estimated 3% to 5% of all school-aged children. The ratio of boys to girls ranges from 3:1 in nonclinical settings to 9:1 in clinical settings (Hechtman, 2005). To avoid overdiagnosis of ADHD, a qualified specialist such as a pediatric neurologist or a child psychiatrist must conduct the evaluation for ADHD. Children who are very active or hard to handle in the classroom can be diagnosed and treated mistakenly for ADHD. Some of these overly active children may suffer from psychosocial stressors at home, inadequate parenting, or other psychiatric disorders. Distinguishing bipolar disorder from ADHD can be difficult but is crucial in order to prescribe the most effective treatment (Faedda & Teicher, 2005).

Onset and Clinical Course

ADHD usually is identified and diagnosed when the child begins preschool or school, although many parents report problems from a much younger age. As infants, children with ADHD are often fussy and temperamental and have poor sleeping patterns. Toddlers may be described as "always on the go" and "into everything," at times dismantling toys and cribs. They dart back and forth, jump and climb on furniture, run through the house, and cannot tolerate sedentary activities such as listening to stories. At this point in a child's development, it can be difficult for parents to distinguish normal active behavior from excessive hyperactive behavior.

By the time the child starts school, symptoms of ADHD begin to interfere significantly with behavior and performance (Raggi & Chronis, 2006). The child fidgets constantly, is in and out of assigned seats, and makes excessive noise by tapping or playing with pencils or other objects.

CLINICAL VIGNETTE: ATTENTION DEFICIT HYPERACTIVITY DISORDER

Scott is 8 years old. At 7 AM, his mother looks into Scott's bedroom and sees Scott playing. "Scott, you know the rules: no playing before you are ready for school. Get dressed and come eat breakfast." Although these rules for a school day have been set for the past 7 months, Scott always tests them. In about 10 minutes, he is still not in the kitchen. His mother checks his room and finds Scott on the floor, still in his pajamas, playing with miniature cars. Once he gets started doing or talking about something, it is often difficult for Scott to stop.

"Scott, you need to get dressed first. Your jeans and shirt are over here on the chair." "Mom, after school today, can we go shopping? There is the coolest new car game that anyone can play. I'd love to try it out." As he is talking, Scott walks over to the chair and begins to pull his shirt over his head. "Scott, you're putting your shirt over your pajamas. You need to take your pajamas off first," his mother reminds him.

Ten minutes later, Scott bounds into the kitchen, still without socks and shoes, and hair tousled. "You forgot your socks, and your hair isn't combed," his mother reminds him. "Oh yeah. What's for breakfast?" he says. "Scott, finish dressing first." "Well, where are my shoes?" "By the back door where you left them." This is the special designated place where Scott is supposed to leave his shoes so he doesn't forget.

Scott starts toward his shoes but spots his younger sister playing with blocks on the floor. He hurries to her. "Wow, Amy, watch this—I can make these blocks into a huge tower, all the way to the ceiling." He grabs the blocks and begins to stack them higher and higher. "Scott makes a better tower than Amy," he chants. Amy shrieks at this intrusion, but she is used to Scott grabbing things from her. The shriek brings their mother into the room. She notices Scott's feet still do not have socks and shoes.

"Scott, get your socks and shoes on now and leave Amy alone!" "Where are my socks?" he asks. "Go to your room and get a clean pair of socks and brush your teeth and hair. Then come eat your breakfast or you'll miss the bus."

"I will in just a minute, Mom." "No! Now! Go get your socks." Scott continues stacking blocks.

Wearily, his mother directs him toward his room. As he is looking for the socks, he is still chattering away. He finds a pair of socks and bolts in the direction of the kitchen, grabbing Amy and pinching her cheek as he swirls by her. Amy shrieks again and he begins to chant, "Amy's just a baby! Amy's just a baby!" "Scott, stop it right now and come eat something! You've got just 10 minutes until the bus comes."

Normal environmental noises such as someone coughing distract the child. He or she cannot listen to directions or complete tasks. The child interrupts and blurts out answers before questions are completed. Academic performance suffers because the child makes hurried, careless mistakes in schoolwork, often loses or forgets homework assignments, and fails to follow directions.

Socially, peers may ostracize or even ridicule the child for his or her behavior. Forming positive peer relationships is difficult because the child cannot play cooperatively or take turns and constantly interrupts others (APA, 2000). Studies have shown that both teachers and peers perceive children with ADHD as more aggressive, more bossy, and less likable (Hechtman, 2005). This perception results from the child's impulsivity, inability to share or take turns, tendency to interrupt, and failure to listen to and follow directions. Thus, peers and teachers may exclude the child from activities and play, may refuse to socialize with the child, or may respond to the child in a harsh, punitive, or rejecting manner.

About two thirds of children diagnosed with ADHD continue to have problems in adolescence. Typical impulsive behaviors include cutting class, getting speeding tickets, failing to maintain interpersonal relationships, and adopting risk-taking behaviors such as using drugs or alcohol, engaging in sexual promiscuity, fighting, and violating curfew. Many adolescents with ADHD have discipline problems serious enough to warrant suspension or expulsion from high school (Hechtman, 2005). The secondary complications of ADHD such as low self-esteem and peer rejection continue to pose serious problems.

Previously, it was believed that children outgrew ADHD, but it is now known that ADHD can persist into adulthood (McGough, 2005). Estimates are that 30% to 50% of children with ADHD have symptoms that continue into adulthood. In one study, adults who had been treated for hyperactivity 25 years earlier were three to four times more likely than their brothers to experience nervousness, restlessness, depression, lack of friends, and low frustration tolerance (McGough, 2005). Adults in whom ADHD was diagnosed in childhood also have higher rates of impulsivity, alcohol and drug use, legal troubles, and personality disorders. Box 20.2 contains a screening questionnaire for ADHD in adults.

Etiology

Although much research is taking place, the definitive causes of ADHD remain unknown. There may be cortical-arousal, information-processing, or maturational abnormalities in the brain (Rowe & Hermens, 2006). A combination of factors such as environmental toxins, prenatal influences, heredity, and damage to brain structure and functions is likely responsible (Hechtman, 2005). Prenatal exposure to alcohol, tobacco, and lead and severe malnutrition in early childhood increase the likelihood of ADHD. Although the relation between ADHD and dietary sugar

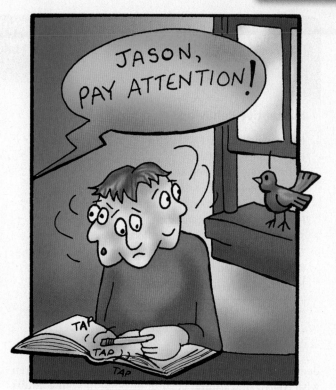

Attention deficit

and vitamins has been studied, results have been inconclusive (Hechtman, 2005).

Brain images of people with ADHD have suggested decreased metabolism in the frontal lobes, which are essential for attention, impulse control, organization, and sustained goal-directed activity. Studies also have shown

Box 20.2   ADULT ADHD SCREENING QUESTIONS

- How often do you have trouble wrapping up the final details of a project once the challenging parts have been done?
- How often do you have difficulty getting things in order when you have to do a task that requires organization?
- How often do you have problems remembering appointments or obligations?
- When you have a task that requires a lot of thought, how often do you avoid or delay getting started?
- How often do you fidget or squirm with your hands or feet when you have to sit down for a long time?
- How often do you feel overly active and compelled to do things, like you were driven by a motor?

Adapted from World Health Organization Composite Diagnostic Interview *(2003).*

DSM-IV-TR DIAGNOSTIC CRITERIA: SYMPTOMS OF ADHD

Inattentive Behaviors

Misses details
Makes careless mistakes
Has difficulty sustaining attention
Doesn't seem to listen
Does not follow-through on chores or homework
Has difficulty with organization
Avoids tasks requiring mental effort
Often loses necessary things
Is easily distracted by other stimuli
Is often forgetful in daily activities

Hyperactive/Impulsive Behaviors

Fidgets
Often leaves seat (e.g., during a meal)
Runs or climbs excessively
Can't play quietly
Is always on the go; driven
Talks excessively
Blurts out answers
Interrupts
Can't wait for turn
Is intrusive with siblings/playmates

Adapted from DSM-IV-TR, 2000.

decreased blood perfusion of the frontal cortex in children with ADHD and frontal cortical atrophy in young adults with a history of childhood ADHD. Another study showed decreased glucose use in the frontal lobes of parents of children with ADHD who had ADHD themselves (Hechtman, 2005). Evidence is not conclusive, but research in these areas seems promising.

There seems to be a genetic link for ADHD that is most likely associated with abnormalities in catecholamine and possibly serotonin metabolism. Having a first-degree relative with ADHD increases the risk for the disorder by four to five times that of the general population (Hechtman, 2005). Despite the strong evidence supporting a genetic contribution, there are also sporadic cases of ADHD with no family history of ADHD; this furthers the theory of multiple contributing factors.

Risk factors for ADHD include family history of ADHD; male relatives with antisocial personality disorder or alcoholism; female relatives with somatization disorder; lower socioeconomic status; male gender; marital or family discord, including divorce, neglect, abuse, or parental deprivation; low birth weight; and various kinds of brain insult (Hechtman, 2005).

Cultural Considerations

ADHD is known to occur in various cultures. It is more prevalent in Western cultures, but that may be the result of different diagnostic practices rather than actual differences in existence (APA, 2000).

The Child Behavior Checklist, Teacher Report Form, and Youth Self Report (for ages 11 to 18 years) are rating scales frequently used to determine problem areas and competencies. These scales are often part of a comprehensive assessment of ADHD in children. They have been deter-

mined to be culturally competent and are widely used in various countries (King et al., 2005).

Pierce and Reid (2004) found that increasing numbers of children from culturally diverse groups are diagnosed with ADHD. They believe this increase may represent over-identification of ADHD in culturally diverse children and urge practitioners to consider cultural context before making the diagnosis.

Yeh and colleagues (2004) studied parental beliefs about the causes of mental illness in their children. They found that African American, Asian/Pacific Islander American, and Latino parents were less likely to endorse biopsychosocial causes of mental illness than non-Hispanic white parents and were more likely to believe in sociologic causes. The authors believe this may affect participation in and compliance with prescribed treatment.

Treatment

No one treatment has been found to be effective for ADHD; this gives rise to many different approaches such as sugar-controlled diets and megavitamin therapy. Parents need to know that any treatment heralded as the cure for ADHD is probably too good to be true (Hechtman, 2005). ADHD is chronic; goals of treatment involve managing symptoms, reducing hyperactivity and impulsivity, and increasing the child's attention so that he or she can grow and develop normally. The most effective treatment combines pharmacotherapy with behavioral, psychosocial, and educational interventions (Raggi & Chronis, 2006).

PSYCHOPHARMACOLOGY

Medications often are effective in decreasing hyperactivity and impulsiveness and improving attention; this enables the child to participate in school and family life. The most common medications are methylphenidate (Ritalin) and an amphetamine compound (Adderall) (Hechtman, 2005; Lehne, 2003). Methylphenidate is effective in 70% to 80% of children with ADHD; it reduces hyperactivity, impulsivity, and mood lability and helps the child to pay attention more appropriately. Dextroamphetamine (Dexedrine) and pemoline (Cylert) are other stimulants used to treat ADHD. The most common side effects of these drugs are insomnia, loss of appetite, and weight loss or failure to gain weight. A methylphenidate, dextroamphetamine, and amphetamine compound is also available in a sustained-release form taken once daily; this eliminates the need for additional doses when the child is at school. Methylphenidate is also available in a daily transdermal patch, marketed as Daytrana. Because pemoline can cause liver damage, it is the last of these drugs to be prescribed.

Giving stimulants during daytime hours usually effectively combats insomnia. Eating a good breakfast with the morning dose and substantial nutritious snacks late in the day and at bedtime helps the child to maintain an adequate dietary intake. When stimulant medications are not effective or their side effects are intolerable, antidepressants are the second choice for treatment (see Chapter 2). Atomoxetine (Strattera) is a nonstimulant drug approved in 2002 by the U.S. Food and Drug Administration for treatment of ADHD. It is an antidepressant, specifically a selective norepinephrine reuptake inhibitor. The most common side effects in children during clinical trials were decreased appetite, nausea, vomiting, tiredness, and upset stomach. In adults, side effects were similar to those of other antidepressants, including insomnia, dry mouth, urinary retention, decreased appetite, nausea, vomiting, dizziness, and sexual side effects. In addition, atomoxetine can cause liver damage, so individuals taking the drug need to have liver function tests periodically (Federal Drug Administration, 2004). Table 20.1 lists drugs, dosages, and nursing considerations for clients with ADHD.

STRATEGIES FOR HOME AND SCHOOL

Medications do not automatically improve the child's academic performance or ensure that he or she makes friends. Behavioral strategies are necessary to help the child to master appropriate behaviors. Environmental strategies at school and home can help the child to succeed in those settings. Educating parents and helping them with parenting strategies are crucial components of effective treatment of ADHD. Effective approaches include providing consistent rewards and consequences for behavior, offering consistent praise, using time-out, and giving verbal reprimands. Additional strategies are issuing daily report cards for behavior and using point systems for positive and negative behavior (Hechtman, 2005).

In **therapeutic play**, play techniques are used to understand the child's thoughts and feelings and to promote communication. This should not be confused with play therapy, a psychoanalytic technique used by psychiatrists. Dramatic

Table 20.1   DRUGS USED TO TREAT ADHD

Generic (Trade) Name	Dosage (mg/day)	Nursing Considerations
Stimulants		
Methylphenidate (Ritalin)	10–60 in 3–4 divided doses	Monitor for appetite suppression or growth delays.
Sustained release (Ritalin-SR, Concerta, Metadate-CD)	20–60 in the morning	Give regular tablets after meals. Alert client that full drug effect takes 2 days.
Transdermal patch (Daytrana)	15	Wear patch for 9 hours—drug effects last 3 hours after removal.
Dextroamphetamine (Dexedrine)	5–40 in 2–3 divided doses	Monitor for insomnia.
Sustained release (Dexedrine-SR)	10–30 in the morning	Give last dose in early afternoon. Monitor for appetite suppression. Alert client that full drug effect takes 2 days.
Amphetamine (Adderall)	5–40 in 2–3 divided doses	See *Dextroamphetamine*.
Sustained release (Adderall-XR)	10–30 in the morning	
Pemoline (Cylert)	37.5–112.5 in the morning	Monitor for elevated liver function tests and appetite suppression. Alert client that drug may take 2 weeks for full effect.
Antidepressant (SNRI)		
Atomoxetine (Strattera)	1.2 mg/kg/day in 1 or 2 divided doses (children < 70 kg) 40–80 in 1 or 2 divided doses (children > 70 kg and adults)	Give with food. Monitor for appetite suppression. Use calorie-free beverages to relieve dry mouth. Monitor for elevated liver function tests.

Adapted from *Lexi-comp's Psychotropic Drug Information Handbook* (2005).

play is acting out an anxiety-producing situation such as allowing the child to be a doctor or use a stethoscope or other equipment to take care of a patient (a doll). Play techniques to release energy could include pounding pegs, running, or working with modeling clay. Creative play techniques can help children to express themselves, for example, by drawing pictures of themselves, their family, and peers. These techniques are especially useful when children are unable or unwilling to express themselves verbally.

APPLICATION OF THE NURSING PROCESS: ATTENTION DEFICIT HYPERACTIVITY DISORDER

Assessment

During assessment, the nurse gathers information through direct observation and from the child's parents, day care providers (if any), and teachers. Assessing the child in a group of peers is likely to yield useful information because the child's behavior may be subdued or different in a focused one-to-one interaction with the nurse. It is often helpful to use a checklist when talking with parents to help focus their input on the target symptoms or behaviors their child exhibits.

HISTORY

Parents may report that the child was fussy and had problems as an infant. Or they may not have noticed the hyperactive behavior until the child was a toddler or entered day care or school. The child probably has difficulties in all major life areas such as school or play, and he or she likely displays overactive or even dangerous behavior at home. Often, parents say the child is "out of control," and they feel unable to deal with the behavior. Parents may report many largely unsuccessful attempts to discipline the child or to change the behavior.

GENERAL APPEARANCE AND MOTOR BEHAVIOR

The child cannot sit still in a chair and squirms and wiggles while trying to do so. He or she may dart around the room with little or no apparent purpose. Speech is unimpaired, but the child cannot carry on a conversation: he or she interrupts, blurts out answers before the question is finished, and fails to pay attention to what has been said. Conversation topics may jump abruptly. The child may appear immature or lag behind in developmental milestones.

MOOD AND AFFECT

Mood may be labile, even to the point of verbal outbursts or temper tantrums. Anxiety, frustration, and agitation are common. The child appears to be driven to keep moving or talking and appears to have little control over movement or speech. Attempts to focus the child's attention or redirect the child to a topic may evoke resistance and anger.

THOUGHT PROCESS AND CONTENT

There are generally no impairments in this area, although assessment can be difficult depending on the child's activity level and age or developmental stage.

SENSORIUM AND INTELLECTUAL PROCESSES

The child is alert and oriented with no sensory or perceptual alterations such as hallucinations. Ability to pay attention or to concentrate is markedly impaired. The child's attention span may be as little as 2 or 3 seconds with severe ADHD or 2 or 3 minutes in milder forms of the disorder. Assessing the child's memory may be difficult; he or she frequently answers, "I don't know," because he or she cannot pay attention to the question or stop the mind from racing. The child with ADHD is very distractible and rarely able to complete tasks.

JUDGMENT AND INSIGHT

Children with ADHD usually exhibit poor judgment and often do not think before acting. They may fail to perceive harm or danger and engage in impulsive acts such as running into the street or jumping off high objects. Although assessing judgment and insight in young children is difficult, children with ADHD display more lack of judgment when compared with others of the same age. Most young children with ADHD are totally unaware that their behavior is different from that of others and cannot perceive how it harms others. Older children might report, "No one at school likes me," but they cannot relate the lack of friends to their own behavior.

SELF-CONCEPT

Again, this may be difficult to assess in a very young child, but generally the self-esteem of children with ADHD is low. Because they are not successful at school, may not develop many friends, and have trouble getting along at home, they generally feel out of place and bad about themselves. The negative reactions their behavior evokes from others often cause them to see themselves as bad or stupid.

ROLES AND RELATIONSHIPS

The child is usually unsuccessful academically and socially at school. He or she frequently is disruptive and intrusive at home, which causes friction with siblings and parents. Until the child is diagnosed and treated, parents often believe that the child is willful, stubborn, and purposefully misbehaving. Generally, measures to discipline have limited success; in some cases, the child becomes physically out of control, even hitting parents or destroying family possessions. Parents find themselves chronically exhausted mentally and physically. Teachers often feel the same frustration as parents, and day care providers or baby-sitters may refuse to care for the child with ADHD, which adds to the child's rejection.

PHYSIOLOGIC AND SELF-CARE CONSIDERATIONS

Children with ADHD may be thin if they do not take time to eat properly or cannot sit through meals. Trouble settling down and difficulty sleeping are problems as well. If the child engages in reckless or risk-taking behaviors, there also may be a history of physical injuries.

Data Analysis and Planning

Nursing diagnoses commonly used when working with children with ADHD include the following:
- Risk for Injury
- Ineffective Role Performance
- Impaired Social Interaction
- Compromised Family Coping

Outcome Identification

Treatment outcomes for clients with ADHD may include the following:
- The client will be free of injury.
- The client will not violate the boundaries of others.
- The client will demonstrate age-appropriate social skills.
- The client will complete tasks.
- The client will follow directions.

Intervention

Interventions described in this section can be adapted to various settings and used by nurses and other health professionals, teachers, and parents or caregivers.

ENSURING SAFETY

Safety of the child and others is always a priority. If the child is engaged in a potentially dangerous activity, the first step is to stop the behavior. This may require physical intervention if the child is running into the street or attempting to jump from a high place. Attempting to talk to or reason with a child engaged in a dangerous activity is unlikely to succeed because his or her ability to pay attention and to listen is limited. When the incident is over and the child is safe, the adult should talk to the child directly about the expectations for safe behavior. Close supervision may be required for a time to ensure compliance and to avoid injury.

Explanations should be short and clear, and the adult should not use a punitive or belittling tone of voice. The adult should not assume that the child knows acceptable behavior but instead should state expectations clearly. For example, if the child was jumping down a flight of stairs, the adult might say,

"It is unsafe to jump down stairs. From now on, you are to walk down the stairs, one at a time."

> ### NURSING INTERVENTIONS FOR ADHD
>
> - Ensuring the child's safety and that of others
>   Stop unsafe behavior.
>   Provide close supervision.
>   Give clear directions about acceptable and unacceptable behavior.
> - Improved role performance
>   Give positive feedback for meeting expectations.
>   Manage the environment (e.g., provide a quiet place free of distractions for task completion).
> - Simplifying instructions/directions
>   Get child's full attention.
>   Break complex tasks into small steps.
>   Allow breaks.
> - Structured daily routine
>   Establish a daily schedule.
>   Minimize changes.
> - Client/family education and support
>   Listen to parent's feelings and frustrations.

If the child crowded ahead of others, the adult would walk the child back to the proper place in line and say,

"It is not okay to crowd ahead of others. Take your place at the end of the line."

To prevent physically intrusive behavior, it also may be necessary to supervise the child closely while he or she is playing. Again, it often is necessary to act first to stop the harmful behavior by separating the child from the friend, such as stepping between them or physically removing the child. Afterward, the adult should clearly explain expected and unacceptable behavior. For example, the adult might say,

"It is not okay to grab other people. When you are playing with others, you must ask for the toy."

IMPROVING ROLE PERFORMANCE

It is extremely important to give the child specific positive feedback when he or she meets stated expectations. Doing so reinforces desired behaviors and gives the child a sense of accomplishment. For example, the adult might say,

"You walked down the stairs safely" or "You did a good job of asking to play with the guitar and waited until it was your turn."

Managing the environment helps the child to improve his or her ability to listen, pay attention, and complete tasks. A quiet place with minimal noise and distraction is desirable. At school, this may be a seat directly facing the teacher at the front of the room and away from the distraction of a window or door. At home, the child should have a quiet area for homework away from the television or radio.

SIMPLIFYING INSTRUCTIONS

Before beginning any tasks, adults must gain the child's full attention. It is helpful to face the child on his or her level and use good eye contact. The adult should tell the child what needs to be done and break the task into smaller steps if necessary. For example, if the child has 25 math problems, it may help to give him or her 5 problems at a time, then 5 more when those are completed, and so on. This approach prevents overwhelming the child and provides the opportunity for feedback about each set of problems he or she completes. With sedentary tasks, it is also important to allow the child to have breaks or opportunities to move around.

Adults can use the same approach for tasks such as cleaning or picking up toys. Initially, the child needs the supervision or at least the presence of the adult. The adult can direct the child to do one portion of the task at a time; when the child shows progress, the adult can give only occasional reminders and then allow the child to complete the task independently. It helps to provide specific, step-by-step directions rather than give a general direction such as "Please clean your room." The adult could say,

"Put your dirty clothes in the hamper."

After this step is completed, the adult gives another direction:

"Now make the bed."

The adult assigns specific tasks until the child has completed the overall chore.

PROMOTING A STRUCTURED DAILY ROUTINE

A structured daily routine is helpful. The child will accomplish getting up, dressing, doing homework, playing, going to bed, and so forth much more readily if there is a routine time for these daily activities. Children with ADHD do not adjust to changes readily and are less likely to meet expectations if times for activities are arbitrary or differ from day to day.

PROVIDING CLIENT AND FAMILY EDUCATION AND SUPPORT

Including parents in planning and providing care for the child with ADHD is important. The nurse can teach parents the approaches described previously for use at home. Parents feel empowered and relieved to have specific strategies that can help both them and their child be more successful.

The nurse must listen to parents' feelings. They may feel frustrated, angry, or guilty and blame themselves or the school system for their child's problems. Parents need to hear that neither they nor their child are at fault and that techniques and school programs are available to help. Children with ADHD qualify for special school services under the Individuals With Disabilities Education Act.

Because raising a child with ADHD can be frustrating and exhausting, it often helps parents to attend support groups that can provide information and encouragement from other parents with the same problems. Parents must learn strategies to help their child improve his or her social and academic abilities, but they also must understand how to help rebuild their child's self-esteem. Most of these children have low self-esteem because they have been labeled as having behavior problems and have been corrected continually by parents and teachers for not listening, not paying attention, and misbehaving. Parents should give positive comments as much as possible to encourage the child and acknowledge his or her strengths. One technique to help parents to achieve a good balance is to ask them to count the numbers of times they praise or criticize their child each day or for several days.

Although medication can help reduce hyperactivity and inattention and allow the child to focus during school, it is by no means a cure-all. The child needs strategies and practice to improve social skills and academic performance. Because these children often are not diagnosed until the second or third grade, they may have missed much basic learning for reading and math. Parents should know that it takes time for them to catch up to other children of the same age.

Evaluation

Parents and teachers are likely to notice positive outcomes of treatment before the child does. Medications are often effective in decreasing hyperactivity and impulsivity and improving attention relatively quickly, if the child responds to them. Improved sociability, peer relationships, and academic achievement happen more slowly and gradually but are possible with effective treatment.

CONDUCT DISORDER

Conduct disorder is characterized by persistent antisocial behavior in children and adolescents that significantly impairs their ability to function in social, academic, or occupational areas. Symptoms are clustered in four areas: aggression to people and animals, destruction of property, deceitfulness and theft, and serious violation of rules (Thomas, 2005). People with conduct disorder have little empathy for others; they have low self-esteem, poor frustration tolerance, and temper outbursts. Conduct disorder frequently is associated with early onset of sexual behavior, drinking, smoking, use of illegal substances, and other reckless or risky behaviors. It occurs three times more often in boys than in girls. As many as 30% to 50% of these children are diagnosed with antisocial personality disorder as adults.

Onset and Clinical Course

Two subtypes of conduct disorder are based on age at onset. The childhood-onset type involves symptoms before 10 years of age, including physical aggression toward others and disturbed peer relationships. These children are more likely to have persistent conduct disorder and to develop antisocial personality disorder as adults. Adolescent-onset type is defined by no behaviors of conduct disorder until after 10 years of age. These adolescents are less likely to be aggressive, and they have more normal peer relationships. They are less likely to have persistent conduct disorder or antisocial personality disorder as adults (APA, 2000).

Conduct disorders can be classified as mild, moderate, or severe (APA, 2000):

- Mild: The person has some conduct problems that cause relatively minor harm to others. Examples include lying, truancy, and staying out late without permission.
- Moderate: The number of conduct problems increases as does the amount of harm to others. Examples include vandalism and theft.
- Severe: The person has many conduct problems that cause considerable harm to others. Examples include forced sex, cruelty to animals, use of a weapon, burglary, and robbery.

The course of conduct disorder is variable. People with the adolescent-onset type or mild problems can achieve adequate social relationships and academic or occupational success as adults. Those with the childhood-onset type or more severe problem behaviors are more likely to develop antisocial personality disorder as adults. Even those who do not have antisocial personality disorder may lead troubled lives with difficult interpersonal relationships, unhealthy lifestyles, and an inability to support themselves (Thomas, 2005).

Etiology

Researchers generally accept that genetic vulnerability, environmental adversity, and factors such as poor coping interact to cause the disorder. Risk factors include poor parenting, low academic achievement, poor peer relationships, and low self-esteem; protective factors include resilience, family support, positive peer relationships, and good health (Thomas, 2005).

There is a genetic risk for conduct disorder, although no specific gene marker has been identified (Thomas, 2005). The disorder is more common in children who have a sibling with conduct disorder or a parent with antisocial personality disorder, substance abuse, mood disorder, schizophrenia, or ADHD (APA, 2000).

A lack of reactivity of the autonomic nervous system has been found in children with conduct disorder; this nonresponsiveness is similar to adults with antisocial personality disorder. The abnormality may cause more aggression in social relationships as a result of decreased normal avoidance or social inhibitions. Research into the role of neurotransmitters is promising (Thomas, 2005).

Poor family functioning, marital discord, poor parenting, and a family history of substance abuse and psychiatric problems are all associated with the development of conduct disorder. Child abuse is an especially significant risk factor. The specific parenting patterns considered ineffective are inconsistent parental responses to the child's demands and giving in to demands as the child's behavior escalates. Exposure to violence in the media and community is a contributing factor for the child at risk in other areas. Socioeconomic disadvantages such as inadequate housing, crowded conditions, and poverty also increase the likelihood of conduct disorder in at-risk children (McGuinness, 2006).

(text continues on p. 446)

Nursing Care Plan

Attention Deficit Hyperactivity Disorder

Nursing Diagnosis

Impaired Social Interaction: *Insufficient or excessive quantity or ineffective quality of social exchange.*

ASSESSMENT DATA

- Short attention span
- High level of distractibility
- Labile moods
- Low frustration tolerance
- Inability to complete tasks
- Inability to sit still or fidgeting
- Excessive talking
- Inability to follow directions

EXPECTED OUTCOMES

Immediate
The client will
- Successfully complete tasks or assignments with assistance
- Demonstrate acceptable social skills while interacting with staff or family members

Stabilization
The client will
- Participate successfully in the educational setting
- Demonstrate the ability to complete tasks with reminders
- Demonstrate successful interactions with family members

Community
The client will
- Verbalize positive statements about himself or herself
- Complete tasks independently

IMPLEMENTATION

Nursing Interventions *denotes collaborative interventions	**Rationale**
Identify the factors that aggravate and alleviate the client's performance.	The external stimuli that exacerbate the client's problems can be identified and minimized. Likewise, ones that positively influence the client can be effectively used.
Provide an environment as free from distractions as possible. Institute interventions on a one-to-one basis. Gradually increase the amount of environmental stimuli.	The client's ability to deal with external stimulation is impaired.
Engage the client's attention before giving instructions (i.e., call the client's name and establish eye contact).	The client must hear instructions as a first step toward compliance.
Give instructions slowly, using simple language and concrete directions.	The client's ability to comprehend instructions (especially if they are complex or abstract) is impaired.
Ask the client to repeat instructions before beginning tasks.	Repetition demonstrates that the client has accurately received the information.
Separate complex tasks into small steps.	The likelihood of success is enhanced with less complicated components of a task.

Nursing Care Plan: Attention Deficit Hyperactivity Disorder, cont.

IMPLEMENTATION

Nursing Interventions *denotes collaborative interventions	Rationale
Provide positive feedback for completion of each step.	The client's opportunity for successful experiences is increased by treating each step as an opportunity for success.
Allow breaks, during which the client can move around.	The client's restless energy can be given an acceptable outlet, so he or she can attend to future tasks more effectively.
State expectations for task completion clearly.	The client must understand the request before he or she can attempt task completion.
Initially, assist the client to complete tasks.	If the client is unable to complete a task independently, having assistance will allow success and will demonstrate how to complete the task.
Progress to prompting or reminding the client to perform tasks or assignments.	The amount of intervention gradually is decreased to increase client independence as the client's abilities increase.
Give the client positive feedback for performing behaviors that come close to task achievement.	This approach, called *shaping,* is a behavioral procedure in which successive approximations of a desired behavior are positively reinforced. It allows rewards to occur as the client gradually masters the actual expectation.
Gradually decrease reminders.	Client independence is promoted as staff participation is decreased.
Assist the client to verbalize by asking sequencing questions to keep on the topic ("Then what happens?" and "What happens next?").	Sequencing questions provide a structure for discussions to increase logical thought and decrease tangentiality.
*Teach the client's family or caregivers to use the same procedures for the client's tasks and interactions at home.	Successful interventions can be instituted by the client's family or caregivers by using this process. This will promote consistency and enhance the client's chances for success.
*Explain and demonstrate "positive parenting" techniques to family or caregivers, such as *time-in* for good behavior or being vigilant in identifying and responding positively to the child's first bid for attention; *special time,* or guaranteed time spent daily with the child with no interruptions and no discussion of problem-related topics; *ignoring minor transgressions* by immediate withdrawal of eye contact or physical contact and cessation of discussion with the child to avoid secondary gains.	It is important for parents or caregivers to engage in techniques that will maintain their loving relationship with the child while promoting, or at least not interfering with, therapeutic goals. Children need to have a sense of being lovable to their significant others that is not crucial to the nurse–client therapeutic relationship.

Adapted from Schultz, J. M., and Videbeck, S. L. (2005). Lippincott's manual of psychiatric nursing care plans (7th ed.). Philadelphia: Lippincott Williams & Wilkins.

DSM-IV-TR DIAGNOSTIC CRITERIA:
SYMPTOMS OF CONDUCT DISORDER

Aggression to people and animals
Bullies, threatens, or intimidates others
Physical fights
Use of weapons
Forced sexual activity
Cruelty to people or animals
Destruction of property
Fire setting
Vandalism
Deliberate property destruction
Deceitfulness and theft
Lying
Shoplifting
Breaking into house, building, or car
Cons others to avoid responsibility
Serious violation of rules
Stays out overnight without parental consent
Runs away from home overnight
Truancy from school

Adapted from DSM-IV-TR, 2000.

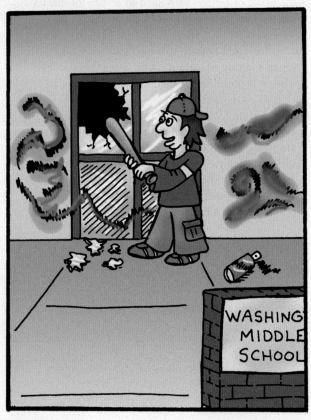

Conduct disorder

Academic underachievement, learning disabilities, hyperactivity, and problems with attention span are all associated with conduct disorder. Children with conduct disorder have difficulty functioning in social situations. They lack the abilities to respond appropriately to others and to negotiate conflict, and they lose the ability to restrain themselves when emotionally stressed. They often are accepted only by peers with similar problems (Thomas, 2005).

Cultural Considerations

Concerns have been raised that "difficult" children may be mistakenly labeled as having conduct disorder. Knowing the client's history and circumstances is essential for accurate diagnosis. In high-crime areas, aggressive behavior may be protective and not necessarily indicative of conduct disorder. In immigrants from war-ravaged countries, aggressive behavior may have been necessary for survival, so these individuals should not be diagnosed with conduct disorder (APA, 2000).

Treatment

Many treatments have been used for conduct disorder with only modest effectiveness. Early intervention is more effective, and prevention is more effective than treatment. Dramatic interventions such as "boot camp" or incarceration have not proved effective and may even worsen the situation (Thomas, 2005). Treatment must be geared toward the client's developmental age; no one treatment is suitable for all ages. Preschool programs such as Head Start result in lower rates of delinquent behavior and conduct disorder through use of parental education about normal growth and development, stimulation for the child, and parental support during crises.

For school-aged children with conduct disorder, the child, family, and school environment are the focus of treatment. Techniques include parenting education, social skills training to improve peer relationships, and attempts to improve academic performance and increase the child's ability to comply with demands from authority figures. Family therapy is considered to be essential for children in this age group (Thomas, 2005).

Adolescents rely less on their parents and more on peers, so treatment for this age group includes individual therapy. Many adolescent clients have some involvement with the legal system as a result of criminal behavior, and they may have restrictions on their freedom as a result. Use of alcohol and other drugs plays a more significant role for this age group; any treatment plan must address this issue. The most promising treatment approach includes keeping the client in his or her environment with family and individual therapies. The plan usually includes conflict resolution, anger management, and teaching social skills.

Medications alone have little effect but may be used in conjunction with treatment for specific symptoms. For

CLINICAL VIGNETTE: CONDUCT DISORDER

Tom, 14 years of age, leaves the principal's office after being involved in a physical fight in the hall. He knows his parents will be furious because he is suspended for 1 week. "It wasn't my fault," he thinks to himself. "What am I supposed to do when someone calls me names?" Tom is angry that he even came to school today; he'd much rather spend time hanging out with his friends and having a few drinks or smoking pot.

On his way home, Tom sees a car parked next to the grocery store, and it is unlocked and running. Tom jumps in, thinking, "This is my lucky day!" He speeds away, but soon he can hear police sirens as a patrol car closes in on him. He is eventually stopped and arrested. As he waits for his parents at the station,

he's not sure what to do next. He tells the police officer that the car belongs to a friend and he just borrowed it. He promises never to get into trouble again if the officer will let him go. But the officer has Tom's record, which includes school truancy, underage drinking, suspicion in the disappearance of a neighbor's pet cat, and shoplifting.

When Tom's father arrives, he smacks Tom across the face and says, "You stupid kid! I told you the last time you'd better straighten up. And look at you now! What a sorry excuse for a son!" Tom slumps in his chair with a sullen, defiant look on his face. "Go ahead and hit me! Who cares? I'm not gonna do what you say, so you might as well give up!"

example, the client who presents a clear danger to others may be prescribed an antipsychotic medication, or a client with a labile mood may benefit from lithium or another mood stabilizer such as carbamazepine (Tegretol) or valproic acid (Depakote) (Thomas, 2005).

APPLICATION OF THE NURSING PROCESS: CONDUCT DISORDER

Assessment

HISTORY

Children with conduct disorder have a history of disturbed relationships with peers, aggression toward people or animals, destruction of property, deceitfulness or theft, and serious violation of rules (e.g., truancy, running away from home, staying out all night without permission). The behaviors and problems may be mild to severe.

GENERAL APPEARANCE AND MOTOR BEHAVIOR

Appearance, speech, and motor behavior are typically normal for the age group but may be somewhat extreme (e.g., body piercings, tattoos, hairstyle, clothing). These clients often slouch and are sullen and unwilling to be interviewed. They may use profanity, call the nurse or physician names, and make disparaging remarks about parents, teachers, police, and other authority figures.

MOOD AND AFFECT

Clients may be quiet and reluctant to talk or openly hostile and angry. Their attitude is likely to be disrespectful toward parents, the nurse, or anyone in a position of authority. Irritability, frustration, and temper outbursts are common. Clients may be unwilling to answer questions or to cooperate with the interview; they believe they do not need help

or treatment. If a client has legal problems, he or she may express superficial guilt or remorse, but it is unlikely that these emotions are sincere.

THOUGHT PROCESS AND CONTENT

Thought processes are usually intact—that is, clients are capable of logical rational thinking. Nevertheless, they perceive the world to be aggressive and threatening, and they respond in the same manner. Clients may be preoccupied with looking out for themselves and behave as though everyone is "out to get me." Thoughts or fantasies about death or violence are common.

SENSORIUM AND INTELLECTUAL PROCESSES

Clients are alert and oriented with intact memory and no sensory-perceptual alterations. Intellectual capacity is not impaired, but typically these clients have poor grades because of academic underachievement, behavioral problems in school, or failure to attend class and to complete assignments.

JUDGMENT AND INSIGHT

Judgment and insight are limited for developmental stage. Clients consistently break rules with no regard for the consequences. Thrill-seeking or risky behavior is common, such as use of drugs or alcohol, reckless driving, sexual activity, and illegal activities such as theft. Clients lack insight and usually blame others or society for their problems; they rarely believe their behavior is the cause of difficulties.

SELF-CONCEPT

Although these clients generally try to appear tough, their self-esteem is low. They do not value themselves any more than they value others. Their identity is related to their behaviors, such as being cool if they have had many sexual encounters or feeling important if they have stolen expensive merchandise or been expelled from school.

ROLES AND RELATIONSHIPS

Relationships with others, especially those in authority, are disruptive and may be violent. This includes parents, teachers, police, and most other adults. Verbal and physical aggression is common. Siblings may be a target for ridicule or aggression. Relationships with peers are limited to others who display similar behaviors; these clients see peers who follow rules as dumb or afraid. Clients usually have poor grades, have been expelled, or have dropped out. It is unlikely that they have a job (if old enough) because they would prefer to steal. Their idea of fulfilling roles is being tough, breaking rules, and taking advantage of others.

PHYSIOLOGIC AND SELF-CARE CONSIDERATIONS

Clients are often at risk for unplanned pregnancy and sexually transmitted diseases because of their early and frequent sexual behavior. Use of drugs and alcohol is an additional risk to health. Clients with conduct disorders are involved in physical aggression and violence including weapons; this results in more injuries and deaths than compared with others of the same age.

Data Analysis and Planning

Nursing diagnoses commonly used for clients with conduct disorders include the following:
- Risk for Other-Directed Violence
- Noncompliance
- Ineffective Coping
- Impaired Social Interaction
- Chronic Low Self-Esteem

Outcome Identification

Treatment outcomes for clients with conduct disorders may include the following:
- The client will not hurt others or damage property.
- The client will participate in treatment.
- The client will learn effective problem-solving and coping skills.
- The client will use age-appropriate and acceptable behaviors when interacting with others.
- The client will verbalize positive, age-appropriate statements about self.

Intervention

DECREASING VIOLENCE AND INCREASING COMPLIANCE WITH TREATMENT

The nurse must protect others from the manipulative or aggressive behaviors common with these clients. He or she must set limits on unacceptable behavior at the beginning of treatment. **Limit setting** involves three steps:

1. Inform clients of the rule or limit.
2. Explain the consequences if clients exceed the limit.
3. State expected behavior.

Providing consistent limit enforcement with no exceptions by all members of the health team, including parents, is essential. For example, the nurse might say,

"It is unacceptable to hit another person. If you are angry, tell a staff person about your anger. If you hit someone, you will be restricted from recreation time for 24 hours."

For limit setting to be effective, the consequences must have meaning for clients—that is, they must value or desire recreation time (in this example). If a client wanted to be alone in his or her room, then this consequence would not be effective.

The nurse can negotiate with a client a behavioral contract outlining expected behaviors, limits, and rewards to increase treatment compliance. The client can refer to the written agreement to remember expectations, and staff can refer to the agreement if the client tries to change any terms. A contract can help staff to avoid power struggles over requests for special favors or attempts to alter treatment goals or behavioral expectations.

Whether there is a written contract or treatment plan, staff must be consistent with these clients. They will attempt to bend or break rules, blame others for noncompliance, or make excuses for behavior. Consistency in following the treatment plan is essential to decrease manipulation.

Time-out is retreat to a neutral place so clients can regain self-control. It is not a punishment. When a client's behavior begins to escalate, such as when he or she yells at or threatens someone, a time-out may prevent aggression or acting out. Staff may need to institute a time-out for clients if they are unwilling or unable to do so. Eventually, the goal is for clients to recognize signs of increasing agitation and take a self-instituted time-out to control emotions and outbursts. After the time-out, the nurse should discuss the events with the client. Doing so can help clients to recognize situations that trigger emotional responses and to learn more effective ways of dealing with similar situations in the future. Providing positive feedback for successful efforts at avoiding aggression helps to reinforce new behaviors for clients.

It helps for clients to have a schedule of daily activities, including hygiene, school, homework, and leisure time. Clients are more likely to establish positive habits if they have routine expectations about tasks and responsibilities. They are more likely to follow a daily routine if they have input concerning the schedule.

IMPROVING COPING SKILLS AND SELF-ESTEEM

The nurse must show acceptance of clients as worthwhile persons even if their behavior is unacceptable. This means

menting one of the alternatives, and evaluating the results (see Chapter 16). The nurse can help clients to work on actual problems using this process. Problem-solving skills are likely to improve with practice.

PROMOTING SOCIAL INTERACTION

Clients with conduct disorder may not have age-appropriate social skills, so teaching social skills is important. The nurse can role model these skills and help clients to practice appropriate social interaction. The nurse identifies what is not appropriate, such as profanity and name calling, and also what is appropriate. Clients may have little experience discussing the news, current events, sports, or other topics. As they begin to develop social skills, the nurse can include other peers in these discussions. Positive feedback is essential to let clients know they are meeting expectations.

PROVIDING CLIENT AND FAMILY EDUCATION

Parents may also need help in learning social skills, solving problems, and behaving appropriately. Often, parents have their own problems, and they have had difficulties with the client for a long time before treatment was instituted. Parents need to replace old patterns such as yelling, hitting, or simply ignoring behavior with more effective strategies. The nurse can teach parents age-appropriate activities and expectations for clients such as reasonable curfews, household responsibilities, and acceptable behavior at home. The parents may need to learn effective limit setting with appropriate consequences. Parents often need to learn to communicate their feelings and expectations clearly and directly to these clients. Some parents may need to let clients experience the consequences of their behavior rather than rescuing them. For example, if a client gets a speeding ticket, the parents should not pay the fine for him or her. If a client causes a disturbance in school and receives detention, the parents can support the teacher's actions instead of blaming the teacher or school.

Evaluation

Treatment is considered effective if the client stops behaving in an aggressive or illegal way, attends school, and follows reasonable rules and expectations at home. The client will not become a model child in a short period; instead, he or she may make modest progress with some setbacks over time.

COMMUNITY-BASED CARE

Clients with conduct disorder are seen in acute care settings only when their behavior is severe and only for short periods of stabilization. Much long-term work takes place at school and home or another community setting. Some clients are placed outside their parents' home for short or long periods. Group homes, halfway houses, and residential

---

> ### NURSING INTERVENTIONS FOR CONDUCT DISORDER
>
> - Decreasing violence and increasing compliance with treatment
>   Protect others from client's aggression and manipulation.
>   Set limits for unacceptable behavior.
>   Provide consistency with client's treatment plan.
>   Use behavioral contracts.
>   Institute time-out.
>   Provide a routine schedule of daily activities.
> - Improving coping skills and self-esteem
>   Show acceptance of the person, not necessarily the behavior.
>   Encourage the client to keep a diary.
>   Teach and practice problem-solving skills.
> - Promoting social interaction
>   Teach age-appropriate social skills.
>   Role model and practice social skills.
>   Provide positive feedback for acceptable behavior.
> - Providing client and family education

that the nurse must be matter-of-fact about setting limits and must not make judgmental statements about clients. He or she must focus only on the behavior. For example, if a client broke a chair during an angry outburst, the nurse would say,

"John, breaking chairs is unacceptable behavior. You need to let staff know you're upset so you can talk about it instead of acting out."

The nurse must avoid saying things like,

"What's the matter with you? Don't you know any better?"

Comments such as these are subjective and judgmental and do not focus on the specific behavior; they reinforce the client's self-image as a "bad person."

Clients with a conduct disorder often have a tough exterior and are unable or reluctant to discuss feelings and emotions. Keeping a diary may help them to identify and express their feelings. The nurse can discuss these feelings with clients and explore better, safer expressions than through aggression or acting out.

Clients also may need to learn how to solve problems effectively. Problem-solving involves identifying the problem, exploring all possible solutions, choosing and imple-

> **CLIENT/FAMILY EDUCATION FOR CONDUCT DISORDER**
>
> Teach parents social and problem-solving skills when needed.
>
> Encourage parents to seek treatment for their own problems.
>
> Help parents to identify age-appropriate activities and expectations.
>
> Assist parents with direct, clear communication.
>
> Help parents to avoid "rescuing" the client.
>
> Teach parents effective limit-setting techniques.
>
> Help parents identify appropriate discipline strategies.

treatment settings are designed to provide safe, structured environments and adequate supervision if that cannot be provided at home. Clients with legal issues may be placed in detention facilities, jails, or jail-diversion programs. Chapter 4 discusses treatment settings and programs.

MENTAL HEALTH PROMOTION

Parental behavior profoundly influences children's behavior. Parents who engage in risky behaviors such as smoking, drinking, and ignoring their health are more likely to have children who also engage in risky behaviors, including early unprotected sex. Group-based parenting classes are effective to deal with problem behaviors in children and to prevent later development of conduct disorders (Turner & Sanders, 2006; Zubrick et al., 2005).

Rapee and associates (2006) reported that an early intervention program for children at risk for anxiety disorders improved behavior. The program consisted of parent sessions, child anxiety management, parent–child sessions that emphasized coping skills, and graduated exposure to anxiety-provoking situations.

The SNAP-IV Teacher and Parent Rating Scale (Swanson, 2000) is an assessment tool that can be used for initial evaluation in many areas of concern such as ADHD, oppositional defiant disorder, conduct disorder, and depression (Box 20.3). Such tools can identify problems or potential problems that signal a need for further evaluation and follow-up. Early detection and successful intervention are often the key to mental health promotion.

OPPOSITIONAL DEFIANT DISORDER

Oppositional defiant disorder consists of an enduring pattern of uncooperative, defiant, and hostile behavior toward authority figures without major antisocial violations. A certain level of oppositional behavior is common in children and adolescents; indeed, it is almost expected at some phases such as 2 to 3 years of age and in early adolescence. Table 20.2 contrasts acceptable characteristics with abnormal behavior in adolescents. Oppositional defiant disorder is diagnosed only when behaviors are more frequent and intense than in unaffected peers and cause dysfunction in social, academic, or work situations. This disorder is diagnosed in about 5% of the population and occurs equally among male and female adolescents. Most authorities believe that genes, temperament, and adverse social conditions interact to create oppositional defiant disorder. Twenty-five percent of people with this disorder develop conduct disorder; 10% are diagnosed with antisocial personality disorder as adults (Thomas, 2005). Treatment approaches are similar to those used for conduct disorder.

Feeding and Eating Disorders of Infancy and Early Childhood

The disorders of feeding and eating included in this category are persistent in nature and are not explained by underlying medical conditions. They include pica, rumination disorder, and feeding disorder.

PICA

Pica is persistent ingestion of nonnutritive substances such as paint, hair, cloth, leaves, sand, clay, or soil. Pica is commonly seen in children with mental retardation; it occasionally occurs in pregnant women. It comes to the clinician's attention only if a medical complication develops such as a bowel obstruction or an infection or if a toxic condition develops such as lead poisoning. In most instances, the behavior lasts for several months and then remits.

RUMINATION DISORDER

Rumination disorder is the repeated regurgitation and rechewing of food. The child brings partially digested food up into the mouth and usually rechews and reswallows the food. The regurgitation does not involve nausea, vomiting, or any medical condition (APA, 2000). This disorder is relatively uncommon and occurs more often in boys than in girls; it results in malnutrition, weight loss, and even death in about 25% of affected infants. In infants, the disorder frequently remits spontaneously, but it may continue in severe cases.

FEEDING DISORDER

Feeding disorder of infancy or early childhood is characterized by persistent failure to eat adequately, which results in significant weight loss or failure to gain weight. Feeding

(text continues on p. 456)

Box 20.3 THE SNAP-IV TEACHER AND PARENT RATING SCALE

Name: _____ Gender: _____ Age: _____ Grade: _____

Ethnicity (circle one which best applies):   African American   Asian   Caucasian   Hispanic   Other _____

Completed by: _____ Type of Class: _____ Class size: _____

For each item, check the column which best describes this child:	Not at All	Just a Little	Quite a Bit	Very Much
1. Often fails to give close attention to details or makes careless mistakes in schoolwork or tasks	____	____	____	____
2. Often has difficulty sustaining attention in tasks or play activities	____	____	____	____
3. Often does not seem to listen when spoken to directly	____	____	____	____
4. Often does not follow through on instructions and fails to finish schoolwork, chores, or duties	____	____	____	____
5. Often has difficulty organizing tasks and activities	____	____	____	____
6. Often avoids, dislikes, or reluctantly engages in tasks requiring sustained mental effort	____	____	____	____
7. Often loses things necessary for activities (e.g., toys, school assignments, pencils, or books)	____	____	____	____
8. Often is distracted by extraneous stimuli	____	____	____	____
9. Often is forgetful in daily activities	____	____	____	____
10. Often has difficulty maintaining alertness, orienting to requests, or executing directions	____	____	____	____
11. Often fidgets with hands or feet or squirms in seat	____	____	____	____
12. Often leaves seat in classroom or in other situations in which remaining seated is expected	____	____	____	____
13. Often runs about or climbs excessively in situations in which it is inappropriate	____	____	____	____
14. Often has difficulty playing or engaging in leisure activities quietly	____	____	____	____
15. Often is "on the go" or often acts as if "driven by a motor"	____	____	____	____
16. Often talks excessively	____	____	____	____
17. Often blurts out answers before questions have been completed	____	____	____	____
18. Often has difficulty awaiting turn	____	____	____	____
19. Often interrupts or intrudes on others (e.g., butts into conversations/games)	____	____	____	____
20. Often has difficulty sitting still, being quiet, or inhibiting impulses in the classroom or at home	____	____	____	____
21. Often loses temper	____	____	____	____
22. Often argues with adults	____	____	____	____
23. Often actively defies or refuses adult requests or rules	____	____	____	____
24. Often deliberately does things that annoy other people	____	____	____	____
25. Often blames others for his or her mistakes or misbehavior	____	____	____	____
26. Often is touchy or easily annoyed by others	____	____	____	____
27. Often is angry and resentful	____	____	____	____
28. Often is spiteful or vindictive	____	____	____	____
29. Often is quarrelsome	____	____	____	____
30. Often is negative, defiant, disobedient, or hostile toward authority figures	____	____	____	____

continued ⋯→

Box 20.3: The SNAP-IV Teacher and Parent Rating Scale, cont.

For each item, check the column which best describes this child:	Not at All	Just a Little	Quite a Bit	Very Much
31. Often makes noises (e.g., humming or odd sounds)	_____	_____	_____	_____
32. Often is excitable, impulsive	_____	_____	_____	_____
33. Often cries easily	_____	_____	_____	_____
34. Often is uncooperative	_____	_____	_____	_____
35. Often acts "smart"	_____	_____	_____	_____
36. Often is restless or overactive	_____	_____	_____	_____
37. Often disturbs other children	_____	_____	_____	_____
38. Often changes mood quickly and drastically	_____	_____	_____	_____
39. Often easily frustrated if demands are not met immediately	_____	_____	_____	_____
40. Often teases other children and interferes with their activities	_____	_____	_____	_____
41. Often is aggressive to other children (e.g., picks fights or bullies)	_____	_____	_____	_____
42. Often is destructive with property of others (e.g., vandalism)	_____	_____	_____	_____
43. Often is deceitful (e.g., steals, lies, forges, copies the work of others, or "cons" others)	_____	_____	_____	_____
44. Often and seriously violates rules (e.g., is truant, runs away, or completely ignores class rules)	_____	_____	_____	_____
45. Has persistent pattern of violating the basic rights of others or major societal norms	_____	_____	_____	_____
46. Has episodes of failure to resist aggressive impulses (to assault others or to destroy property)	_____	_____	_____	_____
47. Has motor or verbal tics (sudden, rapid, recurrent, nonrhythmic motor or verbal activity)	_____	_____	_____	_____
48. Has repetitive motor behavior (e.g., hand waving, body rocking, or picking at skin)	_____	_____	_____	_____
49. Has obsessions (persistent and intrusive inappropriate ideas, thoughts, or impulses)	_____	_____	_____	_____
50. Has compulsions (repetitive behaviors or mental acts to reduce anxiety or distress)	_____	_____	_____	_____
51. Often is restless or seems keyed up or on edge	_____	_____	_____	_____
52. Often is easily fatigued	_____	_____	_____	_____
53. Often has difficulty concentrating (mind goes blank)	_____	_____	_____	_____
54. Often is irritable	_____	_____	_____	_____
55. Often has muscle tension	_____	_____	_____	_____
56. Often has excessive anxiety and worry (e.g., apprehensive expectation)	_____	_____	_____	_____
57. Often has daytime sleepiness (unintended sleeping in inappropriate situations)	_____	_____	_____	_____
58. Often has excessive emotionality and attention-seeking behavior	_____	_____	_____	_____
59. Often has need for undue admiration, grandiose behavior, or lack of empathy	_____	_____	_____	_____
60. Often has instability in relationships with others, reactive mood, and impulsivity	_____	_____	_____	_____
61. Sometimes for at least a week has inflated self esteem or grandiosity	_____	_____	_____	_____
62. Sometimes for at least a week is more talkative than usual or seems pressured to keep talking	_____	_____	_____	_____

Box 20.3: The SNAP-IV Teacher and Parent Rating Scale, cont.

For each item, check the column which best describes this child:

	Not at All	Just a Little	Quite a Bit	Very Much
63. Sometimes for at least a week has flight of ideas or says that thoughts are racing	____	____	____	____
64. Sometimes for at least a week has elevated, expansive or euphoric mood	____	____	____	____
65. Sometimes for at least a week is excessively involved in pleasurable but risky activities	____	____	____	____
66. Sometimes for at least 2 weeks has depressed mood (sad, hopeless, discouraged)	____	____	____	____
67. Sometimes for at least 2 weeks has irritable or cranky mood (not just when frustrated)	____	____	____	____
68. Sometimes for at least 2 weeks has markedly diminished interest or pleasure in most activities	____	____	____	____
69. Sometimes for at least 2 weeks has psychomotor agitation (even more active than usual)	____	____	____	____
70. Sometimes for at least 2 weeks has psychomotor retardation (slowed down in most activities)	____	____	____	____
71. Sometimes for at least 2 weeks is fatigued or has loss of energy	____	____	____	____
72. Sometimes for at least 2 weeks has feelings of worthlessness or excessive, inappropriate guilt	____	____	____	____
73. Sometimes for at least 2 weeks has diminished ability to think or concentrate	____	____	____	____
74. Chronic low self-esteem most of the time for at least a year	____	____	____	____
75. Chronic poor concentration or difficulty making decisions most of the time for at least a year	____	____	____	____
76. Chronic feelings of hopelessness most of the time for at least a year	____	____	____	____
77. Currently is hypervigilant (overly watchful or alert) or has exaggerated startle response	____	____	____	____
78. Currently is irritable, has anger outbursts, or has difficulty concentrating	____	____	____	____
79. Currently has an emotional (e.g., nervous, worried, hopeless, tearful) response to stress	____	____	____	____
80. Currently has a behavioral (e.g., fighting, vandalism, truancy) response to stress	____	____	____	____
81. Has difficulty getting started on classroom assignments	____	____	____	____
82. Has difficulty staying on task for an entire classroom period	____	____	____	____
83. Has problems in completion of work on classroom assignments	____	____	____	____
84. Has problems in accuracy or neatness of written work in the classroom	____	____	____	____
85. Has difficulty attending to a group classroom activity or discussion	____	____	____	____
86. Has difficulty making transitions to the next topic or classroom period	____	____	____	____
87. Has problems in interactions with peers in the classroom	____	____	____	____
88. Has problems in interactions with staff (teacher or aide)	____	____	____	____
89. Has difficulty remaining quiet according to classroom rules	____	____	____	____
90. Has difficulty staying seated according to classroom rules	____	____	____	____

Developed by James M. Swanson, Ph. D., University of California, Irvine.

Nursing Care Plan *Conduct Disorder*

Nursing Diagnosis

Ineffective Coping: *Inability to form a valid appraisal of the stressors, inadequate choices of practiced responses, and/or inability to use available resources.*

ASSESSMENT DATA

- Few or no meaningful peer relationships
- Inability to empathize with others
- Inability to give and receive affection
- Low self-esteem, masked by "tough" act

EXPECTED OUTCOMES

Immediate
The client will
- Engage in social interaction
- Verbalize feelings
- Learn problem-solving skills

Stabilization
The client will
- Demonstrate effective problem-solving and coping skills
- Assess own strengths and weaknesses realistically

Community
The client will
- Demonstrate development of relationships with peers
- Verbalize real feelings of self-worth that are age appropriate
- Perform at a satisfactory academic level

IMPLEMENTATION

Nursing Interventions *denotes collaborative interventions

Encourage the client to discuss his or her thoughts and feelings.

Give positive feedback for appropriate discussions.

Tell the client that he or she is accepted as a person, although a particular behavior may not be acceptable.

Give the client positive attention when behavior is not problematic.

Teach the client about limit setting and the need for limits. Include time for discussion.

Teach the client the problem-solving process as an alternative to acting out (identify the problem, consider alternatives, select and implement an alternative, evaluate the effectiveness of the solution).

Rationale

Verbalizing feelings is an initial step toward dealing with them in an appropriate manner.

Positive feedback increases the likelihood of continued performance.

Clients with conduct disorders frequently experience rejection. The client needs support to increase self-esteem, while understanding that behavioral changes are necessary.

The client may have been receiving the majority of attention from others when he or she was engaged in problematic behavior, a pattern that needs to change.

This allows the client to hear about the relationship between aberrant behavior and consequences when behavior is not problematic. The client may have no knowledge of the concept of limits and how limits can be beneficial.

The client may not know how to solve problems constructively or may not have seen this behavior modeled in the home.

Nursing Care Plan: Conduct Disorder, cont.

IMPLEMENTATION

Nursing Interventions *denotes collaborative interventions	Rationale
Help the client practice the problem-solving process with situations on the unit, then situations the client may face at home, school, and so forth.	The client's ability and skill will increase with practice. He or she will experience success with practice.
Role model appropriate conversation and social skills for the client.	This allows the client to see what is expected in a nonthreatening situation.
Specify and describe the skills you are demonstrating.	Clarification of expectations decreases the chance for misinterpretation.
Practice social skills with the client on a one-to-one basis.	As the client gains comfort with the skills through practice, he or she will increase their use.
Gradually introduce other clients into the interactions and discussions.	Success with others is more likely to occur once the client has been successful with the staff.
Assist the client to focus on age- and situation-appropriate topics.	Peer relationships are enhanced when the client is able to interact as other adolescents do.
Encourage the client to give and receive feedback with others in his or her age group.	Peer feedback can be influential in shaping the behavior of an adolescent.
Facilitate expression of feelings among clients in supervised group situations.	Adolescents are reluctant to be vulnerable to peers and may need encouragement to share feelings.
Teach the client about transmission of human immunodeficiency virus (HIV) infection and other sexually transmitted diseases (STDs).	Because these clients may act out sexually or use intravenous drugs, it is especially important that they be educated about preventing transmission of HIV and STDs.
*Assess the client's use of alcohol or other substances, and provide referrals as indicated.	Often adolescents with conduct disorders also have substance abuse issues.

Adapted from Schultz, J. M., and Videbeck, S. L. (2005). Lippincott's manual of psychiatric nursing care plans (7th ed.). Philadelphia: Lippincott Williams & Wilkins.

Table 20.2	ACCEPTABLE CHARACTERISTICS AND ABNORMAL BEHAVIOR IN ADOLESCENCE

Acceptable	Abnormal
Occasional psychosomatic complaints	Fears, anxiety, and guilt about sex, health, education
Inconsistent and unpredictable behavior	Defiant, negative, or depressed behavior
Eagerness for peer approval	Frequent hypochondriacal complaints
Competitive in play	Learning irregular or deficient
Erratic work-leisure patterns	Poor personal relationships with peers
Critical of self and others	Inability to postpone gratification
Highly ambivalent toward parents	Unwillingness to assume greater autonomy
Anxiety about lost parental nurturing	Acts of delinquency, ritualism, obsessions
Verbal aggression to parents	Sexual aberrations
Strong moral and ethical perceptions	Inability to work or socialize

Adapted from Pataki, C. (2005). Normal adolescence. In B. J. Sadock & V. A. Sadock (Eds.), *Comprehensive textbook of psychiatry* (8th ed., pp. 3035–3043). Philadelphia: Lippincott Williams & Wilkins.

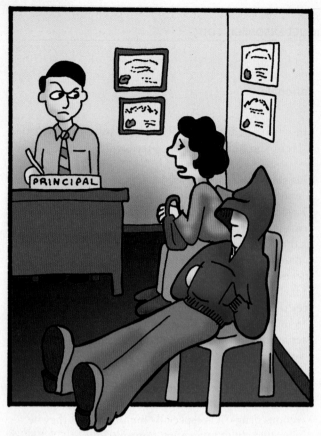

Oppositional defiant disorder

disorder is equally common in boys and in girls and occurs most often during the first year of life. Estimates are that 5% of all pediatric hospital admissions are for failure to gain weight, and up to 50% of those admissions reflect a feeding disorder with no predisposing medical condition. In severe cases, malnutrition and death can result, but most children have improved growth after some time (APA, 2000).

Tic Disorders

A **tic** is a sudden, rapid, recurrent, nonrhythmic, stereotyped motor movement or vocalization (APA, 2000). Tics can be suppressed but not indefinitely. Stress exacerbates tics, which diminish during sleep and when the person is engaged in an absorbing activity. Common simple motor tics include blinking, jerking the neck, shrugging the shoulders, grimacing, and coughing. Common simple vocal tics include clearing the throat, grunting, sniffing, snorting, and barking. Complex vocal tics include repeating words or phrases out of context, coprolalia (use of socially unacceptable words, frequently obscene), palilalia (repeating one's own sounds or words), and echolalia (repeating the last-heard sound, word, or phrase; APA, 2000). Complex motor tics include facial gestures, jumping, or touching or smelling an object.

Tic disorders tend to run in families. Abnormal transmission of the neurotransmitter dopamine is thought to play a part in tic disorders (Scahill & Leckman, 2005). Tic disorders usually are treated with risperidone (Risperdal) or olanzapine (Zyprexa), which are atypical antipsychotics. It is important for clients with tic disorders to get plenty of rest and to manage stress because fatigue and stress increase symptoms.

TOURETTE'S DISORDER

Tourette's disorder involves multiple motor tics and one or more vocal tics, which occur many times a day for more than 1 year. The complexity and severity of the tics change over time, and the person experiences almost all the possible tics described previously during his or her lifetime. The person has significant impairment in academic, social, or occupational areas and feels ashamed and self-conscious. This rare disorder (4 or 5 in 10,000) is more common in boys and is usually identified by 7 years of age. Some people have lifelong problems; others have no symptoms after early adulthood (APA, 2000).

CHRONIC MOTOR OR TIC DISORDER

Chronic motor or vocal tic differs from Tourette's disorder in that either the motor or the vocal tic is seen, but not both. Transient tic disorder may involve single or multiple vocal or motor tics, but the occurrences last no longer than 12 months.

Elimination Disorders

Encopresis is the repeated passage of feces into inappropriate places such as clothing or the floor by a child who is at least 4 years of age either chronologically or developmentally. It is often involuntary, but it can be intentional. Involuntary encopresis usually is associated with constipation that occurs for psychological, not medical, reasons. Intentional encopresis often is associated with oppositional defiant disorder or conduct disorder.

Enuresis is the repeated voiding of urine during the day or at night into clothing or bed by a child at least 5 years of age either chronologically or developmentally. Most often enuresis is involuntary; when intentional, it is associated with a disruptive behavior disorder. Seventy-five percent of children with enuresis have a first-degree relative who had the disorder. Most children with enuresis do not have a coexisting mental disorder.

Both encopresis and enuresis are more common in boys than in girls; 1% of all 5 year olds have encopresis, and 5% of all 5 year olds have enuresis. Encopresis can persist with intermittent exacerbations for years; it is rarely chronic. Most children with enuresis are continent by adolescence; only 1% of all cases persist into adulthood.

Impairment associated with elimination disorders depends on the limitations on the child's social activities, effects on self-esteem, degree of social ostracism by peers, and anger, punishment, and rejection on the part of parents or caregivers (APA, 2000).

Enuresis can be treated effectively with imipramine (Tofranil), an antidepressant with a side effect of urinary retention. Both elimination disorders respond to behavioral approaches such as a pad with a warning bell and to positive reinforcement for continence. For children with a disruptive behavior disorder, psychological treatment of that disorder may improve the elimination disorder (Mikkelsen, 2005).

Other Disorders of Infancy, Childhood, or Adolescence

SEPARATION ANXIETY DISORDER

Separation anxiety disorder is characterized by anxiety exceeding that expected for developmental level related to separation from the home or those to whom the child is attached (APA, 2000). When apart from attachment figures, the child insists on knowing their whereabouts and may need frequent contact with them, such as phone calls. These children are miserable away from home and may fear never seeing their homes or loved ones again. They often follow parents like a shadow, cannot be in a room alone, and have trouble going to bed at night unless someone stays with them. Fear of separation may lead to avoidance behaviors such as refusal to attend school or go on errands. Separation anxiety disorder often is accompanied by nightmares and multiple physical complaints such as headaches, nausea, vomiting, and dizziness.

Separation anxiety disorders are thought to result from an interaction between temperament and parenting behaviors. Inherited temperament traits such as passivity, avoidance, fearfulness, or shyness in novel situations coupled with parenting behaviors that encourage avoidance as a way to deal with strange or unknown situations are thought to cause anxiety in the child (Bernstein & Layne, 2005).

Depending on the severity of the disorder, children may have academic difficulties and social withdrawal if their avoidance behavior keeps them from school or relationships with others. Children may be described as demanding, intrusive, and in need of constant attention, or they may be compliant and eager to please. As adults, they may be slow to leave the family home or overly concerned about and protective of their own spouses and children. They may continue to have marked discomfort when separated from home or family. Parent education and family therapy are essential components of treatment; 80% of children experience remission at 4-year follow-up (Bernstein & Layne, 2005).

SELECTIVE MUTISM

Selective mutism is characterized by persistent failure to speak in social situations where speaking is expected, such as school (APA, 2000). Children may communicate by gestures, nodding or shaking the head, or occasionally one-syllable vocalizations in a voice different from their natural voice. These children are often excessively shy, socially withdrawn or isolated, and clinging; they may have temper tantrums. Selective mutism is rare and slightly more common in girls than in boys. It usually lasts only a few months but may persist for years.

REACTIVE ATTACHMENT DISORDER

Reactive attachment disorder involves a markedly disturbed and developmentally inappropriate social relatedness in most situations. This disorder usually begins before 5 years of age and is associated with grossly pathogenic care such as parental neglect, abuse, or failure to meet the child's basic physical or emotional needs. Repeated changes in primary caregivers, such as multiple foster care placements, also can prevent the formation of stable attachments (APA, 2000). The disturbed social relatedness may be evidenced by the child's failure to initiate or respond to social interaction (inhibited type) or indiscriminate sociability or lack of selectivity in choice of attachment figures (disinhibited type). In the first type, the child will not cuddle or desire to be close to anyone. In the second type, the child's response is the same to a stranger or to a parent.

Initially, treatment focuses on the child's safety, including removal of the child from the home if neglect or abuse is found. Individual and family therapy (either with parents or foster caregivers) is most effective. With early identification and effective intervention, remission or considerable improvements can be attained. Otherwise, the disorder follows a continuous course, with relationship problems persisting into adulthood.

STEREOTYPIC MOVEMENT DISORDER

Stereotypic movement disorder is associated with many genetic, metabolic, and neurologic disorders and often accompanies mental retardation. The precise cause is unknown. It involves repetitive motor behavior that is nonfunctional and either interferes with normal activities or results in self-injury requiring medical treatment (APA, 2000). **Stereotypic movements** may include waving, rocking, twirling objects, biting fingernails, banging the head, biting or hitting oneself, or picking at the skin or body orifices. Generally speaking, the more severe the retardation, the higher the risk for self-injury behaviors. Stereotypic movement behaviors are relatively stable over time but may diminish with age (Shah, 2005).

No specific treatment has been shown effective. Clomipramine (Anafranil) and desipramine (Norpramin) are effective in treating severe nail biting; haloperidol (Haldol) and chlorpromazine (Thorazine) have been effective for stereotypic movement disorder associated with mental retardation and autistic disorder.

SELF-AWARENESS ISSUES

Working with children and adolescents can be both rewarding and difficult. Many disorders of childhood such as severe developmental disorders severely limit the child's abilities. It may be difficult for the nurse to remain positive with the child and parents when the prognosis for improvement is poor. Even in overwhelming and depressing situations, the nurse has an opportunity to positively influence children and adolescents, who are still in crucial phases of development. The nurse often can help these clients to develop coping mechanisms they'll use throughout adulthood.

Working with parents is a crucial aspect of dealing with children with these disorders. Parents often have the most influence on how these children learn to cope with their disorders. The nurse's beliefs and values about raising children affect how he or she deals with children and parents. The nurse must not be overly critical about how parents handle their children's problems until the situation is fully understood: Caring for a child as a nurse is very different from being responsible around the clock. Given their own skills and problems, parents often give their best efforts. Given the opportunity, resources, support, and education, many parents can improve their parenting.

Points to Consider When Working With Children and Adolescents and Their Parents

- Remember to focus on the client's and parents' strengths and assets, not just their problems.
- Support parents' efforts to remain hopeful while dealing with the reality of their child's situation.
- Ask parents how they are doing. Offer to answer questions, and provide support or make referrals to meet their needs as well as those of the client.

Critical Thinking Questions

1. In an effort to protect the fetus from neurologic damage, many states are attempting to enact legislation providing penalties for pregnant women who drink heavily or use drugs. What is your position on this issue? What, if anything, should be done? Why do you believe what you do?
2. What values or beliefs about child rearing and families do you have as a result of your own experiences growing up? Have these values and beliefs changed over time? If so, how?

KEY POINTS

- Psychiatric disorders are more difficult to diagnose in children than in adults because their basic development is incomplete and children may lack the ability to recognize or to describe what they are experiencing.
- Children and adolescents can experience some of the same mental health problems seen in adults, such as depression, bipolar disorder, and anxiety.
- The disorders of childhood and adolescence most often encountered in mental health settings include pervasive developmental disorders, ADHD, and disruptive behavior disorders.
- Mental retardation involves below-average intellectual functioning (IQ below 70) and is accompanied by significant limitations in adaptive functioning such as communication, self-care, self-direction, academic achievement, work, and health and safety. The degree of impairment is directly related to the IQ.
- Learning disorders include categories for substandard achievement in reading, mathematics, and written expression. They are treated through special education in schools.
- Communication disorders may be expressive or receptive and expressive. They primarily involve articulation or stuttering and are treated by speech and language therapists.
- Pervasive developmental disorders are characterized by severe impairment of reciprocal social interaction skills, communication deviance, and restricted stereotyped behavioral patterns.
- Children with autism, the best known of the pervasive developmental disorders, seem detached and make little eye contact with and few facial expressions toward others. They do not relate to peers or parents, lack spontaneous enjoyment, and cannot engage in play or make-believe with toys. Autism often is treated with behavioral approaches. Months or years of treatment may be needed before positive outcomes appear.
- The essential feature of ADHD is a persistent pattern of inattention and/or hyperactivity and impulsivity. ADHD, the most common disorder of childhood, results in poor academic performance, strained family relations, and rejection by peers.
- Interventions for ADHD include a combination of medication, behavioral interventions, and parental education. Often, special educational assistance is needed to help with academic achievement.
- Conduct disorder, the most common disruptive behavior disorder, is characterized by aggression to people and animals, destruction of property, deceitfulness and theft, and serious violation of rules.
- Interventions for conduct disorder include decreasing violent behavior, increasing compliance, improving cop-

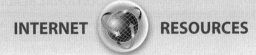

INTERNET RESOURCES

RESOURCE	INTERNET ADDRESS
• Administration on Developmental Disabilities	http://www.acf.dhhs.gov/programs/add
• American Academy of Child and Adolescent	http://www.aacap.org/Psychiatry
• Center for the Study of Autism	http://www.autism.com
• Children and Adults With Attention Deficit	http://www.chadd.org/Disorders (CHADD)
• Conduct and Oppositional Defiant Disorders	http://www.conductdisorders.com
• National Attention Deficit Disorder Association	http://www.add.org
• National Center for Learning Disabilities	http://www.ncld.org
• Tourette Spectrum Disorder Association, Inc.	http://www.tourettesyndrome.org

ing skills and self-esteem, promoting social interaction, and educating and supporting parents.

- Feeding and eating disorders of infancy and childhood include pica, rumination, and feeding disorders. Pica and rumination often improve with time, and most cases of feeding disorders can be successfully treated.

- Tic disorders involve various combinations of involuntary vocal and/or motor tics. Tourette's disorder is most common. Tic disorders are usually treated successfully with atypical antipsychotic medications.

- Elimination disorders cause impairment for the child based on the response of parents, the level of self-esteem, and the degree of ostracism by peers.

REFERENCES

American Psychiatric Association. (2000). *Diagnostic and statistical manual of mental disorders* (4th ed., text revision). Washington, DC: American Psychiatric Association.

Bernstein, G. A., & Layne, A. E. (2005). Separation anxiety disorder and other anxiety disorders. In B. J. Sadock & V. A. Sadock (Eds.), *Comprehensive textbook of psychiatry* (8th ed., pp. 3292–3302). Philadelphia: Lippincott Williams & Wilkins.

Cashin, A. J. (2005). Autism: Understanding conceptual processing deficits. *Journal of Psychosocial Nursing, 43*(4), 22–30.

Faedda, G. L., & Teicher, M. H. (2005). Objective measures of activity and attention in the differential diagnosis of psychiatric disorders of childhood. *Essential Psychopharmacology, 6*(5), 239–249.

Federal Drug Administration. (2004). New warning for Strattera. Retrieved January 23, 2005, from http://www.fda.gov/topics/ANSWERS/2004/ANS01335.html.

Hechtman, L. (2005). Attention deficit disorders. In B. J. Sadock & V. A. Sadock (Eds.), *Comprehensive textbook of psychiatry* (8th ed., pp. 3183–3198). Philadelphia: Lippincott Williams & Wilkins.

Johnson, C. J., & Beitchman, J. H. (2005). Communication disorders. In B. J. Sadock & V. A. Sadock (Eds.), *Comprehensive textbook of psychiatry* (8th ed., pp. 3136–3154). Philadelphia: Lippincott Williams & Wilkins.

King, B. H., Hodapp, R. M., & Dykens, E. M. (2005). Mental retardation. In B. J. Sadock & V. A. Sadock (Eds.), *Comprehensive textbook of psychiatry* (8th ed., pp. 3076–3106). Philadelphia: Lippincott Williams & Wilkins.

Lehne, R. A. (2006). *Pharmacology for nursing care* (6th ed.). Philadelphia: W. B. Saunders.

McGough, J. J. (2005). Adult manifestations of attention deficit/hyperactivity disorder. In B. J. Sadock & V. A. Sadock (Eds.), *Comprehensive textbook of psychiatry* (8th ed., pp. 3198–3198). Philadelphia: Lippincott Williams & Wilkins.

McGuinness, T. M. (2006). Update on conduct disorder. *Journal of Psychosocial Nursing, 44*(12), 21–25.

Mikkelsen, E. J. (2005). Elimination disorders. In B. J. Sadock & V. A. Sadock (Eds.), *Comprehensive textbook of psychiatry* (8th ed., pp. 3237–3246). Philadelphia: Lippincott Williams & Wilkins.

National Institute of Child Health and Human Development. (2006). Available: http://www.nichd.nih.gov/publications/pubs/autismfacts.pdf.

Pataki, C. S. (2005). Normal adolescence. In B. J. Sadock & V. A. Sadock (Eds.), *Comprehensive textbook of psychiatry* (8th ed., pp. 3035–3043). Philadelphia: Lippincott Williams & Wilkins.

Pataki, C. S., & Spence, S. J. (2005). Motor skills disorder: Developmental coordination disorder. In B. J. Sadock & V. A. Sadock (Eds.), *Comprehensive textbook of psychiatry* (8th ed., pp. 3130–3135). Philadelphia: Lippincott Williams & Wilkins.

Pierce, C. D., & Reid, R. (2004). Attention deficit hyperactivity disorder: Assessment and treatment of children from culturally different groups. *Seminars in Speech and Language, 25*(3), 233–240.

Raggi, V. L., & Chronis, A. M. (2006). Interventions to address the academic impairment of children and adolescents with ADHD. *Clinical Child and Family Psychology Review, 9*(2), 85–111.

Rapee, R. M., Kennedy, S., Ingram, M., et al. (2005). Prevention and early intervention of anxiety disorders in inhibited preschool children. *Journal of Consulting and Clinical Psychology, 73*(3), 488–497.

Rowe, D. L., & Hermens, D. F. (2006). Attention-deficit/hyperactivity disorder: Neurophysiology, information processing, arousal, and drug development. *Expert Review of Neurotherapeutics, 6*(11), 1721–1734.

Scahill, L., & Leckman, J. F. (2005). Tic disorders. In B. J. Sadock & V. A. Sadock (Eds.), *Comprehensive textbook of psychiatry* (8th ed., pp. 3228–3236). Philadelphia: Lippincott Williams & Wilkins.

Shah, B. G. (2005). Stereotypic movement disorder of infancy. In B. J. Sadock & V. A. Sadock (Eds.), *Comprehensive textbook of psychiatry* (8th ed., pp. 3254–3257). Philadelphia: Lippincott Williams & Wilkins.

Swanson, J. M. (2000). The SNAP-IV Teacher and Parent Rating Scale. Available: http://www.adhd.net/snap-iv-form.pdf.

Thomas, C. R. (2005). Disruptive behavior disorders. In B. J. Sadock & V. A. Sadock (Eds.), *Comprehensive textbook of psychiatry* (8th ed., pp. 3205–3216). Philadelphia: Lippincott Williams & Wilkins.

Turner, K. M., & Sanders, M. R. (2006). Help when it's needed first: A controlled evaluations of brief, preventive behavioral family intervention in a primary care setting. *Behavior Therapy, 37*(2), 131–142.

Volkmar, F. R., Klin, A., & Schultz, R. T. (2005). Pervasive developmental disorders. In B. J. Sadock & V. A. Sadock (Eds.), *Comprehensive textbook of psychiatry* (8th ed., pp. 3164–3182). Philadelphia: Lippincott Williams & Wilkins.

Yeh, M., Hough, R. L., McCabe, K., et al. (2004). Parental beliefs about the causes of child problems: Exploring racial/ethnic patterns. *Journal of the American Academy of Child and Adolescent Psychiatry, 43*(5), 605–612.

Zubrick, S. R., Ward, K. A., Silburn, S. A., et al. (2005). Prevention of child behavior problems through implementation of a group behavioral family intervention. *Prevention Science, 6*(4), 287–304.

ADDITIONAL READINGS

Ambrosini, P. J. (2000). A review of pharmacotherapy of major depression in children and adolescents. *Psychiatric Services, 51*(5), 627–633.

Gordon, M. F. (2005). Normal child development. In B. J. Sadock & V. A. Sadock (Eds.), *Comprehensive textbook of psychiatry* (8th ed., pp. 3018–3035). Philadelphia: Lippincott Williams & Wilkins.

Pataki, C. S. (2005). Child psychiatry: Introduction and overview. In B. J. Sadock & V. A. Sadock (Eds.), *Comprehensive textbook of psychiatry* (8th ed., pp. 3015–3017). Philadelphia: Lippincott Williams & Wilkins.

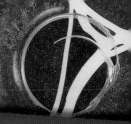

Chapter Study Guide

MULTIPLE-CHOICE QUESTIONS

Select the best answer for each of the following questions.

1. A child is taking pemoline (Cylert) for ADHD. The nurse must be aware of which of the following side effects?
   A. Decreased thyroid-stimulating hormone
   B. Decreased red blood cell count
   C. Elevated white blood cell count
   D. Elevated liver function tests

2. Teaching for methylphenidate (Ritalin) should include which of the following?
   A. Give the medication after meals.
   B. Give the medication when the child becomes overactive.
   C. Increase the child's fluid intake when he or she is taking the medication.
   D. Take the child's temperature daily.

3. The nurse would expect to see all the following symptoms in a child with ADHD except
   A. Easily distracted and forgetful
   B. Excessive running, climbing, and fidgeting
   C. Moody, sullen, and pouting behavior
   D. Interrupts others and can't take turns

4. Which of the following is normal adolescent behavior?
   A. Critical of self and others
   B. Defiant, negative, and depressed behavior
   C. Frequent hypochondriacal complaints
   D. Unwillingness to assume greater autonomy

5. Which of the following is used to treat enuresis?
   A. Imipramine (Tofranil)
   B. Methylphenidate (Ritalin)
   C. Olanzapine (Zyprexa)
   D. Risperidone (Risperdal)

6. An effective nursing intervention for the impulsive and aggressive behaviors that accompany conduct disorder is
   A. Assertiveness training
   B. Consistent limit setting
   C. Negotiation of rules
   D. Open expression of feelings

7. The nurse recognizes which of the following as a common behavioral sign of autism?
   A. Clinging behavior toward parents
   B. Creative imaginative play with peers
   C. Early language development
   D. Indifference to being hugged or held

FILL-IN-THE-BLANK QUESTIONS

Identify the disorder associated with the following behaviors.

_____ Ingestion of paint, clay, sand, or soil

_____ Repeated regurgitation and rechewing of food

_____ Disturbed and developmentally inappropriate social relatedness

_____ Persistent failure to speak in specific social situations

SHORT-ANSWER QUESTIONS

1. Define the steps in limit setting.

2. Explain the therapeutic use of time-out.

CLINICAL EXAMPLE

Dixie, 7 years of age, has been brought by her parents to the mental health center because she has been very rough with her 18-month-old brother. She cannot sit still at school or at meals and is beginning to fall behind academically in the first grade. Her parents report that they have "tried everything," but Dixie will not listen to them. She cannot follow directions, pick up toys, or get ready for school on time.

   After a thorough examination of Dixie and a lengthy interview with the parents, the psychiatrist diagnoses ADHD and prescribes methylphenidate (Ritalin), 10 mg in the morning, 5 mg at noon, and 5 mg in the afternoon. The nurse meets with the parents to provide teaching and to answer questions before they go home.

1. What teaching will the nurse include about methylphenidate?

2. What information will the nurse provide about ADHD?

3. What suggestions for managing the home environment might be helpful for the parents?

4. What referrals can the nurse make for Dixie and her parents?

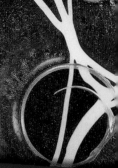

Chapter

21

Cognitive Disorders

Key Terms

- agnosia
- Alzheimer's disease
- amnestic disorder
- aphasia
- apraxia
- confabulation
- Creutzfeldt-Jakob disease
- delirium
- dementia
- distraction
- echolalia
- executive functioning
- going along
- Huntington's disease
- Korsakoff's syndrome
- palilalia
- Parkinson's disease
- Pick's disease
- reframing
- reminiscence therapy
- supportive touch
- time away
- vascular dementia

Learning Objectives

After reading this chapter, you should be able to

1. Describe the characteristics of and risk factors for cognitive disorders.

2. Distinguish between delirium and dementia in terms of symptoms, course, treatment, and prognosis.

3. Apply the nursing process to the care of clients with cognitive disorders.

4. Identify methods for meeting the needs of people who provide care to clients with dementia.

5. Provide education to clients, families, caregivers, and community members to increase knowledge and understanding of cognitive disorders.

6. Evaluate your feelings, beliefs, and attitudes regarding clients with cognitive disorders.

Visit the Point http://thePoint.lww.com for NCLEX-style questions, journal articles, and more!

Cognition is the brain's ability to process, retain, and use information. Cognitive abilities include reasoning, judgment, perception, attention, comprehension, and memory. These cognitive abilities are essential for many important tasks, including making decisions, solving problems, interpreting the environment, and learning new information.

A cognitive disorder is a disruption or impairment in these higher-level functions of the brain. Cognitive disorders can have devastating effects on the ability to function in daily life. They can cause people to forget the names of immediate family members, to be unable to perform daily household tasks, and to neglect personal hygiene (Davis, 2005).

The primary categories of cognitive disorders are delirium, dementia, and amnestic disorders. All involve impairment of cognition, but they vary with respect to cause, treatment, prognosis, and effect on clients and family members or caregivers. This chapter focuses on delirium and dementia. It emphasizes not only the care of clients with cognitive disorders but also the needs of their caregivers.

DELIRIUM

Delirium is a syndrome that involves a disturbance of consciousness accompanied by a change in cognition. Delirium usually develops over a short period, sometimes a matter of hours, and fluctuates, or changes, throughout the course of the day. Clients with delirium have difficulty paying attention, are easily distracted and disoriented, and may have sensory disturbances such as illusions, misinterpretations, or hallucinations. An electrical cord on the floor may appear to them to be a snake (illusion). They may mistake the banging of a laundry cart in the hallway for a gunshot (misinterpretation). They may see "angels" hovering above when nothing is there (hallucination). At times, they also experience disturbances in the sleep–wake cycle, changes

in psychomotor activity, and emotional problems such as anxiety, fear, irritability, euphoria, or apathy (American Psychiatric Association [APA], 2000).

An estimated 10% to 15% of people in the hospital for general medical conditions are delirious at any given time. Delirium is common in older acutely ill clients. An estimated 30% to 50% of acutely ill older adult clients become delirious at some time during their hospital stay. Risk factors for delirium include increased severity of physical illness, older age, and baseline cognitive impairment such as that seen in dementia (Samuels & Neugroschl, 2005). Children may be more susceptible to delirium, especially that related to a febrile illness or certain medications such as anticholinergics (APA, 2000).

Etiology

Delirium almost always results from an identifiable physiologic, metabolic, or cerebral disturbance or disease or from drug intoxication or withdrawal. The most common causes are listed in Box 21.1. Often, delirium results from multiple causes and requires a careful and thorough physical examination and laboratory tests for identification.

Cultural Considerations

People from different cultural backgrounds may not be familiar with the information requested to assess memory, such as the name of former U.S. presidents. Other cultures may consider orientation to placement and location differently. Also, some cultures and religions, such as Jehovah's Witnesses, do not celebrate birthdays, so clients may have difficulty stating their date of birth. The nurse should not mistake failure to know such information for disorientation (APA, 2000).

CLINICAL VIGNETTE: DELIRIUM

On a hot and humid August afternoon, the 911 dispatcher received a call requesting an ambulance for an elderly woman who had collapsed on the sidewalk in a residential area. According to neighbors gathered at the scene, the woman had been wandering around the neighborhood since early morning. No one recognized her and several people had tried to approach her to offer help or give directions. She would not or could not give her name or address; much of her speech was garbled and hard to understand. She was not carrying a purse or identification. She finally collapsed and appeared unconscious, so they called emergency services.

The woman was taken to the emergency room. She was perspiring profusely, was found to have a fever of 103.2°F, and was grossly dehydrated. Intravenous therapy was started to

replenish fluids and electrolytes. A cooling blanket was applied to lower her temperature, and she was monitored closely over the next several hours. As the woman began to regain consciousness, she was confused and could not provide any useful information about herself. Her speech remained garbled and confused. Several times she attempted to climb out of the bed and remove her intravenous tube, so restraints were used to prevent injury and to allow treatment to continue.

By the end of the second day in the hospital, she could accurately give her name, address, and some of the circumstances surrounding the incident. She remembered she had been gardening in her back yard in the sun and felt very hot. She remembered thinking she should go back in the house to get a cold drink and rest. That was the last thing she remembered.

DSM-IV-TR DIAGNOSTIC CRITERIA:
SYMPTOMS OF DELIRIUM

- Difficulty with attention
- Easily distractible
- Disoriented
- May have sensory disturbances such as illusions, mis-interpretations, or hallucinations
- Can have sleep–wake cycle disturbances
- Changes in psychomotor activity
- May experience anxiety, fear, irritability, euphoria, or apathy

Adapted from DSM-IV-TR, 2000.

Treatment and Prognosis

The primary treatment for delirium is to identify and treat any causal or contributing medical conditions. Delirium is almost always a transient condition that clears with successful treatment of the underlying cause. Nevertheless, some causes such as head injury or encephalitis may leave clients with cognitive, behavioral, or emotional impairments even after the underlying cause resolves.

PSYCHOPHARMACOLOGY

Clients with quiet, hypoactive delirium need no specific pharmacologic treatment aside from that indicated for the causative condition. Many clients with delirium, however, show persistent or intermittent psychomotor agitation that can interfere with effective treatment or pose a risk to safety. Sedation to prevent inadvertent self-injury may be indicated. An antipsychotic medication such as haloperidol (Haldol) may be used in doses of 0.5 to 1 mg to decrease agitation. Sedatives and benzodiazepines are avoided because they may worsen delirium (Samuels & Neugroschl, 2005). Clients with impaired liver or kidney function could have difficulty metabolizing or excreting sedatives. The exception is delirium induced by alcohol withdrawal, which usually is treated with benzodiazepines (see Chapter 17).

OTHER MEDICAL TREATMENT

While the underlying causes of delirium are being treated, clients also may need other supportive physical measures. Adequate nutritious food and fluid intake speed recovery. Intravenous fluids or even total parenteral nutrition may be necessary if a client's physical condition has deteriorated and he or she cannot eat and drink.

If a client becomes agitated and threatens to dislodge intravenous tubing or catheters, physical restraints may be necessary so that needed medical treatments can continue. Restraints are used only when necessary and stay in place no longer than warranted because they may increase the client's agitation.

APPLICATION OF THE NURSING PROCESS: DELIRIUM

Nursing care for clients with delirium focuses on meeting their physiologic and psychological needs and maintaining their safety. Behavior, mood, and level of consciousness of these clients can fluctuate rapidly throughout the day. Therefore, the nurse must assess them continuously to recognize changes and to plan nursing care accordingly.

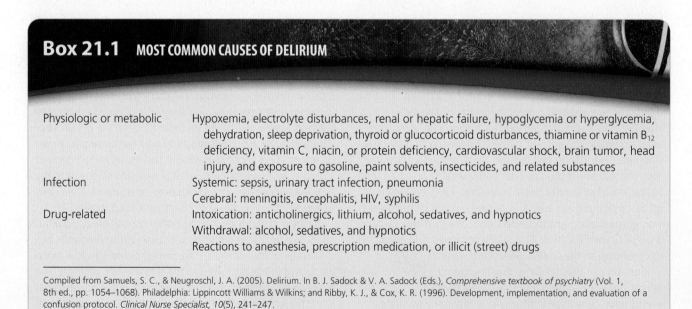

Box 21.1   MOST COMMON CAUSES OF DELIRIUM

Physiologic or metabolic	Hypoxemia, electrolyte disturbances, renal or hepatic failure, hypoglycemia or hyperglycemia, dehydration, sleep deprivation, thyroid or glucocorticoid disturbances, thiamine or vitamin B_{12} deficiency, vitamin C, niacin, or protein deficiency, cardiovascular shock, brain tumor, head injury, and exposure to gasoline, paint solvents, insecticides, and related substances
Infection	Systemic: sepsis, urinary tract infection, pneumonia
	Cerebral: meningitis, encephalitis, HIV, syphilis
Drug-related	Intoxication: anticholinergics, lithium, alcohol, sedatives, and hypnotics
	Withdrawal: alcohol, sedatives, and hypnotics
	Reactions to anesthesia, prescription medication, or illicit (street) drugs

Compiled from Samuels, S. C., & Neugroschl, J. A. (2005). Delirium. In B. J. Sadock & V. A. Sadock (Eds.), *Comprehensive textbook of psychiatry* (Vol. 1, 8th ed., pp. 1054–1068). Philadelphia: Lippincott Williams & Wilkins; and Ribby, K. J., & Cox, K. R. (1996). Development, implementation, and evaluation of a confusion protocol. *Clinical Nurse Specialist, 10*(5), 241–247.

Assessment

HISTORY

Because the causes of delirium are often related to medical illness, alcohol, or other drugs, the nurse obtains a thorough history of these areas. The nurse may need to obtain information from family members if a client's ability to provide accurate data is impaired.

Information about drugs should include prescribed medications, alcohol, illicit drugs, and over-the-counter medications. Although many people perceive prescribed and over-the-counter medications as relatively safe, combinations or standard doses of medications can produce delirium, especially in older adults. Box 21.2 lists types of drugs that can cause delirium. Combinations of these drugs significantly increase risk.

GENERAL APPEARANCE AND MOTOR BEHAVIOR

Clients with delirium often have a disturbance of psychomotor behavior. They may be restless and hyperactive, frequently picking at bedclothes or making sudden, uncoordinated attempts to get out of bed. Conversely, clients

---

Box 21.2 DRUGS CAUSING DELIRIUM

Anesthesia
Anticonvulsants
Anticholinergics
Antidepressants
Antihistamines
Antihypertensives
Antineoplastics
Antipsychotics
Aspirin
Barbiturates
Benzodiazepines
Cardiac glycosides
Cimetidine (Tagamet)
Hypoglycemic agents
Insulin
Narcotics
Propranolol (Inderal)
Reserpine
Steroids
Thiazide diuretics

Adapted from Samuels, S. C., & Neugroschl, J. A. (2005). Delirium. In B. J. Sadock and V. A. Sadock (Eds.), *Comprehensive Textbook of Psychiatry* (Vol. 1, 8th ed., pp. 1068–1093). Philadelphia: Lippincott Williams and Wilkins.

---

may have slowed motor behavior, appearing sluggish and lethargic with little movement.

Speech also may be affected, becoming less coherent and more difficult to understand as delirium worsens. Clients may perseverate on a single topic or detail, may be rambling and difficult to follow, or may have pressured speech that is rapid, forced, and usually louder than normal. At times, clients may call out or scream, especially at night.

MOOD AND AFFECT

Clients with delirium often have rapid and unpredictable mood shifts. A wide range of emotional responses is possible, such as anxiety, fear, irritability, anger, euphoria, and apathy. These mood shifts and emotions usually have nothing to do with the client's environment. When clients are particularly fearful and feel threatened, they may become combative to defend themselves from perceived harm.

THOUGHT PROCESS AND CONTENT

Although clients with delirium have changes in cognition, it is difficult for the nurse to assess these changes accurately and thoroughly. Marked inability to sustain attention makes it difficult to assess thought process and content. Thought content in delirium often is unrelated to the situation, or speech is illogical and difficult to understand. The nurse may ask how clients are feeling, and they will mumble about the weather. Thought processes often are disorganized and make no sense. Thoughts also may be fragmented (disjointed and incomplete). Clients may exhibit delusions, believing that their altered sensory perceptions are real.

SENSORIUM AND INTELLECTUAL PROCESSES

The primary and often initial sign of delirium is an altered level of consciousness that is seldom stable and usually fluctuates throughout the day. Clients usually are oriented to person but frequently disoriented to time and place. They demonstrate decreased awareness of the environment or situation and instead may focus on irrelevant stimuli such as the color of the bedspread or the room. Noises, people, or sensory misperceptions easily distract them.

Clients cannot focus, sustain, or shift attention effectively, and there is impaired recent and immediate memory (APA, 2000). This means the nurse may have to ask questions or provide directions repeatedly. Even then, clients may be unable to do what is requested.

Clients frequently experience misinterpretations, illusions, and hallucinations. Both misperceptions and illusions are based on some actual stimuli in the environment: clients may hear a door slam and interpret it as a gunshot or see the nurse reach for an intravenous bag and believe the nurse is about to strike them. Examples of common illusions include clients believing that intravenous tubing or an electrical cord is a snake and mistaking the nurse for a family member. Hallucinations are most often visual: clients "see" things for which there is no stimulus in reality. Some clients, when more lucid, are aware that they are experiencing sensory misperceptions. Others, however, actually believe their misinterpretations are correct and cannot be convinced otherwise.

JUDGMENT AND INSIGHT

Judgment is impaired. Clients often cannot perceive potentially harmful situations or act in their own best interests. For example, they may try repeatedly to pull out intravenous tubing or urinary catheters; this causes pain and interferes with necessary treatment.

Insight depends on the severity of the delirium. Clients with mild delirium may recognize that they are confused, are receiving treatment, and will likely improve. Those with severe delirium may have no insight into the situation.

ROLES AND RELATIONSHIPS

Clients are unlikely to fulfill their roles during the course of delirium. Most regain their previous level of functioning, however, and have no longstanding problems with roles or relationships.

SELF-CONCEPT

Although delirium has no direct effect on self-concept, clients often are frightened or feel threatened. Those with some awareness of the situation may feel helpless or powerless to do anything to change it. If delirium has resulted from alcohol, illicit drug use, or overuse of prescribed medications, clients may feel guilt, shame, and humiliation or think, "I'm a bad person; I did this to myself." This would indicate possible long-term problems with self-concept.

PHYSIOLOGIC AND SELF-CARE CONSIDERATIONS

Clients with delirium most often experience disturbed sleep–wake cycles that may include difficulty falling asleep, daytime sleepiness, nighttime agitation, or even a complete reversal of the usual daytime waking/nighttime sleeping pattern (APA, 2000). At times, clients also ignore or fail to perceive internal body cues such as hunger, thirst, or the urge to urinate or defecate.

Data Analysis

The primary nursing diagnoses for clients with delirium are as follows:
- Risk for Injury
- Acute Confusion

    Additional diagnoses that are commonly selected based on client assessment include the following:
- Disturbed Sensory Perception
- Disturbed Thought Processes
- Disturbed Sleep Pattern
- Risk for Deficient Fluid Volume
- Risk for Imbalanced Nutrition: Less Than Body Requirements

Outcome Identification

Treatment outcomes for the client with delirium may include the following:
- The client will be free of injury.
- The client will demonstrate increased orientation and reality contact.
- The client will maintain an adequate balance of activity and rest.
- The client will maintain adequate nutrition and fluid balance.
- The client will return to his or her optimal level of functioning.

Intervention

PROMOTING THE CLIENT'S SAFETY

Maintaining the client's safety is the priority focus of nursing interventions. Medications should be used judiciously because sedatives may worsen confusion and increase the risk for falls or other injuries (Samuels & Neugroschl, 2005).

    The nurse teaches clients to request assistance for activities such as getting out of bed or going to the bathroom. If clients cannot request assistance, they require close supervision to prevent them from attempting activities they cannot perform safely alone. The nurse responds promptly

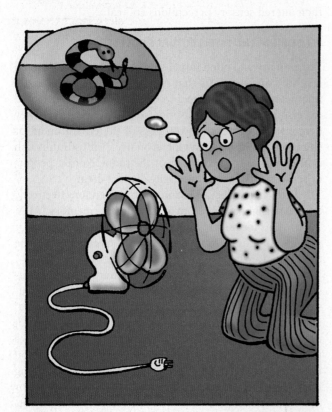

Illusion

to calls from clients for assistance and checks clients at frequent intervals.

If a client is agitated or pulling at intravenous lines or catheters, physical restraints may be necessary. Use of restraints, however, may increase the client's fears or feelings of being threatened, so restraints are a last resort. The nurse first tries other strategies such as having a family member stay with the client to reassure him or her.

MANAGING THE CLIENT'S CONFUSION

The nurse approaches these clients calmly and speaks in a clear low voice. It is important to give realistic reassurance to clients, such as

> *"I know things are upsetting and confusing right now, but your confusion should clear as you get better"* (validating/giving information).

Facing clients while speaking helps to capture their attention. The nurse provides explanations that clients can comprehend, avoiding lengthy or too detailed discussions. The nurse phrases questions or provides directions to clients in short, simple sentences, allowing adequate time for clients to grasp the content or to respond to a question. He or she permits clients to make decisions as they are able and takes care not to overwhelm or frustrate them.

The nurse provides orienting cues when talking with clients, such as calling them by name and referring to the time of day or expected activity. For example, the nurse might say,

> *"Good morning, Mrs. Jones. I see you are awake and look ready for breakfast"* (giving information).

Reminding the client of the nurse's name and role repeatedly may be necessary, such as

> *"My name is Sheila, and I'm your nurse today. I'm here now to walk in the hall with you"* (reality orientation).

Orienting objects such as a calendar and clock in the client's room are useful.

Often, the use of touch reassures clients and provides contact with reality. It is important to evaluate each client's response to touch rather than to assume all clients welcome it. A client who smiles or draws closer to the nurse when touched is responding positively. The fearful client may perceive touch as threatening rather than comforting and startle or draw away.

Clients with delirium can experience sensory overload, which means more stimulation is coming into the brain than they can handle. Reducing environmental stimulation is helpful because these clients are distracted and overstimulated easily. Minimizing environmental noises, including television or radio, should calm them. It is also important to monitor response to visitors. Too many visitors or more than one person talking at once may increase the client's confusion. The nurse can explain to visitors that the client will best tolerate quiet talking with one person at a time.

The client's room should be well lit to minimize environmental misperceptions. When clients experience illusions or misperceptions, the nurse corrects them matter-of-factly. It is important to validate the client's feelings of anxiety or fear generated by the misperception but not to reinforce that misperception. For example, a client hears a loud noise in the hall and asks the nurse, *"Was that an explosion?"* The nurse might respond,

> *"No, that was a cart banging in the hall. It was really loud, wasn't it? It startled me a little when I heard it"* (presenting reality/validating feelings).

PROMOTING SLEEP AND PROPER NUTRITION

The nurse monitors the client's sleep and elimination patterns and food and fluid intake. Clients may require prompting or assistance to eat and drink adequate food and fluids. It may be helpful to sit with clients at meals or to frequently offer fluids. Family members also may be able to help clients to improve their intake. Assisting clients to the bathroom periodically may be necessary to promote elimination if clients do not make these requests independently.

Promoting a balance of rest and sleep is important if clients are experiencing a disturbed sleep pattern. Discouraging or limiting daytime napping may improve ability to sleep at night. It is also important for clients to have some exercise during the day to promote nighttime sleep. Activ-

---

CLIENT/FAMILY EDUCATION FOR DELIRIUM

Monitor chronic health conditions carefully.
Visit physician regularly.
Tell all physicians and health care providers what medications are taken, including over-the-counter medications, dietary supplements, and herbal preparations.
Check with physician before taking any nonprescription medication.
Avoid alcohol and recreational drugs.
Maintain a nutritious diet.
Get adequate sleep.
Use safety precautions when working with paint solvents, insecticides, and similar products.

ities could include sitting in a chair, walking in the hall, or engaging in diversional activities (as possible).

Evaluation

Usually, successful treatment of the underlying causes of delirium returns clients to their previous levels of functioning. Clients and caregivers or family must understand what health care practices are necessary to avoid a recurrence. This may involve monitoring a chronic health condition, using medications carefully, or abstaining from alcohol or other drugs.

COMMUNITY-BASED CARE

Even when the cause of delirium is identified and treated, clients may not regain all cognitive functions, or problems with confusion may persist. Because delirium and dementia frequently occur together, clients may have dementia. A thorough medical evaluation can confirm dementia, and appropriate treatment and care can be initiated (see the following section).

When delirium has cleared and any other diagnoses have been eliminated, it may be necessary for the nurse or other health care professionals to initiate referrals to home health, visiting nurses, or a rehabilitation program if clients continue to experience cognitive problems. Various community programs provide such care, including adult day care or residential care. Clients who have ongoing cognitive deficits after an episode of delirium may have difficulties similar to those of clients with head injuries or mild dementia. Clients and family members or caregivers might benefit from support groups to help them deal with the changes in personality and remaining cognitive or motor deficits.

DEMENTIA

Dementia is a mental disorder that involves multiple cognitive deficits, primarily memory impairment, and at least one of the following cognitive disturbances (APA, 2000):

- **Aphasia,** which is deterioration of language function
- **Apraxia,** which is impaired ability to execute motor functions despite intact motor abilities
- **Agnosia,** which is inability to recognize or name objects despite intact sensory abilities
- Disturbance in **executive functioning,** which is the ability to think abstractly and to plan, initiate, sequence, monitor, and stop complex behavior

These cognitive deficits must be sufficiently severe to impair social or occupational functioning and must represent a decline from previous functioning.

Dementia must be distinguished from delirium; if the two diagnoses coexist, the symptoms of dementia remain even when the delirium has cleared. Table 21.1 compares delirium and dementia.

Memory impairment is the prominent early sign of dementia. Clients have difficulty learning new material and forget previously learned material. Initially, recent memory is impaired—for example, forgetting where certain objects were placed or that food is cooking on the stove. In later stages, dementia affects remote memory; clients forget the

---

NURSING INTERVENTIONS FOR DELIRIUM

- **Promoting client's safety**
  Teach client to request assistance for activities (getting out of bed, going to bathroom).
  Provide close supervision to ensure safety during these activities.
  Promptly respond to client's call for assistance.
- **Managing client's confusion**
  Speak to client in a calm manner in a clear low voice; use simple sentences.
  Allow adequate time for client to comprehend and respond.
  Allow client to make decisions as much as able.
  Provide orienting verbal cues when talking with client.
  Use supportive touch if appropriate.
- **Controlling environment to reduce sensory overload**
  Keep environmental noise to minimum (television, radio).

Monitor client's response to visitors; explain to family and friends that client may need to visit quietly one on one.
Validate client's anxiety and fears, but do not reinforce misperceptions.
- **Promoting sleep and proper nutrition**
  Monitor sleep and elimination patterns.
  Monitor food and fluid intake; provide prompts or assistance to eat and drink adequate amounts of flood and fluids.
  Provide periodic assistance to bathroom if client does not make requests.
  Discourage daytime napping to help sleep at night.
  Encourage some exercise during day like sitting in a chair, walking in hall, or other activities client can manage.

Nursing Care Plan

Delirium

Nursing Diagnosis

Acute Confusion: *Abrupt onset of a cluster of global, transient changes and disturbances in attention, cognition, psychomotor activity, level of consciousness, and/or sleep–wake cycle.*

ASSESSMENT DATA

- Poor judgment
- Cognitive impairment
- Impaired memory
- Lack of or limited insight
- Loss of personal control
- Inability to perceive harm
- Illusions
- Hallucinations
- Mood swings

EXPECTED OUTCOMES

Immediate
The client will
- Engage in a trust relationship with staff and caregiver
- Be free of injury
- Increase reality contact
- Cooperate with treatment

Stabilization
The client will
- Establish or follow a routine for activities of daily living
- Demonstrate decreased confusion, illusions, or hallucinations
- Experience minimal distress related to confusion
- Validate perceptions with staff or caregiver before taking action

Community
The client will
- Return to optimal level of functioning
- Manage health conditions, if any, effectively
- Seek medical treatment as needed

IMPLEMENTATION

Nursing Interventions *denotes collaborative interventions	Rationale
Do not allow the client to assume responsibility for decisions or actions if he or she is unsafe.	The client's safety is a priority. He or she may be unable to determine harmful actions or situations.
If limits on the client's actions are necessary, explain limits and reasons clearly, within the client's ability to understand.	The client has the right to be informed of any restrictions and the reasons limits are needed.
Involve the client in making plans or decisions as much as he or she is able to participate.	Compliance with treatment is enhanced if the client is emotionally invested in it.
In a matter-of-fact manner give the client factual feedback on misperceptions, delusions, or hallucinations (e.g., "That is a chair.") and convey that others do not share his or her interpretations (e.g., "I don't see anyone else in the room.").	When given feedback in a nonjudgmental way, the client can feel validated for his or her feelings, while recognizing that his or her perceptions are not shared by others.
Assess the client daily or more often if needed for his or her level of functioning.	Clients with organically based problems tend to fluctuate frequently in terms of their capabilities.
Allow the client to make decisions as much as he or she is able.	Decision making increases the client's participation, independence, and self-esteem.

continued ⋯▶

Nursing Care Plan: Delirium, cont.

IMPLEMENTATION

Nursing Interventions *denotes collaborative interventions

Rationale

Assist the client to establish a daily routine, including hygiene, activities, and so forth.

Teach the client about underlying cause(s) of confusion and delirium.

Routine or habitual activities do not require decisions about whether or not to perform a particular task.

Knowledge about the cause(s) of confusion can help the client seek assistance when indicated.

Adapted from Schultz, J. M., & Videbeck, S. L. (2005). Lippincott's manual of psychiatric nursing care plans (7th ed.). Philadelphia: Lippincott Williams & Wilkins.

names of adult children, their lifelong occupations, and even their names.

Aphasia usually begins with the inability to name familiar objects or people and then progresses to speech that becomes vague or empty with excessive use of terms such as *it* or *thing*. Clients may exhibit **echolalia** (echoing what is heard) or **palilalia** (repeating words or sounds over and over) (APA, 2000). Apraxia may cause clients to lose the ability to perform routine self-care activities such as dressing or cooking. Agnosia is frustrating for clients: they may look at a table and chairs but are unable to name them. Disturbances in executive functioning are evident as clients lose the ability to learn new material, solve problems, or carry out daily activities such as meal planning or budgeting.

Clients with dementia also may underestimate the risks associated with activities or overestimate their ability to function in certain situations. For example, while driving, clients may cut in front of other drivers, sideswipe parked cars, or fail to slow down when they should.

Onset and Clinical Course

When an underlying, treatable cause is not present, the course of dementia is usually progressive. Dementia often is described in stages:

- *Mild:* Forgetfulness is the hallmark of beginning, mild dementia. It exceeds the normal, occasional forgetfulness experienced as part of the aging process. The person has difficulty finding words, frequently loses objects, and begins to experience anxiety about these losses. Occupational and social settings are less enjoyable, and the person may avoid them. Most people remain in the community during this stage.
- *Moderate:* Confusion is apparent, along with progressive memory loss. The person no longer can perform com-

Table 21.1 COMPARISON OF DELIRIUM AND DEMENTIA

Indicator	Delirium	Dementia
Onset	Rapid	Gradual and insidious
Duration	Brief (hours to days)	Progressive deterioration
Level of consciousness	Impaired, fluctuates	Not affected
Memory	Short-term memory impaired	Short- then long-term memory impaired, eventually destroyed
Speech	May be slurred, rambling, pressured, irrelevant	Normal in early stage, progressive aphasia in later stage
Thought processes	Temporarily disorganized	Impaired thinking, eventual loss of thinking abilities
Perception	Visual or tactile hallucinations, delusions	Often absent, but can have paranoia, hallucinations, illusions
Mood	Anxious, fearful if hallucinating; weeping, irritable	Depressed and anxious in early stage, labile mood, restless pacing, angry outbursts in later stages

Adapted from American Psychiatric Association. (2000). *Diagnostic and statistical manual of mental disorders* (4th ed., text revision). Washington, DC: APA; and Ribby, K. J., and Cox, K. R. (1996). Development, implementation, and evaluation of a confusion protocol. *Clinical Nurse Specialist, 10*(5), 241–247.

plex tasks but remains oriented to person and place. He or she still recognizes familiar people. Toward the end of this stage, the person loses the ability to live independently and requires assistance because of disorientation to time and loss of information such as address and telephone number. The person may remain in the community if adequate caregiver support is available, but some people move to supervised living situations.

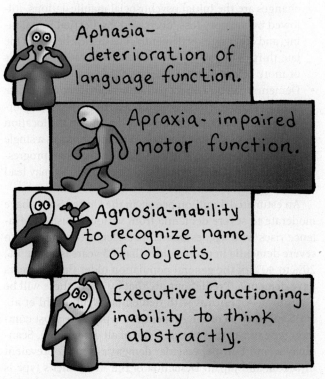

Aphasia— deterioration of language function.

Apraxia— impaired motor function.

Agnosia—inability to recognize name of objects.

Executive functioning— inability to think abstractly.

Multiple cognitive deficits of dementia

- *Severe:* Personality and emotional changes occur. The person may be delusional, wander at night, forget the names of his or her spouse and children, and require assistance in activities of daily living (ADLs). Most people live in nursing facilities when they reach this stage unless extraordinary community support is available.

Etiology

Causes vary, although the clinical picture is similar for most dementias. Often, no definitive diagnosis can be made until completion of a postmortem examination. Metabolic activity is decreased in the brains of clients with dementia; it is not known whether dementia causes decreased metabolic activity or if decreased metabolic activity results in dementia. A genetic component has been identified for some dementias such as Huntington's disease. An abnormal *APOE* gene is known to be linked with Alzheimer's disease. Other causes of dementia are related to infections such as human immunodeficiency virus (HIV) infection or Creutzfeldt-Jakob disease. The most common types of dementia and their known or hypothesized causes follow (APA, 2000; Neugroschl et al., 2005):

- **Alzheimer's disease** is a progressive brain disorder that has a gradual onset but causes an increasing decline in functioning, including loss of speech, loss of motor function, and profound personality and behavioral changes such as paranoia, delusions, hallucinations, inattention to hygiene, and belligerence. It is evidenced by atrophy of cerebral neurons, senile plaque deposits, and enlargement of the third and fourth ventricles of the brain. Risk for Alzheimer's disease increases with age, and average duration from onset of symptoms to death is 8 to 10 years. Dementia of the Alzheimer's type, especially with late onset (after 65 years of age), may have a genetic component. Research has shown linkages to chromosomes 21, 14, and 19 (APA, 2000).
- **Vascular dementia** has symptoms similar to those of Alzheimer's disease, but onset is typically abrupt, followed by rapid changes in functioning; a plateau, or leveling-off period; more abrupt changes; another leveling-off period; and so on. Computed tomography or magnetic resonance imaging usually shows multiple vascular lesions of the cerebral cortex and subcortical structures resulting from the decreased blood supply to the brain.
- **Pick's disease** is a degenerative brain disease that particularly affects the frontal and temporal lobes and results in a clinical picture similar to that of Alzheimer's disease. Early signs include personality changes, loss of social skills and inhibitions, emotional blunting, and language abnormalities. Onset is most commonly 50 to 60 years of age; death occurs in 2 to 5 years.
- **Creutzfeldt-Jakob disease** is a central nervous system disorder that typically develops in adults 40 to 60 years

CLINICAL VIGNETTE: DEMENTIA

Jack Smith, 74, and his wife, Marion, 69, have been living in their home and managing fairly well until lately. The Smiths have two grown children who both live out of town but visit about every 2 months and at holidays and birthdays. Jack recently had a stroke and entered a rehabilitation facility to try to learn to walk and talk again. Marion wanted to stay at home and wait for his return, but when the children would call to check on her, she would often be crying and confused or frightened. On one visit, they found her looking very tired, dressed in a wrinkled dress that looked soiled. She looked as if she had lost weight, and she couldn't remember what she had eaten for breakfast or lunch.

Marion's daughter remembered that before her father had the stroke, she noticed that Jack had taken over several routine tasks her mother had always done, such as making the grocery list and planning and helping to cook their meals. Her mother seemed more forgetful and would ask the same questions over and over and often related the same story several times during their visit.

A few weeks after Jack entered the rehab center and Marion was living at home alone, the neighbors found Marion wander-

ing around the neighborhood one morning lost and confused. It was now clear to her children that their mother could not remain in her home alone and take care of herself. It was uncertain how long Jack would need to remain at the rehabilitation center, and they were not sure what his physical capabilities would be when he did return.

Her daughter decided that Marion (and eventually Jack) would come to live with her family. They moved her in with them, but even after getting settled at her daughter's home, Marion continued to be confused and often did not know where she was. She kept asking where Jack was and forgot her grandchildren's names. At times, she grew agitated and would accuse them of stealing her purse or other possessions. Later, she would always find them. Marion would sometimes forget to go to the bathroom and would soil her clothes. She would forget to brush her hair and teeth and take a bath and often needed help with these activities. When her daughter came home from work in the evening, the sandwich she had made for her mother was often left untouched in the refrigerator. Marion spent much of her time packing her bags to go home and "see Jack."

of age. It involves altered vision, loss of coordination or abnormal movements, and dementia that usually progresses rapidly (a few months). The cause of the encephalopathy is an infectious particle resistant to boiling, some disinfectants (e.g., formalin, alcohol), and ultraviolet radiation. Pressured autoclaving or bleach can inactivate the particle.

- HIV infection can lead to dementia and other neurologic problems; these may result directly from invasion of nervous tissue by HIV or from other acquired immunodeficiency syndrome–related illnesses such as toxoplasmosis and cytomegalovirus. This type of dementia can result in a wide variety of symptoms ranging from mild sensory impairment to gross memory and cognitive deficits to severe muscle dysfunction.

- **Parkinson's disease** is a slowly progressive neurologic condition characterized by tremor, rigidity, bradykinesia, and postural instability. It results from loss of neurons of the basal ganglia. Dementia has been reported in approximately 20% to 60% of people with Parkinson's disease and is characterized by cognitive and motor slowing, impaired memory, and impaired executive functioning.

- **Huntington's disease** is an inherited, dominant gene disease that primarily involves cerebral atrophy, demyelination, and enlargement of the brain ventricles. Initially,

there are choreiform movements that are continuous during waking hours and involve facial contortions, twisting, turning, and tongue movements. Personality changes are the initial psychosocial manifestations, followed by memory loss, decreased intellectual functioning, and other signs of dementia. The disease begins in the late thirties or early forties and may last 10 to 20 years or more before death.

- Dementia can be a direct pathophysiologic consequence of head trauma. The degree and type of cognitive impairment and behavioral disturbance depend on the location and extent of the brain injury. When it occurs as a single injury, the dementia is usually stable rather than progressive. Repeated head injury (e.g., from boxing) may lead to progressive dementia.

An estimated 5 million people in the United States have moderate to severe dementia from various causes. Prevalence rises with age: estimated prevalence of moderate to severe dementia in people older than 65 years is about 5%; 20% to 40% of the general population older than 85 years have dementia. Predictions are that by 2050, there will be 18 million Americans with dementia (Neugroschl et al., 2005). Dementia of the Alzheimer's type is the most common type in North America (60% of all dementias), Scandinavia, and Europe; vascular dementia is more prevalent in Russia and Japan. Dementia of the Alzheimer's type is more common in women; vascular dementia is more common in men.

Cultural Considerations

Clients from other cultures may find the questions used on many assessment tools for dementia difficult or impossible to answer. Examples include the names of former U.S. presidents. To avoid drawing erroneous conclusions, the nurse must be aware of differences in the person's knowledge base.

The nurse also must be aware of different culturally influenced perspectives and beliefs about elderly family members. In many Eastern countries and among Native Americans, elders hold a position of authority, respect, power, and decision making for the family; this does not change despite memory loss or confusion. For fear of seeming disrespectful, other family members may be reluctant to make decisions or plans for elders with dementia. The nurse must work with family members to accomplish goals without making them feel they have betrayed the revered elder.

Treatment and Prognosis

Whenever possible, the underlying cause of dementia is identified so that treatment can be instituted. For example, the progress of vascular dementia, the second most common type, may be halted with appropriate treatment of the underlying vascular condition (e.g., changes in diet, exercise, control of hypertension or diabetes). Improvement of cerebral blood flow may arrest the progress of vascular dementia in some people (Neugroschl et al., 2005).

The prognosis for the progressive types of dementia may vary as described earlier, but all prognoses involve progressive deterioration of physical and mental abilities until death. Typically, in the later stages, clients have minimal cognitive and motor function, are totally dependent on caregivers, and are unaware of their surroundings or people in the environment. They may be totally uncommunicative or make unintelligible sounds or attempts to verbalize.

For degenerative dementias, no direct therapies have been found to reverse or retard the fundamental pathophysiologic processes. Levels of numerous neurotransmitters such as acetylcholine, dopamine, norepinephrine, and serotonin are decreased in dementia. This has led to attempts at replenishment therapy with acetylcholine precursors, cholinergic agonists, and cholinesterase inhibitors. Tacrine (Cognex), donepezil (Aricept), rivastigmine (Exelon), and galantamine (Reminyl) are cholinesterase inhibitors and have shown modest therapeutic effects and temporarily slow the progress of dementia (Table 21.2). They have no effect, however, on the overall course of the disease. Tacrine elevates liver enzymes in about 50% of clients using it; therefore, liver function is assessed every 1 to 2 weeks.

Clients with dementia demonstrate a broad range of behaviors that can be treated symptomatically. Doses of medications are one half to two thirds lower than usually prescribed. Antidepressants are effective for significant depressive symptoms. Antipsychotics such as haloperidol (Haldol), olanzapine (Zyprexa), risperidone (Risperdal), and quetiapine (Seroquel) may be used to manage psychotic symptoms of delusions, hallucinations, or paranoia. Lithium carbonate, carbamazepine (Tegretol), and valproic acid (Depakote) help to stabilize affective lability and to diminish aggressive outbursts. Benzodiazepines are used cautiously because they may cause delirium and can worsen already compromised cognitive abilities (Neugroschl et al., 2005). These medications are discussed in Chapter 2.

APPLICATION OF THE NURSING PROCESS: DEMENTIA

This section focuses on caring for clients with progressive dementia, which is the most common type. The nurse can use these guidelines as indicated for clients with dementia that is not progressive.

Table 21.2   DRUGS USED TO TREAT DEMENTIA

Name	Dosage Range and Route	Nursing Considerations
Tacrine (Cognex)	40–160 mg orally per day divided into 4 doses	Monitor liver enzymes for hepatotoxic effects. Monitor for flu-like symptoms.
Donepezil (Aricept)	5–10 mg orally per day	Monitor for nausea, diarrhea, and insomnia. Test stools periodically for GI bleeding.
Rivastigmine (Exelon)	3–12 mg orally per day divided into 2 doses	Monitor for nausea, vomiting, abdominal pain, and loss of appetite.
Galantamine (Reminyl)	16–32 mg orally per day divided into 2 doses	Monitor for nausea, vomiting, loss of appetite, dizziness, and syncope.

Adapted from *Drug facts and comparisons.* (2007). 61st ed. St. Louis: A Wolters Kluwer Company.

Assessment

The assessment process may seem confusing and complicated to clients with dementia. They may not know or may forget the purpose of the interview. The nurse provides simple explanations as often as clients need them, such as "I'm asking these questions so the staff can see how your health is." Clients may become confused or tire easily, so frequent breaks in the interview may be needed. It helps to ask simple rather than compound questions and to allow clients ample time to answer.

A mental status examination can provide information about the client's cognitive abilities such as memory, concentration, and abstract information processing. Typically, the client is asked to interpret the meaning of a proverb, perform subtraction of figures without paper and pencil, recall the names of objects, make a complete sentence, and copy two intersecting pentagons. Although this does not replace a thorough assessment, it gives a cursory evaluation of the client's cognitive abilities. It is important to remember that people with severe depression or psychosis may also be unable to perform some of these cognitive tasks correctly.

HISTORY

Considering the impairment of recent memory, clients may be unable to provide an accurate and thorough history of the onset of problems. Interviews with family, friends, or caregivers may be necessary to obtain data.

GENERAL APPEARANCE AND MOTOR BEHAVIOR

Dementia progressively impairs the ability to carry on meaningful conversation. Clients display aphasia when they cannot name familiar objects or people. Conversation becomes repetitive because they often perseverate on one idea. Eventually, speech may become slurred, followed by a total loss of language function.

The initial finding with regard to motor behavior is the loss of ability to perform familiar tasks (*apraxia*) such as dressing or combing one's hair, although actual motor abilities are intact. Clients cannot imitate the task when others demonstrate it for them. In the severe stage, clients may experience a gait disturbance that makes unassisted ambulation unsafe, if not impossible.

Some clients with dementia show uninhibited behavior, including making inappropriate jokes, neglecting personal hygiene, showing undue familiarity with strangers, or disregarding social conventions for acceptable behavior. This can include the use of profanity or making disparaging remarks about others when clients have never displayed these behaviors before.

MOOD AND AFFECT

Initially, clients with dementia experience anxiety and fear over the beginning losses of memory and cognitive functions. Nevertheless, they may not express these feelings to anyone. Mood becomes more labile over time and may shift rapidly and drastically for no apparent reason. Emotional outbursts are common and usually pass quickly. Clients may display anger and hostility, sometimes toward other people. They begin to demonstrate catastrophic emotional reactions in response to environmental changes that clients may not perceive or understand accurately or when they cannot respond adaptively. These catastrophic reactions may include verbal or physical aggression, wandering at night, agitation, or other behaviors that seem to indicate a loss of personal control.

Clients may display a pattern of withdrawal from the world they no longer understand. They are lethargic, look apathetic, and pay little attention to the environment or the people in it. They appear to lose all emotional affect and seem dazed and listless.

THOUGHT PROCESS AND CONTENT

Initially, the ability to think abstractly is impaired, resulting in loss of the ability to plan, sequence, monitor, initiate, or stop complex behavior (APA, 2000). The client loses the ability to solve problems or to take action in new situations because he or she cannot think about what to do. The ability to generalize knowledge from one situation to another is lost because the client cannot recognize similarities or differences in situations. These problems with cognition make it impossible for the employed client to continue working. The client's ability to perform tasks such as planning activities, budgeting, or planning meals is lost.

As the dementia progresses, delusions of persecution are common. The client may accuse others of stealing objects he or she has lost or may believe he or she is being cheated or pursued.

SENSORIUM AND INTELLECTUAL PROCESSES

Clients lose intellectual function, which eventually involves the complete loss of their abilities. Memory deficits are the initial and essential feature of dementia. Dementia first affects recent and immediate memory and then eventually impairs the ability to recognize close family members and even oneself. In mild and moderate dementia, clients may make up answers to fill in memory gaps (**confabulation**). Agnosia is another hallmark of dementia. Clients lose visual spatial relations, which is often evidenced by deterioration of the ability to write or draw simple objects.

Attention span and ability to concentrate are increasingly impaired until clients lose the ability to do either. Clients are chronically confused about the environment, other people, and eventually themselves. Initially, they are disoriented to time in mild dementia, time and place in moderate dementia, and finally to self in the severe stage.

Hallucinations are a frequent problem. Visual hallucinations are most common and generally unpleasant. Clients are likely to believe the hallucination is reality.

JUDGMENT AND INSIGHT

Clients with dementia have poor judgment in light of the cognitive impairment. They underestimate risks and unrealistically appraise their abilities, which result in a high risk for injury. Clients cannot evaluate situations for risks or danger. For example, they may wander outside in the winter wearing only thin nightclothes and not consider this to be a risk.

Insight is limited. Initially, the client may be aware of problems with memory and cognition and may worry that he or she is "losing my mind." Quite quickly, these concerns about the ability to function diminish, and clients have little or no awareness of the more serious deficits that have developed. In this context, clients may accuse others of stealing possessions that the clients themselves have actually lost or forgotten.

SELF-CONCEPT

Initially, clients may be angry or frustrated with themselves for losing objects or forgetting important things. Some clients express sadness at their bodies for getting old and at the loss of functioning. Soon, though, clients lose that awareness of self, which gradually deteriorates until they can look in a mirror and fail to recognize their own reflections.

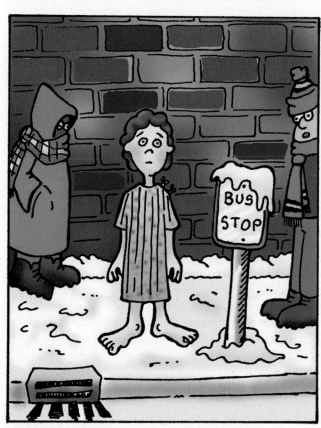

Judgment

ROLES AND RELATIONSHIPS

Dementia profoundly affects the client's roles and relationships. If the client is still employed, work performance suffers, even in the mild stage of dementia, to the point that work is no longer possible given the memory and cognitive deficits. Roles as spouse, partner, or parent deteriorate as clients lose the ability to perform even routine tasks or recognize familiar people. Eventually, clients cannot meet even the most basic needs.

Inability to participate in meaningful conversation or social events severely limits relationships. Clients quickly become confined to the house or apartment because they are unable to venture outside unassisted. Close family members often begin to assume caregiver roles; this can change previously established relationships. Grown children of clients with dementia experience role reversal; that is, they care for parents who once cared for them. Spouses or partners may feel as if they have lost the previous relationship and now are in the role of custodian.

PHYSIOLOGIC AND SELF-CARE CONSIDERATIONS

Clients with dementia often experience disturbed sleep–wake cycles; they nap during the day and wander at night. Some clients ignore internal cues such as hunger or thirst; others have little difficulty with eating and drinking until dementia is severe. Clients may experience bladder and even bowel incontinence or have difficulty cleaning themselves after elimination. They frequently neglect bathing and grooming. Eventually, clients are likely to require complete care from someone else to meet these basic physiologic needs.

Data Analysis

Many nursing diagnoses can be appropriate because the effects of dementia on clients are profound; the disease touches virtually every part of their lives. Commonly used nursing diagnoses include the following:

- Risk for Injury
- Disturbed Sleep Pattern
- Risk for Deficient Fluid Volume
- Risk for Imbalanced Nutrition: Less Than Body Requirements
- Chronic Confusion
- Impaired Environmental Interpretation Syndrome
- Impaired Memory
- Impaired Social Interaction
- Impaired Verbal Communication
- Ineffective Role Performance

In addition, the nursing diagnoses of Disturbed Thought Processes and Disturbed Sensory Perception would be appropriate for a client with psychotic symptoms. Multiple nursing diagnoses related to physiologic status also may be indicated based on the nurse's assessment, such as alterations in nutrition, hydration, elimination, physical mobility, and activity tolerance.

Outcome Identification

Treatment outcomes for clients with progressive dementia do not involve regaining or maintaining abilities to function. In fact, the nurse must reassess overall health status and revise treatment outcomes periodically as the client's condition changes. Outcomes and nursing care that focus on the client's medical condition or deficits are common. Current literature proposes a focus on psychosocial care that maximizes the client's strengths and abilities for as long as possible. Psychosocial care involves maintaining the client's independence as long as possible, validating the client's feelings, keeping the client involved in the environment, and dealing with behavioral disruptions respectfully (Hendry & Douglas, 2003; Mittelman et al., 2004; Yuhas et al., 2006). Treatment outcomes for a client with dementia may include the following:

- The client will be free of injury.
- The client will maintain an adequate balance of activity and rest, nutrition, hydration, and elimination.
- The client will function as independently as possible given his or her limitations.
- The client will feel respected and supported.
- The client will remain involved in his or her surroundings.
- The client will interact with others in the environment.

Intervention

Psychosocial models for care of clients with dementia are based on the approach that each client is a unique person and remains so, even as the disease's progression blocks the client's ability to demonstrate those unique characteristics. Interventions are rooted in the belief that clients with dementia have personal strengths. They focus on demonstrating caring, keeping clients involved by relating to the environment and other people, and validating feelings and dignity of clients by being responsive to them, offering choices, and **reframing** (offering alternative points of view to explain events; Hendry & Douglas, 2003). This is in contrast to medical models of care that focus on progressive loss of function and identity.

Nurses can use the following interventions in any setting for clients with dementia. Education for family members caring for clients at home and for professional caregivers in residential or skilled facilities is an essential component of providing safe and supportive care. The discussion provides examples that apply to various settings.

PROMOTING THE CLIENT'S SAFETY

Safety considerations involve protecting against injury, meeting physiologic needs, and managing risks posed by the environment, including internal stimuli such as delusions and hallucinations. Clients cannot accurately appraise the environment and their abilities; therefore, they do not exercise normal caution in daily life. For example, the client

---

NURSING INTERVENTIONS FOR DEMENTIA

- Promoting client's safety and protecting from injury
  Offer unobtrusive assistance with or supervision of cooking, bathing, or self-care activities.
  Identify environmental triggers to help client avoid them.
- Promoting adequate sleep, proper nutrition and hygiene, and activity
  Prepare desirable foods and foods client can self-feed; sit with client while eating.
  Monitor bowel elimination patterns; intervene with fluids and fiber or prompts.
  Remind client to urinate; provide pads or diapers as needed, checking and changing them frequently to avoid infection, skin irritation, unpleasant odors.
  Encourage mild physical activity such as walking.
- Structuring environment and routine
  Encourage client to follow regular routine and habits of bathing and dressing rather than impose new ones.

- Monitor amount of environmental stimulation, and adjust when needed.
- Providing emotional support
  Be kind, respectful, calm, and reassuring; pay attention to client.
  Use supportive touch when appropriate.
- Promoting interaction and involvement
  Plan activities geared to client's interests and abilities.
  Reminisce with client about the past.
  If client is nonverbal, remain alert to nonverbal behavior.
  Employ techniques of distraction, time away, going along, or reframing to calm clients who are agitated, suspicious, or confused.

living at home may forget food cooking on the stove; the client living in a residential care setting may leave for a walk in cold weather without a coat and gloves. Assistance or supervision that is as unobtrusive as possible protects clients from injury while preserving their dignity.

A family member might say,

"I'll sit in the kitchen and talk to you while you make lunch" (suggesting collaboration) rather than *"You can't cook by yourself because you might set the house on fire."*

In this way, the nurse or caregiver supports the client's desire and ability to engage in certain tasks while providing protection from injury.

Clients with dementia may believe that their physical safety is jeopardized; they may feel threatened or suspicious and paranoid. These feelings can lead to agitated or erratic behavior that compromises safety. Avoiding direct confrontation of the client's fears is important. Clients with dementia may struggle with fears and suspicion throughout their illness. Triggers of suspicion include strangers, changes in the daily routine, or impaired memory. The nurse must discover and address these environmental triggers rather than confront the paranoid ideas.

For example, a client reports that his belongings have been stolen. The nurse might say,

"Let's go look in your room and see what's there"

and help the client to locate the misplaced or hidden items (suggesting collaboration). If the client is in a room with other people and says, "They're here to take me away!" the nurse might say,

"Those people are here visiting with someone else. Let's go for a walk and let them visit" (presenting reality/distraction).

The nurse then can take the client to a quieter and less stimulating place, which moves the client away from the environmental trigger.

PROMOTING ADEQUATE SLEEP AND PROPER NUTRITION, HYGIENE, AND ACTIVITY

Clients require assistance to meet basic physiologic needs. The nurse monitors food and fluid intake to ensure adequacy. Clients may eat poorly because of limited appetite or distraction at mealtimes. The nurse addresses this problem by providing foods clients like, sitting with clients at meals to provide cues to continue eating, having nutritious

snacks available whenever clients are hungry, and minimizing noise and undue distraction at mealtimes. Clients who have difficulty manipulating utensils may be unable to cut meat or other foods into bite-sized pieces. The food should be cut up when it is prepared, not in front of clients, to deflect attention from their inability to do so. Food that can be eaten without utensils, or finger foods such as sandwiches and fresh fruit, may be best. In contrast, clients may eat too much, even ingesting inedible items. Providing low-calorie snacks such as carrot and celery sticks can satisfy the desire to chew and eat without unnecessary weight gain. Enteral nutrition often becomes necessary when dementia is most severe, although not all families choose to use tube feedings.

Adequate intake of fluids and food is also necessary for proper elimination. Clients may fail to respond to cues indicating constipation, so the nurse or caregiver monitors the client's bowel elimination patterns and intervenes with increased fluids and fiber or prompts as needed. Urinary elimination can become a problem if clients do not respond to the urge to void or are incontinent. Reminders to urinate may be helpful when clients are still continent but not initiating use of the bathroom. Sanitary pads can address dribbling or stress incontinence; adult diapers, rather than indwelling catheters, are indicated for incontinence. The nurse checks disposable pads and diapers frequently and changes soiled items promptly to avoid infection, skin irritation, and unpleasant odors. It is also important to provide good hygiene to minimize these risks.

Balance between rest and activity is an essential component of the daily routine. Mild physical activity such as walking promotes physical health but is not a cognitive challenge. Daily physical activity also helps clients to sleep at night. The nurse provides rest periods so clients can conserve and regain energy, but extensive daytime napping may interfere with nighttime sleep. The nurse encourages clients to engage in physical activity because they may not initiate such activities independently; many clients tend to become sedentary as cognitive abilities diminish. Clients often are quite willing to participate in physical activities but cannot initiate, plan, or carry out those activities without assistance.

STRUCTURING THE ENVIRONMENT AND ROUTINE

A structured environment and established routines can reassure clients with dementia. Familiar surroundings and routines help to eliminate some confusion and frustration from memory loss. Providing routines and structure, however, does not mean forcing clients to conform to the structure of the setting or routines that other people determine. Rather than impose new structure, the nurse encourages clients to follow their usual routines and habits of bathing and dressing (Yuhas et al., 2006). For example, it is important to know whether a client prefers a tub bath or shower and washes at night or in the morning and to include those preferences in the client's care. Research has shown that attempting to change the dressing behavior of clients may result in physical aggression as clients make ineffective attempts to resist unwanted changes. Monitoring response to daily routines and making needed adjustments are important aspects of care.

The nurse needs to monitor and manage the client's tolerance of stimulation. Generally, clients can tolerate less stimulation when they are fatigued, hungry, or stressed. Also, with the progression of dementia, tolerance for environmental stimuli decreases. As this tolerance diminishes, clients need a quieter environment with fewer people and less noise or distraction.

PROVIDING EMOTIONAL SUPPORT

The therapeutic relationship between client and nurse involves "empathic caring" (Hendry & Douglas, 2003), which includes being kind, respectful, calm, and reassuring and paying attention to the client. Nurses use these same qualities with many different clients in various settings. In most situations, clients give positive feedback to the nurse or caregiver, but clients with dementia often seem to ignore the nurse's efforts and may even respond with negative behavior such as anger or suspicion. This makes it more difficult for the nurse or caregiver to sustain caring behavior. Nevertheless, nurses and caregivers must maintain all the qualities of the therapeutic relationship even when clients do not seem to respond.

Because of their disorientation and memory loss, clients with dementia often become anxious and require much patience and reassurance. The nurse can convey reassurance by approaching the client in a calm, supportive manner, as if nurse and client are a team—a "we can do it together" approach. The nurse reassures the client that he or she knows what is happening and can take care of things when the client is confused and cannot do so. For example, if the client is confused about getting dressed, the nurse might say,

"I'll be glad to help you with that shirt. I'll hold it for you while you put your arms in the sleeves" (offering self/suggesting collaboration).

Supportive touch is effective with many clients. Touch can provide reassurance and convey caring when words may not be understood. Holding the hand of the client who is tearful and sad and tucking the client into bed at night are examples of ways to use supportive touch. As with any use of touch, the nurse must evaluate each client's response. Clients who respond positively will smile or move closer toward the nurse. Those who are threatened by physical touch will look frightened or pull away from the nurse, especially if the touch is sudden or unexpected or if the client misperceives the nurse's intent.

PROMOTING INTERACTION AND INVOLVEMENT

In a psychosocial model of dementia care, the nurse or caregiver plans activities that reinforce the client's identity and keep him or her engaged and involved in the business of living (Yuhas et al., 2006). The nurse or caregiver tailors these activities to the client's interests and abilities: They should not be routine group activities that "everyone is supposed to do." For example, a client with an interest in history may enjoy documentary programs on television; a client who likes music may enjoy singing. Clients often need the involvement of another person to sustain attention in the activity and to enjoy it more fully. Those who have long periods without anything to engage their interest are more likely to become restless and agitated. Clients engaged in activities are more likely to stay calm.

Reminiscence therapy (thinking about or relating personally significant past experiences) is an effective intervention for clients with dementia (Woods et al., 2005). Rather than lamenting that the client is "living in the past," this therapy encourages family and caregivers also to reminisce with the client. Reminiscing uses the client's remote memory, which is not affected as severely or quickly as recent or immediate memory. Photo albums may be useful in stimulating remote memory, and they provide a focus on the client's past. Sometimes clients like to reminisce about local or national events and talk about their roles or what they were doing at the time. In addition to keeping clients involved in the business of living, reminiscence also can build self-esteem as clients discuss accomplishments. Engaging in active listening, asking questions, and providing cues to continue promote successful use of this technique.

Clients have increasing problems interacting with others as dementia progresses. Initially, clients retain verbal language skills, but other people may find them difficult to understand as words are lost or content becomes vague. The nurse must listen carefully to the client and try to determine the meaning behind what is being said. The nurse might say,

"Are you trying to say you want to use the bathroom?" or *"Did I get that right, you are hungry?"* (seeking clarification).

It is also important not to interrupt clients or to finish their thoughts. If a client becomes frustrated when the nurse cannot understand his or her meaning, the nurse might say,

"Can you show me what you mean or where you want to go?" (assisting to take action).

When verbal language becomes less coherent, the nurse should remain alert to the client's nonverbal behavior. When nurses or caregivers consistently work with a particular client, they develop the ability to determine the client's meaning through nonverbal behavior. For example, if the client becomes restless, it may indicate that he or she is hungry if it is close to mealtime or tired if it is late in the evening. Sometimes it is impossible to determine exactly what the client is trying to convey, but the nurse can still be responsive. For example, a client is pacing and looks upset but cannot indicate what is bothering her. The nurse says,

"You look worried. I don't know what's wrong, but let's go for a walk" (making an observation/ offering self).

Interacting with clients with dementia often means dealing with thoughts and feelings that are not based in reality but arise from the clients' suspicion or chronic confusion. Rather than attempting to explain reality or allay suspicion or anger, it is often helpful to use the techniques of distraction, time away, or going along to reassure the client.

Distraction involves shifting the client's attention and energy to a more neutral topic. For example, the client may display a catastrophic reaction to the current situation, such as jumping up from dinner and saying, "My food tastes like poison!" The nurse might intervene with distraction by saying,

"Can you come to the kitchen with me and find something you'd like to eat?" or "You can leave that food. Can you come and help me find a good program on television?" (redirection/distraction).

Clients usually calm down when the nurse directs their attention away from the triggering situation.

Time away involves leaving clients for a short period and then returning to them to re-engage in interaction. For example, the client may get angry and yell at the nurse for no discernible reason. The nurse can leave the client for about 5 or 10 minutes and then return without referring to the previous outburst. The client may have little or no memory of the incident and may be pleased to see the nurse on his or her return.

Going along means providing emotional reassurance to clients without correcting their misperception or delusion. The nurse does not engage in delusional ideas or reinforce them, but he or she does not deny or confront their existence. For example, a client is fretful, repeatedly saying, "I'm so worried about the children. I hope they're okay," and speaking as though his adult children were small and needed protection. The nurse could reassure the client by saying,

"There's no need to worry; the children are just fine" (going along),

which is likely to calm the client. The nurse has responded effectively to the client's worry without addressing the reality of the client's concern. Going along is a specific intervention for clients with dementia and should not be used with those experiencing delusions whose conditions are expected to improve.

The nurse can use reframing techniques to offer clients different points of view or explanations for situations or events. Because of their perceptual difficulties and confusion, clients frequently interpret environmental stimuli as threatening. Loud noises often frighten and agitate them. For example, one client may interpret another's yelling as a direct personal threat. The nurse can provide an alternative explanation such as

"That lady has many family problems, and she yells sometimes because she's frustrated" (reframing).

Alternative explanations often reassure clients with dementia and help them become less frightened and agitated.

Evaluation

Treatment outcomes change constantly as the disease progresses. For example, in the early stage of dementia, maintaining independence may mean that the client dresses with minimal assistance. Later, the same client may keep some independence by selecting what foods to eat. In the late stage, the client may maintain independence by wearing his or her own clothing rather than an institutional nightgown or pajamas.

The nurse must assess clients for changes as they occur and revise outcomes and interventions as needed. When a client is cared for at home, this includes providing ongoing education to family members and caregivers while supporting them as the client's condition worsens. See the sections that follow on the role of the caregiver and community-based care.

COMMUNITY-BASED CARE

At least half of all nursing home residents have Alzheimer's disease or some other illness that causes dementia. In addition, for every person with dementia in a nursing home, two or three with similar impairments are receiving care in the community by some combination of family members, friends, and paid caregivers.

Programs and services for clients with dementia and their families have increased with the growing awareness of Alzheimer's disease, the increasing numbers of older adults in the United States, and the fundraising efforts for education by noted figures (e.g., the family of former president Ronald Reagan). Home care is available through home health agencies, public health agencies, and visiting nurses. These services offer assistance with bathing, food preparation, and transportation as well as with other support. Periodic nursing assessment ensures that the level of care provided is appropriate to the client's current needs.

Adult day care centers provide supervision, meals, support, and recreational activities in group settings. Clients may attend the center a few hours a week or full-time on weekdays if needed. Respite care offers in-home supervision for clients so that family members or caregivers can run errands or have social time of their own.

Residential facilities are available for clients who do not have in-home caregivers or whose needs have progressed beyond the care that could be provided at home. These clients usually require assistance with ADLs such as eating and taking medications. Clients in residential facilities are often referred for skilled nursing home placement as dementia progresses.

The physician, nurse, or family can initiate referrals for community-based services. Families can contact the local public health department or the department of human or social services listed in the phone book. If the client has been admitted to the hospital, social services also can assist in making an appropriate referral.

MENTAL HEALTH PROMOTION

Research continues to identify risk factors for dementia. People with elevated levels of plasma homocysteine are at increased risk for dementia. As levels of plasma homocysteine increase, so does the risk for dementia (Herrmann, 2006). Because folate, vitamin B_{12}, and betaine are known to reduce plasma homocysteine levels, potential therapeutic strategies using these substances may modify or diminish the risk for dementia. Clinical trials currently are in progress to see if lowering homocysteine levels actually decreases the risk for dementia and whether taking high supplemental doses of B vitamins slows the progression of Alzheimer's disease.

People who regularly participate in brain-stimulating activities such as reading books and newspapers or doing crossword puzzles are less likely to develop Alzheimer's disease than those who do not. Engaging in leisure-time physical activity during midlife (Rovio et al., 2005) and having a large social network (Bennett et al., 2006) are both associated with a decreased risk for Alzheimer's disease in later life.

ROLE OF THE CAREGIVER

Most family caregivers are women (72%) who are either adult daughters (29%) or wives (23%) of clients with cognitive disorders. Husbands account for 13% of all caregivers. The trend toward caring for family members with dementia at home is largely the result of the high costs of institutional care, dissatisfaction with institutional care, and difficulty locating suitable placements for clients with behaviors that are sometimes disruptive and difficult to manage. Family members identify many other reasons for becoming primary caregivers, including the desire to reciprocate for past assistance, to provide love and affection, to uphold family values

or loyalty, to meet duty or obligation, and to avoid feelings of guilt.

Caregivers need to know about dementia and the required client care as well as how client care will change as the disease progresses. Caregivers also may be dealing with other family members who may or may not be supportive or who may have differing expectations. Many caregivers have other demands on their time, such as their own families, careers, and personal lives. Caregivers must deal with their feelings of loss and grief as the health of their loved ones continually declines (Mittelman et al., 2004).

Caring for clients with dementia can be emotionally and physically exhausting and stressful. Caregivers may need to drastically change their own lives, such as quitting a job, to provide care. Caregivers may have young children as well. They often feel exhausted and as if they are "on duty" 24 hours a day. Caregivers caring for parents may have difficulty "being in charge" of their mothers or fathers (role reversal). They may feel uncomfortable or depressed about having to bathe, feed, or change diapers for parents.

Role strain is identified when the demands of providing care threaten to overwhelm a caregiver. Indications of role strain include constant fatigue that is unrelieved by rest, increased use of alcohol or other drugs, social isolation, inattention to personal needs, and inability or unwillingness to accept help from others. Caregivers may feel unappreciated by other family members, as indicated by statements such as "No one ever asks how I am!" (Mittelman et al., 2004). In some situations, role strain can contribute to the neglect or abuse of clients with dementia (see Chapter 11).

Supporting the caregiver is an important component of providing care at home to clients with dementia. Caregivers must have an ongoing relationship with a knowledgeable health professional; the client's physician can make referrals to other health care providers. Depending on the situation, that person may be a nurse, care manager, or social worker. He or she can provide information, support, and assistance during the time that home care is provided. Caregivers need education about dementia and the type of care that clients need. Caregivers should use the interventions previously discussed to promote the client's well-being, deal with deficits and limitations, and maximize the quality of the client's life. Because the care that clients need changes as the dementia progresses, this education by the nurse, care manager, or social worker is ongoing.

Caregivers need outlets for dealing with their own feelings. Support groups can help them to express frustration, sadness, anger, guilt, or ambivalence; all these feelings are common. Attending a support group regularly also means that caregivers have time with people who understand the many demands of caring for a family member with dementia. The client's physician can provide information about support groups, and the local chapter of the National Alzheimer's Disease Association is listed in the phone book. Area hospitals and public health agencies also can help caregivers to locate community resources.

Caregivers should be able to seek and accept assistance from other people or agencies. Often, caregivers believe that others may not be able to provide care as well as they do, or they say they will seek help when they "really need it." Caregivers must maintain their own well-being and not wait until they are exhausted before seeking relief. Sometimes family members disagree about care for the client. The primary caregiver may believe other family members should volunteer to help without being asked, but other family members may believe that the primary caregiver chose to take on the responsibility and do not feel obligated to help out regularly. Whatever the feelings are among family members, it is important for them all to express their feelings and ideas and to participate in caregiving according to their own expectations. Many families need assistance to reach this type of compromise.

Finally, caregivers need support to maintain personal lives. They need to continue to socialize with friends and to engage in leisure activities or hobbies rather than focus solely on the client's care. Caregivers who are rested, happy, and have met their own needs are better prepared to manage the rigorous demands of the caregiver role. Most caregivers need to be reminded to take care of themselves; this act is not selfish but really is in the client's best long-term interests.

RELATED DISORDERS

Amnestic disorders are characterized by a disturbance in memory that results directly from the physiologic effects of a general medical condition or the persisting effects of a substance such as alcohol or other drugs (APA, 2000). The memory disturbance is sufficiently severe to cause marked impairment in social or occupational functioning and represents a significant decline from previous functioning. Confusion, disorientation, and attentional deficits are common. Clients with amnestic disorders are similar to those with dementia in terms of memory deficits, confusion, and problems with attention. They do not, however, have the multiple cognitive deficits seen in dementia such as aphasia, apraxia, agnosia, and impaired executive functions.

Several medical conditions can cause brain damage and result in an amnestic disorder—for example, stroke or other cerebrovascular events, head injuries, and neurotoxic exposures such as carbon monoxide poisoning, chronic alcohol ingestion, and vitamin B_{12} or thiamine deficiency. Alcohol-induced amnestic disorder results from a chronic thiamine or vitamin B deficiency and is called **Korsakoff's syndrome.**

The main difference between dementia and amnestic disorders is that once the underlying medical cause is treated or removed, the client's condition no longer deteriorates. Treatment of amnestic disorders focuses on eliminating the underlying cause and rehabilitating the client and includes preventing further medical problems. Some amnestic disorders improve over time when the underlying cause is stabilized. Other clients have persistent impairment of memory and attention with minimal improvement; this can occur in cases of chronic alcohol ingestion or malnutrition (Grossman, 2005). Nursing diagnoses and interventions are similar to those used when dealing with the memory loss, confusion, and impaired attention abilities of clients with dementia or delirium (see Nursing Interventions for Dementia).

SELF-AWARENESS ISSUES

Working with and caring for clients with dementia can be exhausting and frustrating for both nurse and caregiver. Teaching is a fundamental role for nurses, but teaching clients who have dementia can be especially challenging and frustrating. These clients do not retain explanations or instructions, so the nurse must repeat the same things continually. The nurse must be careful not to lose patience and not to give up on these clients. The nurse may begin to feel that repeating instructions or explanations does no good because clients do not understand or remember them. Discussing these frustrations with others can help the nurse to avoid conveying negative feelings to clients and families or experiencing professional and personal burnout.

The nurse may get little or no positive response or feedback from clients with dementia. It can be difficult to deal with feelings about caring for people who will never "get better and go home." As dementia progresses, clients may seem not to hear or respond to anything the nurse does. It is sad and frustrating for the nurse to see clients decline and eventually lose their abilities to manage basic self-care activities and to interact with others. Remaining positive and supportive to clients and family can be difficult when the outcome is so bleak. In addition, the progressive decline may last months or years, which adds to the frustration and sadness. The nurse may need to deal with personal feelings of depression and grief as the dementia progresses; he or she can do so by discussing the situation with colleagues or even a counselor.

Points to Consider When Working With Clients With Dementia

- Remember how important it is to provide dignity for the client and family as the client's life ends.
- Remember that death is the last stage of life. The nurse can provide emotional support for the client and family during this period.
- Clients may not notice the caring, patience, and support the nurse offers, but these qualities will mean a great deal to the family for a long time.

Nursing Care Plan *Dementia*

Nursing Diagnosis

Impaired Memory: *Inability to remember or recall bits of information or behavioral skills.*

ASSESSMENT DATA

- Inability to recall factual information or events
- Inability to learn new material or recall previously learned material
- Inability to determine whether a behavior was performed
- Agitation or anxiety regarding memory loss

EXPECTED OUTCOMES

Immediate
The client will
- Respond positively to memory cues
- Demonstrate decreased agitation or anxiety

Stabilization
The client will
- Attain an optimal level of functioning with routine tasks
- Use long-term memory effectively as long as it remains intact
- Verbalize or demonstrate decreased frustration with memory loss

Community
The client will
- Maintain an optimal level of functioning
- Feel respected and supported

IMPLEMENTATION

Nursing Interventions *denotes collaborative interventions

Provide opportunities for reminiscence or recall of past events, on a one-to-one basis or in a small group.

Encourage the client to use written cues such as a calendar, lists, or a notebook.

Minimize environmental changes. Determine practical locations for the client's possessions, and return items to this location after use. Establish a usual routine and alter the routine only when necessary.

Provide single step instructions for the client when instructions are needed.

Provide verbal connections about using implements. For example, "Here is a washcloth to wash your face," "Here is a spoon you can use to eat your dessert."

Integrate reminders of previous events into current interactions such as "Earlier you put some clothes in the washing machine; it's time to put them in the dryer."

Rationale

Long-term memory may persist after loss of recent memory. Reminiscence is usually an enjoyable activity for the client.

Written cues decrease the client's need to recall appointments, activities, and so on from memory.

There is less demand on memory function when structure is incorporated in the client's environment and daily routine.

Clients with memory impairment cannot remember multistep instructions.

The client may not remember what an implement is for; stating its related function is an approach that compensates for memory loss.

Providing links with previous behaviors helps the client to make connections that he or she may not be able to make independently.

Nursing Care Plan: Dementia, cont.

IMPLEMENTATION

Nursing Interventions *denotes collaborative interventions	**Rationale**
Assist with tasks as needed, but do not "rush" to do things for the client that he or she can still do independently.	It is important to maximize independent function, yet assist the client when memory has deteriorated further.
Use a matter-of-fact approach when assuming tasks the client can no longer perform. Do not allow the client to work unsuccessfully at a task for an extended time.	It is important to preserve the client's dignity and minimize his or her frustration with progressive memory loss.

Adapted from Schultz, J. M., & Videbeck, S. L. (2005). Lippincott's manual of psychiatric nursing care plans (7th ed.). Philadelphia: Lippincott Williams & Wilkins.

Critical Thinking Questions

1. The nurse is working in a long-term care setting with clients with dementia. One of the ancillary staff makes a joke about a client in the client's presence. The nurse tells the staff person that is unacceptable behavior. The staff person replies, "Oh, he can't understand what I'm saying, and besides, he was laughing too. What's the big deal?" How should this nurse respond?
2. A client is newly diagnosed with dementia in the early stages. Can the client make decisions about advance medical directives? Why or why not? At what point in the progression of dementia can the client no longer make quality-of-life decisions?

KEY POINTS

- Cognitive disorders involve disruption or impairment in the higher functions of the brain. They include delirium, dementia, and amnestic disorders.
- Delirium is a syndrome that involves disturbed consciousness and changes in cognition. It usually is caused by an underlying, treatable medical condition such as physiologic or metabolic imbalances, infections, nutritional deficits, medication reactions or interactions, drug intoxication, or alcohol withdrawal.
- The primary goals of nursing care for clients with delirium are protection from injury, management of confusion, and meeting their physiologic and psychological needs.

- Dementia is a disease involving memory loss and multiple cognitive deficits such as language deterioration (aphasia), motor impairment (apraxia), or inability to name or recognize objects (agnosia).
- Dementia is usually progressive, beginning with prominent memory loss (mild stage) and confusion and loss of independent functioning (moderate), followed by total disorientation and loss of functioning (severe).
- Medications used to treat dementia, tacrine and donepezil, slow disease progression for about 6 months. Other medications such as antipsychotics, antidepressants, and benzodiazepines help manage symptoms but do not affect the course of dementia.
- A psychosocial model for providing care for people with dementia addresses needs for safety, structure, support, interpersonal involvement, and social interaction.
- Many clients with dementia receive care at home rather than in institutional settings (e.g., nursing homes). The caregiver role (often assumed by a spouse or adult child) can be physically and emotionally exhausting and stressful; this contributes to caregiver role strain. To deal with the exhausting demands of this role, family caregivers need ongoing education and support from a health care professional such as a nurse, social worker, or case manager.
- Caregivers must learn how to meet the client's physiologic and emotional needs and to protect him or her from injury. Areas for teaching include monitoring the client's health, avoiding alcohol and recreational drugs, ensuring adequate nutrition, scheduling regular checkups, getting adequate rest, promoting activity and socialization, and helping the client to maintain independence as much as possible.
- The therapeutic relationship with clients with dementia is supportive and protective and recognizes the client's individuality and dignity.

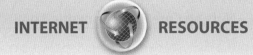

INTERNET RESOURCES

RESOURCE	INTERNET ADDRESS
• Alzheimer's Association	http://www.alz.org
• Alzheimer's Disease Education and Referral	http://www.alzheimers.org
• Alzheimer's Info Links	http://www.alzheimer-info.com/links_info.html
• Alzheimer's Disease International	http://www.alz.co.uk
• Alzheimer Society of Canada	http://www.alzheimer.ca
• Support and Education for Patients, Caregiver, Doctors, and Others	http://www.alzwell.com

REFERENCES

American Psychiatric Association. (2000). *Diagnostic and statistical manual of mental disorders* (4th ed., text revision). Washington, DC: American Psychiatric Association.

Bennett, D. A., Schneider, J. A., Tang, Y., et al. (2006). The effect of social networks on the relation between Alzheimer's disease pathology and level of cognitive function in old people: A longitudinal cohort study. *Lancet Neurology, 5*(5), 406–412.

Davis, K. L. (2005). Cognitive disorders: Introduction and overview. In B. J. Sadock & V. A. Sadock (Eds.), *Comprehensive textbook of psychiatry* (Vol. 1, 8th ed., pp. 1053–1054). Philadelphia: Lippincott Williams & Wilkins.

Grossman, H. (2005). Amnestic disorders. In B. J. Sadock & V. A. Sadock (Eds.), *Comprehensive textbook of psychiatry* (Vol. 1, 8th ed., pp. 1093–1106). Philadelphia: Lippincott Williams & Wilkins.

Hendry, K. C., & Douglas, D. H. (2003). Promoting quality of life for clients diagnosed with dementia. *Journal of the American Psychiatric Nurses Association, 9*(3), 96–102.

Herrmann, W. (2006). Significance of hyperhomocysteinemia. *Clinical Laboratory, 52*(7–8), 367–374.

Mittelman, M. S., Roth, D. L., Coon, D. W., et al. (2004). Sustained benefit of supportive intervention for depressive symptoms in caregivers of patients with Alzheimer's disease. *American Journal of Psychiatry, 161*(5), 850–856.

Neugroschl, J. A., Kolevzon, A., Samuels, S. C., et al. (2005). Dementia. In B. J. Sadock & V. A. Sadock (Eds.), *Comprehensive textbook of psychiatry* (Vol. 1, 8th ed., pp. 1068–1093). Philadelphia: Lippincott Williams & Wilkins.

Rovio, S., Kareholt, I., Helkala, E. L., et al. (2005). Leisure-time physical activity at midlife and the risk of dementia and Alzheimer's disease. *Lancet Neurology, 4*(11), 705–711.

Samuels, S. C., & Neugroschl, J. A. (2005). Delirium. In B. J. Sadock & V. A. Sadock (Eds.), *Comprehensive textbook of psychiatry* (Vol. 1, 8th ed., pp. 1054–1068). Philadelphia: Lippincott Williams & Wilkins.

Schultz, J. M., & Videbeck, S. L. (2005). *Lippincott's manual of psychiatric nursing care plans* (7th ed.). Philadelphia: Lippincott Williams & Wilkins.

Woods, B., Spector, A., Jones, C., et al. (2005). Reminiscence therapy for dementia. *Cochrane database of systematic reviews (online), 2*(CD001120)

Yuhas, N., McGowan, B., Fintaine, T., et al. (2006). Psychosocial interventions for disruptive symptoms of dementia. *Journal of Psychosocial Nursing, 44*(11), 34–42.

ADDITIONAL READINGS

Kolanowski, A., Fick, D., Waller, J. L., & Ahern, F. (2006). Outcomes of antipsychotic drug use in community-dwelling elders with dementia. *Archives of Psychiatric Nursing, 20*(5), 217–225.

Sorensen, S., Duberstein, P., Gill, D., & Pinquart, M. (2006). Dementia care: Mental health effects, intervention strategies, and clinical implications. *Lancet Neurology, 5*(11), 961–973.

Whitlatch, C. J., Judge, K., Zarit, S. H., & Femia, E. (2006). Dyadic intervention for family caregivers and care receivers in early-stage dementia. *Gerontologist, 46*(5), 688–694.

Chapter Study Guide

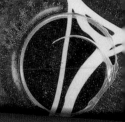

MULTIPLE-CHOICE QUESTIONS

Select the best answer for each of the following questions.

1. The nurse is talking with a woman who is worried that her mother has Alzheimer's disease. The nurse knows that the first sign of dementia is
   A. Disorientation to person, place, or time
   B. Memory loss that is more than ordinary forgetfulness
   C. Inability to perform self-care tasks without assistance
   D. Variable with different people

2. The nurse has been teaching a caregiver about donepezil (Aricept). The nurse knows that teaching has been effective by which of the following statements?
   A. "Let's hope this medication will stop the Alzheimer's disease from progressing any further."
   B. "It is important to take this medication on an empty stomach."
   C. "I'll be eager to see if this medication makes any improvement in concentration."
   D. "This medication will slow the progress of Alzheimer's disease temporarily."

3. When teaching a client about tacrine (Cognex), the nurse will include which of the following?
   A. Taking tacrine can increase the risk for elevated liver enzymes.
   B. Tacrine causes agranulocytosis in some clients.
   C. The most common side effect is skin rash.
   D. Tacrine has no known serious side effects.

4. Which of the following statements by the caregiver of a client newly diagnosed with dementia requires further intervention by the nurse?
   A. "I will remind Mother of things she has forgotten."
   B. "I will keep Mother busy with favorite activities as long as she can participate."
   C. "I will try to find new and different things to do every day."
   D. "I will encourage Mother to talk about her friends and family."

5. A client with delirium is attempting to remove the intravenous tubing from his arm, saying to the nurse, "Get off me! Go away!" The client is experiencing which of the following?
   A. Delusions
   B. Hallucinations
   C. Illusions
   D. Disorientation

6. Which of the following statements indicates the caregiver's accurate knowledge about the needs of a parent at the onset of the moderate stage of dementia?
   A. "I need to give my parent a bath at the same time every day."
   B. "I need to postpone any vacations for 5 years."
   C. "I need to spend time with my parent doing things we both enjoy."
   D. "I need to stay with my parent 24 hours a day for supervision."

7. Which of the following interventions is most appropriate in helping a client with early-stage dementia complete activities of daily living (ADLs)?
   A. Allow enough time for the client to complete ADLs as independently as possible.
   B. Provide the client with a written list of all the steps needed to complete ADLs.
   C. Plan to provide step-by-step prompting to complete the ADLs.
   D. Tell the client to finish ADLs before breakfast or the nursing assistant will do them.

8. A client with late moderate stage dementia has been admitted to a long-term care facility. Which of the following nursing interventions will help the client to maintain optimal cognitive function?
   A. Discuss pictures of children and grandchildren with the client.
   B. Do word games or crossword puzzles with the client.
   C. Provide the client with a written list of daily activities.
   D. Watch and discuss the evening news with the client.

FILL-IN-THE-BLANK QUESTIONS

Identify each of the following behaviors as occurring primarily in delirium or dementia.

_____ Change in level of consciousness

_____ Sudden acute confusion

_____ Loss of long-term memory

_____ Tactile hallucinations

_____ Slurred speech

_____ Loss of language abilities

_____ Change in personality traits

_____ Chronic confusion

SHORT-ANSWER QUESTIONS

Describe each of the following interventions for a client with dementia, and give an example.

Distraction

Time away

Going along

Reminiscence

CLINICAL EXAMPLE

Martha Smith, a 79-year-old widow with Alzheimer's disease, was admitted to a nursing home. The disease has progressed during the past 4 years to the point that she can no longer live alone in her own house. Martha has poor judgment and no short-term memory. She had stopped paying bills, preparing meals, and cleaning her home. She had become increasingly suspicious of her visiting nurse and home health aide, finally refusing to allow them in the house.

After her arrival at the facility, Martha has been sleeping poorly and frequently wanders from her room in the middle of the night. She seems agitated and afraid in the dining room at mealtimes, is eating very little, and has lost weight. If left alone, Martha would wear the same clothing day and night and would not attend to her personal hygiene.

1. What additional assessments would the nurse want to make to plan care for this client?

2. What nursing diagnoses would the nurse identify for this client?

3. Write an expected outcome and at least two interventions for each nursing diagnosis.

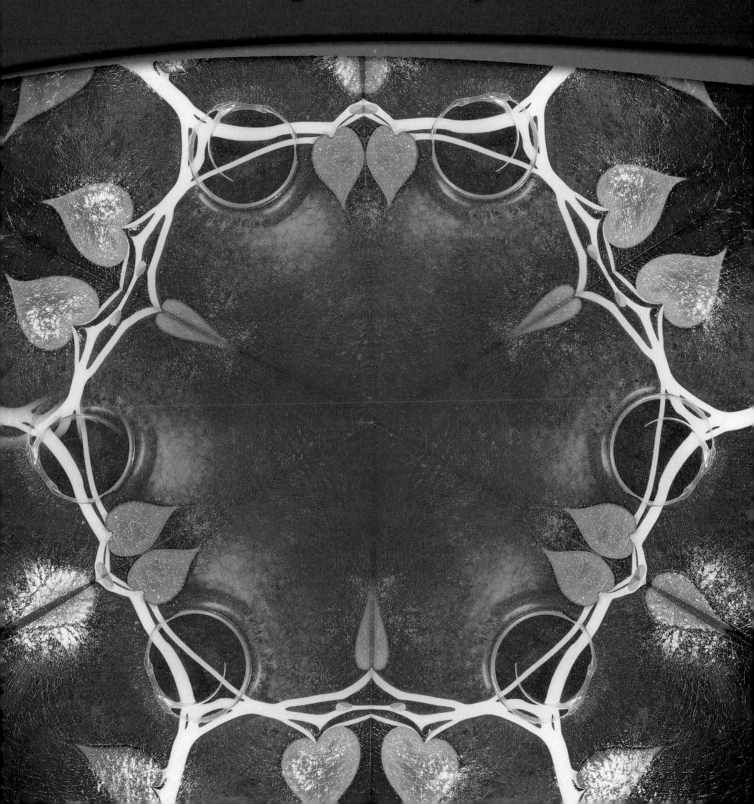

Answers to
Chapter Study Guides

ANSWER KEY

CHAPTER 1

Multiple-Choice Questions

1. C
2. B
3. A
4. D
5. C

Fill-in-the-Blank Questions

Axis I: All major psychiatric disorders except mental retardation and personality disorders

Axis II: Mental retardation, personality disorders, prominent maladaptive personality features, defense mechanisms

Axis III: Current medical conditions, contributing medical conditions

Axis IV: Psychosocial and environmental problems

Axis V: Global Assessment of Functioning (GAF) score

Short-Answer Questions

1. The standards are used to guide nursing practice in psychiatric settings and to determine safe and acceptable practices in legal disputes.
2. Cost containment and managed care, population diversity, community-based care
3. Examples of fears include saying the wrong thing, not knowing what to do, being rejected by clients, handling bizarre or inappropriate behavior, maintaining physical safety, and seeing a friend or acquaintance as a client.

CHAPTER 2

Multiple-Choice Questions

1. A
2. B
3. D
4. C
5. B
6. B
7. C
8. B

Fill-in-the-Blank Questions

1. Atypical antipsychotic
2. SSRI antidepressant
3. Tricyclic antidepressant
4. Anticholinergic
5. Stimulant
6. Anticonvulsant used as mood stabilizer
7. Benzodiazepine
8. Atypical antipsychotic

Short-Answer Questions

1. Abrupt cessation results in a rebound effect (return of symptoms), recurrence of the original symptoms, or possible withdrawal symptoms. Tapering gradually alleviates or minimizes these problems.
2. A radioactive substance will be injected into the bloodstream. The client will be asked to perform "thinking" tasks while the camera takes scans of the brain working. The procedure will take 2 to 3 hours.
3. Just as kindling is used to start a larger fire, mild or small manic mood swings can eventually trigger a major, acute manic episode.

CHAPTER 3

Multiple-Choice Questions

1. D
2. D
3. C
4. B
5. A
6. C
7. A
8. A
9. A

Fill-in-the-Blank Questions

1. Carl Rogers
2. Erik Erikson
3. Ivan Pavlov
4. Albert Ellis
5. B. F. Skinner
6. Carl Rogers
7. Frederick Perls
8. Abraham Maslow
9. Viktor Frankl
10. Albert Ellis
11. William Glasser

Short-Answer Questions

1. Clients participate in group sessions with members who have the shared purposes of benefiting one another and making some change. An example is family therapy to learn conflict resolution.
2. Members gather to learn about a particular topic from someone who has expertise. An example is an assertiveness training group.
3. Members help themselves and one another to cope with some life stress, event, illness, or problem. An example is Survivors of Suicide (for family members of someone who has committed suicide).
4. This group is structured around a common experience that all members share and is run by the group members. An example is Alcoholics Anonymous.

CHAPTER 4

Multiple-Choice Questions

1. B
2. B
3. C
4. B
5. C
6. C
7. C
8. D

Fill-in-the-Blank Questions

Psychiatric social worker
Occupational therapist
Psychiatrist
Vocational rehabilitation specialist

Short-Answer Questions

1. Double stigma, lack of family or social support, co-morbidity, adjustment problems, boundary issues
2. The evolving consumer household is a group-living situation intended to transform itself into a residence where the residents fulfill their own responsibilities and function without on-site supervision from paid staff. It is intended to be a permanent residence for the client.
3. Deinstitutionalization, more rigid criteria for civil commitment, lack of adequate support, attitudes of police and society

CHAPTER 5

Multiple-Choice Questions

1. A
2. A
3. C
4. B

Fill-in-the-Blank Questions

Empirical
Aesthetic
Personal
Ethical

Short-Answer Questions

1. Congruence: Nurse faces client, makes eye contact, and says, "My name is Mary Day, and I will be your nurse today." (Verbal and nonverbal components match.)
Positive regard: Nurse sits next to client, makes eye contact, leans forward, and says, "Rosie, I am glad we have this opportunity to work on some of your problems together." (Verbal and nonverbal components provide the client with a message of personal regard.)

Acceptance: Client shakes nurse's hand very hard. Nurse says, in a normal tone of voice, "Tom, I'm always pleased to shake hands when we meet, but you don't need to squeeze so hard!" (Lets client know nurse likes to meet him, but places boundary)
2. Nurse: "You seem unsure of your doctor's abilities. Would you like to tell me about this concern?" Rationale: attempts to get client to expand on the comment.
Nurse: "No, I clearly stated 6 weeks, but do you wish it were 8?" Rationale: clarifies timing with client and addresses possible underlying issue of nurse's leaving.

Clinical Example

Mr. V: "I like to choose my student nurses; otherwise, I don't get chosen."
Nurse: "I am honored that you chose me, Mr. V. My name is Sandy Moore, and I will be your student nurse for the next 6 weeks. You seem to have some experience with other groups of students." (Nurse clearly states information about herself and her role and acknowledges client's previous experience.)
Mr. V: "Oh, yeah, I've seen 'em come and go, but I never get picked to be their patient. I guess I'm too crazy for them!" (laughs nervously)
Nurse: "Well, I'm delighted you chose me. It makes me feel honored." (Nurse makes it clear she is glad to be with client.)
Mr. V: "Are you sure?"
Nurse: "Yes. I will be here on Tuesdays from 10 AM to 3 PM for the next 6 weeks. I hope we can identify and work on some issues together." (provides clear parameters for the relationship)

CHAPTER 6

Multiple-Choice Questions

1. C
2. A
3. B
4. B
5. B
6. C
7. A

Short-Answer Questions

1. Knowledge, values, and beliefs transmitted down through generations
2. Distance between people during interaction
3. Behavior that is inconsistent with words
4. Belief about one's place in the universe
5. Facial expression, eye contact, silence, body posture and movements
6. Trite phrase
7. Describing an object or situation by comparing it to something familiar

8. The nurse uses the self as a tool to relate to the client in a therapeutic communication, identifies with a client-centered issue, and works toward the goal of guiding the client to determine socially acceptable problem resolution.

Cues and Responses

1. Cue: I feel good.
   "What is one way you feel good?"
   "When did you start feeling good?"
   "What was going on around you just before you realized you felt good?"
2. Cue: I can't take it anymore.
   "What is it you can't take?"
   "How long have you had to take it?"
   "What is going on that you believe you have to take?"
3. Cues: two children, my wife, my girlfriend
   Nurse: "What are the children's names and ages?"
   Client: "Taylor is 4, and Anita is 1."
   Nurse: "Tell me about the relationship between you and Taylor." After discussion concludes, try, "Tell me about your relationship with Anita."
4. Cues: we, standing, corner
   "Who do you mean by 'we'?"
   "On what corner were you standing?"
   "What were you doing at the corner?"
5. Cues: my son, never going to understand, way his wife is ruining them
   Nurse: "What is your son's name?"
   Client: "Paul."
   Nurse: "What is his wife's name?"
   Client: "Susan."
   Nurse: "How do you perceive Susan is ruining herself and Paul?"
   "How did you arrive at the conclusion that Paul will never understand something Susan is doing that appears perfectly clear to you?"

CHAPTER 7

Multiple-Choice Questions

1. A
2. B
3. A
4. A
5. D
6. B
7. C
8. B

Fill-in-the-Blank Questions

Trust vs. Mistrust
Industry vs. Inferiority
Identity vs. Role diffusion
Intimacy vs. Isolation
Ego Integrity vs. Despair

Short-Answer Questions

1. Culturally competent nursing care means being sensitive to issues related to culture, race, gender, sexual orientation, social class, economic situation, and other factors that affect client care. It means that the nurse promotes the client's practice of his or her beliefs (e.g., spiritual practices), uses nonverbal communication that is congruent with the client, and so forth.
2. Failure to successfully complete the developmental tasks at a given stage results in a negative outcome for that stage—such as mistrust rather than trust—and impedes successful completion of future tasks. Successful completion of tasks sets the stage for further success at the next developmental stage.
3. *Hardiness* describes the individual's ability to resist illness when under stress. *Resilience* refers to having healthy responses under stressful circumstances or at-risk situations.

CHAPTER 8

Multiple-Choice Questions

1. B
2. D
3. C
4. B
5. B
6. C
7. A
8. C

Fill-in-the-Blank Questions

1. Automatisms
2. Thought broadcasting
3. Psychomotor retardation
4. Word salad

Short-Answer Questions

1. What does the saying "A rolling stone gathers no moss" mean to you?
2. What led you to come to the clinic?
3. How would you describe yourself as a person?
4. If you were lost downtown, what would you do?
5. In general, how are you feeling?
6. Can you tell me today's date? (time)
   Can you tell me where you are? (place)
   Can you tell me your name? (person)

Clinical Example

1. Give positive feedback for coming to the clinic to get help. Tell her it is all right to cry.
   Tell the client that the nurse will sit with her until she's ready to talk.

Validate the client's feelings (i.e., "I can see you're very upset").

2. What is the problem as the client sees it (to gain the client's perception of the situation)?

   Has the client ever felt this way before (to determine if this is a new occurrence, or recurrent)?

   Does the client have thoughts of harming herself or others (to determine safety)?

   Has the client been drinking alcohol, using drugs, or taking medication (to assess client's ability to think clearly or if there is impairment)?

   What kind of help does the client need (to see what kind of help the client wants, e.g., someone to listen, help to solve a specific problem, a referral)?

3. The client is in crisis.

   The client is seeking help/treatment.

   The client is not currently stable.

4. Tell the client that the nurse needs to know if the client is safe (from suicidal ideas or self-harm urges). If the client is safe, she can leave the clinic. If she is not safe, the nurse must ask her to stay or must call emergency services (911) if necessary.

CHAPTER 9

Multiple-Choice Questions

1. A
2. A
3. B
4. D
5. D

Fill-in-the-Blank Questions

Veracity
Nonmaleficence
Fidelity
Beneficence
Justice
Autonomy

Short-Answer Questions

1. The client has the right to be treated in the environment with the least restriction that meets his or her needs, such as providing outpatient treatment that meets the client's needs rather than hospitalization.

2. The mentally ill client makes a specific threat of harm to a third party who is identifiable.

3. Gathering information, clarifying values, identifying options, identifying legal considerations and practical restraints, building consensus, and reviewing/analyzing the decision

4. *Standard of care* means care provided to the client meets set expectations and is what any nurse in a similar situation would do.

5. Malpractice liability involves an existing duty, a breach of that duty, and harm or injury that is a direct result of the breach of duty.

CHAPTER 10

Multiple-Choice Questions

1. B
2. B
3. B
4. C
5. B

Short-Answer Questions

1. The cocktail method involves giving two medications, usually haloperidol and lorazepam, in successive doses at the time of the behavior, 30 minutes to 1 hour later, and 1 to 2 hours after the behavior, until sedation is achieved. The chaser method involves giving lorazepam at the time of the behavior, 30 minutes to 1 hour later, and 1 to 2 hours after the behavior, until the client is sedated. Then, an antipsychotic medication, such as haloperidol, is offered.

2. Remove or direct clients to a safe area, summon additional staff and/or security as needed to direct client to quiet area or to physically stop client's aggression, and offer to provide medication.

CHAPTER 11

Multiple-Choice Questions

1. B
2. C
3. C
4. C
5. D
6. B
7. A
8. A

Fill-in-the-Blank Questions

Child neglect
Elder self-neglect
Financial abuse
Psychological or emotional abuse

Short-Answer Questions

A repeated pattern of violence in which an abusive episode is followed by a period of remorse (honeymoon period); then, tension builds until the next abusive episode. *Example:* A man beats his wife, then apologizes and is loving for a few weeks, and then beats her again.

Assigning responsibility for the abuse or rape to the victim rather than to the abuser or rapist. *Example:* A woman walking alone at night is raped. Some say, "What did she expect? She should have been more careful."

When the person surviving a trauma feels ashamed or guilty about surviving. *Example:* The driver involved in a car crash in which two friends were killed blames himself for their deaths and says, "Why didn't I die with the others?"

Violence in families is learned by role modeling from one generation to the next. *Example:* A man who witnessed his father beating his mother finds himself beating his own wife when he gets angry.

CHAPTER 12

Multiple-Choice Questions

1. C
2. B
3. C
4. D
5. A

Fill-in-the-Blank Questions

Emotional dimension
Behavioral dimension
Cognitive dimension
Spiritual dimension
Physiologic dimension

Short-Answer Questions

1. Styles of grieving: when a person moves from high to low distress over time in his or her grieving process
   Adequate support: when the bereaved can identify a person or persons who are able and willing to be supportive while he or she is grieving for a loss
   Emotional response during numbing phase of grieving: a feeling of being stunned
2. Nurse: "This is really a shock for you, and it's difficult to believe it has happened."
   Rationale: This reflection acknowledges the client's feelings and directs those feelings back to the client as a way to convey understanding as well as to encourage further verbalization of feelings.
   Nurse: "Tell me more about that."
   Rationale: This statement encourages exploration of the client's feelings, and a description of the client's perception can assist the nurse in understanding the client's experience. As the client speaks, feelings and perceptions shift toward a healthy integration of loss.
   Nurse: "You're feeling all alone."
   Rationale: This reflective statement encourages the client to express more.
   Nurse: "There's absolutely no one who cares about what is happening to you?"

Rationale: Voicing doubt implies that the client's beliefs are exaggerated or false perceptions.
Nurse: "Who could we get who would be helpful to you right now?"
Rationale: This acknowledges that the client's anger is normal and most likely not a personal attack on the nurse. Using "we" suggests collaboration with the client, and focusing on the client's statement about help is a way to stay engaged and give the client the opportunity to say more.

CHAPTER 13

Multiple-Choice Questions

1. C
2. D
3. D
4. B
5. D
6. C
7. C
8. D

Fill-in-the-Blank

1. Severe
2. Mild
3. Panic
4. Moderate

Short-Answer Questions

1. Primary gain is the relief of anxiety, for example, the person with social phobia avoids eating in restaurants with others. Secondary gain is the attention received from others, for example, the person who just had a panic attack gets support and comfort from friends.
2. The client is exposed to increasing anxiety-provoking situations associated with the phobic object while using techniques to manage the anxiety response.

Clinical Example

1. The nurse should have Mrs. Noe come up with suggestions. She is more likely to take responsibility for and act on her own solutions to problems than on the suggestions of others.
2. Mrs. Noe receives secondary gain from the attention and focus Mr. Noe gives her. He is her phobic partner. The nurse could recommend that both Mr. and Mrs. Noe attend an agoraphobic self-help group in the community. Mr. Noe would benefit from attending such a group to learn about his counter-phobic partner behaviors that enable his wife to continue her agoraphobia.
3. Behavior therapy, relaxation techniques, or other measures designed to help her manage the anxiety response

are available, so referral to a therapist is indicated. Also, medications can reduce agoraphobic behaviors, so referral to a psychiatrist is appropriate.

CHAPTER 14

Multiple-Choice Questions

1. C
2. D
3. B
4. D
5. C
6. A
7. B
8. D

Fill-in-the-Blank Questions

1. Neologism
2. Verbigeration
3. Word salad
4. Clang association

Short-Answer Questions

1. Client believes the FBI is spying on him.
2. Client hears voices saying "You're no good."
3. Client sees electrical cord on the floor and thinks it is a snake, but on second glance sees it is a cord.
4. *Response:* "It sounds like you're scared."
   Rationale: Focus on feeling without challenging delusion.
5. *Response:* "Tell me why you think you're in the hospital."
   Rationale: Focus on client's perceptions.
6. *Response:* "That would be very unusual."
   Rationale: Casting doubt without challenging client.
7. *Response:* "What is God telling you to do?"
   Rationale: Essential to discover content of command hallucination.

Clinical Example

1. Additional assessment data (examples): discover content of any command hallucinations; ask about preferences for hygiene (for example, shower or bath); determine whether there is a thing or place that makes him feel safe and secure.
2. Disturbed thought processes: client will have 5-minute interactions that are reality-based; client will express feelings and emotions.
   Ineffective therapeutic regimen management (medication refusal): client will take medication as prescribed; client will verbalize difficulties in following medication regimen.
   Self-care deficit: client will shower or bathe, wash hair, and clean clothes every other day; client will wear appropriate clothing for the weather or activity.

3. Disturbed thought processes: engage client in present, here-and-now topics not related to delusional ideas; focus on client's emotions and feelings.
   Ineffective therapeutic regimen management: offer scheduled medications in matter-of-fact manner; allow client to open unit-dose packets; assess for side effects and give medications or provide nursing interventions to relieve side effects; provide factual information to the client: "This medication will decrease the voices you're hearing." Self-care deficit: provide supplies and privacy for hygiene activities; give feedback about body odor, dirty clothes, and so forth; help client store extra clothing where he has access to it and believes it is safe.
4. John might benefit from a case manager in the community and a community support program or a clinic for possible depot injections of his medication.

CHAPTER 15

Multiple-Choice Questions

1. D
2. A
3. A
4. C
5. A
6. D
7. B
8. D
9. A

Short-Answer Questions

1. Proper medication administration, salt and water needs, symptoms of lithium toxicity, need for periodic serum lithium monitoring
2. "You've been a good friend;" "I can't do this anymore;" "This is where I keep my important papers;" and "I'd like you to have my chess set, the one you always admired."

Clinical Example

(These are examples of correct answers; others are possible.)

1. It is essential that the nurse ask if June is having suicidal thoughts. If so, the nurse would assess June's lethality by finding out if she has a plan, if she has access to the means to carry out the plan, and details of her plan.
2. Ineffective Coping; Ineffective Role Performance; and Impaired Social Interaction.
   Note: Risk for Suicide would be a priority if the nurse determined June was having suicidal thoughts.
3. The client will identify past successful coping strategies; the client will carry out activities of daily living; the client will verbalize her feelings.
4. Spending 1:1 interaction time with June to discuss feelings and past coping strategies; providing encouragement

and support to get up, shower, get dressed, eat, and so forth; educating June about depression and its treatment; assisting June to identify life stressors and possible sources of support

CHAPTER 16

Multiple-Choice Questions

1. C
2. A
3. D
4. B
5. D
6. C
7. A
8. A

Fill-in-the-Blank Questions

Borderline personality disorder
Antisocial personality disorder
Schizoid personality disorder
Avoidant personality disorder

Short-Answer Questions

Harm avoidance: High—fear of uncertainty, social inhibition, shyness with strangers, rapid fatigability, pessimistic worry in anticipation of problems

Harm avoidance: Low—carefree, energetic, outgoing, optimistic

Novelty seeking: High—quick-tempered, curious, easily bored, impulsive, extravagant, disorderly

Novelty seeking: Low—slow-tempered, stoic, reflective, frugal, reserved, orderly, tolerant of monotony

Reward dependence: High—tenderhearted, sensitive, sociable, socially dependent

Reward dependence: Low—practical, tough-minded, cold, socially insensitive, irresolute, indifferent if alone

Persistence: High—hard-working, persevering, ambitious, overachieving

Persistence: Low—inactive, indolent, unstable, erratic

Clinical Example

(These are examples of correct answers; others are possible.)

1. Risk for Self-Mutilation, Ineffective Coping
2. Risk for Self-Mutilation: The client will be safe and free of significant injury.
   Ineffective Coping: The client will demonstrate increased control of impulsive behavior.
3. Risk for Self-Mutilation: Discuss presence and intensity of self-harm urges with client; negotiate a no self-harm contract with the client; help the client to identify triggers for self-harm behavior.

Ineffective Coping: Help the client to identify feelings by keeping a journal; discuss ways the client can use distraction when gratification must be delayed; discuss alternative ways the client can express feelings without an exaggerated response.

4. Outpatient therapist, community support services, vocational/career counseling, self-help group

CHAPTER 17

Multiple-Choice Questions

1. B
2. A
3. B
4. B
5. A
6. C
7. A
8. C

Fill-in-the-Blank Questions

(These are examples of correct answers; others are possible.)

Stimulants: cocaine, amphetamines
Opioids: morphine, heroin
Hallucinogens: peyote, LSD
Inhalants: paint thinner, gasoline fumes

Short-Answer Questions

1. Increased reporting of "pharmacy errors"; excessive amounts of narcotics are "wasted"; damaged or torn packaging on controlled substances; reports of ineffective pain relief by patients, when the same medication had previously relieved pain
2. Medications are given in decreasing doses over a period of time to detoxify the user slowly and safely. The dose of medication is decreased every 2 or 3 days, until the client is no longer receiving any of the medication.

Clinical Example

1. Ineffective Denial: Ineffective Coping
2. Ineffective Denial: The client will abstain from alcohol or drug use.
   Ineffective Coping: The client will identify two non-chemical ways of coping with life stressors.
3. Ineffective Denial: Teach the client about the disease of alcoholism; dispel myths about alcoholism; ask the client about recent life events (breakup, arrest) and the role of her drinking in those events.
   Ineffective Coping: Encourage the client to express feelings directly and openly; teach the client relaxation techniques; role-play a situation (of the client's choice) that has been difficult for her to handle.

CHAPTER 18

Multiple-Choice Questions

1. B
2. C
3. A
4. B
5. A
6. B
7. D
8. A

Fill-in-the-Blank Questions

Bulimia
Both
Both
Anorexia
Bulimia

Short-Answer Questions

1. Self-induced vomiting; fasting; use of laxatives, diuretics, enemas; excessive exercise
2. Body image is how one sees oneself, a mental picture of the physical body. Body image disturbance involves an extreme discrepancy between one's own perception of body image and the perceptions of others. There is also extreme dissatisfaction with one's body image.

Clinical Example

(These are examples of correct answers; others are possible.)

1. Imbalanced Nutrition: Less Than Body Requirements and Ineffective Coping
2. (Nutrition) The client will eat all of her meals and snacks with no purging behaviors. (Coping) The client will identify two non–food-related mechanisms.
3. (Nutrition) Sit with the client while eating; monitor client 1 to 2 hours after meals and snacks; supervise client's use of the bathroom. (Coping) Ask the client how she is feeling, and continue to focus on feelings if the client gives a somatic response; have the client keep a journal including emotions, feelings, and food eaten; teach the client the use of relaxation and distraction, such as music and activities.

CHAPTER 19

Multiple-Choice Questions

1. B
2. C
3. D
4. B
5. A
6. A

7. A
8. C

Fill-in-the-Blank Questions

Body dysmorphic disorder
Somatization disorder
Conversion disorder
Pain disorder
Hypochondriasis

Short-Answer Questions

Primary gain is the direct benefit clients experience, such as relief from anxiety, conflict, or distress. *Example:* If the client is physically sick, she doesn't have to deal with problems with the children.

Secondary gain is the personal benefit derived from illness, such as special attention or comfort received from others. *Example:* When the client has physical symptoms, she gets breakfast in bed.

La belle indifference is the indifference about physical symptoms seen in clients with a conversion disorder. *Example:* A man who is paralyzed and cannot walk is cheerful and seems unconcerned about the paralysis.

Clinical Example

(These are examples of correct answers; others are possible.)

1. Ineffective Coping, Pain, Anxiety
2. The client will identify the relationship between stress and increased pain; the client will be able to perform activities of daily living.
3. Have the client keep a journal about emotional feelings and the quality or intensity of pain; teach the client relaxation exercises; help the client make a daily schedule of activities, beginning with simple tasks; encourage the client to listen to music or engage in other distracting activities she may enjoy; talk with the client about her feelings of frustration and anxiety in a sensitive and supportive manner.
4. Physical therapy, vocational rehabilitation, nutrition services
5. Support group for persons with chronic pain/pain disorder, exercise group, social or volunteer opportunities

CHAPTER 20

Multiple-Choice Questions

1. D
2. A
3. C
4. A
5. A
6. B
7. D

Fill-in-the-Blank Questions

Pica
Rumination disorder
Reactive attachment disorder
Selective mutism

Short-Answer Questions

1. Limit setting involves informing the client of the rule or limit; explaining the consequences if the limit is exceeded; and consistently enforcing the limit, with no exceptions.
2. Time-out is a retreat to a neutral place so the client can regain control. It is not a punishment. It can be initiated by staff until the client can institute it for him- or herself.

Clinical Example

(These are examples of correct answers; others are possible.)

1. Ritalin is a stimulant medication that is effective for 70% to 80% of children with ADHD by decreasing hyperactivity and impulsivity and improving the child's attention. Ritalin can cause appetite suppression and should be given after meals to encourage proper nutrition. Substantial, nutritious snacks between meals are helpful. Giving the medication in the daytime helps avoid the side effect of insomnia. Parents should notice improvements in a day or two. Notify the physician or return to the clinic if no improvements in behavior are noted.
2. The exact cause of ADHD is not known, but it is not due to faulty parenting or anything the parents have done. Taking medications will be helpful with behavioral symptoms, but other strategies are needed as well. The medication will help control symptoms so Dixie can participate in school, make friends, and so forth.
3. Provide supervision when Dixie is with her brother, and help her learn to play gently with him. Do not forbid her to touch him, but teach her the proper ways to do so. Give Dixie directions in a clear, step-by-step manner, and assist her to follow through and complete tasks. Provide a quiet place with minimal distraction for activities that require concentration, such as homework. Try to establish a routine for getting up and dressing, eating meals, going to school, doing homework, and playing; don't change the routine unnecessarily. Structured expectations will be easier for Dixie to follow. Remember to recognize Dixie's strengths and provide positive feedback frequently to boost her self-esteem and foster continued progress.
4. The parents should contact Dixie's teacher, principal, and guidance counselor to inform them of this diagnosis so that special education classes or tutoring can be made available. It would also be helpful to meet with the school nurse who will be giving Dixie her medication at noon on school days. The nurse can refer the parents to a local support group for parents of children with ADHD and provide pamphlets, books, or other written materials, as well as Internet addresses if the parents have access to a computer.

CHAPTER 21

Multiple-Choice Questions

1. B
2. D
3. A
4. C
5. B
6. C
7. A
8. A

Fill-in-the-Blank Questions

Delirium
Delirium
Dementia
Delirium
Delirium
Dementia
Dementia
Dementia

Short-Answer Questions

Distraction: shifting the client's attention and energy to a more neutral topic. *Example:* The client is yelling at someone. The nurse says, "How would you like to see the new picture in the dining room?"

Time away: leaving the client for a short time. *Example:* The client says, "Leave me alone!" The nurse leaves and then returns a short time later, not mentioning the client's request.

Going along: providing emotional reassurance without correcting the delusion or misinterpretation. *Example:* The client is expecting her dead husband to visit. The nurse says, "He'll be here later."

Reminiscence: encouraging the client to discuss pleasant memories. *Example:* Encourage a client to talk about her childhood and wedding day.

Clinical Example

(These are examples of correct answers; others are possible.)

1. What does she like to eat? What were her usual personal hygiene practices? What are her favorite activities? What personal items does she value?
2. Chronic Confusion, Impaired Socialization, Disturbed Sleep Pattern, Self-Care Deficits, and Risk for Imbalanced Nutrition: Less Than Body Requirements
3. The client will experience as little frustration as possible. *Interventions:* Point out objects, people, and the time

of day to prompt the client and decrease confusion. Do not ask the client to make decisions when she is unable to; offer choices only when she can make them.

The client will interact with the nurse. The client will participate in going for a walk with the group. *Interventions:* Involve the client in solitary activities with the nurse initially. Structure group activities that focus on intact physical abilities rather than those requiring cognition.

The client will eat 50% of meals and snacks. *Interventions:* Provide foods the client likes, and provide those foods in an environment where she will be likely to eat, such as her room or a table alone.

The client will sleep 6 hours per night. *Interventions:* Provide a soothing nighttime routine every night (for example, offering a beverage, reading aloud, dimming lights). Decrease stimulation after dinner, and discourage daytime naps.

The client will participate in hygiene routines with assistance. *Interventions:* Try to imitate the client's home hygiene routine (bath or shower, morning or evening), and develop a structured routine for hygiene.

Appendix

A

DSM-IV-TR Classification

NOS = Not Otherwise Specified.

An *x* appearing in a diagnostic code indicates that a specific code number is required.

An ellipsis (. . .) is used in the names of certain disorders to indicate that the name of a specific mental disorder or general medical condition should be inserted when recording the name (e.g., 293.0 Delirium Due to Hypothyroidism).

Numbers in parentheses are page numbers.

If criteria are currently met, one of the following severity specifiers may be noted after the diagnosis:

Mild
Moderate
Severe

If criteria are no longer met, one of the following specifiers may be noted:

In Partial Remission
In Full Remission
Prior History

DISORDERS USUALLY FIRST DIAGNOSED IN INFANCY, CHILDHOOD, OR ADOLESCENCE (39)

Mental Retardation (41)

Note: These are coded on Axis II.
317   Mild Mental Retardation (43)
318.0   Moderate Mental Retardation (43)
318.1   Severe Mental Retardation (43)
318.2   Profound Mental Retardation (44)
319   Mental Retardation, Severity Unspecified (44)

Learning Disorders (49)

315.00   Reading Disorder (51)
315.1   Mathematics Disorder (53)
315.2   Disorder of Written Expression (54)
315.9   Learning Disorder NOS (56)

Motor Skills Disorder (56)

315.4   Developmental Coordination Disorder (56)

Communication Disorders (58)

315.31   Expressive Language Disorder (58)
315.32   Mixed Receptive-Expressive Language Disorder (62)
315.39   Phonological Disorder (65)
307.0   Stuttering (67)
307.9   Communication Disorder NOS (69)

Pervasive Developmental Disorders (69)

299.00   Autistic Disorder (70)
299.80   Rett's Disorder (76)
299.10   Childhood Disintegrative Disorder (77)
299.80   Asperger's Disorder (80)
299.80   Pervasive Developmental Disorder NOS (84)

Reprinted with permission from the *Diagnostic and Statistical Manual of Mental Disorders*, 4th ed., Text Revision. © 2000 APA.

Attention-Deficit and Disruptive Behavior Disorders (85)

314.xx   Attention-Deficit/Hyperactivity Disorder (85)
- .01   Combined Type
- .00   Predominantly Inattentive Type
- .01   Predominantly Hyperactive-Impulsive Type

314.9   Attention-Deficit/Hyperactivity Disorder NOS (93)

312.xx   Conduct Disorder (93)
- .81   Childhood-Onset Type
- .82   Adolescent-Onset Type
- .89   Unspecified Onset

313.81   Oppositional Defiant Disorder (100)

312.9   Disruptive Behavior Disorder NOS (103)

Feeding and Eating Disorders of Infancy or Early Childhood (103)

307.52   Pica (103)

307.53   Rumination Disorder (105)

307.59   Feeding Disorder of Infancy or Early Childhood (107)

Tic Disorders (108)

307.23   Tourette's Disorder (111)

307.22   Chronic Motor or Vocal Tic Disorder (114)

307.21   Transient Tic Disorder (115)
Specify if: Single Episode/Recurrent

307.20   Tic Disorder NOS (116)

Elimination Disorders (116)

——.——   Encopresis (116)

787.6   With Constipation and Overflow Incontinence

307.7   Without Constipation and Overflow Incontinence

307.6   Enuresis (Not Due to a General Medical Condition) (118)
Specify type: Nocturnal Only/Diurnal Only/Nocturnal and Diurnal

Other Disorders of Infancy, Childhood, or Adolescence (121)

309.21   Separation Anxiety Disorder (121)
Specify if: Early Onset

313.23   Selective Mutism (125)

313.89   Reactive Attachment Disorder of Infancy or Early Childhood (127)
Specify type: Inhibited Type/Disinhibited Type

307.3   Stereotypic Movement Disorder (131)
Specify if: With Self-Injurious Behavior

313.9   Disorder of Infancy, Childhood, or Adolescence NOS (134)

DELIRIUM, DEMENTIA, AND AMNESTIC AND OTHER COGNITIVE DISORDERS (135)

Delirium (136)

293.0   Delirium Due to . . . *[Indicate the General Medical Condition]* (141)

——.——   Substance Intoxication Delirium (*refer to Substance-Related Disorders for substance-specific codes*) (143)

——.——   Substance Withdrawal Delirium (*refer to Substance-Related Disorders for substance-specific codes*) (143)

——.——   Delirium Due to Multiple Etiologies (*code each of the specific etiologies*) (146)

780.09   Delirium NOS (147)

Dementia (147)

294.xx*   Dementia of the Alzheimer's Type, With Early Onset (*also code 331.0 Alzheimer's disease on Axis III*) (154)
- .10   Without Behavioral Disturbance
- .11   With Behavioral Disturbance

294.xx*   Dementia of the Alzheimer's Type, With Late Onset (*also code 331.0 Alzheimer's disease on Axis III*) (154)
- .10   Without Behavioral Disturbance
- .11   With Behavioral Disturbance

290.xx   Vascular Dementia (158)
- .40   Uncomplicated
- .41   With Delirium
- .42   With Delusions
- .43   With Depressed Mood

Specify if: With Behavioral Disturbance

Code presence or absence of a behavioral disturbance in the fifth digit for Dementia Due to a General Medical Condition:

0 = Without Behavioral Disturbance
1 = With Behavioral Disturbance

294.1x*   Dementia Due to HIV Disease (*also code 042 HIV on Axis III*) (163)

294.1x*   Dementia Due to Head Trauma (*also code 854.00 head injury on Axis III*) (164)

294.1x*   Dementia Due to Parkinson's Disease (*also code 332.0 Parkinson's disease on Axis III*) (164)

294.1x*   Dementia Due to Huntington's Disease (*also code 333.4 Huntington's disease on Axis III*) (165)

294.1x*   Dementia Due to Pick's Disease (*also code 331.1 Pick's disease on Axis III*) (165)

294.1x*   Dementia Due to Creutzfeldt-Jakob Disease (*also code 046.1 Creutzfeldt-Jakob disease on Axis III*) (166)

---

*ICD-9-CM code valid after October 1, 2000.

294.1x*   Dementia Due to . . . *[Indicate the General Medical Condition not listed above] (also code the general medical condition on Axis III)* (167)

——.—   Substance-Induced Persisting Dementia *(refer to Substance-Related Disorders for substance-specific codes)* (168)

——.—   Dementia Due to Multiple Etiologies *(code each of the specific etiologies)* (170)

294.8   Dementia NOS (171)

Amnestic Disorders (172)

294.0   Amnestic Disorder Due to . . . *[Indicate the General Medical Condition]* (175)
    Specify if: Transient/Chronic

——.—   Substance-Induced Persisting Amnestic Disorder *(refer to Substance-Related Disorders for substance-specific codes)* (177)

294.8   Amnestic Disorder NOS (179)

Other Cognitive Disorders (179)

294.9   Cognitive Disorder NOS (179)

MENTAL DISORDERS DUE TO A GENERAL MEDICAL CONDITION NOT ELSEWHERE CLASSIFIED (181)

293.89   Catatonic Disorder Due to . . . *[Indicate the General Medical Condition]* (185)

310.1   Personality Change Due to . . . *[Indicate the General Medical Condition]* (187)
    Specify type: Labile Type/Disinhibited Type/Aggressive Type/Apathetic Type/Paranoid Type/Other Type/ Combined Type/Unspecified Type

293.9   Mental Disorder NOS Due to . . . *[Indicate the General Medical Condition]* (190)

SUBSTANCE-RELATED DISORDERS (191)

The following specifiers apply to Substance Dependence as noted:

[a]With Physiological Dependence/Without Physiological Dependence
[b]Early Full Remission/Early Partial Remission/Sustained Full Remission/Sustained Partial Remission
[c]In a Controlled Environment
[d]On Agonist Therapy

The following specifiers apply to Substance-Induced Disorders as noted:

[I]With Onset During Intoxication/[W]With Onset During Withdrawal

Alcohol-Related Disorders (212)

ALCOHOL USE DISORDERS (213)

303.90   Alcohol Dependence[a,b,c] (213)
305.00   Alcohol Abuse (214)

*ICD-9-CM code valid after October 1, 2000.

ALCOHOL-INDUCED DISORDERS (214)

303.00   Alcohol Intoxication (214)
291.81   Alcohol Withdrawal (215)
    Specify if: With Perceptual Disturbances
291.0   Alcohol Intoxication Delirium (143)
291.0   Alcohol Withdrawal Delirium (143)
291.2   Alcohol-Induced Persisting Dementia (168)
291.1   Alcohol-Induced Persisting Amnestic Disorder (177)
291.x   Alcohol-Induced Psychotic Disorder (338)
  .5   With Delusions[I,W]
  .3   With Hallucinations[I,W]
291.89   Alcohol-Induced Mood Disorder[I,W] (405)
291.89   Alcohol-Induced Anxiety Disorder[I,W] (479)
291.89   Alcohol-Induced Sexual Dysfunction[I] (562)
291.89   Alcohol-Induced Sleep Disorder[I,W] (655)
291.9   Alcohol-Related Disorder NOS (223)

Amphetamine (or Amphetamine-Like)–Related Disorders (223)

AMPHETAMINE USE DISORDERS (224)

304.40   Amphetamine Dependence[a,b,c] (224)
305.70   Amphetamine Abuse (225)

AMPHETAMINE-INDUCED DISORDERS (226)

292.89   Amphetamine Intoxication (226)
    Specify if: With Perceptual Disturbances
292.0   Amphetamine Withdrawal (227)
292.81   Amphetamine Intoxication Delirium (143)
292.xx   Amphetamine-Induced Psychotic Disorder (338)
  .11   With Delusions[I]
  .12   With Hallucinations[I]
292.84   Amphetamine-Induced Mood Disorder[I,W] (405)
292.89   Amphetamine-Induced Anxiety Disorder[I] (479)
292.89   Amphetamine-Induced Sexual Dysfunction[I] (562)
292.89   Amphetamine-Induced Sleep Disorder[I,W] (655)
292.9   Amphetamine-Related Disorder NOS (231)

Caffeine-Related Disorders (231)

CAFFEINE-INDUCED DISORDERS (232)

305.90   Caffeine Intoxication (232)
292.89   Caffeine-Induced Anxiety Disorder[I] (479)
292.89   Caffeine-Induced Sleep Disorder[I] (655)
292.9   Caffeine-Related Disorder NOS (234)

Cannabis-Related Disorders (234)

CANNABIS USE DISORDERS (236)

304.30   Cannabis Dependence[a,b,c] (236)
305.20   Cannabis Abuse (236)

CANNABIS-INDUCED DISORDERS (237)

292.89   Cannabis Intoxication (237)
              Specify if: With Perceptual Disturbances
292.81   Cannabis Intoxication Delirium (143)
292.xx   Cannabis-Induced Psychotic Disorder (338)
    .11   With Delusions[I]
    .12   With Hallucinations[I]
292.89   Cannabis-Induced Anxiety Disorder[I] (479)
292.9   Cannabis-Related Disorder NOS (241)

Cocaine-Related Disorders (241)

COCAINE USE DISORDERS (242)

304.20   Cocaine Dependence[a,b,c] (242)
305.60   Cocaine Abuse (243)

COCAINE-INDUCED DISORDERS (244)

292.89   Cocaine Intoxication (244)
              Specify if: With Perceptual Disturbances
292.0   Cocaine Withdrawal (245)
292.81   Cocaine Intoxication Delirium (143)
292.xx   Cocaine-Induced Psychotic Disorder (338)
    .11   With Delusions[I]
    .12   With Hallucinations[I]
292.84   Cocaine-Induced Mood Disorder[I,W] (405)
292.89   Cocaine-Induced Anxiety Disorder[I,W] (479)
292.89   Cocaine-Induced Sexual Dysfunction[I] (562)
292.89   Cocaine-Induced Sleep Disorder[I,W] (655)
292.9   Cocaine-Related Disorder NOS (250)

Hallucinogen-Related Disorders (250)

HALLUCINOGEN USE DISORDERS (251)

304.50   Hallucinogen Dependence[b,c] (251)
305.30   Hallucinogen Abuse (252)

HALLUCINOGEN-INDUCED DISORDERS (252)

292.89   Hallucinogen Intoxication (252)
292.89   Hallucinogen Persisting Perception Disorder
              (Flashbacks) (253)
292.81   Hallucinogen Intoxication Delirium (143)
292.xx   Hallucinogen-Induced Psychotic Disorder (338)
    .11   With Delusions[I]
    .12   With Hallucinations[I]
292.84   Hallucinogen-Induced Mood Disorder[I] (405)
292.89   Hallucinogen-Induced Anxiety Disorder[I] (479)
292.9   Hallucinogen-Related Disorder NOS (256)

Inhalant-Related Disorders (257)

INHALANT USE DISORDERS (258)

304.60   Inhalant Dependence[b,c] (258)
305.90   Inhalant Abuse (259)

INHALANT-INDUCED DISORDERS (259)

292.89   Inhalant Intoxication (259)
292.81   Inhalant Intoxication Delirium (143)
292.82   Inhalant-Induced Persisting Dementia (168)
292.xx   Inhalant-Induced Psychotic Disorder (338)
    .11   With Delusions[I]
    .12   With Hallucinations[I]
292.84   Inhalant-Induced Mood Disorder[I] (405)
292.89   Inhalant-Induced Anxiety Disorder[I] (479)
292.9   Inhalant-Related Disorder NOS (263)

Nicotine-Related Disorders (264)

NICOTINE USE DISORDER (264)

305.1   Nicotine Dependence[a,b] (264)

NICOTINE-INDUCED DISORDERS (265)

292.0   Nicotine Withdrawal (265)
292.9   Nicotine-Related Disorder NOS (269)

Opioid-Related Disorders (269)

OPIOID USE DISORDERS (270)

304.00   Opioid Dependence[a,b,c,d] (270)
305.50   Opioid Abuse (271)

OPIOID-INDUCED DISORDERS (271)

292.89   Opioid Intoxication (271)
              Specify if: With Perceptual Disturbances
292.0   Opioid Withdrawal (272)
292.81   Opioid Intoxication Delirium (143)
292.xx   Opioid-Induced Psychotic Disorder (338)
    .11   With Delusions[I]
    .12   With Hallucinations[I]
292.84   Opioid-Induced Mood Disorder[I] (405)
292.89   Opioid-Induced Sexual Dysfunction[I] (562)
292.89   Opioid-Induced Sleep Disorder[I,W] (655)
292.9   Opioid-Related Disorder NOS (277)

Phencyclidine (or Phencyclidine-Like)–Related Disorders (278)

PHENCYCLIDINE USE DISORDERS (279)

304.60   Phencyclidine Dependence[b,c] (279)
305.90   Phencyclidine Abuse (279)

PHENCYCLIDINE-INDUCED DISORDERS (280)

292.89   Phencyclidine Intoxication (280)
              Specify if: With Perceptual Disturbances
292.81   Phencyclidine Intoxication Delirium (143)
292.xx   Phencyclidine-Induced Psychotic Disorder (338)
    .11   With Delusions[I]
    .12   With Hallucinations[I]

292.84   Phencyclidine-Induced Mood Disorder[1] (405)
292.89   Phencyclidine-Induced Anxiety Disorder[1] (479)
292.9   Phencyclidine-Related Disorder NOS (283)

Sedative-, Hypnotic-, or Anxiolytic-Related Disorders (284)

SEDATIVE, HYPNOTIC, OR ANXIOLYTIC USE DISORDERS (285)

304.10   Sedative, Hypnotic, or Anxiolytic Dependence[a,b,c] (285)
305.40   Sedative, Hypnotic, or Anxiolytic Abuse (286)

SEDATIVE-, HYPNOTIC-, OR ANXIOLYTIC-INDUCED DISORDERS (286)

292.89   Sedative, Hypnotic, or Anxiolytic Intoxication (286)
292.0   Sedative, Hypnotic, or Anxiolytic Withdrawal (287)
          Specify if: With Perceptual Disturbances
292.81   Sedative, Hypnotic, or Anxiolytic Intoxication Delirium (143)
292.81   Sedative, Hypnotic, or Anxiolytic Withdrawal Delirium (143)
292.82   Sedative-, Hypnotic-, or Anxiolytic-Induced Persisting Dementia (168)
292.83   Sedative-, Hypnotic-, or Anxiolytic-Induced Persisting Amnestic Disorder (177)
292.xx   Sedative-, Hypnotic-, or Anxiolytic-Induced Psychotic Disorder (338)
   .11   With Delusions[I,W]
   .12   With Hallucinations[I,W]
292.84   Sedative-, Hypnotic-, or Anxiolytic-Induced Mood Disorder[I,W] (405)
292.89   Sedative-, Hypnotic-, or Anxiolytic-Induced Anxiety Disorder[W] (479)
292.89   Sedative-, Hypnotic-, or Anxiolytic-Induced Sexual Dysfunction[I] (562)
292.89   Sedative-, Hypnotic-, or Anxiolytic-Induced Sleep Disorder[I,W] (655)
292.9   Sedative-, Hypnotic-, or Anxiolytic-Related Disorder NOS (293)

Polysubstance-Related Disorder (293)

304.80   Polysubstance Dependence[a,b,c,d] (293)

Other (or Unknown) Substance-Related Disorders (294)

OTHER (OR UNKNOWN) SUBSTANCE USE DISORDERS (295)

304.90   Other (or Unknown) Substance Dependence[a,b,c,d] (192)
305.90   Other (or Unknown) Substance Abuse (198)

OTHER (OR UNKNOWN) SUBSTANCE-INDUCED DISORDERS (295)

292.89   Other (or Unknown) Substance Intoxication (199)
          Specify if: With Perceptual Disturbances
292.0   Other (or Unknown) Substance Withdrawal (201)
          Specify if: With Perceptual Disturbances
292.81   Other (or Unknown) Substance-Induced Delirium (143)
292.82   Other (or Unknown) Substance-Induced Persisting Dementia (168)
292.83   Other (or Unknown) Substance-Induced Persisting Amnestic Disorder (177)
292.xx   Other (or Unknown) Substance-Induced Psychotic Disorder (338)
   .11   With Delusions[I,W]
   .12   With Hallucinations[I,W]
292.84   Other (or Unknown) Substance-Induced Mood Disorder[I,W] (405)
292.89   Other (or Unknown) Substance-Induced Anxiety Disorder[I,W] (479)
292.89   Other (or Unknown) Substance-Induced Sexual Dysfunction[I] (562)
292.89   Other (or Unknown) Substance-Induced Sleep Disorder[I,W] (655)
292.9   Other (or Unknown) Substance-Related Disorder NOS (295)

SCHIZOPHRENIA AND OTHER PSYCHOTIC DISORDERS (297)

295.xx   Schizophrenia (298)

The following Classification of Longitudinal Course applies to all subtypes of Schizophrenia:

Episodic With Interepisode Residual Symptoms (*specify if:* With Prominent Negative Symptoms)/Episodic With No Interepisode Residual Symptoms
Continuous (*specify if:* With Prominent Negative Symptoms)
Single Episode In Partial Remission (*specify if:* With Prominent Negative Symptoms)/Single Episode In Full Remission
Other or Unspecified Pattern

   .30   Paranoid Type (313)
   .10   Disorganized Type (314)
   .20   Catatonic Type (315)
   .90   Undifferentiated Type (316)
   .60   Residual Type (316)
295.40   Schizophreniform Disorder (317)
          Specify if: Without Good Prognostic Features/ With Good Prognostic Features
295.70   Schizoaffective Disorder (319)
          Specify type: Bipolar Type/Depressive Type
297.1   Delusional Disorder (323)
          Specify type: Erotomanic Type/Grandiose Type/ Jealous Type/Persecutory Type/Somatic Type/ Mixed Type/Unspecified Type

298.8   Brief Psychotic Disorder (329)
         Specify if: With Marked Stressor(s)/Without Marked
         Stressor(s)/With Postpartum Onset

297.3   Shared Psychotic Disorder (332)

293.xx   Psychotic Disorder Due to . . . *[Indicate the
         General Medical Condition]* (334)
    .81   With Delusions
    .82   With Hallucinations

——.—   Substance-Induced Psychotic Disorder
         *(refer to Substance-Related Disorders for
         substance-specific codes)* (338)
         Specify if: With Onset During Intoxication/With Onset
         During Withdrawal

298.9   Psychotic Disorder NOS (343)

MOOD DISORDERS (345)

*Code current state of Major Depressive Disorder or Bipolar I
Disorder in fifth digit:*

1 = Mild
2 = Moderate
3 = Severe Without Psychotic Features
4 = Severe With Psychotic Features
   Specify: Mood-Congruent Psychotic Features/
   Mood-Incongruent Psychotic Features
5 = In Partial Remission
6 = In Full Remission
0 = Unspecified

*The following specifiers apply (for current or most recent
episode) to Mood Disorders as noted:*

[a]Severity/Psychotic/Remission Specifiers/[b]Chronic/[c]With Catatonic
Features/[d]With Melancholic Features/[e]With Atypical Features/
[f]With Postpartum Onset

The following specifiers apply to Mood Disorders as noted:

[g]With or Without Full Interepisode Recovery/[h]With Seasonal Pattern/
[i]With Rapid Cycling

Depressive Disorders (369)

296.xx   Major Depressive Disorder (369)
    .2x   Single Episode[a,b,c,d,e,f]
    .3x   Recurrent[a,b,c,d,e,f,g,h]

300.4   Dysthymic Disorder (376)
         Specify if: Early Onset/Late Onset
         Specify: With Atypical Features

311   Depressive Disorder NOS (381)

Bipolar Disorders (382)

296.xx   Bipolar I Disorder (382)
    .0x   Single Manic Episode[a,c,f]
         Specify if: Mixed
    .40   Most Recent Episode Hypomanic[g,h,i]
    .4x   Most Recent Episode Manic[a,c,f,g,h,i]
    .6x   Most Recent Episode Mixed[a,c,f,g,h,i]
    .5x   Most Recent Episode Depressed[a,b,c,d,e,f,g,h,i]
    .7   Most Recent Episode Unspecified[g,h,i]

296.89   Bipolar II Disorder[a,b,c,d,e,f,g,h,i] (392)
         Specify (current or most recent episode):
         Hypomanic/Depressed

301.13   Cyclothymic Disorder (398)

296.80   Bipolar Disorder NOS (400)

293.83   Mood Disorder Due to . . . *[Indicate the General
         Medical Condition]* (401)
         Specify type: With Depressive Features/With Major
         Depressive–Like Episode/With Manic Features/
         With Mixed Features

——.—   Substance-Induced Mood Disorder
         *(refer to Substance-Related Disorders for
         substance-specific codes)* (405)
         Specify type: With Depressive Features/With Manic
         Features/With Mixed Features
         Specify if: With Onset During Intoxication/With Onset
         During Withdrawal

296.90   Mood Disorder NOS (410)

ANXIETY DISORDERS (429)

300.01   Panic Disorder Without Agoraphobia (433)

300.21   Panic Disorder With Agoraphobia (433)

300.22   Agoraphobia Without History of
         Panic Disorder (441)

300.29   Specific Phobia (443)
         Specify type: Animal Type/Natural Environment Type/
         Blood-Injection-Injury Type/Situational Type/Other Type

300.23   Social Phobia (450)
         Specify if: Generalized

300.3   Obsessive-Compulsive Disorder (456)
         Specify if: With Poor Insight

309.81   Posttraumatic Stress Disorder (463)
         Specify if: Acute/Chronic
         Specify if: With Delayed Onset

308.3   Acute Stress Disorder (469)

300.02   Generalized Anxiety Disorder (472)

293.84   Anxiety Disorder Due to . . . *[Indicate the
         General Medical Condition]* (476)
         Specify if: With Generalized Anxiety/With Panic Attacks/
         With Obsessive-Compulsive Symptoms

——.—   Substance-Induced Anxiety Disorder
         *(refer to Substance-Related Disorders for
         substance-specific codes)* (479)
         Specify if: With Generalized Anxiety/With Panic Attacks/
         With Obsessive-Compulsive Symptoms/With Phobic
         Symptoms
         Specify if: With Onset During Intoxication/With Onset
         During Withdrawal

300.00   Anxiety Disorder NOS (484)

SOMATOFORM DISORDERS (485)

300.81   Somatization Disorder (486)

300.82   Undifferentiated Somatoform Disorder (490)

300.11   Conversion Disorder (492)
         Specify type: With Motor Symptom or Deficit/
         With Sensory Symptom or Deficit/With Seizures or
         Convulsions/With Mixed Presentation

307.xx   Pain Disorder (498)
  .80   Associated With Psychological Factors
  .89   Associated With Both Psychological Factors
    and a General Medical Condition
    Specify if: Acute/Chronic
300.7   Hypochondriasis (504)
    Specify if: With Poor Insight
300.7   Body Dysmorphic Disorder (507)
300.82   Somatoform Disorder NOS (511)

FACTITIOUS DISORDERS (513)

300.xx   Factitious Disorder (513)
  .16   With Predominantly Psychological Signs
    and Symptoms
  .19   With Predominantly Physical Signs
    and Symptoms
  .19   With Combined Psychological and Physical
    Signs and Symptoms
300.19   Factitious Disorder NOS (517)

DISSOCIATIVE DISORDERS (519)

300.12   Dissociative Amnesia (520)
300.13   Dissociative Fugue (523)
300.14   Dissociative Identity Disorder (526)
300.6   Depersonalization Disorder (530)
300.15   Dissociative Disorder NOS (532)

SEXUAL AND GENDER IDENTITY DISORDERS (535)

Sexual Dysfunctions (535)

The following specifiers apply to all primary Sexual Dysfunctions:

  Lifelong Type/Acquired Type
  Generalized Type/Situational Type
  Due to Psychological Factors/Due to Combined Factors

SEXUAL DESIRE DISORDERS (539)

302.71   Hypoactive Sexual Desire Disorder (539)
302.79   Sexual Aversion Disorder (541)

SEXUAL AROUSAL DISORDERS (543)

302.72   Female Sexual Arousal Disorder (543)
302.72   Male Erectile Disorder (545)

ORGASMIC DISORDERS (547)

302.73   Female Orgasmic Disorder (547)
302.74   Male Orgasmic Disorder (550)
302.75   Premature Ejaculation (552)

SEXUAL PAIN DISORDERS (554)

302.76   Dyspareunia (Not Due to a General Medical
    Condition) (554)
306.51   Vaginismus (Not Due to a General Medical
    Condition) (556)

SEXUAL DYSFUNCTION DUE TO A GENERAL MEDICAL CONDITION (558)

625.8   Female Hypoactive Sexual Desire Disorder
    Due to . . . *[Indicate the General Medical
    Condition]* (558)
608.89   Male Hypoactive Sexual Desire Disorder
    Due to . . . *[Indicate the General Medical
    Condition]* (558)
607.84   Male Erectile Disorder Due to . . . *[Indicate the
    General Medical Condition]* (558)
625.0   Female Dyspareunia Due to . . . *[Indicate the
    General Medical Condition]* (558)
608.89   Male Dyspareunia Due to . . . *[Indicate the
    General Medical Condition]* (558)
625.8   Other Female Sexual Dysfunction Due to . . .
    [Indicate the General Medical Condition] (558)
608.89   Other Male Sexual Dysfunction Due to . . .
    [Indicate the General Medical Condition] (558)
——.—   Substance-Induced Sexual Dysfunction
    *(refer to Substance-Related Disorders for
    substance-specific codes)* (562)
    Specify if: With Impaired Desire/With Impaired Arousal/
    With Impaired Orgasm/With Sexual Pain
    Specify if: With Onset During Intoxication
302.70   Sexual Dysfunction NOS (565)

Paraphilias (566)

302.4   Exhibitionism (569)
302.81   Fetishism (569)
302.89   Frotteurism (570)
302.2   Pedophilia (571)
    Specify if: Sexually Attracted to Males/Sexually Attracted to
    Females/Sexually Attracted to Both
    Specify if: Limited to Incest
    Specify type: Exclusive Type/Nonexclusive Type
302.83   Sexual Masochism (572)
302.84   Sexual Sadism (573)
302.3   Transvestic Fetishism (574)
    Specify if: With Gender Dysphoria
302.82   Voyeurism (575)
302.9   Paraphilia NOS (576)

Gender Identity Disorders (576)

302.xx   Gender Identity Disorder (576)
  .6   in Children
  .85   in Adolescents or Adults
    Specify if: Sexually Attracted to Males/Sexually Attracted
    to Females/Sexually Attracted to Both/Sexually Attracted
    to Neither

302.6   Gender Identity Disorder NOS (582)

302.9   Sexual Disorder NOS (582)

EATING DISORDERS (583)

307.1   Anorexia Nervosa (583)
Specify type: Restricting Type; Binge-Eating/Purging Type

307.51   Bulimia Nervosa (589)
Specific type: Purging Type/Nonpurging Type

307.50   Eating Disorder NOS (594)

SLEEP DISORDERS (597)

Primary Sleep Disorders (598)

DYSSOMNIAS (598)

307.42   Primary Insomnia (599)

307.44   Primary Hypersomnia (604)
Specify if: Recurrent

347   Narcolepsy (609)

780.59   Breathing-Related Sleep Disorder (615)

307.45   Circadian Rhythm Sleep Disorder (622)
Specify type: Delayed Sleep Phase Type/Jet Lag Type/
Shift Work Type/Unspecified Type

307.47   Dyssomnia NOS (629)

PARASOMNIAS (630)

307.47   Nightmare Disorder (631)

307.46   Sleep Terror Disorder (634)

307.46   Sleepwalking Disorder (639)

307.47   Parasomnia NOS (644)

Sleep Disorders Related to Another Mental Disorder (645)

307.42   Insomnia Related to . . . *[Indicate the Axis I or Axis II Disorder]* (645)

307.44   Hypersomnia Related to . . . *[Indicate the Axis I or Axis II Disorder]* (645)

Other Sleep Disorders (651)

780.xx   Sleep Disorder Due to . . . *[Indicate the General Medical Condition]* (651)
.52   Insomnia Type
.54   Hypersomnia Type
.59   Parasomnia Type
.59   Mixed Type

——.——   Substance-Induced Sleep Disorder (*refer to Substance-Related Disorders for substance-specific codes*) (655)
Specify type: Insomnia Type/Hypersomnia Type/
Parasomnia Type/Mixed Type
Specify if: With Onset During Intoxication/With Onset During Withdrawal

IMPULSE-CONTROL DISORDERS NOT ELSEWHERE CLASSIFIED (663)

312.34   Intermittent Explosive Disorder (663)

312.32   Kleptomania (667)

312.33   Pyromania (669)

312.31   Pathological Gambling (671)

312.39   Trichotillomania (674)

312.30   Impulse-Control Disorder NOS (677)

ADJUSTMENT DISORDERS (679)

309.xx   Adjustment Disorder (679)
.0   With Depressed Mood
.24   With Anxiety
.28   With Mixed Anxiety and Depressed Mood
.3   With Disturbance of Conduct
.4   With Mixed Disturbance of Emotions and Conduct
.9   Unspecified
Specify if: Acute/Chronic

PERSONALITY DISORDERS (685)

Note: These are coded on Axis II.

301.0   Paranoid Personality Disorder (690)

301.20   Schizoid Personality Disorder (694)

301.22   Schizotypal Personality Disorder (697)

301.7   Antisocial Personality Disorder (701)

301.83   Borderline Personality Disorder (706)

301.50   Histrionic Personality Disorder (711)

301.81   Narcissistic Personality Disorder (714)

301.82   Avoidant Personality Disorder (718)

301.6   Dependent Personality Disorder (721)

301.4   Obsessive-Compulsive Personality Disorder (725)

301.9   Personality Disorder NOS (729)

OTHER CONDITIONS THAT MAY BE A FOCUS OF CLINICAL ATTENTION (731)

Psychological Factors Affecting Medical Condition (731)

316   . . . *[Specified Psychological Factor] Affecting . . . [Indicate the General Medical Condition]* (731)
Choose name based on nature of factors:
Mental Disorder Affecting Medical Condition
Psychological Symptoms Affecting Medical Condition
Personality Traits or Coping Style Affecting Medical Condition
Maladaptive Health Behaviors Affecting Medical Condition
Stress-Related Physiological Response Affecting Medical Condition
Other or Unspecified Psychological Factors Affecting Medical Condition

Medication-Induced Movement Disorders (734)

332.1	Neuroleptic-Induced Parkinsonism (735)
333.92	Neuroleptic Malignant Syndrome (735)
333.7	Neuroleptic-Induced Acute Dystonia (735)
333.99	Neuroleptic-Induced Acute Akathisia (735)
333.82	Neuroleptic-Induced Tardive Dyskinesia (736)
333.1	Medication-Induced Postural Tremor (736)
333.90	Medication-Induced Movement Disorder NOS (736)

Other Medication-Induced Disorder (736)

995.2	Adverse Effects of Medication NOS (736)

Relational Problems (736)

V61.9	Relational Problem Related to a Mental Disorder or General Medical Condition (737)
V61.20	Parent-Child Relational Problem (737)
V61.10	Partner Relational Problem (737)
V61.8	Sibling Relational Problem (737)
V62.81	Relational Problem NOS (737)

Problems Related to Abuse or Neglect (738)

V61.21	Physical Abuse of Child (738)
	(code 995.54 if focus of attention is on victim)
V61.21	Sexual Abuse of Child (738)
	(code 995.53 if focus of attention is on victim)
V61.21	Neglect of Child (738)
	(code 995.52 if focus of attention is on victim)
—.—	Physical Abuse of Adult (738)
V61.12	(if by partner)
V62.83	(if by person other than partner)
	(code 995.81 if focus of attention is on victim)
—.—	Sexual Abuse of Adult (738)
V61.12	(if by partner)
V62.83	(if by person other than partner)
	(code 995.83 if focus of attention is on victim)

Additional Conditions That May Be a Focus of Clinical Attention (739)

V15.81	Noncompliance With Treatment (739)
V65.2	Malingering (739)
V71.01	Adult Antisocial Behavior (740)
V71.02	Child or Adolescent Antisocial Behavior (740)
V62.89	Borderline Intellectual Functioning (740)
	Note: This is coded on Axis II.
780.9	Age-Related Cognitive Decline (740)
V62.82	Bereavement (740)
V62.3	Academic Problem (741)
V62.2	Occupational Problem (741)
313.82	Identity Problem (741)
V62.89	Religious or Spiritual Problem (741)
V62.4	Acculturation Problem (741)
V62.89	Phase of Life Problem (742)

ADDITIONAL CODES (743)

300.9	Unspecified Mental Disorder (nonpsychotic) (743)
V71.09	No Diagnosis or Condition on Axis I (743)
799.9	Diagnosis or Condition Deferred on Axis I (743)
V71.09	No Diagnosis on Axis II (743)
799.9	Diagnosis Deferred on Axis II (743)

MULTIAXIAL SYSTEM

Axis I	Clinical Disorders/Other Conditions That May Be a Focus of Clinical Attention
Axis II	Personality Disorders/Mental Retardation
Axis III	General Medical Conditions
Axis IV	Psychosocial and Environmental Problems
Axis V	Global Assessment of Functioning

This list represents the NANDA-approved nursing diagnoses for clinical use and testing.

Activity Intolerance
Risk for Activity Intolerance
Impaired Adjustment
Ineffective Airway Clearance
Latex Allergy Response
Risk for Latex Allergy Response
Anxiety
Death Anxiety
Risk for Aspiration
Risk for Impaired Parent/Infant/Child Attachment
Autonomic Dysreflexia
Autonomic Dysreflexia, Risk for
Disturbed Body Image
Risk for Imbalanced Body Temperature
Bowel Incontinence
Effective Breastfeeding
Ineffective Breastfeeding
Interrupted Breastfeeding
Ineffective Breathing Pattern
Decreased Cardiac Output
Caregiver Role Strain
Risk for Caregiver Role Strain
Impaired Verbal Communication
Readiness for Enhanced Communication
Decisional Conflict
Parental Role Conflict
Acute Confusion
Chronic Confusion
Constipation
Perceived Constipation
Risk for Constipation
Ineffective Coping
Defensive Coping
Readiness for Enhanced Coping
Ineffective Community Coping
Readiness for Enhanced Community Coping
Compromised Family Coping

Disabled Family Coping
Readiness for Enhanced Family Coping
Risk for Sudden Infant Death Syndrome
Ineffective Denial
Impaired Dentition
Risk for Delayed Development
Diarrhea
Risk for Disuse Syndrome
Deficient Diversional Activity
Disturbed Energy Field
Impaired Environmental Interpretation Syndrome
Adult Failure to Thrive
Risk for Falls
Dysfunctional Family Processes: Alcoholism
Interrupted Family Processes
Readiness for Enhanced Family Processes
Fatigue
Fear
Readiness for Enhanced Fluid Balance
Deficient Fluid Volume
Excess Fluid Volume
Risk for Deficient Fluid Volume
Risk for Imbalanced Fluid Volume
Impaired Gas Exchange
Anticipatory Grieving
Dysfunctional Grieving
Risk for Dysfunctional Grieving
Delayed Growth and Development
Risk for Disproportionate Growth
Ineffective Health Maintenance
Health-Seeking Behaviors (Specify)
Impaired Home Maintenance
Hopelessness
Hyperthermia
Hypothermia
Disturbed Personal Identity
Functional Urinary Incontinence
Reflex Urinary Incontinence
Stress Urinary Incontinence
Total Urinary Incontinence

Urge Urinary Incontinence
Risk for Urge Urinary Incontinence
Disorganized Infant Behavior
Risk for Disorganized Infant Behavior
Readiness for Enhanced Organized Infant Behavior
Ineffective Infant Feeding Pattern
Risk for Infection
Risk for Injury
Risk for Perioperative-Positioning Injury
Decreased Intracranial, Adaptive Capacity
Deficient Knowledge (Specify)
Readiness for Enhanced Knowledge (Specify)
Sedentary Lifestyle
Risk for Loneliness
Impaired Memory
Impaired Bed Mobility
Impaired Physical Mobility
Impaired Wheelchair Mobility
Nausea
Unilateral Neglect
Noncompliance
Imbalanced Nutrition: Less Than Body Requirements
Imbalanced Nutrition: More Than Body Requirements
Readiness for Enhanced Nutrition
Risk for Imbalanced Nutrition: More Than Body
    Requirements
Impaired Oral Mucous Membrane
Acute Pain
Chronic Pain
Readiness for Enhanced Parenting
Impaired Parenting
Risk for Impaired Parenting
Risk for Peripheral Neurovascular Dysfunction
Risk for Poisoning
Post-Trauma Syndrome
Risk for Post-Trauma Syndrome
Powerlessness
Risk for Powerlessness
Ineffective Protection
Rape-Trauma Syndrome
Rape-Trauma Syndrome: Compound Reaction
Rape-Trauma Syndrome, Silent Reaction
Impaired Religiosity
Readiness for Enhanced Religiosity
Risk for Impaired Religiosity
Relocation Stress Syndrome
Risk for Relocation Stress Syndrome
Ineffective Role Performance
Bathing/Hygiene Self-Care Deficit
Dressing/Grooming Self-Care Deficit
Feeding Self-Care Deficit
Toileting Self-Care Deficit
Readiness for Enhanced Self-Concept
Chronic Low Self-Esteem
Situational Low Self-Esteem
Risk for Situational Low Self-Esteem

Self-Mutilation
Risk for Self-Mutilation
Disturbed Sensory Perception (Specify: Visual, Auditory,
    Kinesthetic, Gustatory, Tactile, Olfactory)
Sexual Dysfunction
Ineffective Sexuality Pattern
Impaired Skin Integrity
Risk for Impaired Skin Integrity
Sleep Deprivation
Disturbed Sleep Pattern
Readiness for Enhanced Sleep
Impaired Social Interaction
Social Isolation
Chronic Sorrow
Spiritual Distress
Risk for Spiritual Distress
Readiness for Enhanced Spiritual Well-Being
Risk for Suffocation
Risk for Suicide
Delayed Surgical Recovery
Impaired Swallowing
Effective Therapeutic Regimen Management
Ineffective Therapeutic Regimen Management
Ineffective Community Therapeutic Regimen Management
Ineffective Family Therapeutic Regimen Management
Ineffective Thermoregulation
Disturbed Thought Processes
Impaired Tissue Integrity
Ineffective Tissue Perfusion (Specify Type: Renal,
    Cerebral, Cardiopulmonary, Gastrointestinal,
    Peripheral)
Impaired Transfer Ability
Risk for Trauma
Impaired Urinary Elimination
Readiness for Enhanced Urinary Elimination
Urinary Retention
Impaired Spontaneous Ventilation
Dysfunctional Ventilatory Weaning Response
Risk for Other-Directed Violence
Risk for Self-Directed Violence
Impaired Walking
Wandering

Drug Classification Under the Controlled Substances Act

Schedule I Drugs	Schedule II Drugs	Schedule III Drugs	Schedule IV Drugs	Schedule V Drugs
OPIOIDS	**OPIOIDS**	**OPIOIDS**	**OPIOIDS**	**OPIOIDS**
Acetylmethadol	Alfentanil	Hydrocodone syrup	Pentazocine	Buprenorphine
Heroin	Codeine	Paregoric	Propoxyphene	Diphenoxylate
Normethadone	Fentanyl			plus atropine
Many others	Hydromorphone			
	Levorphanol			
	Meperidine			
	Methadone			
	Morphine			
	Opium tincture			
	Oxycodone			
	Oxymorphone			
	Sufentanil			
PSYCHEDELICS	**PSYCHOSTIMULANTS**	**STIMULANTS**	**STIMULANTS**	
Bufotenin	Amphetamine	Benzphetamine	Diethylpropion	
Diethyltryptamine	Cocaine	Phendimetrazine	Fenfluramine	
Dimethyltryptamine	Dextroamphetamine		Mazindol	
Ibogaine	Methamphetamine		Pemoline	
d-Lysergic acid	Methylphenidate		Phentermine	
diethylamide (LSD)	Phenmetrazine			
Mescaline				
3,4-Methylenedioxy-				
methamphetamine				
(MDMA)				
Psilocin				
Psilocybin				
CANNABIS DERIVATIVES	**BARBITURATES**	**BARBITURATES**	**BARBITURATES**	
Hashish	Amobarbital	Aprobarbital	Mephobarbital	
Marijuana	Pentobarbital	Butabarbital	Methohexital	
	Secobarbital	Methabarbital	Phenobarbital	
		Talbutal		
		Thiamylal		
		Thiopental		

(continued)

(Continued)

Schedule I Drugs	Schedule II Drugs	Schedule III Drugs	Schedule IV Drugs	Schedule V Drugs
OTHERS Methaqualone Phencyclidine Gammahydroxybutyric 　acid (GHB)	**CANNABINOIDS** Dronabinol (THC) Nabilone	**MISCELLANEOUS** **DEPRESSANTS** Glutethimide Methyprylon **ANABOLIC STEROIDS** Fluoxymesterone Methyltestosterone Nandrolone Oxandrolone Stanozolol Testosterone	**BENZODIAZEPINES** Alprazolam Chlordiazepoxide Clonazepam Clorazepate Diazepam Estazolam Flurazepam Halazepam Lorazepam Midazolam Oxazepam Prazepam Quazepam Temazepam Triazolam **MISCELLANEOUS** **DEPRESSANTS** Chloral hydrate Ethchlorvynol Ethinamate Meprobamate Paraldehyde	

Drugs in Schedule I have a high potential for abuse and have no approved medical use in the United States.

Drugs in Schedules II through V all have approved uses and are classified based on their abuse potential. Schedule II drugs have a higher potential for abuse. Schedule V drugs have the lowest potential for abuse.

Canadian Standards of Psychiatric and Mental Health Nursing Practice (3rd ed.)

BELIEFS/VALUES

Psychiatric and mental health nurses believe
- Psychiatry and mental health is a specialized area of nursing practice, education, and research.
- Practice involves the promotion of mental health and the prevention, treatment, and management of mental disorders.
- The therapeutic relationship, based on trust and mutual respect, is central to practice.
- That alleviation of stigma and discrimination associated with mental illness is of paramount importance.
- In the conduct and utilization of research for improvement in care.
- In social action to promote political and social awareness to influence health and organizational policy.
- In working in collaborative relationships with the individual, family, community, populations, and social agencies.
- That a holistic approach is essential to understanding the unique experience of the client and that outcomes are fundamentally intertwined with all other health and social outcomes.
- In equitable access to culturally competent care.
- In reflective ethical practice and a commitment to continuous learning.
- In the protection of human rights in context to civil commitment and relevant aspects of jurisprudence.
- In advocating for practice environments that facilitate and ensure safe and positive work relationships.
- In fostering a legacy of moral and visionary nursing leaders.
- In the Code of Ethics for Registered Nurses.

From the Standard Committee of the Canadian Federation of Mental Health Nurses. (2005). *Canadian standards of psychiatric mental health nursing practice* (3rd ed.). Ottawa, Ontario: Canadian Nurses Association.

STANDARD I: PROVIDES COMPETENT PROFESSIONAL CARE THROUGH THE DEVELOPMENT OF A THERAPEUTIC RELATIONSHIP

A primary goal of psychiatric and mental health nursing is the promotion of mental health and the prevention or diminution of mental disorder. The development of a therapeutic relationship is the foundation from where the psychiatric and mental health nurse can "enter into partnerships with clients, and through the use of the human sciences, and the art of caring, develop helping relationships" (Canadian Nurses Association [CNA], 1997, p. 43).

The nurse is expected to demonstrate competence in a therapeutic relationship by the following:

1. Assesses and clarifies the influences of personal beliefs, values, and life experience on the therapeutic relationship and distinguishes between social and therapeutic relationships
2. Works in partnership with the client, family, and relevant others to determine goal directed needs and establishes an environment that is conducive to goal achievement
3. Uses a range of therapeutic verbal and non-verbal communication skills that include empathy, active listening, observing, genuineness, and curiosity
4. Recognizes the influence of culture, class, ethnicity, language, stigma, and social exclusion on the therapeutic process and negotiates care that is sensitive to these influences
5. Mobilizes and advocates for resources that increase clients' and families' access to mental health services and that improve community integration
6. Understands and responds to human reactions to distress and loss of control that may be expressed as anger, anxiety, fear, grief, helplessness, hopelessness, and humour

7. Guides the client through behavioural, developmental, emotional, or spiritual change while acknowledging and supporting the client's participation, responsibility, and choices in own care
8. Supports the client's and family's sense of resiliency, self-esteem, power, and hope through continuity of therapeutic relationship, on a 1:1 basis or within a group context
9. Fosters mutuality of the relationship by reflectively critiquing therapeutic effectiveness through client and family responses, clinical supervision, and self-evaluation
10. Understands the nature of chronic illness and applies the principles of health promotion and disease prevention when working with clients and families.

STANDARD II: PERFORMS/REFINES CLIENT ASSESSMENTS THROUGH THE DIAGNOSTIC AND MONITORING FUNCTION

Effective assessment, diagnosis, and monitoring is central to the nurse's role and is dependent upon theory, as well as upon understanding the meaning of the health or illness experience from the perspective of the client. This knowledge, integrated with the nurse's conceptual model of nursing practice, provides a framework for processing client data and for developing client-focused plans of care. The nurse makes professional judgments regarding the relevance and importance of this data and acknowledges the client as a valued and respected partner throughout the decision-making process.

The nurse is expected to demonstrate competence in the mental health assessment tools, e.g., mental status exam and recovery principles, in various workplaces. The nurse explains to the client the assessment process and content and provides feedback for all of the following:

1. Collaborates with clients and with other members of the health care team to gather holistic assessments through observation, examination, interview, and consultation while being attentive to issues of confidentiality and pertinent legal statutes
2. Documents and analyzes baseline data to identify health status, potential for wellness, health care deficits, potential for danger to self and others; alterations in thought content and/or process, affect behaviour, communication, and decision-making abilities; substance use and dependency; and history of trauma and/or abuse (emotional, physical, sexual, or verbal abuse; neglect)
3. Formulates and documents a plan of care in collaboration with the client and with the mental health team, recognizing variability in the client's ability to participate in the process
4. Refines and extends client assessment information by assessing and documenting significant change(s) in the client's status and by comparing new data with the baseline assessment and intermediate client goals

5. Continuously assesses status and anticipates potential problems and risks. Collaborates with the client to examine his/her environment for risk factors: self-care, housing, and nutrition; economic, psychological, and social. Utilizes assessment data to identify potential risks to client and others. Advocates and practices for interventions that are appropriate to risk type and level.
6. Determines most appropriate and available therapeutic modality that will potentially best meet client's needs and assists the client to access these resources

STANDARD III: ADMINISTERS AND MONITORS THERAPEUTIC INTERVENTIONS

Due to the nature of mental health problems and mental disorders, there are unique practice issues confronting the psychiatric and mental health nurse in the assessment phase and the administration of therapeutic interventions. Safety in psychiatric and mental health nursing has unique meaning since many clients are at risk for harm to self and/or others and/or for self-neglect. Clients may not be mentally competent to participate in all aspects of decision making. However, every effort must be made to include the client. In collaboration with the client, the psychiatric mental health (PMH) nurse needs to be alert to adverse reactions, as clients' ability to self-report may be impaired.

The PMH nurse uses evidence-based and experiential knowledge from nursing, health sciences, and related mental health disciplines to both select and tailor nursing interventions. The nurse

1. Utilizes and evaluates evidence-based interventions to provide safe, effective, and efficient nursing care
2. Provides information to clients and families/significant others about care and treatment, ensuring that the client consents to such information being shared on an ongoing basis
3. Assists, educates, and empowers clients to select choices that will support positive changes in their affect, cognition, behavior, and/or relationships, even when some of these choices may involve a level of risk as assessed by the clinical team (CNA, 1997, p. 68)
4. Supports clients to draw on own assets and resources for self-care, activities of daily living, mobilizing resources, and mental health promotion (CNA, 1997, p. 68)
5. Makes discretionary clinical decisions, using knowledge of client's unique responses and paradigm cases, e.g., frequency of client contact in the community, as the basis for the decision
6. Uses appropriate technology to perform safe, effective, and efficient nursing intervention (CNA, 1997, p. 68)
7. Administers medications accurately and safely, monitoring therapeutic responses, reactions, untoward effects, toxicity, and potential incompatibilities with other medications or substances; provides medication education with appropriate content and in accordance with workplace policies

8. Assesses client responses to deficits in activities of daily living and mobilizes resources in response to client's capabilities and offers alternatives when appropriate
9. Provides support and assists with protection for clients experiencing difficulty with self-protection
10. Utilizes therapeutic elements of group process
11. Incorporates knowledge of family dynamics and cultural values and beliefs about families in the provision of care
12. Collaborates with the client, health care providers, and community to access and coordinate resources and seeks feedback from the client and others regarding interventions
13. Incorporates knowledge of community needs or responses in the provision of care
14. Encourages and assists clients to seek out support groups for mutual aid and support
15. Assesses the client's response to, and perception of, nursing and other therapeutic interventions

STANDARD IV: EFFECTIVELY MANAGES RAPIDLY CHANGING SITUATIONS

The effective management of rapidly changing situations is essential in critical circumstances that may be termed *psychiatric emergencies*. These situations include self-harm and assaultive behaviours and rapidly changing mental health states. This domain also includes evidence-based assessment and screening for risk factors and referral related to psychiatric illnesses and social problems, i.e., substance abuse, violence/abuse, and suicide/homicide (Society for Education and Research in Psychiatric-Mental Health Nursing, 1996, p. 41).

The nurse

1. Utilizes the therapeutic relationship throughout the management of rapidly changing situations
2. Assesses the client using a comprehensive holistic approach for actual or potential health problems, issues, risk factors, and or crisis/emergency/catastrophic situations, e.g., psychotic episode, neuroleptic malignant syndrome, acute onset of extra pyramidal side effects, substance abuse, violence/abuse and suicide/homicide, drug toxicity, and delirium
3. Knows resources required to manage actual and potential crisis/emergency/catastrophic situations and plans access to these resources
4. Monitors client safety and utilizes continual assessment to detect early changes in client status and intervenes accordingly
5. Implements timely, age-appropriate, client-specific crisis/emergency/catastrophic interventions as necessary
6. Commences critical procedures, i.e., suicide precautions, emergency restraint, elopement precautions, and infectious disease management, when necessary in an institutional and a community setting by using appro-

priate community support systems, e.g., police, ambulance services, crisis response resources
7. Coordinates care to prevent errors and duplication of efforts where rapid intervention is imperative
8. Utilizes a least-restraint approach to care
9. Develops adequate documentation of the crisis/emergency/catastrophic intervention plan
10. Evaluates the effectiveness of the rapid responses and modifies critical plans as necessary
11. In collaboration with the client, facilitates the involvement of the family and significant others to assist in the identification of the precipitates of the crisis/emergency event and plans to minimize risk of recurrence
12. Participates in "debriefing" process, e.g., reviews critical event and/or emergency situation, with team (including client and family) and other service providers
13. Utilizes safety measures to protect self, colleagues, and clients from potentially abusive situations in the work environment, e.g., harassment, psychological abuse, physical aggression
14. Implements appropriate protocols for disasters
15. Participates in educational, organizational, and institutional activities that improve client safety in the practice setting

STANDARD V: INTERVENES THROUGH THE TEACHING–COACHING FUNCTION

All nurse–client interactions are potentially teaching/learning situations. The PMH nurse attempts to understand the life experience of the client and uses this understanding to support and promote learning related to health and personal development. The nurse provides health promotion information to individuals, families, groups, populations, and communities. The nurse

1. In collaboration with the client, determines clients' learning needs
2. Plans and implements, with the client, health promotion education while considering the context of the client's life experiences; considers readiness, culture, literacy, language, preferred learning style, and resources available
3. Engages with the client to explore available options and resources to build knowledge to make informed choices related to health needs and to navigate the system, as needed
4. Facilitates the client's search for ways to find meaning in his or her experience
5. Incorporates knowledge of a wide variety of learning models and principles, e.g., health promotion models, adult-learning principles, stages of development, cultural competence, health beliefs models, when creating opportunities for clients
6. Provides relevant information, guidance, and support to the client's significant others

7. Documents the teaching/learning process (assessment, plan, implementation, client involvement, and evaluation)
8. Determines, with the client, the effectiveness of the educational process and collaboratively develops or adapts the ways to meet learning needs
9. Engages in teaching/learning opportunities as partners with community agencies and consumer and family groups

STANDARD VI: MONITORS AND ENSURES THE QUALITY OF HEALTH CARE PRACTICES

The nurse has a responsibility to advocate for the client's right to receive the least restrictive form of care and to respect and affirm the client's right to self-determination in a safe, fair, and just (equitable) manner.

Mental health care occurs under the provisions of provincial/territorial Mental Health Acts and related legislation. It is essential for the PMH nurse to be informed regarding the interpretation of relevant legislation and its implications for nursing practice.

The nurse

1. Identifies work place cultures (philosophy, attitudes, values, and beliefs that impact the nurse's ability to perform with skill, safety, and compassion) and takes action as appropriate
2. Explores how the determinates of health that impact on the health of the community, e.g., poverty, malnutrition, unsafe housing, affect mental health nursing practice
3. Understands current and relevant legislation, e.g., privacy laws, and the implications for nursing practice
4. Expands and incorporates knowledge of innovations and changes in mental health and psychiatric nursing practice to ensure safe and effective care
5. Ensures and documents ongoing review and evaluation of psychiatric and mental health nursing care activities
6. Understands and questions the interdependent functions of the team within the overall plan of care
7. Advocates for the client within the context of organizational and professional parameters and family and community interests
8. Advocates for changes and improvements to the system/organizational structures in keeping with the principles of delivering safe, ethical, and competent care
9. Recognizes the dynamic changes in health care locally and globally and, in collaboration with stakeholders, develops strategies to manage these changes, e.g., considers changes in determinants of health that impact the community, terrorism, decline of industries

STANDARD VII: PRACTICES WITHIN ORGANIZATIONAL AND WORK-ROLE STRUCTURE

The PMH nurse role is assumed within organizational structures, in both community and institutional contexts, through the provision of psychiatric mental health care. For the PMH nurse, the ethic of care is based on reflective and evidence-based practice judgments within complex and dynamic situations. The increasing move of mental health/psychiatric treatment into the community necessitates the PMH nurse to be knowledgeable and skilful in collaborative care planning and implementation, mental health promotion, social action, and community consultation.

The nurse

1. Works in collaborative partnerships with clients/families and other stakeholders to facilitate healing environments that ensure the safety, support, and respect for all persons
2. Understands quality outcome indicators and strives for continuous quality improvement
3. Actively participates with nurses to sustain and promote a climate that supports ethical practice and the establishment of a moral community (Varcoe, Rodney, & McCormick, 2003)
4. Participates in supporting a climate of trust that sponsors openness and encourages questioning of the status quo and the reporting of incompetent care (CNA, 2002)
5. Seeks to utilize constructive and collaborative approaches to resolve differences impacting care among members of the health care team (CNA, 2002)
6. Actively participates in developing, implementing, and critiquing mental health policy for community and institutional settings
7. Supports the contribution of leadership, as it occurs within the advanced practice role, to effective care and treatment
8. Practices independently within legislated scope of practice
9. Supports and participates in mentoring and coaching new graduates
10. Utilizes knowledge of collaborative strategies for social action in working with consumer and advocacy groups

REFERENCES

Canadian Nurses Association [CNA]. (1997, June). *National nursing competency project.* Final report. Ottawa, ON: Author.

_____. (2002). *Code of ethics for registered nurses.* Ottawa, ON: Author.

Society for Education and Research in Psychiatric-Mental Health Nursing. (1996). *Educational preparation for psychiatric-mental health nursing practice.* Pensacola, FL: Author.

Varcoe, C., Rodney, P., & McCormick, J. (2003). Health care relationships in context: An analysis of three ethnographies. *Qualitative Health Research, 13*(7), 957–973.

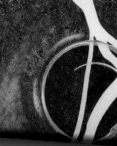

Appendix

E

Canadian Drug Trade Names

SORTED BY DRUG CLASS
*NA means no Canadian Trade Name is available.

ANTIPSYCHOTICS

Generic name	US Trade Name	Canadian Trade Name
Chlorpromazine	Thorazine	Chlorprom, Chlorpromanyl, Largactil, Novo-Chlorpromazine, Apo-Chlorpromazine
Clozapine	Clozaril, Fazaclo	Clozaril, Gen-clozapine, Rhoxal, Clozapine
Droperidol	Inapsine	NA
Fluphenazine	Prolixin	Apo-Fluphenazine, Moditen, PMS-Fluphenazine, Modecate
Haloperidol	Haldol	Apo-Haloperidol, Novo-Peridol, Peridol
Loxapine	Loxitane	Loxapac, PMS-Loxapine, Apo-Loxitane, Nu-Loxitane
Mesoridazine	Serentil	Serentil
Molindone	Moban	Moban
Olanzapine	Zyprexa, Zydis	Zyprexa, Zydis
Perphenazine	Trilafon	Apo-Perphenazine, Phenazine
Prochlorperazine	Compazine, Compro	Stemetil, PMS-Prochlorperazine, Nu-Prochlor, Compazine
Quetiapine	Seroquel	Seroquel
Risperidone	Risperdal	Risperdal
Thioridazine	Mellaril	Apo-Thioridazine, Mellaril
Thiothixene	Navane	Navane
Trifluoperazine	Stelazine	Apo-Trifluoperazine, Novo-Trifluoperazine, PMS-Trifluoperazine, Terfluzine
Ziprasidone	Geodon	Geodon

ANTIDEPRESSANTS

Generic Name	US Trade Name	Canadian Trade Name
Amitriptyline	Elavil	Levate, Novotriptyn
Bupropion	Wellbutrin, Zyban	Wellbutrin, Zyban
Citalopram	Celexa	Celexa
Clomipramine	Anafranil	Apo-Clomipramine, Gen-Clomipramine, Novo-Clopamine, Anafranil
Desipramine	Norpramin, Pertofrane	Apo-Desipramine, Novo-Desipramine, Nu-Desipramine, PMS-Desipramine, Norpramin, Alti-Desipramine
Duloxetine	Cymbalta	NA

(continued)

ANTIDEPRESSANTS (*Continued*)

Generic Name	US Trade Name	Canadian Trade Name
Doxepin	Sinequan, Prudoxin, Zonalon	Alti-Doxepin, Apo-Doxepin, Novo-Doxepin, Triadapin, Zonalon
Escitalopram	Lexapro	NA
Fluoxetine	Prozac, Sarfem	Apo-Fluoxetine, Novo-Fluoxetine, Alti-Fluoxetine, Prozac, PMS-Fluoxetine, FXT, Gen-Fluoxetine, Rhoxal-Fluoxetine
Fluvoxamine	Luvox	Apo-Fluvoxamine, Luvox, Alti-Fluvoxamine, Novo-Fluvoxamine, Nu-Fluvoxamine, Rhoxal-fluvoxamine
Imipramine	Tofranil	Apo-Imipramine, Impril, Tofranil
Isocarboxazid	Marplan	NA
Maprotiline	Ludiomil	Novo-Maprotiline
Mirtazapine	Remeron	Remeron
Nefazodone	Serzone	Apo-Nefazodone, Lin-Nefazodone, Serzone 5HT
Nortriptyline	Aventyl, Pamelor	Apo-Nortriptyline, Norventyl, PMS-Nortriptyline, Gen-Nortriptyline, Nu-Nortriptyline, Aventyl
Paroxetine	Paxil	Paxil
Phenelzine	Nardil	Nardil
Sertraline	Zoloft	Apo-Sertraline, Gen-Sertraline, Novo-Sertraline, Nu-Sertraline, PMS-Sertraline, ratio-Sertraline, Zoloft
Tranylcypromine	Parnate	Parnate
Trazodone	Desyrel	Alti-Trazodone, Apo-Trazodone, Nu-Trazodone, Desyrel, Gen-Trazodone, Novo-Trazodone, PMS-Trazodone
Venlafaxine	Effexor	Effexor

ANTIMANIC AND MOOD STABILIZERS

Generic Name	US Trade Name	Canadian Trade Name
Carbamazepine	Tegretol, Epitol, Equerto	Apo-Carbamazepine, Novo-Carbamaz, Nu-Carbamazepine, PMS-Carbamazepine, Taro-Carbamazepine
Gabapentin	Neurontin	PMS Gabapentin, Neurontin, Apo-Gabapentin, Novo-Gabapentin, Nu-Gabapentin
Lamotrigine	Lamictal	Apo-Lamotrigine, Lamictal, PMS-Lamotrigine, ratio-Lamotrigine
Lithium	Lithane, Eskalith, Lithobid	Carbolith, Duralith, Lithizine, PMS-Lithium Carbonate, Apo-Lithium
Oxcarbazepine	Trileptal	Trileptal
Topiramate	Topamax	Topamax
Valproic acid	Depakote, Valproate, Depakene	Alti-Divalproex, Deproic, Epival, Gen-Divalproex, Novo-Divalproex, Nu-Divalproex, PMS-Valproic acid, Rhoxal-valproic

ANXIOLYTICS

Generic Name	US Trade Name	Canadian Trade Name
Alprazolam	Xanax	Apo-Alpraz, Novo-Alprazol, Nu-Alpraz, Xanax TS
Buspirone	BuSpar	Apo-Buspirone, Buspirex, Gen-Buspirone, Lin-Buspirone, Novo-Buspirone, Nu-Buspirone, PMS-Buspirone, BuSpar

ANXIOLYTICS (Continued)

Generic Name	US Trade Name	Canadian Trade Name
Chlordiazepoxide	Librium	Apo-Chlordiazepoxide, Corax
Clonazepam	Klonopin	Apo-Clonazepam, Clonapam, Gen-Clonazepam, Rivotril, Novo-Clonazepam, Nu-Clonazepam
Clorazepate	Tranxene	Apo-Chlorazepate, Novo-Clopate
Diazepam	Valium, Diastat	Apo-Diazepam, Diazemuls, Valium, Diastat
Estazolam	ProSom	NA
Flurazepam	Dalmane	Somnol
Hydroxyzine	Atarax, Vistaril	Apo-Hydroxyzine, Novo-Hydroxyzine
Lorazepam	Ativan	Apo-Lorazepam, Novo-Lorazem, Nu-Loraz, Ativan, Riva-Lorazepam
Meprobamate	Miltown	Apo-Meprobamate, Novomepro
Midazolam	Versed	Apo-Midazolam
Oxazepam	Serax	Apo-Oxazepam, Novoxapam, Zapex, Oxpram
Temazepan	Restoril	Apo-Temazepam, Novo-Temazepam

DRUGS USED WITH DEMENTIA

Generic Name	US Trade Name	Canadian Trade Name
Donepezil	Aricept	Aricept
Rivastigmine	Exelon	Exelon
Tacrine	Cognex	NA

DRUGS USED FOR ADHD

Generic Name	US Trade Name	Canadian Trade Name
Atomoxetine	Strattera	NA
Amphetamine	Adderall	NA
Amphetamine, long-acting	Adderall XR	NA
Dexmethylphenidate	Focalin	NA
Dextroamphetamine	Dexedrine	Dexedrine
Methylphenidate	Ritalin	PMS-Methylphenidate, Riphenidate
Methylphenidate, long-acting	Concerta, Metadate CD, Ritalin LA	NA
Pemoline	Cylert	NA

DRUGS USED TO TREAT SIDE EFFECTS

Generic name	US Trade Name	Canadian Trade Name
Amantadine	Symmetrel	Endantadine, Gen-Amantadine
Atenolol	Tenormin	Apo-Atenolol, Gen-Atenolol, Novo-Atenol, Tenolin
Benztropine	Cogentin	Apo-Benztropine, Cogentin
Biperiden	Akineton	Akineton
Diphenhydramine	Benadryl (Multiple OTC names)	Allerdryl, Allernix, Benadryl
Procyclidine	Kemadrin	PMS Procyclidine, Procyclid
Trihexyphenidyl	Artane	Apo-Trihex

DRUGS USED IN SUBSTANCE ABUSE

Generic name	US Trade Name	Canadian Trade Name
Clonidine	Catapres	Apo-Clonidine, Dixarit, Nu-Clonidine, Novo-Chonidine, Catapres
Disulfiram	Antabuse	NA
Naltrexone	ReVia, Depade, Trexan	ReVia
Ondansetron	Zofran	NA
Ondansetron Hydrochloride Dihydrate	Zofran	NA

ALPHABETICAL LISTING BY CANADIAN DRUG NAME

Canadian Trade Name	Generic Name
Allerdryl	Diphenhydramine
Allernix	Diphenhydramine
Alti-Desipramine	Desipramine
Alti-Doxepin	Doxepin
Alti-Fluoxetine	Fluoxetin
Alti-Fluvoxamine	Fluvoxamine
Alti-Trazodone	Trazodone
Alti-Valproic	Valproic acid
Anafranil	Clomipramine
Apo-Alpraz	Alprazolam
Apo-Atenolol	Atenolol
Apo-Benztropine	Benztropine
Apo-Buspirone	Buspirone
Apo-Carbamazepine	Carbamazepine
Apo-Chlorazepate	Clorazepate
Apo-Chlordiazepoxide	Chlordiazepoxide
Apo-Chlorpromazine	Chlorpromazine
Apo-Clomipramine	Clomipramine
Apo-Clonazepam	Clonazepam
Apo-Clonidine	Clonidine
Apo-Desipramine	Desipramine
Apo-Diazepam	Diazepam
Apo-Doxepin	Doxepin
Apo-Fluoxetine	Fluoxetine
Apo-Fluphenazine Moditen	Fluphenazine
Apo-Fluvoxamine	Fluvoxamine
Apo-Gabapentin	Gabapentin
Apo-Haloperidol	Haloperidol
Apo-Hydroxyzine	Hydroxyzine
Apo-Imipramine	Imipramine
Apo-Lamotrigine	Lamotrigine
Apo-Lithium	Lithium
Apo-Lorazepam	Lorazepam
Apo-Loxitane	Loxitane
Apo-Midazolam	Midazolam
Apo-Meprobamate	Meprobamate
Apo-Nefazodone	Nefazodone
Apo-Nortriptyline	Nortriptyline
Apo-Oxazepam	Oxazepam
Apo-Perphenazine	Perphenazine
Apo-Sertraline	Sertraline
Apo-Temazepam	Temazepam
Apo-Thioridazine	Thioridazine
Apo-Trazodone	Trazodone
Apo-Trifluoperazine	Trifluoperazine

ALPHABETICAL LISTING BY CANADIAN DRUG NAME (*Continued*)

Canadian Trade Name	Generic Name
Apo-Trihex	Trihexyphenidyl
Aricept	Donepezil
Ativan	Lorazepam
Aventyl	Nortriptyline
BuSpar	Buspirone
Buspirex	Buspirone
Carbolith	Lithium
Chlorprom	Chlorpromazine
Chlorpromanyl	Chlorpromazine
Clonapam	Clonazepam
Clozaril	Clozapine
Cogentin	Benztropine
Compazine	Prochlorperazine
Compro	Prochlorperazine
Corax	Chlordiazepoxide
Deproic	Valproic acid
Desyrel	Trazodone
Dexedrine	Dextroamphetamine
Diastat	Diazepam
Diazemuls	Diazepam
Divalproex	Valproic acid
Dixarit	Clonidine
Duralith	Lithium
Endantadine	Amantadine
Effexor	Venlafaxine
Epitrol	Carbamazepine
Epival	Valproic acid
Equerto	Carbamazepine
Exelon	Rivastigmine
FXT	Fluoxetine
Gen-Amantadine	Amantadine
Gen-Atenolol	Atenolol
Gen-Buspirone	Buspirone
Gen-Clomipramine	Clomipramine
Gen-Clonazepam	Clonazepam
Gen-Clozapine	Clozapine
Gen-Divalproex	Valproic acid
Gen-Fluoxetine	Fluoxetine
Gen-Nortriptyline	Nortriptyline
Gen-Sertraline	Sertraline
Gen-Trazodone	Trazodone
Geodon	Ziprasidone
Impril	Imipramine
Lamictal	Lamotrigine
Largactil	Chlorpromazine
Levate	Amitriptyline
Lin-Buspirone	Buspirone
Lin-Nefazodone	Nefazodone
Lithizine	Lithium
Loxapac	Loxapine
Luvox	Fluvoxamine
Mellaril	Thioridazine
Modecate	Flupheazine
Moditen	Fluphenazine
Nardil	Phenelzine
Navane	Thiothixene
Neurontin	Gabapentin
Norpramin	Desipramine
Norventyl	Nortriptyline

(continued)

ALPHABETICAL LISTING BY CANADIAN DRUG NAME (*Continued*)

Canadian Trade Name	Generic Name
Novo-Alprozol	Alprazolam
Novo-Atenol	Atenolol
Novo-Buspirone	Buspirone
Novo-Carbamaz	Carbamazepine
Novo-Chlorpromazine	Chlorpromazine
Novo-Clonazepam	Clonazepam
Novo-Clopamine	Clomipramine
Novo-Clopate	Clorazepate
Novo-Desipramine	Desipramine
Novo-Divalproex	Valproic acid
Novo-Doxepin	Doxepin
Novo-Fluoxetine	Fluoxetine
Novo-Fluvoxamine	Fluvoxamine
Novo-Gabapentin	Gabapentin
Novo-Hydroxyzine	Hydroxyzine
Novo-Lorazem	Lorazepam
Novo-Maprotiline	Maprotiline
Novomepro	Meprobamate
Novo-Peridol	Haloperidol
Novopramine	Imipramine
Novo-Sertraline	Sertraline
Novo-Temazepam	Temazepam
Novo-Trifluoperazine	Trifluoperazine
Novo-Trazodone	Trazodone
Novotriptyn	Amitriptyline
Novoxapam	Oxazepam
Nu-Alpraz	Alprazolam
Nu-Buspirone	Buspirone
Nu-Carbamazepine	Carbamazepine
Nu-Clonazepam	Clonazepam
Nu-Clonidine	Clonidine
Nu-Desipramine	Desipramine
Nu-Divalproex	Valproic acid
Nu-Fluvoxamine	Fluvoxamine
Nu-Gabapentin	Gabapentin
Nu-Loraz	Lorazepam
Nu-Loxitane	Loxitane
Nu-Nortriptyline	Nortriptyline
Nu-Promchlor	Prochlorperazine
Nu-Sertraline	Sertraline
Nu-Trazodone	Trazodone
Parnate	Tranylcypromine
Paxil	Paroxetine
Peridol	Haloperidol
Phenazine	Perphenazine
PMS Benztropine	Benztropine
PMS-Buspirone	Buspirone
PMS-Carbamazepine	Carbamazepine
PMS-Desipramine	Desipramine
PMS-Fluoxetine	Fluoxetine
PMS-Fluphenazine	Fluphenazine
PMS Gabapentin	Gabapentin
PMS-Lamotrigine	Lamotrigine
PMS-Lithium Carbonate	Lithium
PMS-Loxapine	Loxapine
PMS-Methylphenidate	Methylphenidate
PMS-Nortriptyline	Nortriptyline
PMS-Prochlorperazine	Prochlorperazine
PMS Procyclidine	Procyclidine
PMS-Sertraline	Sertraline
PMS-Trazodone	Trazodone

ALPHABETICAL LISTING BY CANADIAN DRUG NAME (*Continued*)

Canadian Trade Name	Generic Name
PMS-Trifluoperazine	Trifluoperazine
PMS-Valproic acid	Valproic acid
Procyclid	Procyclidine
Prozac	Fluoxetine
ratio-Lamotrigine	Lamotrigine
ratio-Sertraline	Sertraline
Remeron	Mirtazapine
Restoril	Temazepam
Rhoxal-clozapine	Clozapine
Rhoxal-fluoxetine	Fluoxetine
Rhoxal-fluvoxamine	Fluvoxamine
Rhoxal-valproic	Valproic acid
Riphenidate	Methylphenidate
Risperdal	Risperidone
Riva-Lorazepam	Lorazepam
Rivotril	Clonazepam
Serentil	Mesoridazine
Serzone5HT	Nefazodone
Somnol	Flurazepam
Stemetil	Prochlorperazine
Taro-Carbamazepine	Carbamazepine
Tenolin	Atenolol
Terfluzine	Trifluoperazine
Tofranil	Imipramine
Topamax	Topiramate
Triadapin	Doxepin
Trileptal	Oxcarbazepine
Valium	Diazepam
Vivol	Diazepam
Wellbutrin	Bupropion
Xanax TS	Alprazolam
Zapex	Oxazepam
Zoloft	Sertraline
Zonalon	Doxepin
Zyban	Bupropion
Zydis	Olanzapine
Zyprexa	Olanzapine

Mexican Drug Trade Names

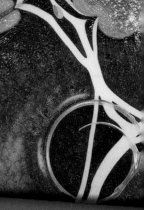

Mexican Trade Name	Generic Name
Abilify	Aripiprazole
Actinium	Oxcarbazepine
Akineton	Biperiden
Alboral	Diazepam
Altruline	Sertraline
Aluprex	Sertraline
Anafranil	Chlomipramine
Ativan	Lorazepam
Aropax	Paroxetine
Carbazep	Carbamazepine
Carbazina	Carbamazepine
Carbolit	Lithium
Clopsine	Clozapine
Clostedol	Carbamazepine
Cryoval	Valproic acid
Dehydrobenzperidol	Droperidol
Depakene	Valproic acid
Dormicum	Midazolam
Efexor	Venlafaxine
Epival	Valproic acid
Eranz	Donepezil
Exelon	Rivastigmine
Fluoxac	Fluoxetine
Flupazine	Trifluoperazine
Haldol	Haloperidol
Haloperil	Haloperidol
Hipokinon	Trihexyphenidyl
Kenoket	Clonazepam
Lamictal	Lamotrigine
Largactil	Chlorpromazine
Leponex	Clozapine
Leptilan	Valproic acid
Leptopsique	Perphenazine
Litheum	Lithium
Luvox	Fluvoxamine
Mellaril	Thiorodazine
Neugeron	Carbamazepine

(continued)

(Continued)

Mexican Trade Name	Generic Name
Neurontin	Gabapentin
Neurosine	Buspirone
Ortopsique	Diazepam
Pacitran	Diazepam
Paxil	Paroxetine
Prozac	Fluoxetine
Remeron	Mirtazapine
Risperdal	Risperidone
Rivotril	Clonazepam
Seropram	Citalopram
Seroquel	Quetiapine
Sinestron	Lorazepam
Siquial	Fluoxetine
Stelazine	Trifluoperazine
Taloprim	Imipramine
Tasedan	Estazolam
Tofranil	Imipramine
Topamax	Topiramate
Tranxene	Chlorazepate
Trileptal	Oxcabazepine
Tzoali	Diphenhydramine
Valium	Diazepam
Valprocid	Valproic acid
Wellbutrin	Bupropion
Zyprexa	Olanzapine

Sleep disorders are organized into four categories: primary sleep disorders; sleep disorder related to another mental disorder; sleep disorder due to a general medical condition; and substance-induced sleep disorder.

Primary sleep disorders are those disorders not attributable to another cause and include dyssomnias and parasomnias.

Dyssomnias are primary disorders of initiating or maintaining sleep or excessive sleepiness and are characterized by abnormalities in the amount, quality, or timing of sleep.

- Primary insomnia—Difficulty initiating or maintaining sleep or of nonrestorative sleep that lasts for one month and causes significant distress or impairment in social, occupational, or other important areas of functioning. Estimates are 1%–10% of the general adult population and up to 25% of the elderly suffer from primary insomnia. Treatment modalities include sleep hygiene measures (see Sleep Hygiene Measures box), cognitive behavioral techniques, and medication.
- Primary hyperinsomnia—Excessive sleepiness for at least one month that involves either prolonged sleep episodes or daily daytime sleeping that causes significant distress or impairment in functioning. Major sleep episodes may be 8–12 hours long, and the person has difficulty waking. Daytime naps leave the person unrefreshed upon awakening. Treatment with stimulant medication is often effective.
- Narcolepsy—Excessive sleepiness characterized by repeated, irresistible sleep attacks. After sleeping 10–20 minutes, the person is briefly refreshed until the next sleep attack. Sleep attacks can occur at inopportune times, such as during important work activities or while driving a car. People with narcolepsy may also experience cataplexy (sudden episodes of bilateral, reversible loss of muscle tone that last for seconds to minutes) or recurrent intrusions of REM sleep in the sleep–wake transitions, manifested by paralysis of voluntary muscles or dream-like hallucinations. Treatment includes stimulant medication, modafinil

(Provigil), and behavioral structuring, such as scheduling naps at convenient times.
- Breathing-related sleep disorders—Sleep disruption leading to excessive sleepiness or, less commonly, insomnia, caused by abnormalities in ventilation during sleep. These disorders include obstructive sleep apnea (repeated episodes of upper airway obstruction), central sleep apnea (episodic cessation of ventilation without airway obstruction), and central alveolar hypoventilation (hypoventilation resulting in low arterial oxygen levels). Central sleep apnea is more common in the elderly while obstructive sleep apnea and central alveolar hypoventilation are commonly seen in obese individuals. The primary treatments for breathing-related sleep disorders are surgical, such as tracheotomy, and use of a continuous positive airway pressure (CPAP) machine during sleep.
- Circadian rhythm sleep disorder (formerly sleep–wake schedule disorder)—Persistent or recurring sleep disruption resulting from altered functioning of circadian rhythm or a mismatch between circadian rhythm and external demands. Subtypes include delayed sleep phase (person's own circadian schedule is incongruent with needed timing of sleep, such as an individual being unable to sleep or remain awake during socially acceptable hours as a result of a work schedule or the like); jet lag (conflict of sleep–wake schedule and a new time zone); shift work (conflict between circadian rhythm and demands of wakefulness for shift work); and unspecified (circadian rhythm pattern is longer than 24 hours despite environmental cues, resulting in varying sleep problems). Sleep hygiene measures (see Sleep Measures Hygiene box), melatonin, and bright light therapy can be effective treatments. Bright light therapy consists of being exposed to bright light when wakefulness is initiated and avoiding bright lights when sleep is desired.

Parasomnias are disorders characterized by abnormal behavioral or psychological events associated with sleep, specific sleep stages, or sleep–wake transition. These disorders involve activation of physiological systems, such as the

SLEEP HYGIENE MEASURES

Establish a regular schedule for going to bed and arising.

Avoid sleep deprivation, and the desire to "catch up" by excessive sleeping.

Do not eat large meals before bedtime; however, a light snack is permissible, even helpful.

Avoid daytime naps, unless necessitated by advanced age or physical condition.

Exercise daily, particularly in the late afternoon or early evening, as exercise before retiring may interfere with sleep.

Minimize or eliminate caffeine and nicotine ingestion.

Do not look at the clock while lying in bed.

Keep the temperature in the bedroom slightly cool.

Do not drink alcohol in an attempt to sleep; it will worsen sleep disturbances and produce poor quality sleep.

Do not use bed for reading, working, watching television, and so forth.

If you are worried about something, try writing it down on paper and assigning a designated time to deal with it—then, let it go.

Soft music, relaxation tapes, or "white noise" may be helpful; experiment with different methods to find those that are beneficial for you.

autonomic nervous system, motor system, or cognitive processes, at inappropriate times, as during sleep.

- Nightmare disorder—Repeated occurrence of frightening dreams that lead to waking from sleep. The dreams are often lengthy and elaborate, provoking anxiety or terror and causing the individual to have trouble returning to sleep and to experience significant distress and,

sometimes, lack of sleep. There is no widely accepted treatment.

- Sleep terror disorder—Repeated occurrence of abrupt awakenings from sleep associated with a panicky scream or cry. Children with sleep terror disorder are confused and upset upon awakening and have no memory of a dream either at the time of awakening or in the morning. Initially, the child is difficult to fully awaken or console. Sleep terror disorder tends to go away in adolescence.
- Sleepwalking disorder—Repeated episodes of complex motor behavior initiated during sleep, including getting out of bed and walking around. Persons appear disoriented and confused and, on occasion, may become violent. Usually they return to bed on their own or can be guided back to bed. Sleepwalking occurs most often in children between 4 and 8 years, and it tends to dissipate by adolescence. No treatment is required.

Sleep disorders related to another mental disorder may involve insomnia or hypersomnia. Mood disorders, anxiety disorders, schizophrenia, and other psychotic disorders are often associated with sleep disturbances. Treatment of the underlying mental disorder is indicated to resolve the sleep disorder.

Sleep disorder due to a general medical condition may involve insomnia, hypersomnia, parasomnias, or a combination of these attributable to a medical condition. These sleep disturbances may result from degenerative neurological illnesses, cerebrovascular disease, endocrine conditions, viral and bacterial infections, coughing, or pain. Sleep disturbances of this type may improve with treatment of the underlying medical condition or may be treated symptomatically with medication for sleep.

Substance-induced sleep disorder involves prominent disturbance in sleep due to the direct physiologic effects of a substance, such as alcohol, other drugs, or toxins. Insomnia and hypersomnia are most common. Treatment of the underlying substance use or abuse generally leads to improvement in sleep.

Adapted from *DSM-IV-TR* (2000) and Mendelson, W. (2005). Sleep disorders. In B. J. Sadock and V. A. Sadock (Eds.). *Comprehensive textbook of psychiatry*, (8th ed., pp. 2022–2034). Philadelphia: Lippincott Williams & Wilkins.

Appendix

H

Sexual and Gender Identity Disorders

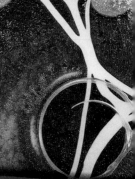

DSM-IV-TR (2000) identifies three groups of sexual and gender identity disorders: sexual dysfunctions (desire, arousal, orgasmic, pain, and dysfunction due to a medical condition); paraphilias (exhibitionism, fetishism, frotteurism, pedophilia, masochism, sadism, transvestic fetishism, and voyeurism), and gender identity disorders. These disorders are usually identified in primary care or outpatient settings and treated with individual, couple/partner, or group psychotherapy. Occasionally, when the diagnosis coincides with behavior defined as criminal, i.e., many of the paraphilias, individuals get involved in the legal system.

SEXUAL DYSFUNCTIONS

Sexual dysfunction is characterized by a disturbance in the processes of the sexual response cycle or by pain associated with sexual intercourse. The sexual response cycle consists of desire, excitement, orgasm, and resolution. Sexual dysfunction may be due to psychological factors alone or a combination of psychological factors and a medical condition.

Sexual desire disorders involve a disruption in the desire phase of the sexual response cycle.
- Hypoactive sexual desire disorder—Characterized by a deficiency or absence of sexual fantasies and desire for sexual activity that causes marked distress or interpersonal difficulty.
- Sexual aversion disorder—Involves aversion to and active avoidance of genital sexual contact with a sexual partner that causes marked distress or interpersonal difficulty. The individual reports anxiety, fear, or disgust when confronted by a sexual opportunity with a partner.

Sexual arousal disorders are a disruption of the excitement phase of the sexual response cycle.
- Female sexual arousal disorder—Persistent or recurrent inability to attain or to maintain, until completion of the sexual activity, an adequate lubrication–swelling

response of sexual excitement, which causes marked distress or interpersonal difficulty.
- Male erectile disorder—Persistent or recurrent inability to attain or maintain, until completion of the sexual activity, an adequate erection, which causes marked distress or interpersonal difficulty.

Orgasmic disorders are disruptions of the orgasm phase of the sexual response cycle.
- Female orgasmic disorders—Persistent or recurrent delay in, or absence of, orgasm following a normal sexual excitement phase, which causes marked distress or interpersonal difficulty.
- Male orgasmic disorder—Persistent or recurrent delay in, or absence of, orgasm following a normal sexual excitement phase, which causes marked distress or interpersonal difficulty.
- Premature ejaculation—Persistent or recurrent onset of orgasm and ejaculation with minimal sexual stimulation before, on, or shortly after penetration and before the person wishes it, causing marked distress or interpersonal difficulty.

Sexual pain disorders involve pain associated with sexual activity.
- Dyspareunia—Genital pain associated with sexual intercourse causing marked distress or interpersonal difficulties. It can occur in both males and females, and symptoms range from mild discomfort to sharp pain.
- Vaginismus—Persistent or recurrent involuntary contractions of the perineal muscles surrounding the outer third of the vagina when vaginal penetration with penis, finger, tampon, or speculum is attempted, causing marked distress or interpersonal difficulties. The contraction may range from mild (tightness and mild discomfort) to severe (preventing penetration).

Sexual dysfunction due to a general medical condition is presence of clinically significant sexual dysfunction that is exclusively due to the physiological effects of a medical condition. It can include pain with intercourse, hypoactive sexual desire, erectile dysfunction, orgasmic problems, or other problems as previously described. The individual experiences marked distress or interpersonal difficulty related to the symptoms.

Substance-induced sexual dysfunction is clinically significant sexual dysfunction resulting in marked distress or interpersonal difficulty caused by the direct physiological effects of a substance (drug of abuse, medication, or toxin). It may involve impaired arousal, impaired orgasm, or sexual pain.

PARAPHILIAS

Paraphilias are recurrent, intensely sexually arousing fantasies, sexual urges, or behaviors generally involving 1) nonhuman objects, 2) the suffering or humiliation of one's self or partner, or 3) children or other nonconsenting persons. For pedophilia, voyeurism, exhibitionism, and frotteurism, the diagnosis is made if the person has acted on these urges or if the urges or fantasies cause marked distress or interpersonal difficulty. For sexual sadism, the diagnosis is made if the person has acted on these urges with a nonconsenting person or if the urges, fantasies, or behaviors cause marked distress or interpersonal difficulty. For the remaining paraphilias, the diagnosis is made if the behavior, sexual urges, or fantasies cause clinically significant distress or impairment in social, occupational, or other important areas of functioning.

- Exhibitionism—Exposure of the genitals to a stranger, sometimes involving masturbation; usually occurs before age 18 and is less severe after age 40.
- Fetishism—Use of nonliving objects (the fetish) to obtain sexual excitement and/or achieve orgasm. Common fetishes include women's underwear, bras, lingerie, shoes, or other apparel. The person might masturbate while holding or rubbing the object. It begins by adolescence and tends to be chronic.
- Frotteurism—Touching and rubbing against a nonconsenting person, usually in a crowded place from which the person with frotteurism can make a quick escape, such as public transportation, a shopping mall, or a crowded sidewalk. The individual rubs his genitals against the victim's thighs and buttocks or fondles her breasts or genitalia with his hands. Acts of frottage occur most often between the ages of 15 and 25; frequency declines after that.
- Pedophilia—Sexual activity with a prepubescent child (generally 13 years or younger) by someone at least 16 years old and 5 years older than the child. It can include an individual undressing the child and looking at the child; exposing him- or herself; masturbating in the presence of the child; touching and fondling the child; fellatio; cunnilingus; or penetration of the child's vagina, anus, or mouth with the individual's fingers or penis or with foreign objects, with varying amounts of force. Contact may involve the individual's own children, stepchildren or relatives, or strangers. Many individuals with pedophilia do not experience distress about their fantasies, urges, or behaviors.

- Sexual masochism—Recurrent, intensely sexually arousing fantasies, sexual urges, or behaviors involving the act of being humiliated, beaten, bound, or otherwise made to suffer. Some individuals act on masochistic urges by themselves, others with a partner.
- Sexual sadism—Recurrent, intensely sexually arousing fantasies, sexual urges, or behaviors involving acts in which the psychological or physical suffering of the victim is sexually arousing to the person. It can involve domination (caging the victim or forcing victim to crawl, beg, plead), restraint, spanking, beating, electrical shock, rape, cutting, and, in severe cases, torture and death. Victims may be consenting (those with sexual masochism) or nonconsenting.
- Transvestic fetishism—Recurrent, intensely sexually arousing fantasies, sexual urges, or behaviors involving cross-dressing by a heterosexual male.
- Voyeurism—Recurrent, intensely sexually arousing fantasies, sexual urges, or behaviors involving the act of observing an unsuspecting person who is naked, in the process of undressing, or engaging in sexual activity. Voyeurism usually begins before age 15, is chronic, and may involve masturbation during the voyeuristic behavior.

GENDER IDENTITY DISORDER

Gender identity disorder is diagnosed when an individual has a strong and persistent cross-gender identification, that is, when an individual has the desire to be, or insists that he or she is of, the other sex, accompanied by the persistent discomfort of his or her assigned sex or a sense of inappropriateness in the gender role of that assigned sex. The person experiences clinically significant distress or impairment in social, occupational, or other important areas of functioning. In boys, there is a preoccupation with traditionally feminine activities, a preference for dressing in girls' or women's clothing, and an expressed desire to be a girl or grow up to be a woman. Girls may resist parental attempts to have them wear dresses or other feminine attire, wear boys' clothing, have short hair, ask to be called by a boy's name, and express the desire to grow a penis and grow up to be a man.

Adapted from *DSM-IV-TR* (2000). American Psychiatric Association. Washington, D.C.

Abnormal Involuntary Movement Scale (AIMS): tool used to screen for symptoms of movement disorders (side effects of neuroleptic medications)

abstract messages: unclear patterns of words that often contain figures of speech that are difficult to interpret

abstract thinking: ability to make associations or interpretations about a situation or comment

abuse: the wrongful use and maltreatment of another person

acceptance: avoiding judgments of the person, no matter what the behavior

ACCESS Demonstration Project: initiated to assess whether or not more integrated systems of service delivery enhance the quality of life of homeless people with serious mental disabilities

acculturation: altering cultural values or behaviors as a way to adapt to another culture

acting out: an immature defense mechanism by which the person deals with emotional conflicts or stressors through actions rather than through reflection or feelings

active listening: concentrating exclusively on what the client says, refraining from other internal mental activities

active observation: watching the speaker's nonverbal actions as he or she communicates

acute stress disorder: diagnosis is appropriate when symptoms appear within the first month after the trauma and do not persist longer than 4 weeks

advocacy: the process of acting in the client's behalf when he or she cannot do so

affect: the outward expression of the client's emotional state

agnosia: inability to recognize or name objects despite intact sensory abilities

agoraphobia: fear of being outside; from the Greek, *fear of the marketplace*

akathisia: intense need to move about; characterized by restless movement, pacing, inability to remain still, and the client's report of inner restlessness

alexithymia: difficulty identifying and expressing feelings

alogia: a lack of any real meaning or substance in what the client says

Alzheimer's disease: a progressive brain disorder that has a gradual onset but causes an increasing decline in functioning, including loss of speech, loss of motor function, and profound personality and behavioral changes such as those involving paranoia, delusions, hallucinations, inattention to hygiene, and belligerence

amnestic disorder: characterized by a disturbance in memory that results directly from the physiologic effects of a general medical condition or from the persisting effects of a substance such as alcohol or other drugs

anergia: lack of energy

anger: a normal human emotion involving a strong, uncomfortable, emotional response to a real or perceived provocation

anhedonia: having no pleasure or joy in life; losing any sense of pleasure from activities formerly enjoyed

anorexia nervosa: an eating disorder characterized by the client's refusal or inability to maintain a minimally normal body weight, intense fear of gaining weight or becoming fat, significantly disturbed perception of the shape or size of the body, and steadfast inability or refusal to acknowledge the existence or seriousness of a problem

anticholinergic effects: dry mouth, constipation, urinary hesitancy or retention, dry nasal passages, and blurred near vision; commonly seen as side effects of medication

anticipatory grieving: when people facing an imminent loss begin to grapple with the very real possibility of the loss or death in the near future

antidepressant drugs: primarily used in the treatment of major depressive illness, anxiety disorders, the depressed phase of bipolar disorder, and psychotic depression

antipsychotic drugs: also known as *neuroleptics;* used to treat the symptoms of psychosis such as the delusions and hallucinations seen in schizophrenia, schizoaffective disorder, and the manic phase of bipolar disorder

antisocial personality disorder: characterized by a pervasive pattern of disregard for and violation of the rights of others and with the central characteristics of deceit and manipulation

anxiety: a vague feeling of dread or apprehension; it is a response to external or internal stimuli that can have behavioral, emotional, cognitive, and physical symptoms

anxiety disorders: a group of conditions that share a key feature of excessive anxiety, with ensuing behavioral, emotional, cognitive, and physiologic responses

anxiolytic drugs: used to treat anxiety and anxiety disorders, insomnia, OCD, depression, posttraumatic stress disorder, and alcohol withdrawal

aphasia: deterioration of language function

apraxia: impaired ability to execute motor functions despite intact motor abilities

assault: involves any action that causes a person to fear being touched, without consent or authority, in a way that is offensive, insulting, or physically injurious

assertive community treatment (ACT): community-based programs that provide many of the services that are necessary for successful community living; includes case management, problem solving, social skills training; support, teaching on a 24/7 basis

assertiveness training: techniques using statements to identify feelings and communicate needs and concerns to others; helps the person negotiate interpersonal situations, fosters self-assurance, and ultimately assists the person to take more control over life situations

asylum: a safe refuge or haven offering protection; in the United States, became a term used to describe institutions for the mentally ill

attachment behaviors: affectional bonds with significant others

attention deficit hyperactivity disorder (ADHD): characterized by inattentiveness, overactivity, and impulsiveness

attentive presence: being with the client and focusing intently on communicating with and understanding him or her

attitudes: general feelings or a frame of reference around which a person organizes knowledge about the world

autistic disorder: a pervasive developmental disorder characterized by impairment of growth and development milestones, such as impaired communication with others, lack of social relationships even with parents, and stereotyped motor behaviors

automatism: repeated, seemingly purposeless behaviors often indicative of anxiety, such as drumming fingers, twisting locks of hair, or tapping the foot; unconscious mannerism

autonomy: the person's right to self-determination and independence

avoidance behavior: behavior designed to avoid unpleasant consequences or potentially threatening situations

avoidant personality disorder: characterized by a pervasive pattern of social discomfort and reticence, low self-esteem, and hypersensitivity to negative evaluation

battery: involves harmful or unwarranted contact with a client; actual harm or injury may or may not have occurred

behavior modification: a method of attempting to strengthen a desired behavior or response by reinforcement, either positive or negative

behaviorism: a school of psychology that focuses on observable behaviors and what one can do externally to bring about behavior changes. It does not attempt to explain how the mind works.

beliefs: ideas that one holds to be true

beneficence: refers to one's duty to benefit or to promote good for others

bereavement: refers to the process by which a person experiences grief

binge eating: consuming a large amount of food (far greater than most people eat at one time) in a discrete period of usually 2 hours or less

Black Box Warning: medication package inserts must have a highlighted box, separate from the text, that contains a warning about the life-threatening or otherwise serious side effect(s) of the medication

blackout: an episode during which the person continues to function but has no conscious awareness of his or her behavior at the time nor any later memory of the behavior; usually associated with alcohol consumption

blunted affect: showing little or a slow-to-respond facial expression; few observable facial expressions

body dysmorphic disorder: preoccupation with an imagined or exaggerated defect in physical appearance

body image: how a person perceives his or her body, i.e., a mental self-image

body image disturbance: occurs when there is an extreme discrepancy between one's body image and the perceptions of others and extreme dissatisfaction with one's body image

body language: a nonverbal form of communication: gestures, postures, movements, and body positions

borderline personality disorder: pervasive and enduring pattern of unstable interpersonal relationships, self-image, affect; marked impulsivity; frequent self-mutilation behavior

breach of duty: The nurse (or physician) failed to conform to standards of care, thereby breaching or failing the existing duty. The nurse did not act as a reasonable, prudent nurse would have acted in similar circumstances.

broad affect: displaying a full range of emotional expressions

bulimia nervosa: an eating disorder characterized by recurrent episodes (at least twice a week for 3 months) of binge eating followed by inappropriate compensatory behaviors to avoid weight gain such as purging (self-induced vomiting or use of laxatives, diuretics, enemas, or emetics), fasting, or excessively exercising

case management: management of care on a case-by-case basis, representing an effort to provide necessary services while containing cost; in the community, case management services include accessing medical and psychiatric services and providing assistance with tasks of daily living such as financial management, transportation, buying groceries

catatonia: psychomotor disturbance, either motionless or excessive motor

catharsis: activities that are supposed to provide a release for strong feelings such as anger, rage

causation: action that constitutes a breach of duty and was the direct cause of the loss, damage, or injury. In other words, the loss, damage, or injury would not have occurred if the nurse had acted in a reasonable, prudent manner.

character: consists of concepts about the self and the external world

child abuse: the intentional injury of a child

circumstantial thinking: term used when a client eventually answers a question but only after giving excessive, unnecessary detail

circumstantiality: the use of extraneous words and long, tedious descriptions

cliché: an expression that has become trite and generally conveys a stereotype

client-centered therapy: focused on the role of the client, rather than the therapist, as the key to the healing process

closed body positions: nonverbal behavior such as crossed legs and arms folded over chest that indicate the listener may be failing to listen, defensive, or not accepting

closed group: structured to keep the same members in the group for a specified number of sessions

clubhouse model: community-based rehabilitation; an "intentional community" based on the belief that men and women with serious and persistent psychiatric disability can and will achieve normal life goals when given the opportunity, time, support, and fellowship

codependence: a maladaptive coping pattern on the part of family members or others that results from a prolonged relationship with the person who uses substances

cognitive behavioral techniques: techniques useful in changing patterns of thinking by helping clients to recognize negative thoughts and to replace them with different patterns of thinking; include positive self-talk, decatastrophizing, positive reframing, thought stopping

cognitive therapy: focuses on immediate thought processing: how a person perceives or interprets his or her experience and determines how he or she feels and behaves

command hallucinations: disturbed auditory sensory perceptions demanding that the client take action, often to harm self or others, and are considered dangerous; often referred to as "voices"

communication: the processes that people use to exchange information

compensatory behaviors: for clients with eating disorders, actions designed to counteract food intake, such as purging (vomiting), excessively exercising, using/abusing laxatives and diuretics

complicated grieving: a response outside the norm and occurring when a person is void of emotion, grieves for prolonged periods, or has expressions of grief that seem disproportionate to the event

compulsions: ritualistic or repetitive behaviors or mental acts that a person carries out continuously in an attempt to neutralize anxiety

computerized tomography (CT): a diagnostic procedure in which a precise x-ray beam takes cross-sectional images (slices) layer by layer

concrete message: words that are as clear as possible when speaking to the client so that the client can understand the message; concrete messages are important for accurate information exchange

concrete thinking: when the client continually gives literal translations; abstraction is diminished or absent

conduct disorder: characterized by persistent antisocial behavior in children and adolescents that significantly impairs their ability to function in social, academic, or occupational areas

confabulation: clients may make up answers to fill in memory gaps; usually associated with organic brain problems

confidentiality: respecting the client's right to keep private any information about his or her mental and physical health and related care

confrontation: technique designed to highlight the incongruence between a person's verbalizations and actual behavior; used to manage manipulative or deceptive behavior

congruence: occurs when words and actions match

congruent message: when communication content and processes agree

content: verbal communication; the literal words that a person speaks

context: the environment in which an event occurs; includes the time and the physical, social, emotional, and cultural environments

contract: includes outlining the care the nurse will give, the times the nurse will be with the client, and acceptance of these conditions by the client.

controlled substance: drug classified under the Controlled Substances Act; includes opioids, stimulants, benzodiazepines, anabolic steroids, cannabis derivatives, psychedelics, and sedatives

conversion disorder: sometimes called conversion reaction; involves unexplained, usually sudden deficits in sensory or motor function related to an emotional conflict the client experiences but does not handle directly

countertransference: occurs when the therapist displaces onto the client attitudes or feelings from his or her past; process that can occur when the nurse responds to the client based on personal, unconscious needs and conflicts

Creutzfeldt-Jakob disease: a central nervous system disorder that typically develops in adults 40 to 60 years of age and involves altered vision, loss of coordination or abnormal movements, and dementia

criminalization of mental illness: refers to the practice of arresting and prosecuting mentally ill offenders, even for misdemeanors, at a rate four times that of the general population in an effort to contain them in some type of institution where they might receive needed treatment

crisis: a turning point in an individual's life that produces an overwhelming emotional response; individual is confronting life circumstance or stressor that cannot be managed through customary coping strategies

crisis intervention: includes a variety of techniques, based on the assessment of the individual in crisis, to assist in resolution or management of the stressor or circumstance

cues (overt and covert): verbal or nonverbal messages that signal key words or issues for the client

culturally competent: being sensitive to issues related to culture, race, gender, sexual orientation, social class, economic situation, and other factors

culture: all the socially learned behaviors, values, beliefs, and customs, transmitted down to each generation, as well as a population's ways of thinking, that guide its members' views of themselves and the world

cycle of violence: a typical pattern in domestic battering: violence; honeymoon or remorseful period; tension-building; and, finally, violence; this pattern continually repeats itself throughout the relationship

date rape (acquaintance rape): sexual assault that may occur on a first date, on a ride home from a party, or when the two people have known each other for some time

day treatment: treatment programs in which clients attend during the day and return home or to the community at night

decatastrophizing: a technique that involves learning to assess situations realistically rather than always assuming a catastrophe will happen

defense mechanisms: cognitive distortions that a person uses unconsciously to maintain a sense of being in control of a situation, to lessen discomfort, and to deal with stress; also called ego defense mechanisms

deinstitutionalization: a deliberate shift in care of the mentally ill from institutional care in state hospitals to care in community-based facilities and through community-based services

delirium: a syndrome that involves a disturbance of consciousness accompanied by a change in cognition

delusion: a fixed, false belief not based in reality

dementia: a mental disorder that involves multiple cognitive deficits, initially involving memory impairment with progressive deterioration that includes all cognitive functioning

denial: defense mechanism; clients may deny directly having any problems or may minimize the extent of problems or actual substance use

deontology: a theory that says ethical decisions should be based on whether or not an action is morally right with no regard for the result or consequences

dependent personality disorder: characterized by a pervasive and excessive need to be taken care of, which leads to submissive and clinging behavior and fears of separation

depersonalization: feelings of being disconnected from himself or herself; the client feels detached from his or her behavior

depot injection: a slow-release, injectable form of antipsychotic medication for maintenance therapy

depressive personality disorder: characterized by a pervasive pattern of depressive cognitions and behaviors in various contexts

derealization: client senses that events are not real, when, in fact, they are

detoxification: the process of safely withdrawing from a substance

Diagnostic and Statistical Manual of Mental Disorders (DSM-IV-TR): taxonomy published by the APA. The *DSM-IV-TR* describes all mental disorders and outlines specific diagnostic criteria for each based on clinical experience and research.

diagnostic axes: the five axes that comprise diagnosis under *DSM-IV-TR* criteria; include major mental illnesses, mental retardation or personality disorders, medical illnesses, psychosocial stressors, and global assessment of functioning (GAF)

directive role: asking direct, yes/no questions and using problem solving to help the client develop new coping mechanisms to deal with present, here-and-now issues

disease conviction: preoccupation with the fear that one has a serious disease

disease phobia: preoccupation with the fear that one will get a serious disease

disenfranchised grief: grief over a loss that is not or cannot be mourned publicly or supported socially

dissociation: a subconscious defense mechanism that helps a person protect his or her emotional self from recognizing the full effects of some horrific or traumatic event by allowing the mind to forget or remove itself from the painful situation or memory

dissociative disorders: have the essential feature of a disruption in the usually integrated functions of consciousness, memory, identity, or environmental perception; include amnesia, fugue, and dissociative identity disorder

distance zones: amount of physical space between people during communication; in the United States, Canada, and many Eastern European nations, four distance zones are generally observed: intimate zone, personal zone, social zone, and public zone

distraction: involves shifting the client's attention and energy to a different topic

dopamine: a neurotransmitter located primarily in the brain stem; has been found to be involved in the control of complex movements, motivation, cognition, and regulation of emotional responses

dream analysis: a primary method used in psychoanalysis; involves discussing a client's dreams to discover their true meaning and significance

dual diagnosis: the client with both substance abuse and another psychiatric illness

duty: existence of a legally recognized relationship, i.e., physician to client, nurse to client

duty to warn: the exception to the client's right to confidentiality; when health care providers are legally obligated to warn another person who is the target of the threats or plan by the client, even if the threats were discussed during therapy sessions otherwise protected by confidentiality

dysfunctional grieving: extended, unsuccessful attempts to working through the grieving process

dysphoric: mood that involves unhappiness, restlessness, and malaise

dystonia: extrapyramidal side effect to antipsychotic medication; includes acute muscular rigidity and cramping, a stiff or thick tongue with difficulty swallowing, and, in severe cases, laryngospasm and respiratory difficulties; also called dystonic reactions

echolalia: repetition or imitation of what someone else says; echoing what is heard

echopraxia: imitation of the movements and gestures of someone an individual is observing

education group: a therapeutic group; provides information to members on a specific issue: for instance, stress management, medication management, or assertiveness training

efficacy: refers to the maximal therapeutic effect a drug can achieve

ego: in psychoanalytic theory, the balancing or mediating force between the id and the superego; represents mature and adaptive behavior that allows a person to function successfully in the world

elder abuse: the maltreatment of older adults by family members or caretakers

electroconvulsive therapy (ECT): used to treat depression in select groups such as clients who do not respond to antidepressants or those who experience intolerable medication side effects at therapeutic doses

emotion-focused coping strategies: techniques to assist clients to relax and reduce feelings of stress

empathy: the ability to perceive the meanings and feelings of another person and to communicate that understanding to that person

enabling: behaviors that seem helpful on the surface but actually perpetuate the substance use of another, e.g., a wife who calls to report her husband has the flu and will miss work when he is actually drunk or hungover

encopresis: the repeated passage of feces into inappropriate places, such as clothing or the floor, by a child who is at least 4 years of age either chronologically or developmentally

enmeshment: lack of clear role boundaries between persons

enuresis: the repeated voiding of urine during the day or at night into clothing or bed by a child at least 5 years of age either chronologically or developmentally

environmental control: refers to a client's ability to control the surroundings or direct factors in the environment

epinephrine: derivative of norepinephrine, the most prevalent neurotransmitter in the nervous system, located primarily in the brain stem, and which plays a role in changes in attention, learning and memory, sleep and wakefulness, and mood regulation

ethical dilemma: a situation in which ethical principles conflict or when there is no one clear course of action in a given situation

ethics: a branch of philosophy that deals with values of human conduct related to the rightness or wrongness of actions and to the goodness and badness of the motives and ends of such actions

ethnicity: concept of people identifying with one another based on a shared heritage

euthymic: normal or level mood

evolving consumer household (ECH): a group-living situation in which the residents make the transition from a traditional group home to a residence where they fulfill their own responsibilities and function without on-site supervision from paid staff

executive functioning: the ability to think abstractly and to plan, initiate, sequence, monitor, and stop complex behavior

exploitation: phase of nurse–client relationship, identified by Peplau, when the nurse guides the client to examine feelings and responses and to develop better coping skills and a more positive self-image; this encourages behavior change and develops independence; part of the working phase

exposure: behavioral technique that involves having the client deliberately confront the situations and stimuli that he or she is trying to avoid

extrapyramidal side effects: reversible movement disorders induced by antipsychotic or neuroleptic medication

eye contact: looking into the other person's eyes during communication

factitious disorders: characterized by physical symptoms that are feigned or inflicted for the sole purpose of drawing attention to oneself and gaining the emotional benefits of assuming the sick role

false imprisonment: the unjustifiable detention of a client, such as the inappropriate use of restraint or seclusion

family therapy: a form of group therapy in which the client and his or her family members participate to deal with mutual issues

family violence: encompasses domestic or partner battering; neglect and physical, emotional, or sexual abuse of children; elder abuse; and marital rape

fear: feeling afraid or threatened by a clearly identifiable, external stimulus that represents danger to the person

fidelity: refers to the obligation to honor commitments and contracts

flat affect: showing no facial expression

flight of ideas: excessive amount and rate of speech composed of fragmented or unrelated ideas; racing, often unconnected, thoughts

flooding: a form of rapid desensitization in which a behavioral therapist confronts the client with the phobic object (either a picture or the actual object) until it no longer produces anxiety

flushing: a reddening of the face and neck as a result of increased blood flow

free association: a method in psychoanalysis used to gain access to subconscious thoughts and feelings in which the therapist tries to uncover the client's true thoughts and feelings by saying a word and asking the client to respond quickly with the first thing that comes to mind

genuine interest: truly paying attention to the client, caring about what he or she is saying; only possible when the nurse is comfortable with himself or herself and aware of his or her strengths and limitations

going along: technique used with clients with dementia; providing emotional reassurance to clients without correcting their misperceptions or delusions

grief: subjective emotions and affect that are a normal response to the experience of loss

grieving: the process by which a person experiences grief

grounding techniques: helpful to use with the client who is dissociating or experiencing a flashback; grounding techniques remind the client that he or she is in the present, as an adult, and is safe

group therapy: therapy during which clients participate in sessions with others. The members share a common purpose and are expected to contribute to the group to benefit others and to receive benefit from others in return.

half-life: the time it takes for half of the drug to be eliminated from the bloodstream

hallucinations: false sensory perceptions or perceptual experiences that do not really exist

hallucinogen: substances that distort the user's perception of reality and produce symptoms similar to psychosis including hallucinations (usually visual) and depersonalization

hardiness: the ability to resist illness when under stress

hierarchy of needs: a pyramid used to arrange and illustrate the basic drives or needs that motivate people; developed by Abraham Maslow

histrionic personality disorder: characterized by a pervasive pattern of excessive emotionality and attention seeking

homeostasis: a state of equilibrium or balance

hostility: an emotion expressed through verbal abuse, lack of cooperation, violation of rules or norms, or threatening behavior; also called verbal aggression

humanism: focuses on a person's positive qualities, his or her capacity to change (human potential), and the promotion of self-esteem

Huntington's disease: an inherited, dominant gene disease that primarily involves cerebral atrophy, demyelination, and enlargement of the brain ventricles

hypertensive crisis: a life-threatening condition that can result when a client taking MAOIs ingests tyramine-containing foods and fluids or other medications

hypochondriasis: preoccupation with the fear that one has a serious disease or will get a serious disease

hypomania: a period of abnormally and persistently elevated, expansive, or irritable mood lasting 4 days; does not impair the ability to function and does not involve psychotic features

hysteria: refers to multiple, recurrent physical complaints with no organic basis

id: in psychoanalytic theory, the part of one's nature that reflects basic or innate desires such as pleasure-seeking behavior, aggression, and sexual impulses. The id seeks instant gratification; causes impulsive, unthinking behavior; and has no regard for rules or social convention.

ideas of reference: client's inaccurate interpretation that general events are personally directed to him or her, such as hearing a speech on the news and believing the message has personal meaning

impulse control: the ability to delay gratification and to think about one's behavior before acting

inappropriate affect: displaying a facial expression that is incongruent with mood or situation; often silly or giddy regardless of circumstances

incongruent message: when the communication content and process disagree

individual psychotherapy: a method of bringing about change in a person by exploring his or her feelings, attitudes, thinking, and behavior. It involves a one-to-one relationship between the therapist and the client.

inhalant: a diverse group of drugs including anesthetics, nitrates, and organic solvents that are inhaled for their effects

injury or damage: the client suffered some type of loss, damage, or injury

insight: the ability to understand the true nature of one's situation and accept some personal responsibility for that situation

interdisciplinary (multidisciplinary) team: treatment group comprised of individuals from a variety of fields or disciplines; the most useful approach in dealing with the multifaceted problems of clients with mental illness

intergenerational transmission process: explains that patterns of violence are perpetuated from one generation to the next through role modeling and social learning

internalization: keeping stress, anxiety, or frustration inside rather than expressing them outwardly

intimate relationship: a relationship involving two people who are emotionally committed to each other. Both parties are concerned about having their individual needs met and helping each other to meet needs as well. The relationship may include sexual or emotional intimacy as well as sharing of mutual goals.

intimate zone: space of 0 to 18 inches between people; the amount of space comfortable for parents with young children, people who mutually desire personal contact, or people whispering. Invasion of this intimate zone by anyone else is threatening and produces anxiety.

intoxication: use of a substance that results in maladaptive behavior

judgment: refers to the ability to interpret one's environment and situation correctly and to adapt one's behavior and decisions accordingly

justice: refers to fairness, or treating all people fairly and equally without regard for social or economic status, race, sex, marital status, religion, ethnicity, or cultural beliefs

kindling process: the snowball-like effect seen when minor seizure activity seems to build up into more frequent and severe seizures

Korsakoff's syndrome: type of dementia caused by long-term, excessive alcohol intake that results in a chronic thiamine or vitamin B deficiency

la belle indifference: a seeming lack of concern or distress; a key feature of conversion disorder

labile: rapidly changing or fluctuating, such as someone's mood or emotions

latency of response: refers to hesitation before the client responds to questions

least restrictive environment: treatment appropriate to meet the client's needs with only necessary or required restrictions

limbic system: an area of the brain located above the brain stem that includes the thalamus, hypothalamus, hippocampus, and amygdala (although some sources differ regarding the structures that this system includes)

limit-setting: an effective technique that involves three steps: stating the behavioral limit (describing the unacceptable behavior); identifying the consequences if the limit is exceeded; and identifying the expected or desired behavior

loose associations: disorganized thinking that jumps from one idea to another with little or no evident relation between the thoughts

magnetic resonance imaging (MRI): diagnostic test used to visualize soft tissue structures; energy field is created with a magnet and radio waves, then converted into a visual image

malingering: the intentional production of false or grossly exaggerated physical or psychological symptoms

malpractice: a type of negligence that refers specifically to professionals such as nurses and physicians

managed care: a concept designed to purposely control the balance between the quality of care provided and the cost of that care

managed care organizations: developed to control the expenditure of insurance funds by requiring providers to seek approval before the delivery of care

mania: a distinct period during which mood is abnormally and persistently elevated, expansive, or irritable

mental disorder: defined by *DSM-IV-TR* as a clinically significant behavioral or psychological syndrome or pattern that occurs in an individual and that is associated with present distress (e.g., a painful symptom) or disability (i.e., impairment in one or more important areas of functioning) or with a significantly increased risk of suffering death, pain, disability, or an important loss of freedom

mental health: a state of emotional, psychological, and social wellness evidenced by satisfying relationships, effective behavior and coping, positive self-concept, and emotional stability

metaphor: a phrase that describes an object or situation by comparing it to something else familiar

mild anxiety: a sensation that something is different and warrants special attention

milieu therapy: the concept involves clients' interactions with one another; i.e., practicing interpersonal relationship skills, giving one another feedback about behavior, and working cooperatively as a group to solve day-to-day problems

moderate anxiety: the disturbing feeling that something is definitely wrong; the person becomes nervous or agitated

mood: refers to the client's pervasive and enduring emotional state

mood disorders: pervasive alterations in emotions that are manifested by depression, mania, or both

mood-stabilizing drugs: used to treat bipolar disorder by stabilizing the client's mood, preventing or minimizing the highs and lows that characterize bipolar illness, and treating acute episodes of mania

mourning: the outward expression of grief

Munchausen's by proxy: when a person inflicts illness or injury on someone else to gain the attention of emergency medical personnel or to be a hero for "saving" the victim

Munchausen's syndrome: a factitious disorder where the person intentionally causes injury or physical symptoms to self to gain attention and sympathy from health care providers, family, and others

narcissistic personality disorder: characterized by a pervasive pattern of grandiosity (in fantasy or behavior), need for admiration, and lack of empathy

negative reinforcement: involves removing a stimulus immediately after a behavior occurs so that the behavior is more likely to occur again

neglect: malicious or ignorant withholding of physical, emotional, or educational necessities for the child's well-being

negligence: an unintentional tort that involves causing harm by failing to do what a reasonable and prudent person would do in similar circumstances

neologisms: invented words that have meaning only for the client

neuroleptic malignant syndrome (NMS): a potentially fatal, idiosyncratic reaction to an antipsychotic (or neuroleptic) drug

neuroleptics: antipsychotic medications

neurotransmitter: the chemical substances manufactured in the neuron that aid in the transmission of information throughout the body

nondirective role: using broad openings and open-ended questions to collect information and help the client to identify and discuss the topic of concern

nonmaleficence: the requirement to do no harm to others either intentionally or unintentionally

nonverbal communication: the behavior that accompanies verbal content, such as body language, eye contact, facial expression, tone of voice, speed and hesitations in speech, grunts and groans, and distance from the listener

norepinephrine: the most prevalent neurotransmitter in the nervous system

no self-harm contract: a client promises to not engage in self-harm and to report to the nurse when he or she is losing control

obsessions: recurrent, persistent, intrusive, and unwanted thoughts, images, or impulses that cause marked anxiety and interfere with interpersonal, social, or occupational function

obsessive-compulsive personality disorder: characterized by a pervasive pattern of preoccupation with perfectionism, mental and interpersonal control, and orderliness at the expense of flexibility, openness, and efficiency

off-label use: a drug will prove effective for a disease that differs from the one involved in original testing and FDA approval

open group: an ongoing group that runs indefinitely; members join or leave the group as they need to

operant conditioning: the theory which says people learn their behavior from their history or past experiences, particularly those experiences that were repeatedly reinforced

opioid: controlled drugs; often abused because they desensitize the user to both physiologic and psychological pain and induce a sense of euphoria and well-being; some are prescribed for analgesic effects but others are illegal in the United States

orientation phase: the beginning of the nurse–client relationship; begins when the nurse and client meet and ends when the client begins to identify problems to examine

pain disorder: has the primary physical symptom of pain, which generally is unrelieved by analgesics and greatly affected by psychological factors in terms of onset, severity, exacerbation, and maintenance

palilalia: repeating words or sounds over and over

panic anxiety: intense anxiety, may be a response to a life-threatening situation

panic attack: between 15 and 30 minutes of rapid, intense, escalating anxiety in which the person experiences great emotional fear as well as physiologic discomfort

panic disorder: composed of discrete episodes of panic attacks, that is, 15 to 30 minutes of rapid, intense, escalating anxiety in which the person experiences great emotional fear as well as physiologic discomfort

paranoid personality disorder: characterized by pervasive mistrust and suspiciousness of others

parataxic mode: begins in early childhood as the child begins to connect experiences in sequence; the child may not make logical sense of the experiences and may see them as coincidence or chance events; the child seeks to relieve anxiety by repeating familiar experiences, although he or she may not understand what he or she is doing

Parkinson's disease: a slowly progressive neurologic condition characterized by tremor, rigidity, bradykinesia, and postural instability

partial hospitalization program (PHP): structured treatment at an agency or facility for clients living in the community; designed to help clients make a gradual transition from being an inpatient to living independently or to avoid hospital admission

participant observer: the therapist's role, meaning that the therapist both participates in and observes the progress of the relationship

passive-aggressive personality disorder: characterized by a negative attitude and a pervasive pattern of passive resistance to demands for adequate social and occupational performance

patterns of knowing: the four patterns of knowing in nursing are empirical knowing (derived from the science of nursing), personal knowing (derived from life experiences), ethical knowing (derived from moral knowledge of nursing), and aesthetic knowing (derived from the art of nursing); provide the nurse with a clear method of observing and understanding every client interaction

personal zone: space of 18 to 36 inches, a comfortable distance between family and friends who are talking

personality: an ingrained, enduring pattern of behaving and relating to self, others, and the environment; includes perceptions, attitudes, and emotions

personality disorders: diagnosed when personality traits become inflexible and maladaptive and significantly interfere with how a person functions in society or cause the person emotional distress.

pervasive developmental disorders: characterized by pervasive and usually severe impairment of reciprocal social interaction skills, communication deviance, and restricted, stereotypical behavioral patterns

phase of disorganization and despair: the point in the grieving process when the bereaved person begins to understand the loss's permanence

phase of numbing: beginning of the grieving process; the common first response to the news of a loss is to be stunned, as though not perceiving reality

phase of reorganization: at the end of the grieving process, when the bereaved person begins to re-establish a sense of personal identity, direction, and purpose for living

phase of yearning and searching: the point in the grieving process when the person begins to recognize the reality of the loss

phenomena of concern: describe the twelve areas of concern that mental health nurses focus on when caring for clients

phobia: an illogical, intense, persistent fear of a specific object or social situation that causes extreme distress and interferes with normal functioning

physical abuse: ranges from shoving and pushing to severe battering and choking and may involve broken limbs and ribs, internal bleeding, brain damage, even homicide

physical aggression: behavior in which a person attacks or injures another person or that involves destruction of property

pica: persistent ingestion of nonnutritive substances such as paint, hair, cloth, leaves, sand, clay, or soil

Pick's disease: a degenerative brain disease that particularly affects the frontal and temporal lobes and results in a clinical picture similar to that of Alzheimer's disease

polydipsia: excessive water intake

polysubstance abuse: abuse of more than one substance

positive reframing: a cognitive behavioral technique involving turning negative messages into positive messages

positive regard: unconditional, nonjudgmental attitude that implies respect for the person

positive reinforcement: a reward immediately following a behavior to increase the likelihood that the behavior will be repeated

positive self-talk: a cognitive behavioral technique in which the client changes thinking about the self from negative to positive

positron emission tomography (PET): a diagnostic test used to examine the function of the brain by monitoring the flow of radioactive substances that are injected into the bloodstream

posttraumatic stress disorder: a disturbing pattern of behavior demonstrated by someone who has experienced a traumatic event: for example, a natural disaster, combat, or an assault; begins 3 or more months following the trauma

potency: describes the amount of a drug needed to achieve maximum effect

preconception: the way one person expects another to behave or speak; often a roadblock to the formation of an authentic relationship

pressured speech: unrelenting, rapid, often loud talking without pauses

primary gain: the relief of anxiety achieved by performing the specific anxiety-driven behavior; the direct external benefits that being sick provides, such as relief of anxiety, conflict, or distress

problem-focused coping strategies: techniques used to resolve or change a person's behavior or situation or to manage life stressors

problem identification: part of the working phase of the nurse–client situation, when the client identifies the issues or concerns causing problems

process: in communication, denotes all nonverbal messages that the speaker uses to give meaning and context to the message

prototaxic mode: characteristic of infancy and childhood that involves brief, unconnected experiences that have no relationship to one another. Adults with schizophrenia exhibit persistent prototaxic experiences.

proverbs: old adages or sayings with generally accepted meanings

proxemics: the study of distance zones between people during communication

pseudoparkinsonism: a type of extrapyramidal side effect of antipsychotic medication; drug-induced parkinsonism; includes shuffling gait, masklike facies, muscle stiffness (continuous) or cogwheeling rigidity (ratchet-like movements of joints), drooling, and akinesia (slowness and difficulty initiating movement)

psychiatric rehabilitation: services designed to promote the recovery process for clients with mental illness; not limited to medication management and symptom control, includes personal growth reintegration into the community, increased independence, and improved quality of life

psychoanalysis: focuses on discovering the causes of the client's unconscious and repressed thoughts, feelings, and conflicts believed to cause anxiety and helping the client to gain insight into and resolve these conflicts and anxieties; pioneered by Sigmund Freud, not commonly seen today

psychoimmunology: examines the effect of psychosocial stressors on the body's immune system

psychological abuse (emotional abuse): includes name-calling, belittling, screaming, yelling, destroying property, and making threats as well as subtler forms such as refusing to speak to or ignoring the victim

psychomotor agitation: increased body movements and thoughts

psychomotor retardation: overall slowed movements; a general slowing of all movements; slow cognitive processing and slow verbal interaction

psychopharmacology: the use of medications to treat mental illness

psychosis: cluster of symptoms including delusions, hallucinations, and grossly disordered thinking and behavior

psychosocial interventions: nursing activities that enhance the client's social and psychological functioning and improve social skills, interpersonal relationships, and communication

psychosomatic: used to convey the connection between the mind (*psyche*) and the body (*soma*) in states of health and illness

psychotherapy: therapeutic interaction between a qualified provider and client or group designed to benefit persons experiencing emotional distress, impairment, or illness; therapist's approach is based on a theory or combination of theories

psychotherapy group: the goal of the group is for members to learn about their behaviors and to make positive changes in their behaviors by interacting and communicating with others as members of a group

psychotropic drugs: drugs that affect mood, behavior, and thinking that are used to treat mental illness

public zone: space of 12 to 25 feet; the acceptable distance between a speaker and an audience, between small groups, and among others at informal functions

purging: compensatory behaviors designed to eliminate food by means of self-induced vomiting

race: a division of mankind possessing traits that are transmitted by descent and sufficient to identify it as a distinct human type

rape: a crime of violence, domination, and humiliation of the victim expressed through sexual means

rebound: temporary return of symptoms; may be more intense than original symptoms

reframing: cognitive behavioral technique in which alternative points of view are examined to explain events

religion: an organized system of beliefs about one or more all-powerful, all-knowing forces that govern the universe and offer guidelines for living in harmony with the universe and others

reminiscence therapy: thinking about or relating personally significant past experiences in a purposeful manner to benefit the client

repressed memories: memories that are buried deeply in the subconscious mind or repressed because they are too painful for the victim to acknowledge; often relate to childhood abuse

residential treatment setting: long-term treatment provided in a living situation; vary according to structure, level of supervision, and services provided

resilience: defined as having healthy responses to stressful circumstances or risky situations

resourcefulness: involves using problem-solving abilities and believing that one can cope with adverse or novel situations

response prevention: behavioral technique that focuses on delaying or avoiding performance of rituals in response to anxiety provoking thoughts

restraining order: legal order of protection obtained to prohibit contact between a victim and perpetrator of abuse

restraint: the direct application of physical force to a person, without his or her permission, to restrict his or her freedom of movement

restricted affect: displaying one type of emotional expression, usually serious or somber

ruminate: to repeatedly go over the same thoughts

satiety: satisfaction of appetite

schizoid personality disorder: characterized by a pervasive pattern of detachment from social relationships and a restricted range of emotional expression in interpersonal settings

schizotypal personality disorder: characterized by a pervasive pattern of social and interpersonal deficits marked by acute discomfort with and reduced capacity for close relationships as well as by cognitive or perceptual distortions and behavioral eccentricities

seasonal affective disorder (SAD): mood disorder with two subtypes. In one, most commonly called winter depression or fall-onset SAD, people experience increased sleep, appetite, and carbohydrate cravings; weight gain; interpersonal conflict; irritability; and heaviness in the extremities beginning in late autumn and abating in spring and summer. The other subtype, called spring-onset SAD, is less common and includes symptoms of insomnia, weight loss, and poor appetite lasting from late spring or early summer until early fall.

seclusion: the involuntary confinement of a person in a specially constructed, locked room equipped with a security window or camera for direct visual monitoring

secondary gain: the internal or personal benefits received from others because one is sick, such as attention from family members, comfort measures, being excused from usual responsibilities or tasks

self-actualized: describes a person who has achieved all the needs according to Maslow's hierarchy and has developed his or her fullest potential in life

self-awareness: the process by which a person gains recognition of his or her own feelings, beliefs, and attitudes; the process of developing an understanding of one's own values, beliefs, thoughts, feelings, attitudes, motivations, prejudices, strengths, and limitations and how these qualities affect others

self-concept: the way one views oneself in terms of personal worth and dignity

self-disclosure: revealing personal information such as biographical information and personal experiences, ideas, thoughts, and feelings about oneself

self-efficacy: a belief that personal abilities and efforts affect the events in our lives

self-help group: members share a common experience, but the group is not a formal or structured therapy group

self-monitoring: a cognitive-behavioral technique designed to help clients manage their own behavior

sense of belonging: the feeling of connectedness with or involvement in a social system or environment of which a person feels an integral part

serotonin: a neurotransmitter found only in the brain

serotonin syndrome: uncommon but potentially life-threatening disorder called serotonin or serotonergic syndrome; characterized by agitation, sweating, fever, tachycardia, hypotension, rigidity, hyperreflexia, confusion, and, in extreme cases, coma and death; most commonly results from a combination of two or more medications with serotonin-enhancing properties, such as taking MAOI and SSRI antidepressants at the same time or too close together

severe anxiety: an increased level of anxiety when more primitive survival skills take over, defensive responses ensue, and cognitive skills decrease significantly; person with severe anxiety has trouble thinking and reasoning

sexual abuse: involves sexual acts performed by an adult on a child younger than 18 years

single photon emission computed tomography (SPECT): a diagnostic test used to examine the function of the brain by following the flow of an injected radioactive substance

social network: groups of people whom one knows and with whom one feels connected

social organization: refers to family structure and organization, religious values and beliefs, ethnicity, and culture, all of which affect a person's role and, therefore, his or her health and illness behavior

social relationship: primarily initiated for the purpose of friendship, socialization, companionship, or accomplishment of a task

social support: emotional sustenance that comes from friends, family members, and even health care providers who help a person when a problem arises

social zone: a space of 4 to 12 feet, which is the distance acceptable for communication in social, work, and business settings

socioeconomic status: refers to one's income, education, and occupation

sodomy: anal intercourse

somatization: the transference of mental experiences and states into bodily symptoms.

somatization disorder: characterized by multiple, recurrent physical symptoms in a variety of bodily systems that have no organic or medical basis

somatoform disorders: characterized as the presence of physical symptoms that suggest a medical condition without a demonstrable organic basis to account fully for them

spirituality: a client's beliefs about life, health, illness, death, and one's relationship to the universe; involves the essence of a person's being and his or her beliefs about the meaning of life and the purpose for living

spontaneous remission: natural recovery that occurs without treatment of any kind

spouse or partner abuse: the mistreatment or misuse of one person by another in the context of an intimate relationship

stalking: repeated and persistent attempts to impose unwanted communication or contact on another person

standards of care: authoritative statements by professional organizations that describe the responsibilities for which nurses are accountable; the care that nurses provide to clients meets set expectations and is what any nurse in a similar situation would do

stereotypic movements: repetitive, seemingly purposeless movements; may include waving, rocking, twirling objects, biting fingernails, banging the head, biting or hitting oneself, or picking at the skin or body orifices

stimulants: drugs that stimulate or excite the central nervous system

stress: the wear and tear that life causes on the body

subconscious: thoughts or feelings in the preconscious or unconscious level of awareness

substance abuse: can be defined as using a drug in a way that is inconsistent with medical or social norms and despite negative consequences

substance dependence: includes problems associated with addiction, such as tolerance, withdrawal, and unsuccessful attempts to stop using the substance

suicidal ideation: thinking about killing oneself

suicide: the intentional act of killing oneself

suicide precautions: removal of harmful items, increased supervision to prevent acts of self-harm

superego: in psychoanalytic theory, the part of a person's nature that reflects moral and ethical concepts, values, and parental and social expectations; therefore, it is in direct opposition to the id

support group: organized to help members who share a common problem to cope with it

supportive touch: the use of physical touch to convey support, interest, caring; may not be welcome or effective with all clients

survivor: view of the client as a survivor of trauma or abuse rather than as a victim; helps to refocus client's view of him- or herself as being strong enough to survive the ordeal, which is a more empowering image than seeing oneself as a victim

syntaxic mode: begins to appear in school-aged children and becomes more predominant in preadolescence; the person begins to perceive him- or herself and the world within the context of the environment and can analyze experiences in a variety of settings

systematic desensitization: behavioral technique used to help overcome irrational fears and anxiety associated with a phobia

tangential thinking: wandering off the topic and never providing the information requested

tapering: administering decreasing doses of a medication leading to discontinuation of the drug

tardive dyskinesia: a late-onset, irreversible neurologic side effect of antipsychotic medications; characterized by abnormal, involuntary movements such as lip smacking, tongue protrusion, chewing, blinking, grimacing, and choreiform movements of the limbs and feet

temperament: refers to the biologic processes of sensation, association, and motivation that underlie the integration of skills and habits based on emotion

termination or resolution phase: the final stage in the nurse–client relationship. It begins when the client's problems are resolved, and it concludes when the relationship ends.

therapeutic communication: an interpersonal interaction between the nurse and client during which the nurse focuses on the client's specific needs to promote an effective exchange of information

therapeutic community or milieu: beneficial environment; interaction among clients is seen as beneficial, and treatment emphasizes the role of this client-to-client interaction

therapeutic nurse–client relationship: professional, planned relationship between client and nurse that focuses on client needs, feelings, problems, and ideas; interaction designed to promote client growth, discuss issues, and resolve problems; includes the three phases of orientation, working (identification and exploitation), and termination (resolution)

therapeutic play: play techniques are used to understand the child's thoughts and feelings and to promote communication

therapeutic relationship: *See* therapeutic nurse–client relationship

therapeutic use of self: nurses use themselves as a therapeutic tool to establish the therapeutic relationship with clients and to help clients grow, change, and heal

thought blocking: stopping abruptly in the middle of a sentence or train of thought; sometimes client is unable to continue the idea

thought broadcasting: a delusional belief that others can hear or know what the client is thinking

thought content: what the client actually says

thought insertion: a delusional belief that others are putting ideas or thoughts into the client's head: that is, the ideas are not those of the client

thought process: how the client thinks

thought stopping: a cognitive-behavioral technique to alter the process of negative or self-critical thought patterns

thought withdrawal: a delusional belief that others are taking the client's thoughts away and the client is powerless to stop it

tic: a sudden, rapid, recurrent, nonrhythmic, stereotyped motor movement or vocalization

time away: involves leaving clients for a short period then returning to them to re-engage in interaction; used in dementia care

time orientation: whether or not one views time as precise or approximate; differs among cultures

time-out: retreat to a neutral place to give the opportunity to regain self-control

tolerance: the need for increased amount of a substance to produce the same effect

tolerance break: very small amounts of a substance will produce intoxication

tort: a wrongful act that results in injury, loss, or damage

Tourette's disorder: involves multiple motor tics and one or more vocal tics, which occur many times a day for more than 1 year

transference: occurs when the client displaces onto the therapist attitudes and feelings that the client originally experienced in other relationships; it is common for the client unconsciously to transfer to the nurse feelings he or she has for significant others

12–step program: based on the philosophy that total abstinence is essential and that alcoholics need the help and support of others to maintain sobriety

unknowing: when the nurse admits she does not know the client or the client's subjective world, this opens the way for a truly authentic encounter. The nurse in a state of unknowing is open to seeing and hearing the client's views without imposing any of his or her values or viewpoints.

utilitarianism: a theory that bases ethical decisions on the "greatest good for the greatest number"; primary consideration is on the outcome of the decision

utilization review firms: developed to control the expenditure of insurance funds by requiring providers to seek approval before the delivery of care

values: abstract standards that give a person a sense of right and wrong and establish a code of conduct for living

vascular dementia: has symptoms similar to those of Alzheimer's disease, but onset is typically abrupt and followed by rapid changes in functioning, a plateau or leveling-off period, more abrupt changes, another leveling-off period, and so on

veracity: the duty to be honest or truthful

verbal communication: the words a person uses to speak to one or more listeners

waxy flexibility: maintenance of posture or position over time even when it is awkward or uncomfortable

withdrawal: new symptoms resulting from discontinuation of drug or substance

withdrawal syndrome: refers to the negative psychological and physical reactions that occur when use of a substance ceases or dramatically decreases

word salad: flow of unconnected words that convey no meaning to the listener

working phase: in the therapeutic relationship, the phase where issues are addressed, problems identified, solutions explored; nurse and client work to accomplish goals; contains Peplau's phases of problem identification and exploitation

Index

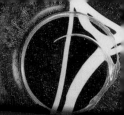

Page numbers followed by b indicate box; those followed by f indicate figure; those followed by t indicate table.